# Pregnancy
## DAY BY DAY

An illustrated daily countdown to motherhood,
from conception to childbirth and beyond

# Pregnancy
## DAY BY DAY

Consultant Editor **Paula Amato, MD**
Adjunct Associate Professor, Department of Obstetrics & Gynecology,
Oregon Health & Science University

Editor-In-Chief **Maggie Blott, MB BS**

# LONDON, NEW YORK, MUNICH, MELBOURNE, DELHI

**Project Editors** Dawn Bates, Claire Cross
**Project Designers** Emma Forge, Tom Forge, Peggy Sadler
**Senior Editors** Andrea Bagg, Anne Yelland, Emma Woolf
**US Editors** Shannon Beatty, Jane Perlmutter
**US Consultant Editors** Lisa Fields, Patricia Bontekoe
**Senior Art Editors** Sarah Ponder, Nicola Rodway, Liz Sephton
**Production Editor** Ben Marcus
**Production Controller** Alice Holloway
**Creative Technical Support** Sonia Charbonnier
**Illustrators** Debbie Maizels, Medi-Mation
**New Photography** Ruth Jenkinson
**Art Direction for Photography** Emma Forge
**Picture Researcher** Sarah Smithies
**Managing Editors** Esther Ripley, Penny Warren
**Managing Art Editors** Glenda Fisher, Marianne Markham
**Publisher** Peggy Vance

Every effort has been made to ensure that the information in this book is complete and accurate. However, neither the publisher nor the author is engaged in rendering professional advice or services to the individual reader. The ideas, procedures, and suggestions contained in this book are not intended as a substitute for consultng with your health-care provider. All matters regarding the health of you and your baby require medical supervision. Neither the publishers nor the author shall be liable or responsible for any loss or damage allegedly arising from any information or suggestion in this book.

First American Edition, 2009
Published in the United States by
DK Publishing
375 Hudson Street
New York, New York 10014

09 10 11  10 9 8 7 6 5 4 3 2

Published in Great Britain by Dorling Kindersley Limited

A catalog record for this book is available from the Library of Congress.

ISBN: 978-0-7566-5041-4

DK books are available at special discounts when purchased in bulk for sales promotions, premiums, fund-raising, or educational use. For details, contact: DK Publishing Special Markets, 375 Hudson Street, New York, New York 10014 or SpecialSales@dk.com.

Color reproduction by MDP, Bath, UK
Printed and bound by Star Standard, Singapore

Discover more at **www.dk.com**

## US consultant editor

**Dr. Paula Amato** is a fertility consultant and an adjunct associate professor at the Oregon Health and Science University in Portland, Oregon. She received her medical degree from the University of Toronto in 1989, where she also completed her residency in obstetrics and gynecology. She subsequently completed a fellowship in reproductive endocrinology and infertility at the University of California, San Diego. Dr. Amato was awarded an American Obstetricians and Gynecologists Foundation Fellowship (1997–2000) and was a recipient of the Berlex Scholar Award in Basic Science Research in 2001. She is board certified in both obstetrics and gynecology and reproductive endocrinology and infertility. As an academician, she has held faculty appointments at the University of California, San Diego, and at Baylor College of Medicine.

Dr. Amato is a former associate editor of *Sexuality, Reproduction, & Menopause*, a vice chair of the American Society of Reproductive Medicine (ASRM) Sexuality Special Interest Group, and a member of the ASRM Ethics Committee. She was the US medical consultant for DK's bestselling title, *I'm Pregnant!*

## Editor-in-chief

**Dr. Maggie Blott MB BS, FRCOG** is Consultant Obstetrician at University College Hospital, London, where she jointly manages a multidisciplinary high-risk prenatal clinic and runs the labor ward. She is also spokesperson for The Royal College of Obstetricians and Gynaecologists, London. Dr. Blott is a regular columnist for *Top Santé* magazine and writes for a number of other pregnancy-related publications.

## Contributors

**Dr. Carol Cooper** MA, MB, BChir (Cantab), MRCP General Practitioner, London; Tutor at Imperial College School of Medicine, London ■ **Ms. Friedericke Eben** FRCOG Consultant Obstetrician and Gynaecologist, Whittington NHS Trust and Portland Hospitals, London ■ **Dr. Katrina Erskine** MD, MRCP, MRCOG Consultant Obstetrician and Gynaecologist, The Homerton Hospital, London ■ **Dr. Laura Goetzl** MD, MPH Associate Professor, Department of Obstetrics and Gynecology, Division of Maternal Fetal Medicine, Medical University of South Carolina, Charleston, South Carolina ■ **Dr. Belinda Green** PhD Midwife, University College London Hospitals, NHS Foundation Trust, London ■ **Dr. Deirdre Guerin** MB BCh, BAO, LRCP and SI, FFA, or CSI Medical Director of Resident Obstetric Services and Consultant Anesthetist, The Portland Hospital for Women and Children, London ■ **Amanda Hutcherson** DipHeMid, RM, PGCert Ed, MA Midwife Practitioner, London ■ **Dr. Philippa Kaye** MB BS Hons, MA Hons (Cantab), DCH, DRCOG, DFSRH Works in general practice ■ **Dr. Su Laurent** MRCP, FRCPCH Consultant Paediatrician, Barnet Hospital, London ■ **Mr. Andrew Loughney** PhD, MRCOG Consultant Obstetrician, Royal Victoria Infirmary, Newcastle upon Tyne ■ **Dr. Paul Moran** MD, MRCOG Consultant Obstetrician, Head of Fetal Medicine, Royal Victoria Infirmary, Newcastle upon Tyne ■ **Melinda Nicci** BA (Psych), HDipEd Fitness and lifestyle coach and founder of baby2body: pregnancy and post pregnancy health and fitness ■ **Catharine Parker-Littler** SRN, RSCN, SCM, DPSM (Advanced midwifery), BScMid (Hons) Practicing midwife; founder and midwifery director of midwivesonline.com, a website for midwives, health-care professionals, and parents-to-be ■ **Dr. Hope Ricciotti** MD Associate Professor of Obstetrics, Gynecology, and Reproductive Biology, Harvard Medical School, Beth Israel Deaconess Medical Center, Boston, Massachussetts ■ **Dr. Vincent M. Reid** PhD Lecturer in Developmental Psychology, Durham University ■ **Dr. Mary Steen** RGN, RM, BHSc PGCRM, PGDipHE, MCGI, PhD Reader in Midwifery and Reproductive Health, University of Chester ■ **Karen Sullivan** ASET, VTCT, BSc Developmental Psychology; Child-care expert and author ■ **Sally Watkin** Pregnancy and parenting author

# Contents

# Introduction

Pregnancy is an exceptional time when you enter one of your most significant life stages and need to quickly assimilate knowledge and understanding of the process of pregnancy and birth. In the past, when women traditionally gave birth at home, cared for by midwives and female relatives, pregnancy and birth was a familiar event. Today, it's unusual to have such firsthand experience and a woman's knowledge of pregnancy and birth is often nonexistent or limited to that which she gained in her first pregnancy. As a result, many, if not all, women contemplate pregnancy with a mixture of trepidation and curiosity. These feelings are often compounded by the recognition that their own lifestyle choices can have an enormous influence on their own and their baby's health. For all these reasons, there is a great need for women to be able to access information about pregnancy that is accurate, balanced, and accessible.

In *Pregnancy Day by Day*, information is gathered from a wide body of professionals, each with his or her own area of expertise. The midwives, doctors, obstetricians, and pediatricians who have contributed the core information in this book have between them cared for thousands of women at each stage of pregnancy and labor, delivered thousands of babies, and provided care and support for women and their babies after the birth. The exhaustive record of pregnancy, birth, and the postpartum period provided by their combined expertise is complemented by specialized knowledge on diet and exercise from a nutritionist and a lifestyle and exercise coach. The information presented—at once practical, detailed, and full of simple explanations and advice—will provide the vital tools women need to help them plan for pregnancy, negotiate the many changes they will experience, and develop a safe and appropriate birth plan.

Most pregnancy books are written for women. Today many men also want to follow closely the development of their unborn child, but have little information and often feel excluded. Within the book, there are reassuring explanations for partners about the changes that occur during pregnancy as well as advice for women on how to include partners during pregnancy and the early days of parenthood.

*Margaret J. Blott*

Dr. Maggie Blott

# How this book is organized

This book starts with guidance on how to enjoy a healthy and safe pregnancy, with lifestyle advice that often applies to the preconceptual period too. The core section of the book gives a day-by-day account of pregnancy with detailed explanations of the physical and emotional changes that take place in your body along with fascinating insights into how your baby develops within the uterus. A labor and birth chapter takes you through the delivery of your baby, followed by a summary of the first two weeks with your new baby. A final chapter deals with concerns and complications in the mother and baby in pregnancy, labor, and the postpartum period.

## A healthy pregnancy

This chapter provides the information you need to make lifestyle choices that will maximize your own health throughout pregnancy and give your baby the best possible start in life. It includes guidelines for exercising safely, eating healthily, avoiding hazards, and dealing with illnesses. It also addresses concerns you may have about how the emotional and physical changes of pregnancy may impact your relationships.

## Pregnancy day by day

Here, the book takes you day by day through the extraordinary story of conception and pregnancy, counting down each of the 280 days until the onset of labor. Each day reveals how your baby is developing and the changes that are occurring in your body. The 280 days, or 40 weeks, of pregnancy are divided into three trimesters, each of which comprises around a third of the pregnancy. Beyond being a simple measure of time, each trimester represents a distinct phase in the development of the baby and in the pregnancy.

**The first trimester** The definition of the first trimester is given here as weeks 1–12, though you may also see weeks 13 and 14 included elsewhere. This trimester covers the time from the beginning of the menstrual period to the moment of conception, which is usually around two weeks. Because the exact moment of conception is unknown, pregnancy is counted from the one definite date, the beginning of the menstrual cycle. Although technically your pregnancy may not begin until two weeks into your menstrual cycle, these two weeks are very important in helping your body achieve a healthy pregnancy. Here, we explain day by day the changes that take place in your uterus to prepare it for conception and implantation of the early embryo, and offer dietary advice and recommendations from fertility experts to boost your chances of conceiving.

The first trimester is a period of extraordinary development, when all your baby's major organs form, and he or she will grow faster than at any other period in life. A day-by-day account is given of the changes that you and your baby undergo, and advice offered on how to cope with the exhausting changes that occur in early pregnancy. There's also an honest appraisal of the emotional feelings you're likely to experience, reassuring you that negative as well as positive emotions are normal. Practical information on accessing prenatal care and detailed explanations of the choices that are available help you begin to plan your pregnancy and think about your options for the birth.

**The second trimester** In the second trimester, which is designated as weeks 13–25, your baby's organs mature further and growth continues. This is an exciting time as your body starts to change shape to accommodate your growing baby and you feel your baby move for the first time. However, it is also a time when women can experience symptoms that are often due to quite normal pregnancy changes but that can occasionally indicate a problem. For example, abdominal pain can be due to ligaments being stretched or to constipation; however, it could also indicate a problem with the placenta. Symptoms such as these are discussed at the relevant point in pregnancy, with detailed explanations that will provide reassurance or alert you to the possibility of something more serious that should be brought to the attention of your doctor.

**The third trimester** In the third trimester, designated as weeks 26–40, your baby continues to grow and mature and, if born early, could survive life outside the uterus. During this time, your body starts to prepare itself for labor. We describe the changes taking place and explain why they occur, as well as providing pointers to what is normal and which symptoms need to be reported to your doctor. Women recount their experiences, and questions that are presented daily to doctors are reproduced to provide a bank of vital knowledge. Practical guidance on all matters, from maternity leave entitlement information to reassurance

that having sex won't harm the growing baby, helps you navigate your way through the final weeks of pregnancy.

## Labor and birth
One of the best ways to cope with labor is to understand its stages. In the labor and birth chapter, a team of professionals covers in detail the progress of labor, each providing their own expert insight. A doctor writes about normal births and discusses natural pain relief. An anesthesiologist gives the options available for medical pain relief, including detailed descriptions of how epidurals are given and their pros and cons. While most women have a normal birth without complications, 30 percent have a cesarean section, and around 5 percent have an assisted delivery, with either forceps or vacuum extraction. An obstetrician writes about difficult births, describing complications and the medical interventions that may be required.

## The first two weeks
Here, the early days as you adjust to life with your new baby are charted in the day-by-day format. A pediatrician addresses the practical issues of baby care. Also discussed are the emotional and physical renewal you undergo as your body recovers from the birth and you begin the new tasks of nurturing and feeding your baby.

## Concerns and complications
This reference section is a concise guide to conditions in pregnancy and labor, and postpartum concerns in the mother and baby. Clear explanations enable you to digest medical information, understand which symptoms are not of concern, and feel reassured about how more serious conditions are managed in pregnancy, labor, and the postpartum period.

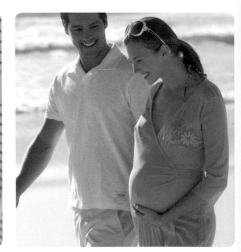

In pregnancy, feelings of awe and excitement are often mingled with concerns about your own and your baby's well-being. With an ever-growing body of knowledge on how a mother's behavior in pregnancy impacts her baby's short- and long-term health, women today have the opportunity to ensure that their lifestyle choices positively benefit their babies. Eating healthily, exercising regularly, and avoiding hazards will all help give your baby the best possible start in life.

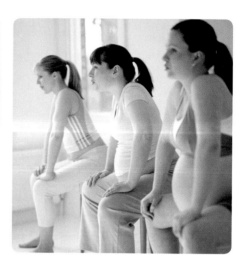

# A healthy pregnancy

# Your pregnancy diet

You can optimize your own health and your baby's future health by eating a nutritious, balanced diet throughout pregnancy.

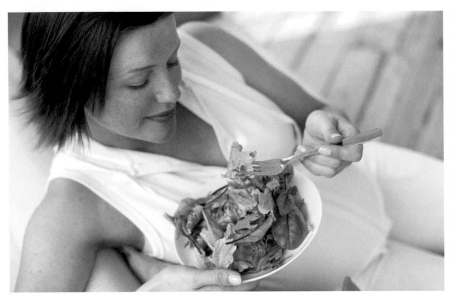

**Eating regular nutritious meals and snacks** throughout the day is vital during pregnancy to keep your energy levels up, and to provide your growing baby with all he needs to develop well.

In recent years, much has been learned about what constitutes a healthy diet in pregnancy. In addition to the importance of nutrients such as folic acid (see p.16), there is mounting evidence that a person's health may be influenced by the mother's diet in pregnancy, including whether particular nutrients were received at certain times. Current thinking is that good nutrition in pregnancy may reduce a baby's future risk of diseases such as obesity, diabetes, and heart disease.

In addition to influencing your baby's health, good nutrition in pregnancy also optimizes your health, helping you to deal with the demands of pregnancy.

## A healthy diet

Getting the right balance of protein, carbohydrates, and fats in pregnancy is simple, since the ratios are the same in pregnancy as at other times: 45–65 percent of your calories should come from carbohydrates; 20–35 percent from fats; and 10–35 percent from protein. The components of these nutrients don't need to be in this exact ratio for each meal, or even every day, but you should aim to achieve this balance over the course of a week. A diet that includes plenty of vegetables, fruits, whole grains, and good proteins and fats will automatically contain the proper mix of nutrients.

## Carbohydrates

Carbohydrates are an important source of fuel for you and for your baby since they are broken down into glucose, which passes easily across the placenta. Try to get six servings a day, a serving being equivalent to a slice of bread, 2 oz (60 g) of cereal, or five crackers.

Carbohydrates are divided into two subgroups: refined and unrefined. In general, white is bad when it comes to carbohydrates, since refined foods such as white rice and white breads are rapidly broken down and enter the bloodstream in the form of a spike of glucose. It is thought that this spike may have health risks for mother and baby, producing larger babies with a subsequent risk of obesity later in life.

Unrefined carbohydrates are less processed, so they break down more slowly in the bloodstream and release glucose steadily. They are also a good source of fiber, which helps prevent constipation. These are a healthier choice, and at least half, if not all, of your carbohydrates should come from unrefined (whole grain) sources. such as whole-wheat or multigrain bread; brown rice, whole-wheat pasta, and cereals.

## Protein

Protein is essential for the growth of the baby and the placenta, as well as for your health. Pregnant women need around 6-6½ oz each day. Aim for two to three servings of protein-rich foods a day, a typical serving being 3 oz (85 g) red meat, or 5 oz (150 g) fish. Since most adults get about 3½ oz (100 g) of protein daily, there is usually no need to increase your intake, especially if you have protein at each meal. If you're vegetarian, in addition to protein at each meal, you should have a protein-containing snack. If you're having twins or more, ask your doctor how much protein to consume and when breast-feeding, 6½ oz (185 g) daily.

Choose protein sources that contain less saturated fat, such as skinless chicken, lean beef and pork, tofu, low-fat cheese and yogurt, and skim milk. Fish, nuts, and seeds contain healthier unsaturated fats (see below), although your intake of some fish should be limited since they contain mercury, which could be harmful to your baby (see p.17).

## Fats

Fats contain vitamins and contribute to the healthy development of cells. However, although fats make a useful contribution to overall nutrition, their intake needs to be limited. Choose healthier unsaturated fats, found in foods such as fish and some types of oil, over unhealthy saturated fats found in whole milk dairy products, meat, or trans fats found in processed foods.

**Omega 3 fatty acids** Studies suggest that the development of the baby's nervous system may be boosted by omega 3 fatty acids, the richest source of which is found in fatty fish. Avoid fish that are high in mercury (see p.17) and opt instead for salmon and anchovies, which are good, safe sources of omega 3 fatty acids. Wild salmon is very rich in omega 3, but farm-raised salmon is also a good source. Other sources include omega 3-enriched eggs, flaxseed, flaxseed oil, walnuts, canola oil, and omega 3 supplements and prenatal vitamins containing omega 3 fatty acids.

## Dairy products

These are an important component of the diet since they provide a good supply of proteins and fats, as well as calcium and some vitamins. Calcium is essential for the healthy development of bones and teeth. Opt for low-fat dairy products and low-fat or skim milk. Aim for 2–3 servings each day, a typical serving being 1 oz (30 g) of hard cheese, or 1 cup (200 ml) milk.

## Vitamins and minerals

In pregnancy, you need to ensure a rich supply of vitamins and minerals, since these are important for your own health and for your developing baby. They support the healthy functioning of body systems and contain antioxidants, which protect the body against the effects of

## YOUR RECOMMENDED DAILY INTAKE

**Eating a healthy, balanced diet** is of paramount importance during pregnancy to help you deal with the additional demands on your body and to provide your developing baby with essential nutrients. By eating a wide variety of healthy foods, you will be ensuring that you and your baby are receiving the correct balance of nutrients. Try to include a range of foods each day from each of the major food groups (see opposite) and eat plenty of fresh fruit and vegetables.

**Include 2–3 portions each day of protein-rich foods,** such as fish, lean meat, chicken, legumes, cheese, and nuts to ensure the healthy growth of body structures.

**Try to include 3 servings of dairy products** each day. Ideally, these should be low-fat products, such as low-fat milk and low-fat cheese and yogurts.

**Have 3 servings of whole grain carbohydrates,** such as brown rice and whole-wheat breads and and pasta, to keep up energy levels and ensure a supply of fiber.

**4–5 servings of vegetables** each day will ensure a good supply of essential vitamins and minerals. Try to eat different colored produce and don't overcook vegetables.

**3–4 portions of fresh fruit** daily will also provide a wide range of vitamins and minerals, many of which contain important protective antioxidants.

**1–2 servings daily of iron-rich foods** such as eggs or dark leafy green vegetables will help maintain healthy iron levels during pregnancy when demands are increased.

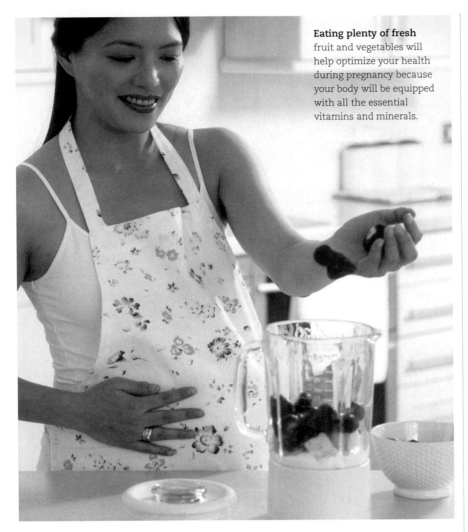

**Eating plenty of fresh** fruit and vegetables will help optimize your health during pregnancy because your body will be equipped with all the essential vitamins and minerals.

harmful chemicals called free radicals. Good sources of the most important vitamins and minerals are given below. As long as you eat a varied diet that includes plenty of fruits and vegetables, you should be getting all you need, with a couple of exceptions. It can be hard to get enough iron in your diet to meet the demands of pregnancy. Your iron levels will be checked during pregnancy and supplements may be recommended. You'll also need a folic acid supplement before conceiving and in early pregnancy (see right).

**Vitamin A** This is important for healthy eyes, skin, and hair; it's found in orange fruit and vegetables, such as apricots, peppers, carrots, and tomatoes.

**Vitamin B** This contributes to the healthy functioning of body systems, and helps the body fight infection. Good sources include bananas, milk, whole grains, cheese, and cabbage.

**Vitamin C** This aids the absorption of iron and helps fight infection. Rich sources include citrus fruits, kiwis, peppers, broccoli, and spinach.

**Vitamin D** This helps the absorption of calcium. Food sources include eggs and dark leafy green vegetables, and it is also obtained from sunlight. Women with limited exposure to sunlight, who are housebound, predominantly covered when outdoors, or from Africa, South Asia, the Middle East, or the Caribbean should take a 10 mg vitamin D supplement daily.

**Vitamin E** This vitamin contains antioxidants and keeps skin, hair, and muscles healthy. Good sources of vitamin E include nuts and seeds.

**Folate and folic acid** Studies have shown that sufficient amounts of the B vitamin folic acid, or its natural form folate, can help reduce the risk of neural tube defects, such as spina bifida, by up to 50 percent. In these defects, the embryonic neural tube fails to close properly during the first four weeks of pregnancy, leading to incomplete development of the brain and spinal cord. Folate helps the neural tube close and pregnant women are advised to eat a folate-rich diet. Foods high in folate include green leafy vegetables, legumes; and fortified cereals. It may not be possible to get sufficient folate through diet alone, so women are also advised to take a folic acid supplement of 400 micrograms before conception and during the first trimester.

**Iron** This is needed for hemoglobin production in red blood cells. Sources include meat, fish, chicken, eggs, dried apricots, spinach, and broccoli.

**Calcium** This is essential for healthy bones and teeth. Sources include dairy products, eggs, fortified cereals, and leafy green vegetables.

**Zinc** This helps maintain a healthy immune system. Sources include seafood and nuts.

## A vegetarian diet

A vegetarian diet, and vegan diets where dairy products are excluded, can be safe and healthy during pregnancy as long as you ensure a good balance of nutrients and sufficient protein (see p.126). Babies born to vegetarians are in a healthy weight range, although vegans do need to be vigilant about obtaining adequate protein, as well as reliable sources of B12 and zinc. Vegans can discuss with their doctors whether they'll be able to meet their vitamin B12 needs through diet alone. Since vitamin B12 is found primarily in animal sources, a supplement may be required. Non-animal sources of B12 may be unreliable.

## A low GI diet

Glucose, the product of carbohydrates, serves as the primary fuel for your growing baby. A new concept in nutrition is the glycemic index (GI), which looks at how much a food will raise the level of glucose in the bloodstream. Foods that release glucose gradually, such as unrefined carbohydrates (see p.14), and thus have a low GI, appear to be healthier.

**Benefits of a low GI diet** Evidence suggests that a low GI diet has health benefits for both the mother and baby. Maternal carbohydrate intake can affect glucose levels in the bloodstream, which in turn can affect the baby's growth. Higher glucose levels, even those in the normal range, can make for a bigger baby—above the 90th percentile (the top

end of a baby's growth chart, see p.284). There are health risks later in life linked to a high birth weight, such as obesity, diabetes, and heart disease. One study found that women who consumed a low GI diet had infants that were a normal size, but had less body fat than those from women who consumed a high GI diet.

A low GI diet can also help control glucose levels in mothers with gestational diabetes (see p.473), in turn reducing complications of labor and birth associated with this condition.

## Your calorie intake

During pregnancy, most women need to increase their calorie intake by 100–300 calories a day for proper nutrition and weight gain. Your energy needs may vary depending on your pre-pregnancy weight and your activity levels.

Gaining the correct amount of weight in pregnancy has benefits for both mother and baby. You're more likely to return to your pre-pregnancy weight if you gain weight within the recommended guidelines (see p.99). Gaining too much weight is linked with bigger babies, which carries future risks to the baby's health (see above). Conversely, gaining too little weight is also not ideal for a baby's future health.

---

**YOUR BODY MASS INDEX**

**At the start of pregnancy, your doctor may tell you your body mass index, or BMI.** This is an estimate of your body fat based on your weight and height. By calculating your BMI, your doctor can establish whether you are a healthy weight for your height or whether your weight could cause problems during pregnancy.

Your BMI is calculated by multiplying your weight in pounds by 703, dividing the answer by your height in inches, then dividing the answer by your height in inches again. A BMI of 18.5–24.9 is considered normal; 25–29.9 is

considered overweight; 30–39.9 is classified as obese; and over 39 is very obese. If you have A BMI of below 18.5, you are thought to be underweight.

Being underweight in pregnancy can make you more likely to give birth prematurely, or have a "small-for-dates" baby. Being overweight means that you are at a higher risk of problems such as high blood pressure, preeclampsia (see p.474), and gestational diabetes (see p.473), and are more likely to have a larger baby. These factors increase the risk of complications at the time of delivery.

---

**WHAT TO AVOID**

# Dietary precautions

Certain foods should be avoided or their intake limited since they may pose a risk to your unborn baby. Simple cooking and hygiene measures are also important to limit the risks.

Listeria is a food-borne bacteria to which pregnant women are more susceptible. It is found in unpasteurized dairy products, as well as refrigerated, ready-to-eat foods like meat, poultry, and seafood. To avoid it, thoroughly reheat hot dogs, lunch meats, or prepared deli foods and avoid unpasteurized dairy products and check soft cheeses labels to be sure they're made with pasteurized milk.

Nearly all seafood contains at least trace amounts of mercury which can affect the development of the fetal nervous system. Pregnant women should avoid swordfish, shark, king mackerel, and tilefish. To stay within safe limits, eat up to 12 ounces per week of lower-mercury seafood like shrimp, salmon, pollock, catfish, and canned light tuna

Toxoplasmosis is a parasite spread through cat feces or undercooked beef, pork, or lamb that can harm the fetus. Avoid changing cat litter and practice careful hygiene in the kitchen when preparing raw meat, being careful not to contaminate other foods such as lettuce or vegetables. Beef, pork, and lamb all need to be well cooked.

Salmonella bacteria are found in chicken and eggs. Infection with salmonella can cause severe vomiting, but doesn't directly affect the baby. Avoid any products containing raw or undercooked eggs, and make sure all poultry is thoroughly cooked through, since cooking kills the bacteria.

# Exercising safely

Staying fit in pregnancy has many benefits for you and your baby and increases your stamina for labor and birth.

**Stay well hydrated** by drinking plenty of water before, during, and after your workout.

If you had an exercise program before you became pregnant, you can continue with this in the first trimester as long as you have the all clear from your doctor. As your pregnancy goes on, you may need to adapt your program.

If you didn't have a regular exercise program before, now is the ideal time to adopt a new, healthier way of life from which you will reap the rewards for years to come. If you do start exercising now, build up gently; listen to your body and do only what feels comfortable.

Regular gentle exercise is much better than intense irregular bouts of exercise (which aren't advisable in pregnancy), since your body responds more postively to consistent, moderate exercise.

## How exercise helps

In addition to increasing your energy levels, exercise helps you maintain a positive outlook and feel confident about your changing body image. Exercise can also ease common pregnancy discomforts such as nausea, leg cramps, swollen feet, varicose veins, constipation, insomnia, and back pain. By keeping muscles strong and toned, exercise makes it easier for your body to deal with changes in posture during pregnancy. There is also evidence that increased fitness helps shorten labor and your postpartum recovery time and lessens your overall anxiety about the birth.

## Food for fuel

A nutritious, balanced diet is vital in pregnancy. If you're exercising too, eating well to keep energy levels balanced is doubly important. Eat regular, nutritious meals, ensuring that your calories come from wholesome, fresh foods, and avoid high-calorie sugary snacks.

---

### DO'S AND DON'TS

**Exercise is safe in pregnancy** as long as you follow the simple guidelines listed below. As your pregnancy progresses, you will probably need to adapt and moderate your exercise program.

**Do:**
- Warm up and cool down properly.
- Drink enough water before, during, and after exercising.
- Wear comfortable clothes that don't restrict your rib cage.
- Exercise regularly and consistently.
- Adjust your expectations; pregnancy is not a time to go for personal bests.

- Build your strength, but do this gradually. Focus on your back, shoulders, chest, and lower body.
- Practice Kegel exercises (see p.69) daily to maintain the pelvic floor tone.
- Breathe properly while exercising, especially when lifting weights.
- Protect your back when getting up from a lying position: roll onto your left side and sit up using your legs.
- Avoid exercises that feel awkward or uncomfortable.
- Focus on posture and alignment.
- Stop immediately and seek advice if you feel severe localized pain, vaginal bleeding, or general unwellness.
- Eat frequent small meals and snacks to maintain energy and avoid having your blood sugar levels fall.

**Don't:**
- Exercise in a hot or humid environment.
- Do jerky or bouncy moves or twist or rotate your abdomen.
- Lift weights that are too heavy.
- Do sports where you risk falling, such as skiing or horseback riding.
- Overstretch: the pregnancy hormone relaxin can make you feel more supple than you are.
- Exercise to exhaustion. If you're tired, decrease the intensity or duration. Get an hour's rest for each hour of exercise.

# Sex and relationships

You may find that you and your partner need to adapt to the emotional and physical changes that accompany pregnancy.

In a low-risk pregnancy, sex is perfectly safe, although your levels of desire may fluctuate throughout pregnancy. Most women report that their interest in sex is the same or slightly reduced in the first trimester. In the second trimester, it varies from woman to woman, and in the third trimester libido often falls.

## Sex during pregnancy

During the first trimester, the hormonal changes that cause nausea, vomiting, and fatigue can naturally result in a reduced interest in sex. However, other pregnancy changes may increase your desire, such as an increased blood flow, which produces swelling in the clitoris and labia and extra vaginal secretions. In the second trimester especially, vaginal lubrication and intensity of orgasm can increase, which may be accompanied by gentle contractions; these are normal and are nothing to worry about. Many women find that their libido falls toward the end of pregnancy since a bigger belly makes sex more awkward and uncomfortable, and they may also feel increasingly anxious about the birth.

**How your partner feels** As with women, men display a range of feelings toward sex in pregnancy. While some may find their partner's new, fuller shape particularly sensuous, others may feel apprehensive about sex, fearing that they may harm the baby. Some men may feel a combination of these emotions. Unless there are concerns about your pregnancy (see right), it's generally thought that sex won't cause harm, since your baby is well protected by the amniotic fluid and your uterus.

**Spending time touching and caressing** can help you and your partner maintain feelings of closeness and intimacy.

## When to seek advice

Some women experience vaginal bleeding after sex in pregnancy. This is most likely to be harmless and is often caused by the increased blood flow to the cervix in pregnancy, which can cause it to bleed on contact with your partner's penis. If this is the cause, the bleeding should resolve after the birth. However, since there are other possible causes, report any bleeding to your doctor.

In addition to the size of your belly causing discomfort during sex, some women experience pain during sex toward the end of pregnancy as the baby moves farther into the pelvis; or they may find that the contractions that can accompany orgasm become increasingly uncomfortable. These symptoms are unlikely to be a cause for concern, but it's worth mentioning them to your doctor for reassurance.

There are some circumstances in late pregnancy when intercourse may not be safe. This can be the case if you've had a previous premature labor or risk factors for premature labor, such as a weak cervix, or if you have placenta previa (see p.473), or leakage of amniotic fluid, which can mean your water has broken.

If you have any concerns, don't be afraid to ask your doctor for advice. Being able to enjoy sex in pregnancy will help you and your partner feel close during this time of transition. Indeed, psychologists have found that couples who enjoy sex in pregnancy are more tender toward each other and communicate better after the birth.

---

**WHAT TO DO**

### An intimate pregnancy

During pregnancy, fatigue, feelings of insecurity about your new shape, and concerns about the safety of sex can all take their toll on your relationship. Allowing yourself time to adjust and keeping the channels of communication open will help you and your partner enjoy this new stage in your relationship.

■ **Talk to each other about your feelings** and be aware that, for both of you, levels of interest may fluctuate.

■ **If your belly makes some positions uncomfortable,** experiment with alternative ones that accommodate your size, such as side-by-side, rear entry, or woman-on-top positions.

■ **Enjoy other ways to maintain intimacy** besides intercourse, such as touching and massage.

# Illnesses and medication

## Knowing how to manage illness and what medications are safe to take is important to protect your own and your baby's health.

Whether you have a preexisting medical condition, or acquire an illness or infection during pregnancy, always consult your doctor before taking medication or before stopping any prescribed medication.

### Preexisting conditions

If you have a condition such as high blood pressure or diabetes prior to pregnancy, your pregnancy will be classified as high risk and you'll need to be monitored carefully. If you become pregnant while taking medication for a condition, don't stop taking the medication, but consult your doctor as soon as possible. You may find that your existing medication is safe, or you may need to change to another type of medication. The most important thing is to control your condition during pregnancy to minimize the risks to you and your baby, which will usually mean continuing with medication.

**Diabetes** If you have diabetes and are planning to conceive, you need to get advice on how to manage your condition. Meet with your doctor while you're thinking about conceiving to discuss the best way to control your blood sugar levels and talk about how diabetes will be managed in pregnancy. Women with diabetes are advised to take a prenatal vitamin with folic acid before trying to conceive and for the first three months of pregnancy. Diabetic women who are overweight may be advised to lose weight before getting pregnant, and they'll likely be told to monitor their blood sugar more frequently and take their medications on time during their pregnancy. Babies

born to diabetic women also have a greater risk of other problems, such as having a large birth weight, respiratory problems at birth, jaundice, and low blood sugar at birth.

As soon as you're pregnant, you should be referred to an obstetrician who specializes in pregnancy and diabetes where you'll receive extra care. You will have more frequent prenatal visits, additional scans, and extra blood tests to monitor your blood sugars. You may need diabetes medication and/or insulin injections each day; the dose usually changes throughout pregnancy and needs to be monitored. The better your blood sugar control, the less likely you or your baby is to experience problems during pregnancy.

Since diabetic women have an increased risk of late pregnancy problems such as preeclampsia (see p.474) and premature labor (see p.431), you may be advised to have an induction of labor a week or so before your due date (see p.432).

Once in labor, your blood sugar levels will be closely monitored, and you will probably be given an insulin IV. After the birth, your baby's blood sugar levels will be closely monitored too for around 24 hours. If you're planning to breast-feed, which is recommended, your insulin dose may need to be changed after the birth.

**Epilepsy** If you have epilepsy, it's very important to discuss pregnancy with your doctor before you become pregnant, since certain drugs carry a small risk of causing harm to the developing baby. Nonetheless, it's also important that your epilepsy is controlled, so your doctor will try to ensure that you're on

**Diabetes is controlled** with daily insulin injections in pregnancy. As the skin on your abdomen becomes taut, you may find it easier to inject into the fatty tissue of the thigh (left). **Continuing with asthma medication** is important to keep symptoms under control in pregnancy (right).

the lowest possible dose of medication before you get pregnant. When you are pregnant, the anomaly scan at around 20 weeks (see p.214) will check for problems such as cleft palate, which are slightly more common with certain medications. If your condition worsens in pregnancy, contact your doctor.

### Systemic lupus erythematosus

This is an autoimmune disorder that can affect many parts of the body, including the kidneys, joints, skin, nervous system, heart, and lungs. The condition is more common in women, and particularly in those of childbearing age. Some women find that the symptoms for this condition ease during pregnancy, however for some they can worsen. It's important to control the condition during pregnancy since it can affect the developing baby, with an increased risk of miscarriage, poor growth, premature labor, and stillbirth. Most medications for lupus are safe to use during pregnancy, but some aren't, so you need to check with your doctor about whether you need to change your current medication. From around 32 weeks, your baby will be closely monitored and his growth and well-being will be checked. If there are concerns about you or your baby, labor may be induced early, or you may have a planned cesarean.

**High blood pressure** If you have high blood pressure that requires medication, check with your doctor that the medication you are on is safe to use during pregnancy. It's important to continue your medication so that your blood pressure is controlled, because high blood pressure can be dangerous both for you and your baby. Your doctor will frequently check your blood pressure, and will test your urine to check for the presence of protein, because high blood pressure and protein in the urine are symptoms of the condition preeclampsia (see p.474).

---

**COMMON WORRIES**

#### I'm asthmatic. Can I use my inhalers during pregnancy?

It's essential that you keep asthma under control in pregnancy, which means continuing to use your inhalers, since the risks from uncontrolled asthma are greater than any risk from taking asthma medication. If asthma is uncontrolled, it can mean that not enough oxygen gets to the baby, leading to a low birth weight or other problems. One of the best ways to control asthma, in addition to taking medication, is to avoid asthma triggers such as pet fur and dust mites. Use air filters, vacuum often, and damp dust, and use duvet, mattress, and pillow protectors. Sometimes, pregnancy reduces the severity of asthma, but if you feel wheezier than usual, talk to your doctor about reviewing your medication.

#### Homeopathy seems to be a popular form of therapy. How effective is it and is it safe?

Homeopathy works on the principle of treating like with like to stimulate the body's natural healing mechanisms. There has been debate about the efficacy of homeopathy and the scientific opinion is that there is insufficient evidence to show that homeopathy has any effect beyond that of a placebo. But talk to your doctor before using any homeopathic products or remedies during pregnancy, since homeopathy is an area of complementary and alternative medicine that's associated with much debate and scientific controversy. If your doctor gives you the okay, a certified homeopath may be able to provide treatment.

#### What's the verdict on taking herbal remedies and teas during pregnancy?

The US Food and Drug Administration does not regulate herbs and other dietary supplements, and there's not much research about the health effects of many herbs on pregnant women, so it's best to avoid them while you're pregnant, including herbal teas. Decaffeinated black teas are your best bet, but if you want a fruit or ginger tea, read the ingredient label on the package carefully to be sure that no herbs are present. If you want to use an herbal remedy, talk to your doctor first.

---

Your doctor may also recommend additional scans to check that your baby is growing well.

**Thyroid problems** If you have an underactive thyroid gland for which you are taking thyroxine, you'll need to have a blood test to ensure that your thyroid is functioning well and that you're taking the correct dose, since sometimes the thyroxine requirement increases in pregnancy. It's important that you are not lacking in thyroxine, because this may affect the baby. If you are being treated for an overactive thyroid gland, check with your doctor that you're taking a thyroid medication that is safe in pregnancy. Your thyroid function will be monitored to check that your medication doesn't need to change.

**Bowel disease** Women with inflammatory bowel conditions, such as ulcerative colitis or Crohn's disease, usually find that their condition improves during pregnancy, although you may relapse after the baby is born. Although it's unusual for bowel conditions to cause major problems during pregnancy, it is important to check that you are not anemic, which can be a side effect of some bowel conditions, and your doctor may recommend extra scans to check that the baby is growing well.

WHAT TO DO

## Exposure to chickenpox or rubella

Chickenpox in pregnancy can cause problems for the baby and can be severe in a pregnant woman, possibly leading to pneumonia. If you contract rubella for the first time in early pregnancy, it can cause miscarriage or severe problems in the fetus.

**If you encounter chickenpox,** contact your doctor who can check your immunity. If you aren't immune, your doctor may advise an injection to protect you from severe chickenpox.

**Your rubella status is checked** at the start of pregnancy. If you aren't immune, you can be vaccinated after the birth. Meanwhile you need to be extra careful.

**If you develop chickenpox or suspect rubella** because of a rash, contact your doctor immediately, but don't go to the doctor's office, where you may spread the infection to other pregnant women.

## Infections during pregnancy

When you're pregnant, your immune system is slightly suppressed. This is necessary to stop you from rejecting the baby, who is genetically half the father's! This means that you may be slightly more susceptible to common problems such as colds, coughs, a sore throat, or food poisoning, and that the illness may last longer.

**Colds and coughs** Most women get a cough or cold at some stage during their pregnancy. However, you should avoid taking cold medications since these can contain ingredients that are not safe in pregnancy, especially during the first three months (see opposite). Steam inhalations can ease congestion and hot honey drinks help to soothe a sore throat. Saline nasal sprays can also help relieve congestion.

**Flu** If you get the flu during pregnancy, call your doctor to get advice or make an appointment. Drink plenty of liquids and get plenty of rest. Don't take any flu or cold medications without talking to your doctor first. Flu complications can include dehydration and pneumonia, and complications are more common in pregnant women. The US Centers for Disease Control and Prevention recommend that all pregnant women should get flu vaccinations. However, the CDC says they should not get the nasal-spray flu vaccine, which is not approved for pregnant women.

**Food poisoning and stomach upsets** A severe episode of food poisoning can cause problems for you and your baby and could trigger an early miscarriage, so it's vital to practice good kitchen hygiene (see p.17). If you do develop food poisoning or a stomach upset, try to drink plenty of fluids, and if it continues for more than 24 hours, see your doctor (see also Gastroenteritis, p.468)

**Yeast** If you have an abnormal discharge, talk to your doctor since this may be yeast (candidiasis), which is common in pregnancy. A swab may be taken to confirm the diagnosis, and an appropriate local antifungal treatment prescribed (see opposite). Eating natural yogurt may help restore the bacterial balance in your vagina. Wearing cotton underwear and avoiding tight clothing is also recommended.

**Urinary infections** Many pregnant women get urinary infections because the hormone progesterone relaxes all of the smooth muscle, allowing the bacteria that normally live in your vagina to travel up the urethra (the tube that leads to the bladder) where they may cause an infection. The symptoms of an urinary infection may be slightly different in pregnancy. You may have the classic symptoms of burning when urinating and frequent passing of urine, or you may have different symptoms such as back pain, lower abdominal pain, nausea, or vomiting. These are usually easily treated with antibiotics, most of which are safe in pregnancy.

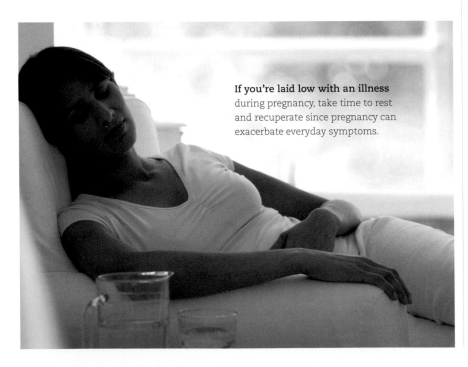

**If you're laid low with an illness** during pregnancy, take time to rest and recuperate since pregnancy can exacerbate everyday symptoms.

# Taking medications during pregnancy

**During the first three months of pregnancy,** it's best to avoid all over-the-counter medications. Once you are past the first trimester, some other medications are considered safe, but always consult your doctor if you are in any doubt. The following provides guidance on medications used for treating common pregnancy complaints and minor illnesses.

**Antacids** Heartburn and indigestion are common problems in pregnancy, particularly during the third trimester when the increased size of the baby puts pressure on your stomach. Some antacids are safe to use during pregnancy, although you should avoid sodium bicarbonate because it may increase fluid retention. Consult your doctor or pharmacist about which ones are recommended.

**Antibiotics** Many antibiotics used to treat infection are safe for use during pregnancy. This includes antibiotics containing penicillin, although there are safe alternatives if you're allergic to penicillin. The following antibiotics should be avoided during pregnancy:
■ Streptomycin. This can damage the ears of the fetus as it develops and may result in hearing loss in the baby.
■ Sulphonamides. These can cause jaundice in the newborn baby.
■ Tetracyclines. These drugs shouldn't be taken because they can affect the development of the baby's bone and teeth and can cause discoloration in the teeth.

**Antiemetics** If you have severe nausea and vomiting and natural remedies such as gingersnaps or ginger tea don't relieve the problem, your doctor may recommend an antiemetic medication that is safe to use during pregnancy.

**Antifungal remedies** You should avoid over-the-counter antifungal remedies, including oral and local remedies, for treating yeast. Consult your doctor, who can recommend an antifungal medication that is appropriate for use in pregnancy.

**Cold remedies** Remedies for coughs and colds often contain a range of ingredients, such as caffeine, antihistamines, and other decongestants, many of which aren't safe in pregnancy. Ideally, avoid all cold remedies and instead have steam inhalations and hot caffeine-free drinks. If you need relief, talk to your doctor before using any over-the-counter treatments.

**Diuretics** It's normal to experience some swelling in the hands and feet during pregnancy, and you shouldn't attempt to deal with this by taking diuretics, including herbal diuretics. If you have sudden swelling in the face, hands, or feet, you should consult your doctor immediately because this can be a sign of preeclampsia (see p.474)

**Laxatives** The first step in dealing with constipation is to take dietary measures by increasing your intake of fiber and drinking plenty of fluids. If this isn't enough to ease constipation, then some over-the-counter laxatives may be safe to take during pregnancy, including laxatives that contain bulking agents. Those containing castor oil may cause uterine contractions. Check with your doctor before taking any laxatives.

**Analgesics** The general advice is to avoid all analgesics during pregnancy, especially during the first trimester. Before using pain medication for a common problem, such as a headache or backache, first try natural remedies; massage or a warm bath are often effective in relieving aches and pains. If these aren't sufficient, call your doctor for advice. Aspirin and anti-inflammatories such as ibuprofen should be avoided throughout pregnancy. The pain medicine codeine can sometimes be used for a short period to treat specific pain, but should only be taken on the advice of a doctor.

**Rehydration solutions** If you have a stomach upset resulting in a severe bout of diarrhea that lasts for an extended period, your doctor may recommend a rehydration solution that is safe to use in pregnancy.

**Steroids** If you have eczema, or find that this condition develops or worsens during pregnancy, talk to your doctor about appropriate medications. Corticosteroids, which are used to treat eczema, aren't associated with birth defects, but they are known to cross the placenta, so both topical and oral corticosteroids aren't recommended during pregnancy.

Steroid inhalers used to treat asthma are safe in pregnancy, and it's important to control your asthma while your're pregnant.

Oral steroids may also be prescribed for certain other conditions, and these may be safe to continue with under the guidance of your doctor. Anabolic steroids should not be taken during pregnancy.

# Lifestyle hazards

Pregnancy can be beset with anxiety about potential hazards. Being aware of exactly what to avoid will help to allay fears.

Whether you're pregnant or are planning to conceive, now is the time to do a safety check on your social habits and home and work environment. Anything that could affect your well-being could affect your baby too, especially in the first trimester. However, don't become overly anxious. Instead, arm yourself with the facts so that you can avoid hazards, but also relax and enjoy your pregnancy.

## Your social habits

The decision to have a baby may inspire you to review your social habits and, if necessary, make changes.

**Alcohol consumption** You should stop drinking alcohol while trying to get pregnant and once you're pregnant according to the US Surgeon General. There is no known safe consumption level for pregnant women, so abstaining from drinking is the safest option. What isn't in doubt is the damage caused to the fetus by excessive alcohol intake. Continuous heavy drinking in pregnancy can lead to a condition known as fetal alcohol syndrome. The effects of this include retarded growth, facial and joint abnormalities, and heart problems.

If you drank in the weeks before you knew you were pregnant, try not to worry, but stop now. Many women also decide to give up alcohol while they're trying to conceive to optimize fertility.

**Smoking** Ideally, you should stop smoking before you get pregnant. If you're still smoking once you conceive, try to stop right away. If your partner or friends smoke, ask them not to smoke in your home or anywhere near you. Inhaled cigarette smoke interferes

**Wearing rubber gloves** when using household cleaning products will reduce your exposure to chemicals (left). **Opt for "greener" paints** and keep rooms ventilated while decorating (right).

with the supply of oxygen to the baby, which can lead to a low birthweight and increases the risk of stillbirth or the death of a baby in the first month of life.

**Recreational drug use** In addition to damaging your own health, recreational drugs are not advised in pregnancy since some pose dangers for the fetus and others carry a range of possible hazards.

Heroin and cocaine are damaging both to a pregnant woman and her unborn baby. These drugs stunt fetal growth, affect the placenta, and can cause miscarriage or premature birth, as well as health problems in the newborn. Babies born to women who use heroin often show drug withdrawal symptoms. A report on ecstasy linked the use of this in pregnancy to a rise in birth defects, such as limb abnormalities. The specific effects on the fetus of amphetamines and LSD are unclear, but it's safest to avoid them.

The direct effects on the fetus of the active chemicals in marijuana are not

clear, but smoking the drug involves the same risks as tobacco smoking.

## Hazards at home

Many of us use chemicals daily in and around the home. In addition to personal products, such as bath oils, deodorants, and hairsprays, we also keep dozens of other substances around the home, including cleaning fluids, detergents, bleach, and air fresheners.

When products are used in accordance with the manufacturers' instructions, there is little chance of them causing harm in pregnancy. However, minute traces of chemicals can enter the bloodstream, either through the skin or by inhalation, and cross the placenta. While there is no hard evidence to show that this has an ill effect, it makes sense to minimize the chances of chemicals from reaching a developing baby.

When using products, wear rubber gloves to prevent skin contact and ventilate rooms. To avoid inhaling mists or vapors, choose nonaerosol products. Also, choose products recommended for their low environmental impact, which contain fewer chemicals. Where possible, use natural alternatives to chemicals.

**Painting and decorating** It's important to stay safe while doing home projects. Don't climb up ladders or stand on tables to reach high places since your belly alters your center of balance. Also avoid skin contact or inhalation if you use oil-based paints; spray paints; paint strippers; floor varnishes; and sealant adhesives. Make sure rooms are well ventilated while decorating, and, ideally, get someone else to do the decorating.

**Pets and infections** Certain infections that could harm the fetus can be picked up from pets. The parasitic infection toxoplasmosis is spread through contact with cat feces. It may produce flulike symptoms, or no symptoms at all, and many unknowingly acquire immunity through previous exposure. However, although it rarely happens, contracting toxoplasmosis for the first time in pregnancy can cause serious problems, such as miscarriage or birth defects. Other pets, such as dogs, caged birds, and turtles can carry salmonella bacteria. Salmonella infection doesn't directly harm the baby, but can make a pregnant woman ill.

Being scrupulous about hygiene helps you avoid such infections. Wear rubber gloves when handling a cat litter box, cleaning cages where animals are kept, or disposing of dog feces, then wash your hands (and the gloves) afterward. Wear gloves also for digging or weeding in case animals have defecated in the garden. Or get someone else to do these tasks.

Toxoplasmosis and salmonella can also be contracted from eating undercooked or raw meat or eggs, so be careful with kitchen hygiene and cooking (see p.17).

## Workplace hazards
It's the legal responsibility of your employer to provide a safe environment.

In pregnancy, being aware of your rights can help protect you and your baby.

In recent decades, women worried about whether working at a computer screen put their babies at risk. It's now clear that using a VDT (as well as photocopiers and printers) is safe. Some environments do pose possible dangers. If you work in a health-care setting with ionizing radiation or cancer-treatment drugs, inform your department that you're pregnant, so that if necessary, you're given alternative duties.

Women employed in places such as hairdressers, manicure salons, labs, and craft workshops may be exposed to toxic chemicals. Working around some dry cleaning solvents has been linked to miscarriage. It's up to employers to ensure protection from hazards. If you're unhappy about conditions, talk to your boss or HR manager.

Standing on your feet all day and physical work that involves heavy lifting can be exhausting in pregnancy. If your work involves either of these, ask if it's possible to switch to less tiring tasks.

**If your job involves handling chemicals,** ensure that a risk assessment is done and that you are able to avoid harmful substances.

### COMMON WORRIES

**Is it safe to use a cell phone during pregnancy? I've read that phones emit radiation.**
The radiation emitted by cell phones is "non-ionizing." This is not the same as the radiation received from X-rays, which can be harmful in large doses. There is no evidence to show that using a cell phone is a health risk to either you or your baby.

**I go swimming twice a week and love the feeling of having the weight taken off my belly! But is the chlorine in the pool bad for my baby?**
In the past there has been some debate about whether it's safe to swim in chlorinated pools during pregnancy. However, now most experts believe that swimming in chlorinated water does not pose any health risks for pregnant women and their developing babies. You may find that the smell of chlorine might add to your nausea if you are suffering from morning sickness, although this is less of a problem in an outdoor pool. Try not to swallow the water, and shower when you come out of the pool. Swimming has great benefits during pregnancy. It has a low risk of injury while providing a good cardiovascular workout and improving muscle tone, so don't be put off by unnecessary worries.

**Is it OK to use nicotine patches or gum while I'm pregnant?**
Nicotine is known to decrease the blood supply to the fetus. This could affect the baby's growth, especially in early pregnancy. Although tobacco substitutes such as patches, gum, and lozenges deliver less nicotine to your body than smoking, you should never use them without a doctor's advice. Ask your doctor for information on safer ways to beat cigarette and nicotine cravings.

# Skin, hair, and teeth

In addition to affecting what happens to you internally, hormonal changes in pregnancy can also affect your external appearance.

Many women look and feel better than ever during pregnany, while those less fortunate report that there is a downturn in their appearance. However pregnancy affects you, the changes will be temporary and you'll be back to your normal self soon after the birth.

## Skin

You may find that your skin looks better in pregnancy due to hormonal changes, mild fluid retention, and increased blood flow. These can all result in smoother skin and are responsible for the famous "pregnancy glow." On the other hand, you may find that your skin gets drier and more pimply and you may need to take extra care of it during pregnancy.

Skin also tends to darken during pregnancy, although the cause for this is unknown. One possible explanation is the increased levels of estrogen and melanocyte-stimulating hormone, which stimulate skin pigmentation.

### Stretch marks (striae gravidarum)

Many women develop stretch marks during pregnancy, which can occur on bellies, breasts, hips, or legs. These initially appear as pink or purple lines and may be quite itchy. After pregnancy they fade into pale wrinkles. Nobody knows for sure why these occur, but they probably result from a combination of pregnancy hormones and your skin stretching. You're more likely to get stretch marks if you're very young, if you gain a lot of weight in pregnancy, or if you have a very big baby. There is less agreement about the role of other factors such as a family history, being very overweight before pregnancy or belonging to a particular ethnic group.

Many creams, lotions, and oils have been marketed for the prevention or treatment of stretch marks but none has been proven to work. Studies have shown that some creams containing ingredients such as vitamin E, elastin, collagen-elastin hydrolysates, and menthol can reduce the development of stretch marks; but other trials have shown that creams containing vitamin E had no effect. If you want to use a commercially recommended cream, lotion, or oil, they are safe to use and may help prevent stretch marks, but unfortunately there is no guarantee.

**Chloasma** This describes the increased pigmentation of the cheeks, nose, and chin that affects around 50–70 percent of pregnant women. Using a protective sunscreen and avoiding the use of any photosensitizing skin-care products may reduce chloasma. A recent study found that using a highly protective sunscreen (SPF 50 and UVA-PF 28) prevented most pregnant women from developing chloasma.

## Hair and nails

Hair stays longer in the growth phase during pregnancy, meaning that your scalp hair is likely to grow and thicken. Not so welcome is the fact that facial and body hair may also increase. After the birth, many women find that they suddenly lose a lot of hair as the growth phase stops. You should find that your hair is back to normal within six months.

Fingernails may also change, often becoming stronger, although some find that they become softer and brittle. Nails may develop white spots or

**Applying moisturizing creams** to relieve dry, itchy skin, or ones recommended to reduce stretch marks, is safe during pregnancy (left). **Taking good care of your teeth and gums** is important during pregnancy, when you're more susceptible to dental problems (right).

I am 18 weeks' pregnant and due to go on a beach vacation. My facial and body hair has grown and become very unsightly. How can I safely remove it?
You can safely tweeze, wax, and shave new stray hair. Skin bleaching and hair removal creams are probably safe during pregnancy, but there has been insufficient research to clear them since they can be absorbed through the skin and their effects on the baby are unknown. Permanent hair-removal techniques, such as laser and electrolysis, are thought to be safe in pregnancy. Both techniques penetrate the skin no deeper than a few millimeters. Consult your doctor to see if this is okay.

I've been using topical cream to treat acne and I've just found out that I'm pregnant. Will it harm my baby?
Tretinoin belongs to a group of medications called retinoids that contain vitamin A and may be associated with birth defects. Studies have looked at the effects of this cream in pregnancy and have found that babies whose mothers used it, even in the first trimester, had no increase in birth defects. However doctors recommend avoiding tretinoin cream in pregnancy.

Another similar medication, isotretinoin, which is taken orally, may increase the risk of birth defects and is therefore contraindicated in pregnancy.

I'm in the first trimester and will be going to my sister's wedding. Can I have highlights put in my hair?
Although the research into the safety of hair dyes if used in the first trimester may seem conflicting, the amount of chemicals used is small and it's unlikely that hair dyes cause harm. Also, if your hairdresser uses foil, the dye is kept off your skin.

I've heard that nail polish needs to be removed if you have a cesarean. Why is this?
Previously, women were encouraged to remove nail polish before surgery. One of the reasons was that the "pulse oximeter," a device attached to your finger to measure the oxygen in your blood during surgery, may give lower readings if placed over nail polish. However the device works as intended with nail polish or long nails if it's mounted sideways on a finger. Therefore there's no need to remove your polish.

# Beauty treatments and cosmetics

The following advises which products and treatments are safe in pregnancy.

**Hair and nail products** Shampoos, conditioners, manicures, and pedicures are safe. Minute amounts of hair dye may be absorbed through the skin, but there's no evidence that this affects the baby. Chemical hair straighteners and curlers are also thought to be safe.

**Piercing** Facial piercing or piercing the belly button, nipples, or genitalia isn't advised since you're at a higher risk of infection. If you have a navel piercing already, you can change a metallic ring for a flexible plastic retainer made from PTFE (polytetrafluoroethylene). Nipple rings can affect breast-feeding, so remove a ring before birth so the skin can heal. Vaginal or vulval piercings are best removed to avoid damage at birth.

**Tanning** Tanning beds aren't advised because of harmful UV rays. Tanning beds can cause your body to overheat, which can harm your baby, and UV rays may break down folic acid. Tanning lotions are safe.

**Body wraps/ Hot tubs** These raise body temperature, which is unsafe for you and your baby. Heat exposure from a hot tub in the first three months can increase the risk of a baby developing spina bifida.

**Facials** The cosmetics used for facials are thought to be safe.

**Botox** The Food and Drug Administration recommends that women who are pregnant or breast-feeding should not use Botox. Although it's used for cosmetic reasons, it is a drug and should be considered as such. Doctors also advise avoiding Botox during pregnancy.

---

transverse grooves, but these are rarely anything to worry about and don't mean that you're lacking in vitamins.

## Teeth

Pregnant women are more prone to tooth decay (dental caries), bleeding gums, and chronic gum infection (periodontal disease). Poor dental health not only affects you, but can also have an impact on your baby. Studies have linked infection of the gums in pregnant women to premature birth, and if a woman has ongoing tooth decay after the birth, her baby may acquire bacteria directly from her saliva, leading to tooth decay in the child later on. It's therefore important that you take care of your teeth during pregnancy and visit your dentist and dental hygienist regularly.

To keep your mouth healthy during pregnancy, brush twice a day with fluoride toothpaste and floss every day. Routine dental treatment and some local anesthetics are safe in pregnancy, although it's better to postpone elective dental treatments until after pregnancy or take care of them before pregnancy. Many women worry about having their teeth x-rayed in pregnancy. The radiation exposure from dental X-rays is minimal and the risk to your baby probably negligible. However, dentists will take every precaution to minimize your radiation exposure, covering you with a leaded apron before the X-rays.

# Traveling in pregnancy

Your growing belly shouldn't put a stop to travel plans. Just a bit of extra planning is required to help your vacation run smoothly.

## Trimester-by-trimester travel guide

Think about the implications of traveling at different times in your pregnancy when planning a trip.

### 1st trimester (weeks 1–12)

■ Period of highest risk for miscarriage and development problems in the baby. Be extra careful to avoid extremes of temperature and overly vigorous activities.
■ Motion sickness could make morning sickness worse.
■ Flying is allowed, provided you have no pregnancy complications.
■ Insurance is unlikely to be a problem.

### 2nd trimester (weeks 13–25)

■ You are likely to be feeling your best, and the chances of miscarriage or fetal development problems are greatly reduced.
■ Flying is allowed, but check to see whether you need to carry a doctor's letter stating your due date.
■ Check with individual travel insurance companies to see if you can get coverage—policies vary.

### 3rd trimester (weeks 26–40)

■ Your belly is huge and travel may be very uncomfortable now.
■ Some airlines may not allow you to fly after 36 weeks without a letter from your doctor written within 72 hours of your flight that includes your due date and confirms your fitness to fly.

Provided your pregnancy is normal, going to faraway places is perfectly possible. However, discomforts such as extreme heat, high altitude, and makeshift accommodations may be less tolerable, and in some cases may compromise the safety of your baby.

## The best time to travel

In the first trimester, you may find that morning sickness and fatigue lessen your enthusiasm for travel. Most women feel at their best in the second trimester and this is also seen as the safest time to travel since your risk of miscarriage is low, energy levels are increased, and your due date is still some way off. After 28 weeks, the size of your belly, fatigue, and the looming birth date are likely to make home seem the best place to be.

**You've found your passport and put the tickets in your bag. However, when you're pregnant you may also need to take the following items:**
■ A note from your doctor stating your due date and giving you the all-clear to travel (helpful if you're over 28 weeks).
■ Any special medical records regarding your pregnancy or general health.
■ A list of numbers for health-care facilities at your destination.
■ Remedies for heartburn or other minor pregnancy problems, such as hemorrhoids. You may not be able to buy your usual products abroad.

## Making plans

A little extra planning is the key to successful travel in pregnancy. However tempting brochures look, think carefully before you book. How will you get there and how long will it take? Pregnancy adds to the stress of a long-haul trip. If you want to fly, check with the airline about its policy. Some require a current letter from your doctor confirming your due date and your fitness to fly after 36 weeks. This is largely because of the possibility of going into labor mid-flight.

**Taking precautions** Unless you have no choice, avoid visiting countries where disease is a high risk factor. Many doctors agree that protective drugs, such as certain vaccines and antimalarial pills, are not advisable in pregnancy

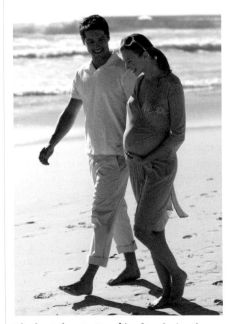

**The best time to travel** is often during the second trimester when nausea has abated and your belly size is not yet uncomfortable.

or when trying to conceive. Check the internet for information about an area's health hazards and local hospitals. If you have a condition such as diabetes that could cause complications, make sure you can get treatment while away.

Before you leave, try to get travel insurance. Some companies consider pregnancy a preexisting condition and won't provide coverage for your trip.

## Avoiding bugs

Pregnancy reduces the efficiency of your immune system, increasing your risk of an infection. When you're traveling, "stomach bugs" caused by contaminated food and water are more likely to strike.

If you're unsure about local tap water, buy bottled water (make sure the seal is unbroken) and use it when brushing your teeth as well as for drinking. Avoid drinks with ice and don't eat salads or fruit you can't peel since they may have been washed in contaminated water. A less obvious danger is fruit such as melon, which may have been injected with water to increase its weight.

Avoid outdoor stalls or cafés where food might have been prepared hours in advance. Try to find restaurants where food is freshly cooked and standards seem high. Be scrupulous about hygiene, and carry moist wipes in case hand-washing facilities are inadequate.

## On the trip

Sitting in a cramped seat for hours can cause your ankles and feet to swell. If you're traveling by car, stop every hour to stretch your legs, have a snack, or find a bathroom. On a train or airplane, keep your circulation moving with foot and ankle exercises, and get up regularly to walk down the aisle when it's safe to do so. Stay hydrated by drinking lots of water or juice, even if you do need to empty your bladder frequently. A few comforts, such as a cushion to tuck behind your back or a cooling water spritzer, can make a trip more bearable.

---

**COMMON WORRIES**

I am five months pregnant and about to go on a beach vacation. I know that too much sunbathing causes skin damage, but can hot sun also harm my baby? Experts are investigating a link between prolonged exposure to the sun and damage to the fetus. There is a possibility that ultraviolet rays could cause a deficiency of folic acid—a vitamin that helps prevent defects in the baby's nervous system leading to spina bifida. Nothing is yet proven, but it's not worth taking the risk. Enjoy the sun in moderation but don't bake yourself or use tanning beds before you go on vacation.

---

I'm worried about flying, because someone told me there is a high risk of DVT in pregnancy. Is this true? Deep vein thrombosis (DVT), the formation of a blood clot in a vein (often in a leg), is sometimes caused by long periods of immobility, such as sitting on a plane (see p.186). Although the risk factor may be slightly increased in pregnant women, because their blood tends to clot more easily, the chance of your developing DVT is still very low. To minimize the risk even further, you could purchase some special support socks, which are designed to improve blood flow in the legs.

**The position of your seatbelt** may need adjusting to accommodate your belly.

Are car seatbelts and airbags safe to use in pregnancy? In the event of an accident, these appliances are far more likely to prevent injury than cause it—never travel without fastening your seatbelt. For comfort, position the straps above and below your belly rather than across it. Being hit by an inflated airbag will not hurt you or the baby, but to lessen the impact you should position your seat as far back as possible.

## Vacation activities

There are some activities to forego in pregnancy, such as water skiing or horse riding, where a fall could harm your baby. Scuba diving is particularly dangerous because of the risk of air bubbles forming in the bloodstream. If you have children, ignore pleas to join them on amusement park rides.

If you're used to exercising, there is no reason not to go swimming or walking, just don't overdo it—hiking up hills under a blazing sun could send your temperature soaring, which is a bad thing in pregnancy. In the first trimester especially, extreme heat can affect fetal development. You might also become dehydrated, which later on can increase the risk of premature labor.

Be cautious also about less energetic activities. Hot tubs and saunas are best avoided since the heat could make you feel faint and may be harmful to your baby. An aromatherapy massage sounds like a treat, but some oils may be toxic to the baby, especially in the early months. If you want pampering, look for spas with treatments for pregnant moms.

In pregnancy, your skin becomes more sensitive to the sun, so whatever you're doing be careful to protect against overexposure to the sun.

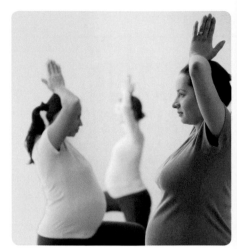

The 40 weeks, or 280 days, of pregnancy are a time of constant change as your body continually adapts to accommodate the new life growing inside you. This extensive chapter guides you through the physical and emotional changes you'll experience and offers reassurance, advice, and practical tips. Your baby's progress is charted in fascinating detail with scans and day-by-day insights into how your baby grows and develops within your uterus.

# Pregnancy
# day by day

# Welcome to your first trimester

| WEEK | 1 | 2 | 3 | 4 | 5 |
|------|---|---|---|---|---|

**Pre-conception care** A daily prental vitamin supplement before and during early pregnancy helps protect your baby from spinal cord defects.

**Avoid alcohol** Drinking soft drinks rather than alcohol may help you to conceive; add fruit to drinks for extra benefit.

**The release of an egg** At ovulation, an enlarged follicle in the ovary ruptures to release the mature egg, ready to be fertilized in a fallopian tube by your partner's sperm.

**It's official!** By the time you discover you're pregnant, your baby has reached the embryonic period and the brain, heart, and other organs are starting to form.

**Early growth** In the crucial first weeks, the baby's vital organs begin to develop and the neural tube, which becomes the brain and spinal cord, is forming.

**At first,** only you are aware of subtle body changes. By three months, changes may be visible.

**The path to conception** Sexual intercourse timed to coincide with ovulation is most likely to lead to a successful pregnancy.

**First trimester** Your baby is developing rapidly and you may have a whole host of symptoms, but outwardly there's little sign that you're pregnant. **Starting to show** By the end of this trimester, your waistline may start to expand.

**Facts and figures** You have a 3.5 in 1000 chance of having identical twins.

# You're at the beginning of an incredible stage of life that will see your body undergo dramatic changes.

| 6 | 7 | 8 | 9 | 10 | 11 | 12 |

**At 6 weeks**, budlike structures can be seen on the embryo that will develop into your baby's limbs.

**By 8 weeks**, the head has grown rapidly, giving an unbalanced appearance, and the limbs are lengthening.

**At 9 weeks**, the fetus is starting to have a recognizable form, with facial features beginning to develop.

**Feeling exhausted** A classic symptom of early pregnancy is a feeling of complete exhaustion, thought to be due to rising hormone levels and the dramatic physiological changes your body undergoes as your baby grows rapidly.

**Facts and figures** At 7 weeks, your baby measures just ⅓ in (8 mm) crown to rump.

**Dating the pregnancy** Between 10 and 14 weeks, your first ultrasound will confirm the gestational age of your baby. Your original due date may be revised as a result of this scan and the timing of future tests will be based on its findings.

**Parents-to-be** As the realization sinks in that you're facing parenthood, you may discover a new dimension to your relationship and an enhanced sense of togetherness.

**Soothing foods** Early pregnancy can often be marred by nausea and vomiting, especially in the mornings; eating crackers or sipping a decaf tea can help quell the symptoms.

# Your 1st week

**THE 280-DAY COUNTDOWN BEGINS HERE—EVEN THOUGH YOU HAVEN'T YET CONCEIVED**

It's business as usual for your body this week. You're having a period, so you know you're not pregnant. But if you conceive during this menstrual cycle, the first day of your period will count as the first day of pregnancy. It's a good idea to review your lifestyle and to make sure that you understand how everything works "inside." Knowing the facts may help to raise your chances of conceiving.

**The fallopian tube** is the passageway down which a newly released egg travels on its way to the uterus.

**Each ovary** contains eggs at various stages of development. By the end of next week, at the mid-point of your cycle, ovulation may occur. This is when a mature egg is released from its follicle.

**The ovarian ligament** stabilizes the ovary within the abdomen.

**Muscular wall of uterus**

**The thick lining** of the uterus (endometrium) that built up during your last menstrual cycle is shed as you have your period.

**Fallopian tube**

**Ovary**

**The pre-pregnant uterus** is about the size of a plum.

**Bladder**

**YOUR REPRODUCTIVE ORGANS**

**Cervix**

**Vagina**

# 279 days to go...

## WHAT'S HAPPENING INSIDE

The lining of the uterus builds up in the first two weeks of the menstrual cycle to prepare for pregnancy. The yellow and blue areas seen here are cells and the pink area, secretions. If no pregnancy occurs, the lining breaks down and menstruation occurs.

This is day one of your period. If you are trying to conceive during this menstrual cycle, keep a note of this highly significant date.

**Although this is officially the first day of your pregnancy,** you won't conceive until around two weeks from now. This is classified as "day one" because once you conceive your pregnancy will be dated from the first day of your menstrual period. It would be more logical to date a pregnancy from the day of ovulation or conception, but, like most women, you're unlikely to know the day on which you ovulate, let alone conceive. You are, however, far more likely to remember when your last period started, especially if you're hoping to get pregnant and are keeping a record of your menstrual cycle.

While dating a pregnancy in this way is a handy, if slightly baffling, convention, it does mean that your body is getting geared up for pregnancy from today. In around 280 days, or nine months' time, you could be holding your newborn baby in your arms. Good luck and enjoy the journey!

## FOCUS ON... NUTRITION

### Take folic acid

**Start taking this vital supplement now,** from day one, if you haven't already. You should take folic acid as soon as you begin trying to conceive because it will be essential to your baby's development in the first few weeks of pregnancy (see p.16).

The amount of folic acid that has been shown to be effective is a daily supplement of 400 mcg. A diet of foods rich in folate is also advisable so eat plenty of green vegetables, such as green beans, spinach, and broccoli; legumes, such as peas, beans, and chickpeas; fortified cereals; and wheat germ and other fortified grains.

## TIME TO THINK ABOUT

### Having a baby

There's no perfect time to become parents, but you might want to bear in mind the following:

- **While practical matters** such as the state of your finances and the size of your house are considerations, remember that being parents is about more than what you are able to offer your baby materially.
- **This is a decision** only you and your partner can make. Don't act on the advice of family members and friends.
- **You might conceive** immediately or it could take several months, so relax and don't have a set date in mind.

## AS A MATTER OF FACT

**Just 20 percent** of couples actively trying to conceive become pregnant in the first monthly cycle.

For 75 percent of couples it takes six months. So be patient and try not to get too stressed if you don't manage to conceive immediately.

# 278 days to go...

### WHAT'S HAPPENING INSIDE

Your eggs are already developing, as can be seen in this color-enhanced ovary. The small white structures are the immature follicles that contain the eggs at different stages of development. Once one of the follicles matures, the egg will burst out.

## By tracking your menstrual cycle and understanding how it works, you may increase your chances of conceiving.

**This is day two of your period** and day two of your complete menstrual cycle, which starts on the first day of your period and ends on the first day of your next period. A full cycle is, on average, 28 days, but many women have a shorter or longer cycle.

This may be the time when your period is at its heaviest, since the tissue and blood that make up the lining of the uterus (the endometrium) is shed. The average blood loss during menstruation is around two tablespoons (30 ml). While the lining is being sloughed off,

the blood vessels in the uterus constrict, which can cause cramplike period pains. As soon as your period has finished, an egg begins to mature within its follicle in one of your ovaries, ready to be released around mid-cycle. This is called ovulation (see p.49).

Meanwhile, the lining of the uterus starts to build up again under the influence of the hormones progesterone and estrogen, ready to receive a fertilized egg. If the egg is not fertilized, hormone levels fall, the lining sheds, and the cycle begins again.

### AS A MATTER OF FACT

**Periods can synchronize** in women who live or work together.

Scientists claim that pheromones (chemicals that trigger a biological response in someone) waft from one woman to another. Receptors in the nose detect these pheromones and a biological process takes place whereby one woman naturally adjusts her menstrual cycle.

### CHANGES DURING THE MENSTRUAL CYCLE

Inside the ovary

| Menstrual period | Relatively infertile phase | Fertile phase | Infertile phase |

Maturing follicle

Ovulation

Corpus luteum

Endometrium

1 2 3 4 5 6 7 8 9 10 11 12 13 14 15 16 17 18 19 20 21 22 23 24 25 26 27 28
**Days of cycle**

**The monthly cycle of an egg** as it grows to maturity inside an ovary is shown at the top of the chart. It is released from its follicle around day 14. The bottom of the chart shows the corresponding development of the lining of the uterus—shedding at the start of a period, then rebuilding in preparation for the fertilized egg.

The empty egg follicle (called the corpus luteum) secretes progesterone, which is a hormone that helps the endometrium reach a thickness of about 0.2 in (6 mm) over the 28 days of the menstrual cycle, ready to receive a fertilized egg.

# 277 days to go...

## WHAT'S HAPPENING INSIDE

The lining of the uterus, known as the endometrium, can be seen here (pink structure) shedding during menstruation. This happens if a fertilized egg does not implant. The red dots are red blood cells, released when the blood vessels break down.

## When you're trying to get pregnant, it helps to be aware of lifestyle and medical factors that can affect your menstrual cycle.

**You may notice the timing and volume** of your period differs. Your menstrual cycle can be affected by stress as well as by medical conditions, such as an overactive thyroid. In both these cases, periods can become lighter or less frequent. If your periods are erratic, it can be difficult to predict when you might ovulate. Unpredictable or missed periods may mean that ovulation isn't occurring at all. If you know this to be the case because you're monitoring the signs of ovulation (see p.43), or using ovulation predictor tests (see p.43), seek medical advice about your fertility.

You may be able to become pregnant naturally and easily despite problems related to your period, but some conditions that cause long, irregular, or heavy periods are linked to lower fertility. Heavy periods can be caused by conditions such as fibroids (see p.218), which can affect fertility. A higher than average level of blood loss can also make you anemic, which is not the best start for pregnancy for you or your baby, so you may want to look at boosting your iron intake (see p.154).

Painful periods can impact fertility. Endometriosis is a common disorder that can make periods painful and cause discomfort during sex. If you have these symptoms, see your doctor who might arrange a scan or refer you to a specialist. In endometriosis, cells resembling those that line the uterus come to lie outside the uterus on structures such as the ovaries, the fallopian tubes, and walls of the pelvis. There are treatments for endometriosis, including laser surgery, that can boost a woman's chances of conceiving.

### ASK A... DOCTOR

**Should I monitor my menstrual cycle?** Yes, monitoring your cycle is an important part of planning for pregnancy because it can help you figure out roughly which day you're ovulating (see p.49) and thereby improve your chances of conceiving. It means you can ensure you have sexual intercourse at roughly the right time.

It's also helpful to note the length of your cycle, which may vary. The most important thing to note is that from ovulation to the start of your next period is always around 14 days so when you get your next period, you can figure out roughly when you ovulated.

### FOCUS ON... IVF

## Stimulating egg follicles

**IVF (in vitro fertilization) may be an option** if a woman is having trouble conceiving. The first stage with this procedure is to stimulate the ovaries to produce many follicles, so that multiple eggs can be fertilized outside the body.

Starting on around day three of your cycle, you will be given drugs to stimulate your ovaries. You will need to inject yourself (see right) or use a nasal spray to suppress the normal cycle, followed by injections of a follicle-stimulating-like hormone. Egg retrieval will then take place (see p.57).

# 276 days to go...

## WHAT'S HAPPENING INSIDE

In this color 3-D scan of the human brain, the green central structure is the hypothalamus. This controls emotions and body temperature, and releases chemicals that regulate the release of hormones from the pituitary gland (green circle at bottom).

## Like many women, you may sometimes feel ruled by your hormones, and it helps to understand why they fluctuate.

**The hormone build-up to ovulation** starts right now in week one of your menstrual cycle. Your pituitary gland, which lies in the base of your brain, produces follicle-stimulating hormone (FSH). During your period, the level of FSH rises steadily, triggering the development of the follicles (around 15–20 each month) in each ovary. As well as containing each egg, the follicles produce estrogen.

The hormone estrogen circulates, affecting the pituitary gland and causing it to produce luteinizing hormone (LH)—this triggers ovulation (see p.49). This week your estrogen levels are low and steady, but will rise dramatically later in your cycle.

Progesterone levels are low during your period, but start to rise several days afterward and stay high for the second part of the cycle. Under the influence of progesterone, the muscles in the cervix relax, easing open the cervical canal. Changes also affect the mucus, which becomes more fluid, so sperm find it easier to swim through. It is progesterone that enables the lining of the uterus to thicken in preparation for implantation of the fertilized egg.

### AS A MATTER OF FACT

**Men** get PMS too!

Scientists have confirmed there's a male version of PMS—Irritable Male Syndrome. Mood swings, temper tantrums, and loss of libido in men were found to be caused by falling levels of testosterone due to stress.

### THE LOWDOWN

## Fertility rites

Rooted in folklore, these fertility tips require a leap of faith and a good sense of humor!

■ **Use the moon.** Exponents of "lunaception" believe that women whose menstrual cycle aligns with the lunar cycle—so they menstruate during the new moon and ovulate when the moon is full—have more chance of conceiving. It's based on the theory that women's cycles are influenced by natural light.

■ **Dance around the Maypole.** Maypoles are thought to herald the arrival of spring and celebrate fertility.

### CHANGES DURING THE MENSTRUAL CYCLE

**There are four hormones at work** during the menstrual cycle: FSH (follicle-stimulating hormone) causes the egg follicles to start developing in the ovary; estrogen is produced by the developing egg and peaks just before ovulation; LH (luteinizing hormone) triggers ovulation; progesterone thickens the lining of the uterus.

# 275 days to go...

## WHAT'S HAPPENING INSIDE

This cross section through the ovary shows several ovarian follicles. Between each follicle, the connective tissue can be seen. Each month about 15–20 follicles mature, but it is usually only one that will fully mature and release an egg.

Making some lifestyle changes is essential when you're trying to get pregnant and cutting down on alcohol is a good start.

**Even though it's still the week of your period,** and some time before you ovulate, try to ensure you're in the best possible health to maximize fertility. One way is to cut down your alcohol intake.

Heavy drinking can reduce the chances of conceiving and, if you do get pregnant, it can also harm your unborn baby's development. There is plenty of evidence that drinking beyond the recommended amounts is harmful. What's lacking is evidence of the effects on conception and pregnancy of the occasional alcoholic drink. There is no known safe level of alcohol consumption for pregnant women. However, many women decide to err on the side of caution and stop drinking alcohol entirely while trying to conceive and in early pregnancy. Some find that morning sickness (see p.81) naturally reduces desire for alcohol.

Alcohol also affects male fertility. It has adverse effects on the quantity and quality of sperm produced, and drinking large amounts can cause impotence.

You may find a drink helps you and your partner relax and puts you in the mood for sex, thereby increasing your chances of conception, but you may want to rethink having the occasional glass of your favorite tipple. The US Surgeon General recommends that women trying to get pregnant abstain from alcohol to eliminate potential problems.

**Opt for nonalcoholic drinks** if you're trying to get pregnant. A high intake of alcohol can adversely affect your chances of conceiving.

### AS A MATTER OF FACT

**Illicit or "street" drugs** can harm your unborn baby.

You should try to stop using drugs before you conceive. However if you regularly use drugs, or find it hard to manage without them, it is essential to get medical support. Ask your doctor for advice. He or she will be able to help and put you in touch with a support group.

### TIME TO THINK ABOUT

## Medical checkups

Before you try to conceive, speak to your doctor about the following tests:

■ **Rubella:** have a blood test to check that you have antibodies against rubella (German measles). Being infected by the rubella virus for the first time in early pregnancy is associated with an increased risk of the baby developing an abnormality, and increasing the risk of miscarriage. If you were vaccinated against rubella as a child, your antibody level may be high enough to protect your baby. If it isn't high enough, you'll be offered a MMR (measles, mumps, rubella) vaccine and advised not to conceive for three months.

■ **Sexually transmitted infections:** go to your doctor for tests to rule out infections such as chlamydia, genital warts, and herpes. You may also want to consider having an HIV test at your as well. Women with HIV can still bear children, but may be prescribed a medicine to reduce the chances of passing the infection to their child. A cesarean may be recommended.

# 274 days to go...

## WHAT'S HAPPENING INSIDE

In this artwork of the uterus, the green central structure is the pear-shaped uterus itself; the red part is the cavity of the uterus. The blue structures to either side are the fallopian tubes, which each have an ovary, seen in pink here, at the end.

Eating well is an essential part of conception and pregnancy so you and your partner should get into good habits now.

### FOCUS ON... NUTRITION

## Vital B vitamins

**Your diet should include** foods containing B vitamins (see p.16). Take a pregnancy multivitamin if needed.
- **B1** deficiency has been linked to failed ovulation and implantation.
- **B2** deficiency has been linked to infertility and miscarriage.
- **B5** is important for conception and fetal development.
- **B6** is essential for the formation and functioning of sex hormones.
- **B12,** with folate (see p.16), is essential to fetal development.

**Take the time in this first two weeks of your cycle,** before you ovulate, to look at what you eat on a daily basis—if you and your partner (see p.44) make some simple changes to your diet, it might just improve your chances of conception.

Use this opportunity to check your weight ie. your Body Mass Index (BMI) (see p.17) since a BMI of under 19 or over 24 could adversely affect fertility.

If you're overweight, excess fat tissue may affect your metabolism and hormones and you may not ovulate as regularly, or at all. If you need fertility treatment, the chances of success are also lower if you're overweight, because you may respond less well to the drugs that stimulate ovulation. Once you're pregnant, being overweight can also cause an increased risk of complications, decreasing the chance of carrying the pregnancy to full term.

Weighing too little when you're trying to conceive isn't healthy either. Pregnancy takes its toll on a woman's reserves, so a little stored fat is a good thing for mother and baby. Being seriously underweight can affect ovulation and make periods irregular or absent, and conception unlikely.

Your BMI when you conceive is also a good indication of how much weight you should gain once you're pregnant (see p.99) so it's worth getting it checked at this point.

### GET FIT AND FERTILE!

**Regular exercise can increase your chances of conceiving** by allowing your body to work at optimum levels. If you're fit and have a healthy lifestyle, you will reduce the level of toxins in your body and be less stressed, which makes it easier to conceive. Exercise will also regulate your energy and your blood-sugar levels, which assists the body in regulating the hormonal cycle—a key player in the reproductive process. Conversely, overexercising can adversely affect the ovulation process and make conception more difficult.

The guidelines for exercising at this crucial time of conception are to continue weight-bearing exercise, such as walking, running, or aerobics, for 30 minutes five times a week at a moderate intensity. It is important to listen to your body— moderate means exercising within a comfortable range, where the exercise isn't too hard but is pushing your body enough to feel the benefits.

# 273 days to go...

## WHAT'S HAPPENING INSIDE

Here an egg can be seen, in orange, developing in the ovary. The cells of the follicle, in which it is contained, can be seen surrounding the egg. At birth, baby girls have millions of follicles present in their ovaries.

When you're trying to get pregnant, you need to take your age into account because your fertility will change as you get older.

**In about a week's time you are likely to ovulate.** At the start of puberty, you had no more than about 400 eggs in your ovaries, and will have made no new eggs. Your lifetime of eggs were there when you were born. Given these facts, it's hardly a surprise that your fertility falls as you age.

Women 20–24 are generally at their most fertile and although, for most women, periods continue until their early fifties, the rate of fertility gradually lowers in the 30s, 40s, and 50s and the rate of chromosomal abnormalities and miscarriage increases. Nonetheless, every year thousands of babies are born to women in their late thirties and forties. Women can conceive beyond that age, which is why doctors advise menopausal women to use contraception for two years after their last period.

If, however, you're hoping to start a family, it's safe to assume that fertility begins to fall off sharply after age 35. Your age also affects the quality of your eggs. In women in their early 20s, around 17 percent of eggs have a chromosomal abnormality, but the figure rises to over 75 percent in women in their 40s. Chromosomal problems increase the chances of having a child with a disorder such as Down syndrome (see p.476).

**The follicle lies below the surface** of the ovarian wall and protrudes just prior to ovulation. The follicle is most likely to rupture and release an egg mid-cycle, around days 13 and 14 of a 28-day cycle.

If you're concerned about your fertility, it is possible to have a blood test that can give an indication of your remaining ovary function so that you know how much reproductive time you have left. While some tests are based on levels of FSH (see p.38) and estrogen, newer tests use other markers found in the blood, such as anti-Mullerian hormone (AMH) and inhibin B.

But making a baby depends on more than releasing an egg; it must travel down the fallopian tube, be fertilized, implant, and the pregnancy be maintained. There's also the father's contribution to consider (see box, right).

### THE MALE BIOLOGICAL CLOCK?

**A man can continue to make sperm** more or less throughout his life, so you might not expect male fertility to fall significantly. There are plenty of older fathers around that seemingly prove this.

Recent research from France, however, found that men over 35 took a lot longer to get their partner pregnant. For those who conceived, there was a slightly higher risk of miscarrying. This is because sperm from older men is more likely to contain damaged DNA. So although older couples do conceive, it's a fact that men, like women, pass their peak fertility.

### AS A MATTER OF FACT

**Sperm have a long and perilous journey** of 12–16 in (30–40 cm) to reach the egg.

This is why nature is bountiful when it comes to sperm, producing many millions with each ejaculation. On average each ejaculation produces 2–8 ml of semen, with over 40 million sperm in each milliliter.

# Your 2nd week

**YOUR "FERTILE WINDOW" IS APPROACHING AND THIS COULD BE THE TIME YOU CONCEIVE**

Toward the end of this week, one of the eggs in your ovaries is likely to have reached full maturity. Ovulation occurs as the egg, under the influence of hormones, bursts out of its follicle. If it meets a sperm, you may become pregnant. Now is the time to enjoy lots of sex with your partner, so go for it—as often as you like. If you have any anxieties about fertility, try to put them aside and relax.

**Cilia (small hairs) lining the fimbriae** produce currents that help move the egg into the fallopian tube.

**The wall of the fallopian tube** contracts and relaxes to draw the egg into the tube for its journey to the uterus.

**The mature egg** is released from its follicle and breaks through the surface of the ovary. To meet a sperm, and be fertilized, it must enter the fallopian tube.

**Fluid from the egg follicle** is released with the mature egg.

**Fimbriae,** the fingerlike projections at the end of the fallopian tube, reach for the egg and sweep it gently into the tube.

OVULATION

**Inside the ovary,** the empty egg follicle produces the hormone progesterone, which stimulates the lining of the uterus to thicken.

# 272 days to go...

## WHAT'S HAPPENING INSIDE

Here, three developing ovarian follicles can be seen in white. The inner circle of each is the egg. Of the follicles shown, it is likely that only one will fully mature at ovulation (see p.49) and release an egg.

By the end of this week you're likely to have ovulated. It's a good idea to know the signs that indicate you're at your most fertile.

**This is week two of your cycle.**
You will probably ovulate by the end of this week and will therefore be fertile. However, the fertile window can be from 5 days before ovulation to 12–24 hours after as sperm can survive for 5 days inside you. If your periods are regular, ovulation can be easier to track, but you may want to use other methods, such as looking out for natural signs (see box, right) or using an ovulation kit. Remember, however, the best way to conceive is to have sex regularly.

While they are useful, testing kits are expensive and can be counterproductive because they make sex more clinical

and less enjoyable. They work by testing the urine to detect a surge in LH, the hormone that triggers egg release.

Always follow the instructions given. Testing between 10 am and 8 pm should be fine, but try to aim for roughly the same time every day. After a positive test, you should ovulate 12–36 hours later. Results are about 99 percent accurate but occasionally the result is a false positive. Results can occasionally give a false negative, especially if you've drunk a lot of water. If your test was negative, do another one the next day. Once you have a positive result, you can stop testing for that month.

### ARE YOU OVULATING?

**This week, look out for:**
■ **Lower abdominal pain** at ovulation, called mittelschmerz (the German for "pain in the middle")
■ **Basal body temperature** (your temperature when you first wake in the morning) rising slightly.
■ **Cervical mucus**—the cervix produces secretions, which become wetter, clearer in color, and stretchy, resembling raw egg white, just before ovulation. This indicates the start of your fertile phase.

## CHANGES DURING THE MENSTRUAL CYCLE

**Body temperature** can be seen at the top of the chart, rising sharply right after ovulation. The bottom section shows cervical secretions. These begin in the days leading up to ovulation, starting off moist and sticky, then becoming wetter and stretchy at your most fertile time.

**If you feel some of the cervical mucus** with your fingers, you will find you can stretch it out. This is a sign that you are about to ovulate.

# 271 days to go...

## WHAT'S HAPPENING INSIDE

In your partner's body, sperm is constantly being produced. Here the sperm cells can be seen: they consist of a head (green), which contains the genetic material, and fertilizes the egg, and a tail (blue), which propels the sperm along.

While you wait to ovulate, fascinating changes are occurring in your ovaries as your follicles mature to release an egg.

**In the time leading up to ovulation,** which will happen later this week, the most advanced follicle moves to the surface of the ovary, ready to release its precious cargo. While you were having your period, around 15–20 follicles were developing in your ovaries.

Both of your ovaries contribute to follicle growth, but usually only one ovary brings a follicle to ovulation. Which ovary it is seems to depend on chance since ovaries are not on a strict rotation. As the follicles grow, they enlarge greatly, filling with fluid secreted inside the follicle. Some women release more than one egg some months (see p.49) and if both are fertilized, it will mean nonidentical twins are conceived.

By the time of ovulation, the follicle will be about 1 in (2 cm) in diameter, while the egg is just about visible without a microscope.

To mature, follicles need FSH (follicle-stimulating hormone) produced by the brain's pituitary gland (see p.38), but their early growth doesn't appear to rely on it. It may, however, depend on other hormones and chemicals.

## SPECIALIZED MEDICAL ADVICE

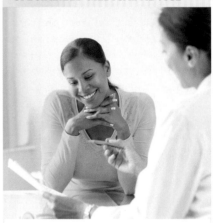

**If you have any ongoing medical problems,** go to see your doctor before you start trying to conceive. Conditions such as diabetes, asthma, high blood pressure, heart trouble, a previous bout of deep vein thrombosis (DVT) (see p.186), thyroid conditions, sickle-cell disease, and epilepsy can all impact a pregnancy.

The effect will depend on the individual condition and a specialist's advice and care will be needed. If you're in any doubt about how your own medical history may affect a pregnancy, check with your doctor before you start trying to conceive.

---

**FOCUS ON...** DADS

## Dads: your diet counts too

**It's never too late to start eating well** if you want to become a dad. But because sperm take some weeks to mature, ideally start eating a healthy diet at least three months before conception. There are supplements, but most vitamins and minerals work better in the form of real food.

■ **Antioxidants** A diet rich in anti-oxidants, including vitamins A, C, and E, selenium, and zinc, helps prevent damage to sperm DNA.

■ **Selenium** may also help sperm penetrate the outer layer of the egg.

Eat tuna, wheatgerm, whole grains, and sesame seeds.

■ **Zinc** is present in large amounts in semen. Eat fish, lean meat, shellfish, turkey, chicken, eggs, whole grains, rye, and oats.

■ **Manganese** is another element that could help male fertility. Eat leafy vegetables (including broccoli) carrots, eggs, whole grains, and ginger.

■ **Essential fatty acids** may improve sperm motility. Eat oily fish, such as mackerel, salmon, and sardines, flaxseed and linseed, and kiwi fruit.

# 270 days to go...

## WHAT'S HAPPENING INSIDE

As ovulation approaches, more cervical mucus is produced. Here it has crystallized to form a "fern leaf" pattern. Around the time of ovulation the mucus becomes clear, slippery, and stretchy, which makes it easier for sperm to swim through.

## You may not care whether you have a boy or a girl, but according to some theories you can influence gender.

**Conceiving is all about having sex at the right time** this week, but if you're hoping to have a child of a specific gender, the timing could be even more important. Some experts claim there is a link between when you have sex and the baby's gender (see below).

Recent research suggests that women who have a high calorie intake (especially if they eat that most phallic of fruit, the banana) are marginally more likely to bear a boy. Those who skip breakfast or have a low calorie intake are more likely to have a girl. One reason for this is thought to be that the extra calories consumed affect vaginal secretions and help to give the Y sperm that makes baby boys a vital boost.

**Research has found that women** with high glucose levels, achieved by eating normally and not skipping breakfast, were more likely to conceive a boy.

### AS A MATTER OF FACT

**If you already have two same-sex** children, you're 75 percent more likely to conceive a child of that sex again.

Although the sex of the baby conceived is random, conceiving children of the same sex could be due to the fact that some men produce better quality X sperm, which makes baby girls, or Y sperm, which makes baby boys.

Statistically, couples who have two children of different sexes are less likely to try for a third child.

### MAKING BABIES... BOYS AND GIRLS

**The Shettles method,** devised by Dr. Landrum Shettles, is based on the fact that Y sperm (for boys) are smaller, faster, and less resilient than X sperm (for girls), and are less able to withstand an acidic environment in the vagina.

**To conceive a boy, the Shettles method advises:**
■ Timing sex as close to ovulation as possible and adopting positions such as rear-entry that promote deep penetration.
■ The woman should orgasm, ideally at the same time as the man to make the vagina less acidic and favor Y sperm.
■ Drinking a cup or two or strong coffee just before sex to give Y-sperm an added kick.

**The Whelan method,** devised by Dr. Elizabeth Whelan, suggests that having sex earlier on in the cycle, some four to six days before ovulation, is more likely to result in a boy. Sex nearer the time of ovulation is more likely to result in a girl. Curiously, the Whelan way is more or less the opposite of the advice given by Shettles.

**But what works?** The mainstream medical view, supported by reports in journals such as the *New England Journal of Medicine*, is that the timing of sex has little or no bearing on gender. The possible exception is that having sex two days before ovulation may be slightly more likely to favor a girl.

# 269 days to go...

## WHAT'S HAPPENING INSIDE

The lining of the fallopian tube, seen here, has a moist mucous membrane. This contains cells (brown) that protect the tube's surface. The hairlike cilia (blue) move the eggs along the tubes following ovulation.

## If this isn't the first month you've been trying to conceive, don't be too disappointed. It's normal for it to take some time.

**Have you been trying for a baby for some time?** It's hard to face the fact that we don't always conceive when we want to. This lack of success may be difficult to handle, especially if you're someone who has achieved in other areas of your life.

With reproduction, there's a large element of chance. Even for young women at their peak of fertility, the odds of conceiving in any one cycle are 50–50. It's not unusual to try for six months, or even 12 months, without success. Around 16 percent of couples take over a year to achieve a pregnancy. So plan for conception over a longer time frame, say 12 months, unless you have any specific reasons to be concerned about your fertility or your health in general.

The main exception is if you are over 30. In this case, see your doctor after trying for about six months. The first step is likely to be a blood test for you, and a semen analysis for your partner. However, be reassured that if you are over 30, you may still get pregnant in the old-fashioned way. The average time taken for a 39-year-old woman to conceive is 15 months. But the snag is that if you do end up needing assisted fertility techniques, it all takes time.

### ASK A... NUTRITIONIST

**I've heard that green tea will help me conceive. Is this true?** So far, studies on green tea and fertility aren't conclusive one way or the other. Overall, it's likely to benefit your health without affecting your fertility. However, although green tea has a host of health benefits, it contains small amounts of caffeine and tannic acid, both of which have (at least in large quantities) been linked to fertility problems and an increased risk of miscarriage.

### STOPPING CONTRACEPTION

**You can get pregnant** as soon as you stop using some contraception.
■ **IUD (coil):** you can get pregnant if you have sex in the week before it's removed since sperm can live 3–5 days.
■ **Pill:** assume you're fertile immediately. Some women seem to be extra fertile after stopping the Pill.
■ **Implants:** fertility can return immediately after removal of the implant, but some women find it takes longer. Occasionally periods can take three to nine months to become regular. This suggests that the effects of the hormone are still lingering, but you may still conceive.
■ **Injections:** irregular bleeding can continue for months, and you may not be able to conceive for several months either. However, as with implants, it's possible to get pregnant before your periods return properly.
■ **IUD or IUS:** you could get pregnant if you have sex in the week before removal of the IUS system, but because the system contains progesterone, conception is less likely than with a regular coil (see left).

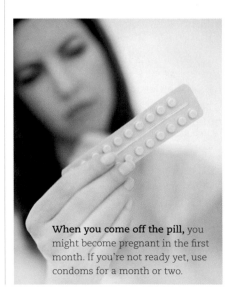

**When you come off the pill,** you might become pregnant in the first month. If you're not ready yet, use condoms for a month or two.

# 268 days to go...

## WHAT'S HAPPENING INSIDE

This mature ovarian follicle contains a fluid-filled cavity (pale pink) known as the follicular antrum. At this stage, just prior to ovulation, one follicle has become much larger than the others, and it is this follicle that will rupture to release an egg.

## As your hormone level rises around this stage of your cycle, so might your libido—it seems nature takes care of everything!

**Estrogen levels are rising and reach their peak today,** based on a 28-day menstrual cycle. The rise in estrogen from the follicles is what stimulates the release of the LH hormone (see p.38), which surges about 24 hours before ovulation. FSH (see p.38) from the pituitary gland starts rising later this week. Progesterone levels are low. There's no call for this hormone until the uterus lining needs to thicken. In fact, high levels would make the cervix hostile to sperm, so they would have trouble getting through to the uterus and the fallopian tubes to fertilize the egg.

Women also produce the male hormone testosterone and this reaches a peak around ovulation. This hormone is responsible for libido in both sexes so, hopefully, you and your partner should find you're both in the mood for making babies at this time.

### ASK A... DOCTOR

**I had a miscarriage four weeks ago. Is it safe to try for another baby right away?** There is no exact advice on when you should try again following a miscarriage. As a general guide, wait until you've had one menstrual period. This will help to date the pregnancy should you conceive quickly. However, your doctor may advise otherwise, especially if your miscarriage was linked with an infection. If you are waiting for tests because you miscarried, it makes sense to have these first.

You and your partner may need time to grieve for the lost pregnancy, so it is unwise to rush into trying to conceive again. Be reassured that the vast majority of women who had a single miscarriage go on to have a baby.

### AS A MATTER OF FACT

**Being stressed** can affect your ability to conceive.

Perhaps it's no surprise that nature makes it more difficult to conceive in stressful circumstances. One reason might be that it reduces the ovary's response to the hormone surge at mid-cycle (see left). There is also a link between stress and the failure of fertility treatments, although the exact reason for this isn't known.

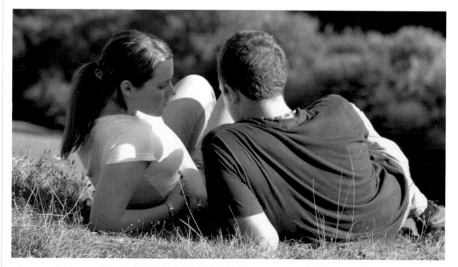

**It's a good idea to talk about and work through your grief** together before trying to get pregnant again. Miscarrying can be extremely tough and may put a strain on your relationship.

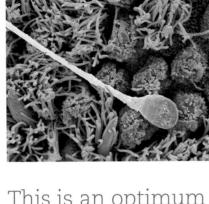

# 267 days to go...

## WHAT'S HAPPENING INSIDE

The sperm cell can be seen here inside the fallopian tube. Since sperm can stay active and alive inside you for up to 72 hours, it's possible to get pregnant even if you don't ovulate for two to three days from now.

## This is an optimum time to conceive, but try not to think too much about when you might be ovulating and just enjoy sex!

### AS A MATTER OF FACT

**Having an orgasm** could boost your chances of conception.

One theory is that the female orgasm is an evolutionary device designed to convey semen into the cervix as the uterus contracts. If the woman climaxes up to a minute before her partner, or she doesn't orgasm, she will retain less semen than if she comes at the same time or after him.

### Use the time around ovulation

to put some excitement and spontaneity back into your sex life. With all the recommendations and restrictions, not to mention old wives' tales, that supposedly maximize conception rates, it's easy to forget that sex is meant to be enjoyable. If you're hell bent on conceiving, then the fun can get forgotten. You might want to try different positions, times, or places for sex. If you and your partner aren't usually that adventurous, this is a good opportunity to try varying things a little.

Try to have sex every 24–48 hours. If your partner ejaculates regularly, it will encourage the production of quality sperm. The benefits of abstaining have been greatly overstated in the past. It is true that not having sex for up to seven days can boost the number of sperm, but research now shows that abstinence can impair the motility (swimming ability) of sperm, especially if the sperm were already borderline. The longer the period of abstinence, the more marked the effect will be. So have fun and if you conceive that's a bonus!

**It may improve your chances of conception** if you lie down for 15–20 minutes after having sex. Lying with your legs in the air will aid gravity further.

### SEXUAL POSITIONS

**It seems that how you have sex can help conception.** Positions that maximize penetration, such as rear entry, may work best since sperm is then deposited as close to the cervix as possible—languishing too long in vaginal secretions can lead to a sperm's early death. If the man is on top, the woman could try placing a pillow under her buttocks to raise her pelvis and aid the movement of sperm toward the cervix. Woman-on-top positions may lead to leakage of sperm. Avoid using lubricants because they can adversely affect sperm.

# 266 days to go...

## WHAT'S HAPPENING INSIDE

The ovary can can be seen here at the end of the fallopian tube. At around this time of the menstrual cycle, a follicle at the surface of the ovary releases an egg, which is swept down the tube by clearly visible fingerlike projections called fimbriae.

You're highly likely to ovulate today, if you haven't already, and if egg meets sperm you may soon be pregnant.

**Typically ovulation occurs around day 14** but it can occur earlier or later. Ovulation is when an egg is released from your ovaries (sometimes two eggs are released—see box, below). LH rises thanks to estrogen output from the growing follicles (see p.47), and it is this rise that triggers the events that now take place in the follicle. LH makes the egg inside the follicle become fully mature, ready for release and fertilization. This is the point at which the egg reduces its number of chromosomes (see p.55) from 46 to 23.

The follicle is rich with fluid by now. Just before ovulation, it is some 1 in (2 cm) or more in diameter. In position, it lies just below the surface of the ovary. If you could see the follicle, it would look like a blister about to burst. Next the follicle produces enzymes that digest its outer layer, releasing the egg on to the surface of the ovary.

Once the egg is released from the follicle, it's soon swept into the nearest fallopian tube by the fingerlike projections that form the end of the tube, where it will hopefully be fertilized.

### AS A MATTER OF FACT

**If you've had nonidentical twins already,** your chance of having another set quadruples.

Nonidentical twins occur when more than one follicle ripens completely and the two eggs released at ovulation are both fertilized. The increased chance of having another set of twins is because most women who conceive nonidentical twins (without fertility drugs) showa pattern of releasing more than one egg per cycle. Your chance of having a second set of twins is about 1 in 3000.

**At ovulation, the follicle ruptures** and the egg breaks through the surface of the ovary. Sometimes two follicles mature to this point, both releasing an egg.

### FOCUS ON... RELATIONSHIPS

## Pressure to conceive

**If you're trying to conceive,** you may have little else on your mind and this can put a strain on your relationship. With the goal of pregnancy in mind, it's easy to become clinical about sex. At this point, you and your partner may be regarding each other not so much as sex objects, but as components of a baby-making machine. Enjoyment can so easily get lost.

Understandably, you may find that your partner becomes aggrieved if he feels pressure to provide sperm; the distress may have an adverse effect on a man's willingness and even ability to have sex. If this happens, it can lead to a downward spiral, which naturally makes conception less likely, and may cause discord.

Make an effort to be loving and work together rather than against each other. Consider taking a break; couples often conceive when they're away on vacation and more relaxed. Make sure you also enjoy some stress-free sex outside of your fertile window.

# Conception

Pregnancy begins with conception, a complex process that involves the release of one or more eggs from the ovary, successful fertilization by a sperm in a fallopian tube, and implantation in the lining of the uterus.

### The release of an egg

Each woman is born with her full quota of follicles that contain immature eggs, some of which will mature and be released in her lifetime. Every month, follicle stimulating hormone (FSH), released from the pituitary gland, encourages a number of the follicles to ripen. These follicles in turn produce the hormone estrogen, rising levels of which encourage the uterus to thicken to prepare for the implantation of a fertilized egg. As the eggs mature, the level of estrogen rises and the pituitary gland receives a message to produce luteinizing hormone (LH). Every month, this surge in LH triggers one follicle (and sometimes more than one) to release a mature egg—the moment of ovulation.

Once the egg leaves the ovary, it enters the fallopian tube, which lies close by, and starts to travel through the tube to the uterus. The fallopian tube is just 4 in (10 cm) long and its lining has many tiny fronds that literally brush the egg in the direction of the uterus. Even so, the journey takes five days or more. In the course of this voyage, the fertilization of the egg takes place.

### The journey of the sperm

During sex, the man releases an abundance of sperm—around 250 million at each ejaculation—into the vagina. Each sperm has a long tail to propel it, so it's well equipped to swim up to the fallopian tube, where fertilization of the egg takes place. The whole distance, from the vagina

**ANATOMY**

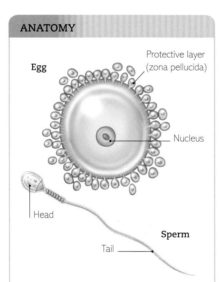

Egg

Protective layer (zona pellucida)

Nucleus

Head

Sperm

Tail

**The mature egg has a diameter of 0.1 mm** and is surrounded by a protective outer layer known as the *zona pellucida*. The far smaller sperm consists of a head, which contains the male genetic material and enzymes to help break down the egg's outer layer, and a tail that propels the sperm up the vagina and uterus to the fallopian tube.

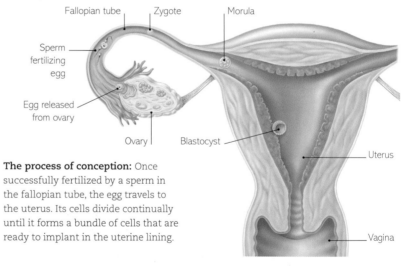

Fallopian tube    Zygote    Morula

Sperm fertilizing egg

Egg released from ovary

Ovary    Blastocyst

Uterus

Vagina

**The process of conception:** Once successfully fertilized by a sperm in the fallopian tube, the egg travels to the uterus. Its cells divide continually until it forms a bundle of cells that are ready to implant in the uterine lining.

**At fertilization,** one sperm penetrates the egg. Once the egg and sperm have merged, they form a single cell called a zygote.

**The zygote** divides into two identical cells, and continues to divide as it travels down through the fallopian tube.

**A morula**—a bundle of around 16 cells—has formed by around three to four days after fertilization of the egg.

**A blastocyst,** a mass of up to 100 cells, hatches out of the egg's protective layer and prepares to implant in the uterus.

through the uterus and up into the fallopian tube can be accomplished in hours. However, the sperm can survive in the vagina and the uterus for 3–5 days, meaning there is a window of around 6 days in which fertilization can take place (an egg lives 12–24 hours after ovulation). Not all of the millions of sperm make it as far as the fallopian tube; in fact, most of them die, seep out of the vagina, or get lost along the way. Around just 200 sperm, only a tiny fraction of the number originally released, arrive at the site of the egg.

## The moment of fertilization

Although many sperm cluster around the egg and try to penetrate its outer layer, only one of them will manage to burrow its way through the surface and fertilize the egg. Once this happens, the egg's outer layer thickens quickly to keep out other competing sperm, so that each egg can be fertilized by only one sperm.

## Implantation in the uterus

By the time the fertilized egg reaches the uterus, it has grown from a single cell into a compact cluster of cells, called a blastocyst. This cluster attaches to the uterine lining very loosely at first, then more deeply and permanently. At this early stage, the blob of cells, which is more than just a fertilized egg, but not quite an embryo, is sometimes referred to as a "conceptus." Although its sex is already determined, it's not remotely baby-shaped yet. The cells produce enzymes that allow it to digest its way into the uterus lining, and lie snugly below the surface.

## Assisting conception

Some couples find that conception takes longer than anticipated. If you haven't become pregnant after two years of trying, your doctor may suggest fertility testing to identify if your fertility or that of your partner is suboptimal. If this is the case, you may want to embark on

# How twins are conceived

**Today in the US, one in every 31 births is a twin birth.** Twins are conceived in two ways that result in either identical or nonidentical twins.

Identical twins occur when one fertilized egg splits into two separate cells. This type of twin is half as common as nonidentical twins. Identical twins have the same genes and are the same sex, so they are very alike, although subtle differences in their environment can mean they're not always identical in every way. Identical twins are known as "monozygotic" twins, since they come from one "zygote," or fertilized egg. Triplets, quads, and higher multiples can be monozygotic too. However, triplets and more can arise from more complex combinations. For example, there may have been two fertilized eggs, one of which split into two.

Nonidentical twins occur when two eggs are released at ovulation. Each twin's genes comes from the parents, but the twins don't share the same mix of genes. Nonidentical twins are also called "fraternal" twins, since they're no more alike than other siblings and can be of a different sex. They're also referred to as "dizygotic" twins, because they come from two separate "zygotes," or fertilized eggs. Nonidentical triplets arise when three eggs are released instead of one. This is more likely to occur when ovulation is induced with drugs during fertility treatment.

A fertilized egg divides into two

Two eggs are fertilized

**Identical twins that result from the division of one fertilized egg** may share a placenta in the uterus. Occasionally, they also share an amniotic sac.

**When two eggs are fertilized at the same time,** nonidentical twins are formed, each with its own placenta and amniotic sac.

fertility treatment to assist conception. The most popular treatment is in vitro fertilization, or IVF. This involves taking fertility drugs to help you produce more eggs. The eggs are harvested and fertilized with your partner's sperm in a laboratory (hence the term "test-tube baby"), and you're given hormone treatment to prepare the uterus to receive the fertilized eggs. If the quality of sperm is poor, a procedure called intracytoplasmic sperm injection, or ICSI may be used, whereby a single sperm is injected directly into an egg and the fertilized egg is transferred to the uterus. Intrauterine insemination, or IUI, involves putting sperm that have been selected for viability directly into the uterus. This is used where sperm has poor motility, or there are problems with ovulation.

# Your 3rd week

**THIS IS THE WEEK A MIRACLE TAKES PLACE—YOUR BABY IS CONCEIVED**

If you ovulated and the egg met a sperm, amazing things will happen fast. It takes just three days from fertilization for a single egg to divide into a ball of 58 cells. By the end of the week, this ball, called the blastocyst, will have reached the uterus, where it will start to implant in the lining. It will be a couple of weeks before you know whether you've conceived, but special hormones kick in now to help maintain the pregnancy.

**Cells surrounding the egg** secrete chemicals that aid egg development.

**The whiplike tail** of the sperm propels it up the fallopian tube to meet the egg.

**The sperm's head** carries genetic material along with enzymes that enable the sperm to penetrate the egg's tough outer layer.

**Maternal blood vessels**

**The outer cells** of the blastocyst anchor into the lining of the uterus.

**Cell cluster** within the blastocyst's fluid-filled cavity forms the beginnings of the embryo.

FERTILIZATION

Egg

Fluid-filled cavity

**Lining of uterus**

START OF IMPLANTATION

Blastocyst

# 265 days to go...

## WHAT'S HAPPENING INSIDE

Here the egg is shown surrounded by sperm. Although only one sperm will fertilize the egg, several hundred are thought to be necessary to break down its defensive layers and enable fertilization to take place.

Your newly released egg will only survive 24 hours, but hopefully in that time it will meet sperm and be fertilized.

**You are likely to have ovulated and your unfertilized egg now begins its journey.** Once it has been released by the ovary, the egg is swept up by one of your fallopian tubes and, moving in the direction of the uterus, comes to rest in the widest portion of the tube, awaiting fertilization.

It is no exaggeration to say that for each sperm released the chance of even reaching the site of fertilization is in the order of one in a million. Around 300 sperm reach the tube but only one will fertilize the egg. Once the sperm has penetrated, it triggers a reaction that makes the surface impenetrable. Each sperm and egg contain 23 chromosomes, half of the total genetic material required. The egg will always contain an X chromosome but the sperm will carry either an X or Y chromosome and therefore determines the sex of the embryo. The sperm and egg chromosomes combine forming the "zygote" and fertilization is complete.

**A few hundred sperm survive** the journey and encounter the egg in the fallopian tube, but it is just one sperm that actually fertilizes the egg.

## FOCUS ON... DADS

## Fit but not fertile?

**If you want to become a dad,** there are many reasons why you should ensure you're in good shape, not least to support your partner as she prepares for pregnancy. However, while a couch potato lifestyle isn't desirable for men who want to conceive, it seems that pulling out all the stops at the gym might not be the best course of action either.

Researchers asked a group of fit young men to exercise intensively four times a week for two weeks.

Afterward, their semen was tested and found to contain fewer sperm and lower levels of the hormones essential for conception. These hormonal changes were temporary and returned to near normal within a few days of the men resuming previous levels of activity.

The concern is that recovery might not be so fast among older men, or in those who have poor sperm counts and/or low hormone levels. So stay in shape but don't overdo it.

## AS A MATTER OF FACT

**The hormones responsible for the production of sperm** are released every 60 to 90 minutes. So a man is constantly producing sperm cells.

In theory, this means that a male is always fertile, but it takes sperm a 72-day period to fully develop. So leading an unhealthy lifestyle during that time will impinge on the quality. For this reason, if you're trying to conceive, your partner should embark on a healthy lifestyle for three months to produce good sperm.

# Genes and inheritance

The genes that parents pass on to their children at least partly determine their children's physical and mental characteristics. In some cases, an abnormal gene may be passed on, resulting in an inherited genetic disorder.

## HOW GENES ARE PASSED ON

## Through the generations

**Through each generation, genes are shuffled and re-shuffled.** Half of a baby's genes come from its father and half from its mother. The baby's parents in turn inherited half each of their genes from each of their own parents. One quarter of each person's genes therefore come from the grandparents. So how does this happen? Instead of containing the full complement of 46 chromosomes, each egg and each sperm has just half, or 23, chromosomes each. When they meet at conception the chromosomes pair up to again make up the full complement that now forms the genetic blueprint for the new individual. One of the 23 pairs of chromosomes are sex chromosomes, so gender is also determined at conception. Each egg carries an X chromosome and each sperm either an X or Y. If two X chromosomes combine, the baby will be a girl; if an X and Y chromosome combine, the baby will be a boy (see right).

**Genetic inheritance** means that successive generations can share certain characteristics.

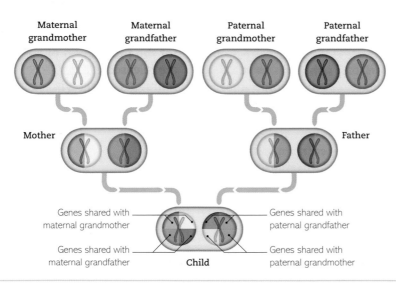

Maternal grandmother    Maternal grandfather    Paternal grandmother    Paternal grandfather

Mother    Father

Genes shared with maternal grandmother

Genes shared with paternal grandfather

Genes shared with maternal grandfather

Genes shared with paternal grandmother

**Child**

## What are genes?

Genes are located on rodlike structures called chromosomes that are found in the nucleus of every cell in the body. Each gene occupies a specific position on a chromosome. Because genes provide instructions for making proteins, and proteins determine the structure and function of each cell in the body, it follows that genes are responsible for all the characteristics you inherit.

The full genetic instructions for each person, known as the human genome, is carried by 23 pairs of chromosomes, and consists of around 20,000–25,000 genes.

## How inheritance works

At conception, the embryo receives 23 chromosomes from the mother's egg and 23 chromosomes from the father's sperm. These pair up to make a total of 46 chromosomes. Pairs 1 to 22 are identical or nearly identical; the 23rd pair consist of the sex chromosomes, which are either X or Y. Each egg and sperm contains a different combination of genes. This is because when egg and sperm cells form, chromosomes join together and randomly exchange genes between each other before the cell divides. This means that, with the exception of identical twins (see p.51), each person has unique characteristics.

## How gender is determined Of

the 23 pairs of chromosomes that are inherited, one pair determines gender. This pair is composed either of two X (female) chromosomes, in which case the baby will be a girl, or of one X and one Y (male) chromosome, in which case the baby will be a boy.

An egg always contains one X chromosome, while a sperm can carry an X or a Y chromosome. Whether your baby is a boy or a girl will therefore always be determined by the father. If a sperm carrying an X chromosome fertilizes the egg, the resulting embryo will be a girl. If a sperm with a Y chromosome fertilizes the egg, the resulting embryo will be a boy. In the male, both the X and Y chromosomes are active. In females, however one of the two X chromosomes is deactivated early in development of the embryo in order to prevent duplicate instructions. This could be the X chromosome from either the mother or the father.

**Gene variations** Each gene within a cell exists in two versions, one inherited from each parent. Often these genes are identical. However, some paired genes occur in slightly different versions, called alleles. There may be two to several hundred alleles of a gene, although each person can only have two. This variation in alleles accounts for the differences between individuals, such as color of eyes or shape of ears. One allele may be dominant and "overpower" the other recessive one (see box, right).

## Why genetic disorders occur

Genes usually exist in a healthy form, but somtimes a gene is faulty. Genetic disorders arise either when an abnormal gene is inherited or when a gene changes, or mutates. Genetic disorders may follow a dominant or recessive pattern of inheritance (see right). They can also be passed on via the X chromosome. Such sex-linked disorders are usually recessive, which means that a woman can carry the faulty gene without being affected, because she has another healthy X chromosome to compensate. If a boy receives an affected X chromosome, he will be affected; a girl will be a healthy carrier like her mother. An affected male could pass on the affected gene only to his daughters.

# Dominant and recessive genes

**Genes come in pairs,** and each gene in a pair may differ slightly. One gene may be dominant, and override the other gene, which is recessive. A recessive gene only has an effect if both genes in a pair are recessive. An example is eye color, although this is not as simple as depicted here.

KEY

 Recessive gene for blue eyes

Dominant gene for brown eyes

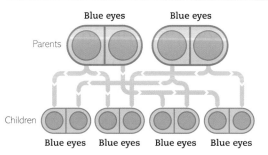

Parents — Blue eyes — Blue eyes
Children — Blue eyes — Blue eyes — Blue eyes — Blue eyes

**Two pairs of recessive genes** When both parents have blue eyes, as shown here, they will both have a pair of recessive genes for blue eye color. All of the children will therefore have blue eyes since there is no dominant gene present to mask the recessive gene.

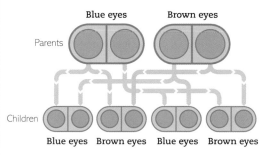

Parents — Blue eyes — Brown eyes
Children — Blue eyes — Brown eyes — Blue eyes — Brown eyes

**Recessive and mixed genes** In this example, each child will inherit at least one recessive blue eye gene from the parents. Depending on whether the other gene is dominant or recessive, the couple's offspring have a 1 in 2 chance of inheriting blue eyes, and a 1 in 2 chance of inheriting brown eyes.

Parents — Brown eyes — Brown eyes
Children — Blue eyes — Brown eyes — Brown eyes — Brown eyes

**Two pairs of mixed genes** Here, each child has a 1 in 4 chance of inheriting two recessive genes and having blue eyes, and a 3 in 4 chance of inheriting a dominant gene for brown eyes. The brown-eyed offspring may have either a pair of dominant genes, or mixed genes.

Parents — Blue eyes — Brown eyes
Children — Brown eyes — Brown eyes — Brown eyes — Brown eyes

**Recessive and dominant genes** In this example, all of the children will have brown eyes. This is because each child receives a recessive gene from one parent and a dominant gene from the other parent. The dominant gene will override the recessive gene on each occasion.

# 264 days to go...

## WHAT'S HAPPENING INSIDE

Here a human egg cell 24 hours after fertilization is artificially colored purple. Around the egg is a thick layer (yellow) that has now become impenetrable. The two red areas, or pro-nuclei, contain genetic material from the mother and father before it has fused.

## When your egg has been fertilized, hormonal changes naturally occur to stop your normal menstrual cycle.

**At this early stage following fertilization of your egg,** the developing embryo will signal its existence to the pituitary gland in your brain and switch off your menstrual cycle. It does this by producing a new hormone, called human chorionic gonadotrophin (hCG). This hormone overrides your usual monthly cycle and maintains the high progesterone levels that are essential for your pregnancy. The hormone progesterone (see p.38) is essential to an embryo's survival in the uterus, and therefore to your baby's well-being and development before birth.

Later, starting around weeks four to five, your embryo will make all the hormones needed to maintain its own life. Of course its nourishment and shelter come from you, but even in the very early weeks of pregnancy the embryo behaves like an independent human, at least as far as its hormones and genes are concerned.

### ASK A... DOCTOR

**I've been doing ovulation tests, but they've all been negative. Does this mean I haven't ovulated this month?** Even if you don't appear to have ovulated this month, you may still have. It's possible to miss the LH surge just by chance. This is more likely if you don't test at the same time each day, or you drink a lot of water.

Remember too that ovulation tests are imperfect, and it's possible to get a false negative. If you had other symptoms of ovulation, such as pain, or changes in your mucus (see p.43), it's likely that you ovulated anyway. However if you have gone two or three months with consistently negative tests, then you might not be ovulating regularly. In that case, it's worth seeking medical advice.

### HEALTHY CONCEPTION

**When you're trying to conceive,** you'll find you are much more aware of your general health. As a rule, colds, flu, and other common infections are unlikely to affect your fertility or your unborn baby if you have conceived. Some infections and viruses, however, can have a more serious impact:

■ **Shingles and chickenpox** (both caused by the same virus) are best avoided around the time of conception if you haven't had chickenpox before.

■ **Food poisoning,** for example caused by listeria bacteria, can be harmful (see p.17).

■ **Toxoplasmosis** can be contracted from handling cat feces (see p.101).

### AS A MATTER OF FACT

**Too much testosterone** can affect a woman's fertility.

Small quantities of testosterone are secreted from the adrenal gland and the ovaries. In low levels it may aid fertility, but too much can affect the menstrual cycle and lead to infertility.

# 263 days to go...

## WHAT'S HAPPENING INSIDE

When the two nuclei have pooled their genetic material to create a cell containing its full complement of 46 chromosomes—23 each from the mother and father—the cell can start dividing, shown here at the first division creating a two-celled body.

## Vital cell divisions are now taking place as the fertilized egg begins its journey toward implantation.

**The chromosomes from the sperm and egg** joined over 24 hours ago. It takes around 30 hours for the resulting zygote to complete its first cell division. The zygote, at only 0.1 mm in diameter goes on to divide into 16 cells, forming a compact ball.

Cell division is such that the ball of cells is hardly any larger than the original zygote. The ball of 16 cells, now known as a "morula" (as it resembles a mulberry), travels toward the uterus, entering on day three after fertilization. Every cell within the morula is totipotent, meaning it is able to form any type of cell. From this point onward the cells will lose this function as they start to specialize.

---

### FOCUS ON... IVF

## From eggs to embryos

**Egg collection will be scheduled (see right),** following the first stage of IVF (see p.37). Not all follicles that were stimulated will contain eggs. Two days after egg retrieval, you will be given progesterone to thicken the uterus lining. Two to five days after fertilization, the most promising embryos are chosen to be transferred.

If you're under 40, you'll have one or two embryos transferred. If you're over 40, you may have up to three or more transferred. The goal is to achieve a pregnancy, yet limit the risks of a multiple pregnancy. Any leftover embryos can be frozen for future treatment cycles. Recent research suggests that frozen embryos are better than fresh ones—this may be

because only the best embryos are selected for freezing and survive the freezing and thawing process.

The outcome of IVF depends to a great extent on the woman's age, but on average each cycle has a 20 percent success rate.

---

### ASK A... DOCTOR

**I've been doing ovulation tests. I've now ovulated so do my partner and I need to keep having sex to make sure I conceive?** You can't be sure that you've conceived already, so the usual advice would be to continue lovemaking. Even if you've been tracking your ovulation by monitoring your temperature or cervical mucus, or by using an ovulation kit (see p.43), you can't be sure exactly when it occurred. It won't be possible for you to pinpoint the exact time of ovulation.

Since the fertile window is several days, you may as well continue having sex for at least a couple of days after what you think is your most fertile time.

Furthermore, since sex says "I love you" more strongly than most other means of communication, it's good for both you and your partner to stay intimate at times you're not trying to conceive.

Remember also that abstention doesn't usually have the hoped-for effect of banking up and improving the quantity and quality of sperm. In fact, the opposite may happen (see p.48).

# 262 days to go...

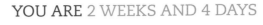

### WHAT'S HAPPENING INSIDE

This is an embryo at the 16-cell stage, when it has changed from a zygote into a morula. It is in the process of dividing into a hollow ball of cells—the blastocyst—which will eventually implant in the lining of the uterus.

## Significant changes are taking place daily within your uterus and within just 72 hours from now, the fertilized egg will implant.

**Around four days following fertilization,** fluid begins to collect within the morula (see p.57). This creates a separate outer cell layer, one cell thick that encapsulates an inner mass of cells. The inner layer will become the embryo, and the outer layer the placenta (see p.76). The whole structure now consists of approximately 58 cells and is termed the "blastocyst."

The blastocyst spends several days within the cavity of the uterus before implanting. The morula had an impenetrable outer surface as it traveled, but this disappears as the blastocyst prepares for implantation.

### ASK A... MOM

**Why are people so interested in whether I've conceived?** I certainly found that once I'd told people I was trying to have a baby, they were inordinately interested in the process. It was difficult, especially in the week when I was waiting to find out if I'd conceived. The best way to deal with it is to respond by saying that you'll let people know if there's news. If you're struggling to conceive, telling people you're having difficulties should help stop them from asking.

### FOCUS ON... HEALTH

## Fertility: the alternative approach

**If you're having difficulty conceiving,** or just want to improve your chances, consider using a complementary therapy. Always inform the practitioner that you might be pregnant.

■ **Reflexology** works by manipulating pressure points in the feet to improve energy flow to specific parts of the body. While there is plenty of anecdotal evidence that reflexology helps conception, this isn't currently backed up by scientific research. However, it may help relieve stress, which can be a factor in couples who have problems conceiving.

■ **Acupuncture** (see right) works on the principle that problems such as infertility are caused by blockages in the body's energy flow or "qi." By inserting tiny needles into energy points that are linked to the reproductive organs, the flow is restored. In 2008, after reviewing seven studies of more than 1,300 women having fertility treatment, researchers concluded that acupuncture given around the time

of embryo transfer increases the chances of pregnancy.

It's not as clear whether acupuncture can improve fertility in couples not undergoing treatment, but it is thought to improve male fertility by improving sperm health and reducing stress, a factor that can impede the chances of conception.

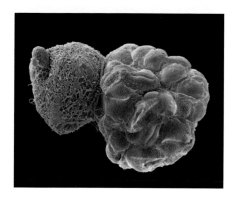

# 261 days to go...

## WHAT'S HAPPENING INSIDE

This is an embryo at the blastocyst stage, five days after fertilization. It is seen hatching from the shell that originally surrounded the unfertilized egg. At this stage, the blastocyst has moved into the uterus and is preparing to implant.

## While playing the waiting game, you may want to consider how you'd feel if there are two fertilized embryos waiting to implant!

**Have you conceived, and might it be twins?** Twins can be nonidentical or identical and each type of twins is conceived differently.

Nonidentical (dizygotic) twins are the result of two separate eggs being fertilized by separate sperm. They may also occur as a result of IVF (see p.37) if two embryos are placed in the uterus.

Identical (monozygotic) twins occur when a single egg is fertilized by a single sperm and divides into two embryos. This split can occur at any stage up to nine days after fertilization and its timing is critical to the way the placenta(s) and amniotic sac(s) are formed. If the zygote (see p.57) splits within the first three days, two separate placentas and amniotic sacs develop. If the split occurs at blastocyst stage (see opposite), four to nine days after fertilization, the fetuses will share a placenta but have separate sacs; when the split occurs after day nine, the fetuses will share a placenta and a sac.

Having nonidentical (fraternal) twins, which come from two separate fertilized eggs, depends a lot on family history. It's often said that twins skip a generation,

**The lining of the uterus**, when fertilization occurs, becomes secretory to nourish an embryo. The lining prepares itself in the same way, no matter how many embryos implant.

which isn't quite true. In fact, your chances of having twins are simply higher if you have a close relative with twins, but twins never become inevitable, however many members of your family have them.

Family history is most relevant with nonidentical twins, and when the twins are on the mother's side. This makes sense because this kind of twin relies on a woman releasing two eggs in any one cycle (see p.49), which may be hereditary. However, for reasons that aren't clear, a family history of twins on the father's side can be important too. It may be that the male of the species can carry a gene which makes his daughter release more than one egg at a time when she ovulates.

### THE LOST TWIN

**Twin conceptions may be more common than they appear.** Without knowing it, some women miscarry one twin in early pregnancy. It is sometimes possible to have symptoms of a miscarriage, yet, confusingly, the pregnancy then appears to continue until term, culminating in the birth of a completely normal singleton baby.

Nobody is quite sure how often this happens, or why. While one in every 31 births in the US today is a twin birth, research using scans in very early pregnancy suggests that at conception the figure is much higher. Some experts believe that 15 percent of all births may start off as twins. Their loss could simply be nature's way of dealing with imperfections.

### AS A MATTER OF FACT

**The odds of having identical twins** are about 3.5 in 1000.

Some estimate that the chances of having twins after fertility-enhancing treatment is as high as 1 in 38.

# 260 days to go...

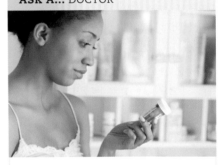

## WHAT'S HAPPENING INSIDE

The blastocyst prepares to embed itself in the lining of the uterus—the endometrium. Once it is completely implanted—usually around seven days after fertilization—the pregnancy will become established.

## Your reproductive organs undergo complex processes that will enable your body to maintain the pregnancy.

**If you have conceived, the ball of cells** known as the blastocyst that will eventually form the fetus will now be preparing to embed in the lining of your uterus, and the placenta will be starting to form.

Before this happens, however, there is another important change going on. After you ovulate, the empty ovarian follicle develops into a structure called the corpus luteum (which means, literally, "yellow body"). This small, fluid-filled sac becomes increasingly "vascular," developing blood vessels and beginning to produce the hormone progesterone. This is required to create mucus to allow your fertilized egg to survive, and build up the lining of your uterus, in which the blastocyst will soon imbed (see opposite).

The corpus luteum also produces a little estrogen. By about 8–12 weeks of pregnancy, your placenta will take over the production of progesterone, but the corpus luteum continues to play a small role in hormone production until about six months, when it usually shrinks away.

### THE MIRACLE OF CONCEPTION

**When you consider the multitude of events** that have to fall neatly into place before a baby is conceived, it's hard to believe that anyone can become pregnant. No wonder they talk about the miracle of life!

To become pregnant the following have to happen:

■ **Your hormone balance** must be correct for the egg to develop.
■ **Ovulation must take place**: if you don't release an egg, there is no way for fertilization to occur.
■ **You need to have sex** at the right time in your menstrual cycle; sperm can last about three days in healthy cervical mucus, but if your timing is off, egg and sperm are unlikely to meet. In some cases there may be only two or three days each month when you can conceive.
■ **Your partner needs to produce** plenty of good, healthy sperm that can penetrate your cervical mucus to reach the egg.
■ **When the egg has been fertilized,** the blastocyst has to implant securely in the lining of the uterus.
■ **The right levels of the hormone** progesterone must be produced by the corpus luteum to maintain the pregnancy.

### ASK A... DOCTOR

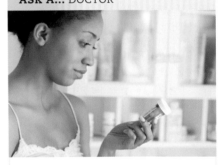

**Should I stop taking medication in case I've conceived?** Many medicines are safe to take, but some are not, or have not been fully evaluated. This last group includes many antihistamines for allergies, over-the-counter sleeping pills, and many analgesics (see p.23).

If you've accidentally taken an over-the-counter remedy that's not considered appropriate for use in pregnancy, you're unlikely to have done any harm with just one dose. However, seek medical advice if you're concerned.

If you need to continue using a medicine in pregnancy, ask if it's safe to do so. While pharmacists are well-informed on all medicines, your doctor is the best person to consult on prescription-only drugs.

# 259 days to go...

## WHAT'S HAPPENING INSIDE

The blastocyst is firmly embedded in the lining of the uterus. Once this has happened, the placenta (the temporary organ that supplies the growing embryo with oxygen and nutrients) will begin to develop.

It's a week since the egg was fertilized and it now implants in your uterus, where it will soon develop into an embryo.

**Around seven days after fertilization,** the blastocyst implants in the lining of the uterus. The outer cell layer, no longer protected, is able to attach to the lining of the uterus. The lining is now more receptive and has undergone changes that make it more "sticky" to aid attachment.

The blastocyst erodes cells to sink beneath the surface.

What was originally a single outer layer of cells now transforms into two layers. The outermost layer of cells creates space by eroding the lining, and it secretes hormones. These hormones inform your body that you're pregnant

and stimulate the uterus to support the pregnancy rather than shed its lining in what would normally be your period. The innermost cell layer will become the placenta and the amniotic sac that encloses the embryo. Within the blastocyst there is an inner cell mass that will form the embryo.

## STRETCH AND UNWIND

**It can help to relax in this interim period,** before you do a pregnancy test. Fill some time by getting in shape with these simple stretches. Getting into the habit of doing these exercises now will help your body deal with the increased demands once you know you're pregnant. Stretch before and after exercising to prevent muscle strain.

**To do a back stretch,** get on all fours and lower your bottom toward your feet while stretching your arms out on the floor in front of you. Lower your forehead as far as you can, keeping your neck and back aligned, and stretch your arms as much as you can. Inhale slowly and then relax your back and arms as you exhale. Inhale and exhale 10 times.

Make sure your neck and back are aligned

Feel the stretch

Keep your hands flat on the floor

**To do a leg stretch,** sit on the floor and stretch your left leg in front of you. Using your left hand take hold of your left foot for a few seconds. If you can't reach your toes, don't worry. Inhale to begin and exhale as you stretch. Repeat with your right leg.

Hold your toes if you can

Feel the stretch down the back of your leg

# Your 4th week

**THIS WEEK, YOU'LL NEED A LITTLE PATIENCE AS YOU WAIT, WONDER, AND HOPE**

The embryo-to-be, now securely implanted in the lining of your uterus, is starting to develop. Although you could do a home pregnancy test this week, you may end up disappointed or uncertain because at this stage a definite result is unlikely. It can be nerve racking, wondering if an unwanted period is about to arrive and dash your hopes. Talk to your partner and share your feelings with him—he may be anxious, too.

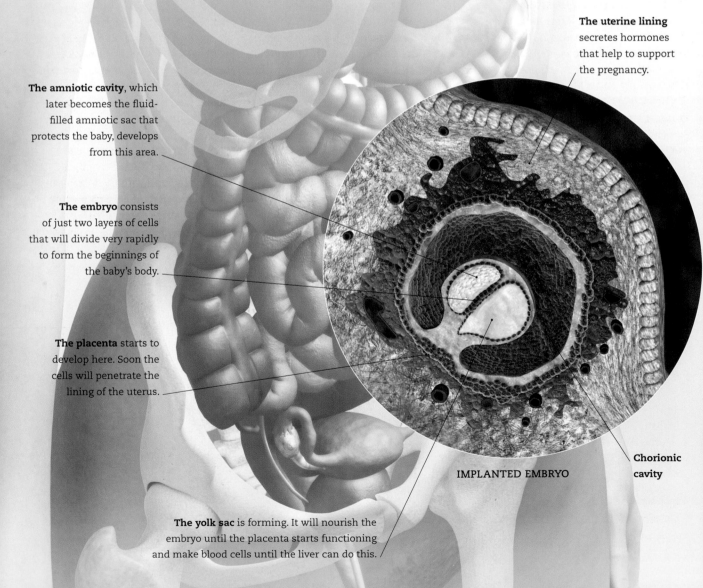

**The uterine lining** secretes hormones that help to support the pregnancy.

**The amniotic cavity**, which later becomes the fluid-filled amniotic sac that protects the baby, develops from this area.

**The embryo** consists of just two layers of cells that will divide very rapidly to form the beginnings of the baby's body.

**The placenta** starts to develop here. Soon the cells will penetrate the lining of the uterus.

**The yolk sac** is forming. It will nourish the embryo until the placenta starts functioning and make blood cells until the liver can do this.

IMPLANTED EMBRYO

**Chorionic cavity**

# 258 days to go...

## YOUR BABY TODAY

This is a cross section of the ball of cells embedded in the uterus at this early stage of pregnancy. It contains fluid in the center and two areas of white cells with a darker streak of cells between them—these will form the embryo, now less than 0.5 mm long.

Pregnancy hormones are being produced, but it may be difficult to detect them accurately, so it's best to wait before you do a test.

**You might be eager to do a pregnancy test** as you enter the fourth week of your cycle. Most women use over-the-counter home pregnancy tests (see p.71). These are simple to use and work by detecting the levels of hCG in your urine—this is the hormone that is produced as soon as the embryo implants in the lining of the uterus (see p.61).

There are home pregnancy tests that claim to detect a pregnancy six days before your period is due. But if you use one of these and test this early, your hCG levels (see above) may not be high enough to give a positive result, even though you might be pregnant.

### ASK A... DOCTOR

**I'm worried about doing a pregnancy test because I think my partner is going to be disappointed if I'm not pregnant.** Feeling pressured to conceive is stressful, and this can affect the hypothalamus (see p.38)—the structure in your brain that governs your menstrual cycle. So your partner's avid interest may actually be counterproductive.

Be honest with your partner about how you feel. Explain to him that you share his enthusiasm for having a baby, but that you're feeling pressured, and that you're worried it will affect your ability to conceive. Conversely, if you aren't entirely sure that you are ready for a baby, now is the time to discuss this, too. Pregnancy is a life-changing event, and both you and your partner need to be fully committed, and also aware that it can, in itself, be stressful.

Have fun together and make sure the pressure to conceive doesn't take the fun and spontaneity out of your lovemaking (see p.49).

### YOUR PREGNANCY DIARY

**Trying to get pregnant is an exciting experience,** so why not keep a written record—it's a good way to pass time in this interim period while you're waiting to take a pregnancy test. Rather than just noting down the dates of your period and signs of ovulation, use it to record the highs and lows so far.

Once you're pregnant, you can continue to use the diary to record your feelings: for example, your emotions when you saw the positive symbol on the pregnancy testing kit; how you broke the news to your partner and his response; what your baby's first kick felt like; the best and worst aspects of being pregnant. You may also find that letting off steam about your partner's quirks or your mother-in-law's idiosyncrasies is surprisingly therapeutic!

Besides providing a unique record of your pregnancy, keeping a journal can also help you in subsequent pregnancies: for example, you may find it reassuring to look back and find that morning sickness was just a phase.

# 257 days to go...

**YOUR BABY TODAY**

In this computer-generated image the entire blastocyst can be seen embedded in the lining of the uterus. The cells that will develop into the embryo are seen as the dark area in the 12 o'clock position.

Adopting a healthy lifestyle and improving your well-being are sensible measures now that you might be pregnant.

## THE LOWDOWN

## Cultural beliefs

**Here's what some cultures believe:**

■ **Hindu fathers** part the hair on their partner's head three times upward from the front to the back to boost the development of the growing baby.

■ **In some countries,** there is great emphasis placed on protecting the unborn baby. In Thailand, the pregnant woman's abdomen may be painted to ward off evil spirits. It is also believed that giving gifts before the birth will attract evil spirits.

### AS A MATTER OF FACT

**There are at least 30 chemicals** in cigarette smoke that can adversely affect fertility.

Because smoking reduces the rate at which cells replicate, it may cause most damage during the first days and weeks of pregnancy. In addition to causing fertility problems in women, smoking can have negative effects on sperm and reduce testosterone in men.

**Once your pregnancy is confirmed** in the next week or so, you'll find you're bombarded with more health information than ever. Is your diet well balanced? Could you cut back on the amount of salt, sugar, and fast food you eat? Are you eating plenty of fruit and vegetables, particularly leafy green vegetables, which are a good

**Get gentle exercise,** such as walking or swimming, which are ideal before, during, and after pregnancy.

source of folic acid. Are you exercising enough and safely? Even though you don't know you're pregnant yet, it's worth being aware of the recommended advice and making some basic dietary and lifestyle changes. Turn to the section on pages 14–29 for some up-to-date information. It's also worth being aware of the early signs of pregnancy so you know what's normal.

If you have a preexisting medical condition or are taking medication, seek medical advice.

### FOCUS ON... YOUR HEALTH

## Lifestyle changes

**If you smoke, you should quit** (so should your partner) for health reasons. Once you're pregnant, not smoking will reduce the risk of miscarriage, stillbirth, premature birth, low birth weight, and sudden infant death.

You should also stop drinking alcohol entirely. The current advice from the US Surgeon General is to avoid drinking alcohol completely while trying to get pregnant and once you are pregnant, since there is no known safe consumption level for pregnant women.

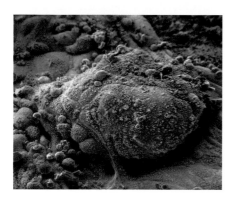

# 256 days to go...

## YOUR BABY TODAY

The embryo is implanted and is 10 days old. The entry point at which the embryo buried into the lining of the uterus is now covered by a clot, and this prevents blood loss and protects the embryo.

Try to stay busy to distract yourself from constantly wondering whether you're pregnant, and think positively.

### ASK A... DOCTOR

**I did an early pregnancy test and have failed to conceive again, for the sixth month. Could it be because I have irregular periods?**
Menstrual cycles that vary more than a few days in length from month to month are considered irregular. An irregular cycle can be troublesome when trying to conceive, but being aware of the signs of ovulation (see p.43) can help you determine when you are approaching your short window of fertility.

Irregular ovulation and menstruation account for around 30–40 percent of fertility problems. Many factors determine how fertile a woman is, such as her age, whether her cervical fluid is wet enough to sustain sperm, or whether her fallopian tubes are open, but the most important factor is whether she ovulates regularly. Sometimes, a condition called anovulation occurs, in which there is irregular menstrual bleeding but no ovulation. If you don't release an egg each month, you won't have as many chances to conceive. You may be given medication to stimulate egg production and boost ovulation.

**Waiting for your period to start**—or better yet, not start—can be quite stressful when you're trying to conceive. If your menstrual cycle is irregular you may not know when your period is due and therefore may not know if you're late and potentially pregnant or not. The uncertainty is likely to make you anxious and every time you go to the bathroom you dread seeing that your period has started.

Whether or not you know you have fertility problems, the wait can be difficult. If you do get your period, the disappointment can be hard. The cycle of having your period, waiting for ovulation, hoping you're pregnant, and then finding out you're not can become very wearing month after month.

If you have been trying to conceive for a year with no luck then you should go to your doctor for tests. Or go at six months if you are over 35 or know that you may have fertility problems, such as blocked fallopian tubes. Try confiding in a good friend about your problems so that you have someone to talk to, but try not to become obsessive and let it dominate all your relationships.

If you've only just started trying, remember there is a only a one in four or five chance that you will conceive each month, so you're unlikely to get pregnant in the first month of trying!

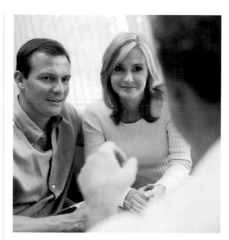

**If you're over 35** and have been trying to conceive for six months, speak to your doctor about fertility tests. You should both be checked because your partner's sperm will need to be tested too. You will be given blood tests.

### AS A MATTER OF FACT

**Around half** of pregnancies in the US could be accidental.

According to the US Centers for Disease Control and Prevention's Pregnancy Risk Assessment Monitoring System, 49 percent of all US pregnancies, and 31 percent of US pregnancies resulting in a live birth, are unintended. Data collected is from 60 percent of US births in 31 states and one city.

# 255 days to go...

**YOUR BABY TODAY**

To embed itself in the lining of the uterus, the embryo-to-be needs the help of progesterone, secreted after ovulation by the empty egg follicle, the corpus luteum (shown in pink in this cross section of an ovary). Progesterone helps the lining thicken.

Do you feel different? You'll find yourself analyzing every twinge in your body as you look for signs that you're pregnant.

## FOCUS ON... NUTRITION

### Diet ban

**If you were dieting before you conceived,** it can be tempting to continue once you find out you're pregnant. Don't: diet, your baby may become undernourished and is more likely to be premature and underweight at birth. Do, however, eat a healthy, balanced diet (see p.15). Don't eat junk food when you're pregnant since this can increase the risk of your baby developing weight problems.

If you are overweight or obese, your doctor may recommend that you gain less weight than other pregnant women. The recommended weight gain for overweight women is 15–25 pounds. And for obese women, the recommended weight gain is at least 15 pounds. (By contrast, normal-weight women should gain 25–35 pounds during pregnancy.)

In an ideal world, you should lose excess weight before conceiving, because obesity makes you more prone to diabetes and high blood pressure and means you're more likely to need a cesarean.

**It's still very early** and you're unlikely to have pregnancy symptoms yet—although you may have some light spotting (see opposite). Some women claim to "feel" pregnant, even before changes to their breasts are noticeable or before they start feeling sick. Some women say that they just "know." You may be very in tune with your body and may notice that your body is changing even before you are able to take a test. Unfortunately, sometimes our minds can play tricks on us: you may want to be pregnant so much that you can sometimes convince yourself that you're feeling different. If you don't feel any different, don't worry, this is also completely normal.

Either way the only definitive way to know whether or not you are pregnant is to take a pregnancy test (see p.71). You don't need to go to your doctor to confirm your pregnancy since the tests that they use are the same as those bought over the counter. If the test is positive, you're pregnant!

## ASK A... NUTRITIONIST

**Should I give up coffee in case I'm pregnant?** The March of Dimes advises pregnant women or those trying to become pregnant to drink no more than 200 mg of caffeine a day (that's a 12-ounce cup of coffee). Going without your caffeine fix is a good thing when you're pregnant, since research shows that, in high doses, it can increase the risk of miscarriage.

One study discovered that pregnant women who consumed two or more cups of coffee (or a caffeine-rich equivalent) were twice as likely to miscarry as those who gave up caffeine. Before switching to decaff, be aware that decaffeinated drinks

may raise cholesterol. The good news is that many women find they naturally stop wanting coffee in early pregnancy.

YOU ARE 3 WEEKS AND 5 DAYS

# 254 days to go...

## YOUR BABY TODAY

The first stage of placental development—your baby's life support system—is shown here. The image shows nuclei (blue) within a continuous network of cells that will become the placental villi. At first the tiny villi are solid; later, they will contain blood vessels.

As the fertilized egg becomes completely embedded in your uterus, it may cause some light bleeding.

**This computer-generated image** shows the ball of cells—the blastocyst—as it appears situated within the uterus. The outer ring of interconnected cells that will eventually form the placenta are clearly seen.

### AS A MATTER OF FACT

**It is thought that around 50 percent** of pregnancies might miscarry before implantation.

Up to a third of pregnancies miscarry up to the fifth week and around a quarter will end in miscarriage between the fifth and seventh week. Thankfully, the risk of miscarriage becomes much lower as the weeks go by, decreasing dramatically after the 12th week of pregnancy.

**The ball of cells, known as the blastocyst,** that will form the embryo has now completely embedded within the lining of the uterus and the lining has regenerated over it.

Unfortunately, in the complex process of conception, only about half of all fertilized eggs progress to become a blastocyst and only about half of these go on to become successfully implanted in the uterus.

When the blastocyst embeds, there may be some bleeding, known as "spotting." This often leads to confusion regarding the dating of the pregnancy, not least because it can occur around the time that you would normally start your period.

The color of the blood can vary. In most cases it is pinkish, although bright red blood (fresh blood) can occur, as can brownish, old blood. As long as it is not profuse, the color really doesn't matter. If the bleeding lasts for a short period, and you don't experience discomfort, it's likely that things are just fine, but do see your doctor for a checkup.

Around 25 percent of women will experience some bleeding in early pregnancy, but most go on to full term. However, in some cases, bleeding does mean a miscarriage is occurring so always report the fact that you've bled to your doctor.

### DOUBLING UP

**As with many parents,** you probably thought long and hard about trying to conceive your second child. There's no ideal age gap between children, but consider:

**The pros:**
- **You are in "baby mode"** and will be used to the routine and all aspects of baby care. You will have all the equipment you need from bottles to a carriage and crib.
- **A two-year-old** might find it easier to accept his new sibling than a four-year-old who is much more conscious of having the sole attention of his parents.
- **There will always be squabbles,** but children close in age tend to play better together.

**The cons:**
- **It's tiring** caring for a one- or two-year-old while pregnant.
- **It can put a strain on your body** to have pregnancies close together.
- **If you have a second baby** before the first one can walk, you could be doing a lot of carrying, increasing the chance of backaches.
- **You won't have as much time** to get to know your first child before your second is on the scene.

Your 4th week

67

# 253 days to go...

## YOUR BABY TODAY

This microscope view of an embedded blastocyst shows the amniotic cavity (semcircular white area at top), with the cells that will develop into the baby just below (dark oval at the 12 o'clock position). The yolk sac is the pink area below.

Complex changes are taking place inside your uterus to create a safe and nourishing environment for your unborn baby.

**The ball of cells embedded in the uterus** is already laying down the foundations for its future life as an embryo. At two layers thick, the germ cells form a flat disk that divides the fluid-filled inner part of the ball of cells into two chambers. The smaller of these fluid-filled chambers will become the amniotic sac. The larger chamber, lying closest to the future placenta, will become the yolk sac that supports the early embryo. The umbilical cord will eventually develop close to the smaller chamber. The inner germ cells have been developing at a slower rate than the rapidly expanding outer cell layers.

At first the umbilical cord is a simple stalk, containing no blood vessels but simply anchoring the embryo to the future placenta (see p.76), which will eventually become your unborn baby's lifeline.

### AS A MATTER OF FACT

**Newborns** are getting heavier.

This is mostly due to improved diet and living standards. However, obesity in the mother is another factor—if the mother is overweight, there is an increased risk of diabetes (see p.473), which can increase the baby's weight.

### ASK A... NUTRITIONIST

**I'm hoping I'm pregnant, but I'm already worrying about the amount of weight I might put on, and am scared I'll never be slim again!**

These days, it is almost impossible to pass a newspaper stand without seeing the latest celebrity who has not only fit right back into her clothes after having her baby, but who actually weighs less than she did before pregnancy. However, this is concerning for health professionals, since a dramatic weight loss after the birth is not good for mother or baby.

The recommended weight gain during pregnancy is 25–35 lb, if you have a Body Mass Index (BMI) (see p.17) within the normal range. Your baby and her support system will make up a good proportion of this (see p.99), as will the increased pregnancy fluids, fats, and an enlarged uterus. Much of this extra weight will be lost as soon as your baby is born. Also, after the birth, some of this extra weight provides nutrients for breast-feeding, which uses up to 500 calories a day.

The most sensible approach to controlling your weight during pregnancy is to eat a healthy diet and get gentle exercise to ensure that weight gain is not too dramatic. You should be aiming to eat around 2,100–2,500 calories a day, increasing this by 200 calories in the last trimester of pregnancy—the equivalent of a banana and a glass of milk.

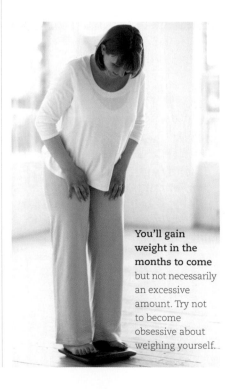

**You'll gain weight in the months to come** but not necessarily an excessive amount. Try not to become obsessive about weighing yourself.

# 252 days to go...

**YOUR BABY TODAY**

This highly magnetized image shows that the embryo consists of two layers of cells—those of the upper, darker layer are more rectangular in shape and lie on the side of the amniotic cavity, and those on the lower layer lie on the side of the yolk sac.

## Are you feeling irritable and tired, and are your breasts tender? Well, you might just be pregnant!

**Nature has a strange way of working.** You might feel low if you have your usual PMS symptoms and think it means that you haven't conceived, but in fact, there are many similarities between the symptoms of premenstrual syndrome (PMS) and those of early pregnancy. This is because the hormones that cause PMS are raised in pregnancy and so can cause the same symptoms. In addition to this, you might be irritable and emotional even without having PMS, just due to the anxiety of wanting to be pregnant and waiting to see whether or not your period arrives.

While you are in the middle of this storm of hormones and raging emotions it can be difficult to remain calm. Talk to your partner about your emotions and anxieties—just expressing that you're finding things stressful can help you get through this tense time.

Alternatively, confide in a female relative or friend, who might be able to relate to how you're feeling.

Frustratingly, at this point it is still a waiting game; all you can do is try to be patient until you take your pregnancy test. If your period was due today—day 28 of your cycle—and hasn't made an appearance, you can take a test as early as today or tomorrow. Good luck!

---

FOCUS ON... YOUR BODY

## Start squeezing!

**It's never too early to start Kegel exercises** and you'll be glad you did once you become pregnant. The pelvic floor is a broad sling of muscles that stretches between your legs and extends from the pubic bone in front to the spine at the rear. It holds and supports your bladder, uterus, and bowel in place and controls the muscles which hold closed the anus, urethra, and vagina.

**Try these simple steps to tone your pelvic floor:**

■ **First** try to locate your pelvic floor: sit on a chair and close your eyes—now visualize the sling of muscles stretching right across your body holding your uterus and bladder.

■ **Next** contract your pelvic floor muscles pulling inward and upward, hold for a count of five, then release. Repeat this exercise at least 10 times a day.

■ **Test:** if you're having trouble identifying the muscles, imagine that you are trying to stop the flow of urine; the muscles you feel contracting are those of the pelvic floor.

Uterus

Bladder

Position of well-toned pelvic floor

Position of sagging pelvic floor

# Your 5th week

**IF YOU HAVE NO PERIOD AND A POSITIVE TEST RESULT, YOU'RE GOING TO HAVE A BABY!**

When your pregnancy is confirmed, it's natural to experience a mixed bag of emotions—excitement, disbelief, joy, and anxiety. Everything is about to change forever for you and your partner. Give yourselves time to take in the big news. You may not feel pregnant yet, but momentous changes are taking place in the hidden world of your uterus. Step by step, the building blocks of life are being set in place.

**The amniotic sac** is a fluid-filled sac that cocoons the developing embryo.

**The chorionic cavity** surrounds the amniotic sac and is bounded by a membrane called the chorion.

**The embryo** now measures 0.09 in (2.5 mm).

**The yolk sac** nourishes the embryo until the placenta is established and can provide nutrients through its blood supply.

**Embryonic tissues** are already forming into a structure that will become the heart.

**The umbilical cord** connects the baby to the developing placenta. At first it is rather short and has yet to develop any coils.

**Chorionic villi** reach into the wall of the uterus to form the placenta. The villi contain blood vessels that tap into your body's blood supply to access nutrients for the baby.

**EMBRYO AT 5 WEEKS**

**A fold down** the back of the embryo marks the beginnings of the spine.

# 251 days to go...

## YOUR BABY TODAY

This is a microscope view of the amniotic cavity with the cells that will become the baby in a close-up. These cells will repeatedly divide and multiply, becoming more and more specialized at each stage of their development.

The waiting is over. If your period hasn't started, take a home pregnancy test to find out whether you've conceived.

### If you've missed your period

(assuming that your normal cycle is no more than 28 days and that your period is therefore late), you may want to do a home pregnancy test today.

A home pregnancy test, available at pharmacists and most supermarkets, contains a chemical that reacts if your urine contains the hormone hCG (human chorionic gonadotrophin). This is produced by an implanting embryo and will be found in your urine if you are pregnant. Levels of hCG are likely to be over 50 mIU/ml on the day your period is due. With between 97 and 99 percent accuracy, the majority of over-the-counter tests are sensitive enough to detect this amount, so they can be used on the first day of your missed period; some can be used earlier (see p.63).

The tests only turn positive once there is a certain level of the hCG hormone present in your urine: if you test too early, the result might be negative even though you are pregnant. Therefore, if you don't get your period but you had a negative result, test again after two to three days. If you are pregnant, the levels of hCG will have risen, giving a positive result.

If you get a positive result but your period starts anyway, it may be that you have suffered a very early miscarriage.

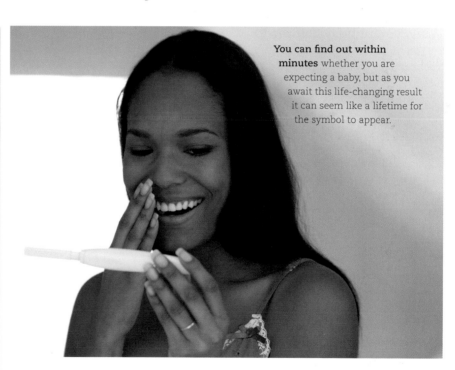

You can find out within minutes whether you are expecting a baby, but as you await this life-changing result it can seem like a lifetime for the symbol to appear.

### HOW TO USE A HOME PREGNANCY TEST

**Always read the instructions,** but most tests work as follows:

■ **You urinate on the stick** and leave it for a specified number of minutes.

■ **A symbol will appear** in the control window to indicate the test is working (if this does not appear, the test is faulty). If a symbol then appears in the results window, you are pregnant.

■ **It is advisable to do the test** first thing in the morning when your urine is most concentrated. By doing this, the hCG levels are likely to be detected more easily

■ **The results symbol** gradually fades, so read it after the specified time, not later. Do another test the next morning if you're unsure of the result.

# 250 days to go...

### YOUR BABY TODAY

The embryo until this stage of development has consisted of two layers of cells. Now, a third layer starts to become visible as a "bulge" between the two—this bulge can be seen in the center of this image.

## In this third week since conception, the cells that will become the embryo move to form the basis of the central nervous system.

**While you're busy coming to terms with being pregnant,** there are incredible changes taking place inside you. The group of cells, that will become your baby is currently shaped as a flat disk and undergoing significant development. A narrow groove begins to form down the middle of the cells. The leading edge of the groove is slightly wider forming a circular "node." The outer edges of the node and groove are slightly raised. The cells move from the rolled edges of these structures downward into the groove to lie between the original two layers of cells. This creates three layers of cells, those on each outer disk surface and those sandwiched between them. The node and groove do not extend along the entire length of the disk.

At the head end, a separate groove forms. Called the neural groove, this ultimately forms the brain and spinal cord (the central nervous system). In four days time, the disk will lengthen and widen at the end that will form your baby's head. In six days time, the neural groove has folds on either side that will later meet to form the neural tube.

**Shown here is the neural tube of an embryo** in the early stages of pregnancy. The brain and spinal cord will develop from the neural tube. If the tube does not fully close, it can lead to birth defects, most commonly spina bifida.

### ASK A... DOCTOR

**I've been having difficulty getting pregnant and have now been diagnosed with polycystic ovary syndrome. What is this?** This condition causes the ovaries to be bigger than normal and they produce a large number of small follicles that never grow to full maturity. Therefore an egg is not released to be fertilized and periods are very irregular.

The condition is a common cause of fertility problems and treatments are aimed at stimulating ovulation and also reducing some of the symptoms, such as increased body hair. Polycystic ovary syndrome appears to run in families.

### FOCUS ON... RELATIONSHIPS

## "You're going to be a dad!"

**It's the positive result you've been waiting for**—hopefully!—but how do you share it with your partner? You could present him with an envelope containing your positive pregnancy test, or explain that you have a "special gift" for him but it won't be ready until about, oh, nine months. It shouldn't take him long to figure it out! Ideally, choose a time when you are both alone and feeling relaxed so that it can be a special moment. You may want to do another test with your partner just to make sure and also so that he feels involved.

Even if you're excited, and even if you can't get in touch with your partner for a day, don't be tempted to tell your mom and close friends first Your partner may be upset, understandably, if others know he's going to be a dad before he does.

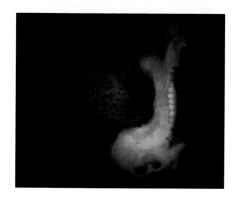

# 245 days to go...

**YOUR BABY TODAY**

The bulge at the lower part of this image will eventually become the baby's head. Segments called somites (seen as bright, round areas running down one side of the embryo), which will form the baby's spine, have started to develop.

At this important stage of development, the building blocks of your baby's spine are being laid down.

**By the end of this 5th week,** individual elements that will form the embryo have begun to develop.

Starting at what will become the head end, individual segments, called "somites," form. Roughly three new pairs of somites appear every day and each forms part of your baby's spine as well as the muscles associated with each segment of the body. Eventually there will be four somites at the head, eight in the region of the neck, 12 at chest level, five in the lumbar region, and five in the pelvic area.

More somites develop in the baby below the pelvis but most disappear. In other mammals, these develop to form the tail.

**FOCUS ON... YOUR BODY**

## Your metabolism

**Regular exercise will increase** your basic metabolic rate, which is the rate at which your body burns calories. During pregnancy your metabolism will already be slightly elevated. When exercising your body will be encouraged to use up excess energy and fat reserves, but will always keep enough reserve energy to facilitate the growth of your baby.

Exercise will also help your body regulate blood sugar (see p.92) and energy levels.

**ASK A... NUTRITIONIST**

**I'm underweight. Could this affect my pregnancy?** You may be more likely to suffer from nutritional deficiencies, which could affect the baby's health; you are also more likely to give birth prematurely, and have a smaller-than-usual baby, who is more vulnerable to health problems.

To gain weight, eat bigger portions and choose healthy foods that have plenty of protein, good-quality fats, and unrefined carbohydrates (see p.92). Opt for nutrient- and calorie-dense foods, such as avocados and whole-milk dairy products; eat lots of leafy greens to ensure you are getting key vitamins and minerals (see pp.15–16). Eat healthy snacks, such as nuts, fruit, and seeds, and don't skip breakfast. Your doctor will refer you to a dietician, if necessary.

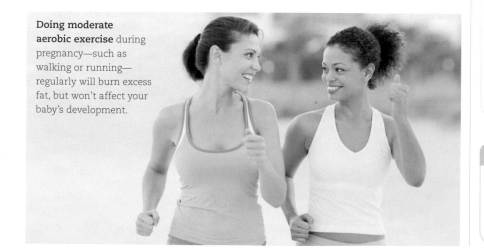

**Doing moderate aerobic exercise** during pregnancy—such as walking or running—regularly will burn excess fat, but won't affect your baby's development.

**ACTUAL SIZE OF YOUR BABY**

**At 5 weeks** of pregnancy, the embryo is 0.09 in (2.5 mm) long.

5 weeks

# Your 6th week

**THIS WEEK YOU MAY NOTICE THE FIRST SYMPTOMS OF PREGNANCY—IF NOT, DON'T WORRY**

Not all women start to feel pregnant this early on. Some experience a twinge of nausea or breast tenderness, while others notice no changes. Of course, it's natural to long for "proof" that your pregnancy is progressing, even if that happens to be morning sickness. But a lack of symptoms doesn't mean something is wrong; it's all really happening and your baby is going through some critical stages of development.

**Small pits** on either side of the baby's head represent the first signs of the developing of eyes.

**The embryo** measures 0.15 in (4 mm) from crown to rump.

**The yolk sac** still provides the majority of your baby's nourishment.

**The baby's head** folds forward over the body.

**Chorionic villi form more branches** as the placenta continues to develop.

**The umbilical cord** contains blood vessels to and from the developing placenta, but they do not yet supply all of your baby's nutrients.

**A curved tail-like extension** has developed.

**Tiny buds** that will grow into arms and legs have started to sprout.

**Your baby's heart** is making its first fluttering beats.

EMBRYO AT 6 WEEKS

**These pharyngeal arches** will develop into various structures in the head and neck, incuding the lower jaw and larynx.

YOU ARE 5 WEEKS AND 1 DAY

# 244 days to go...

## YOUR BABY TODAY

The embryo now has 14 somites—the building blocks of your baby's muscular system. The first nine pairs are shown here. The upper part of the image shows the open end of the neural tube, which, along with the opening at the base of the spine, has closed.

If you've had no symptoms as you enter your 6th week, you may be on the lookout for signs that you are in fact pregnant.

**You and your partner are probably the only people** who know you're pregnant, and you may still be wondering if it's real. At this stage you may not have any symptoms at all, despite the rapidly changing and growing embryo inside you.

This absence of pregnancy signs is completely normal and is not a cause for concern. Try to remember that the majority of pregnancies are without any complications. It's normal for a healthy pregnant woman to have a wide range of side effects or none at all. So don't worry if you're feeling great—in fact count yourself lucky!

### ASK A... NUTRITIONIST

**Since being pregnant, I don't seem to have much of an appetite. Is this normal?** It is common to not especially want food if you have morning sickness (see p.81). You may no longer be able to stomach your favorite foods. If you're not eating much, it's important that what you do eat is nutritious. Choose nutrient-rich dark green leafy vegetables and legumes, and fish (see p.96) since it contains essential fatty acids.

### AS A MATTER OF FACT

**Up to 90 percent** of your supply of vitamin D depends on adequate exposure to sunlight.

Vitamin D helps your body absorb calcium, which is vital for the development of your unborn baby's skeleton. A daily 15-minute walk outside—with the sun on your skin—is sufficient; you can also boost your intake of vitamin D by eating oily fish, eggs, fortified cereals, and bread, and by taking supplements (see p.16).

### EARLY ULTRASOUND SCANS

**Some women will have an early ultrasound scan,** but the majority of women will have one around the 12th week of pregnancy (see p.137). Early scans are usually done vaginally, with a scanning probe inserted gently into the vagina. They are performed for the following reasons:

■ **If there is a history of multiple births** in your family (or you have used IVF or another form of assisted pregnancy), your doctor may want to check the number of fetuses.

■ **If you've had a miscarriage in the past,** or show signs of cramping or spotting, or more profuse bleeding, a scan can be done to check that there is still a heartbeat.

■ **To establish the cause of vaginal bleeding.** Your baby may be healthy, but fibroids or other conditions may be causing you to bleed. This will be addressed by your doctor.

Amniotic fluid

Length of embryo can be measured to estimate pregnancy dates

**Early vaginal scans do not show** a great deal of detail. The sonographer waits until the embryo is in the correct position (left) to be measured.

# 243 days to go...

**YOUR BABY TODAY**

The center of this image shows the baby's developing heart (darker gray), a very primitive structure at this stage. The baby's head is to the right of the image. The embryo is almost completely transparent.

There won't be any visible signs of pregnancy on the outside for some time, but there are many changes taking place inside.

**At this early stage, all your unborn baby's needs** will be met by the yolk sac. Attached to the embryo by a connecting stalk, this essential balloonlike structure indicates the site of your pregnancy and can usually be seen as early as this week as a sphere 0.1–0.2 in (3–4 mm) across. At first the yolk sac is as large as the disk of embryonic cells that will eventually become your baby.

Containing cells that perform a similar function to the liver, the yolk sac releases several pregnancy hormones and produces the embryo's first red blood cells. After week 9 the liver will take over these functions as the yolk sac gradually disappears and the placenta takes over, by around the 10th week of pregnancy.

Over the next seven days, a primitive circulatory system develops, well before any blood circulates to the placenta in the 10th week. And, by the end of this week, using the highest quality ultrasound equipment, it is just possible to see the embryo's heartbeat. At this early stage, the heart is simply a tube.

**If you can't stomach big plates** of food, try eating a combination of small portions at mealtimes and as snacks.

**ASK A... NUTRITIONIST**

**Should I be eating for two?**
Unfortunately, pregnancy is by no means a licence to eat anything and everything you'd like. "Eating for two" is a myth, and if you do so, you'll end up consuming too many calories and gaining too much weight. The best advice is to use your common sense. Studies show that pregnant women who eat according to their appetite naturally eat the proper amount and gain a healthy amount of weight.

Caloric needs in pregnancy vary greatly from woman to woman, depending upon pre-pregnancy weight and physical activity. In general, energy needs increase by approximately 300–500 calories per day during pregnancy. In the first trimester, caloric needs are a bit less, more at the lower end of the range.

In the first trimester, when up to 80 percent of women are nauseous or vomiting, getting enough calories can sometimes be a challenge. Like many pregnant women, you may feel most nauseous when your stomach is empty. One good trick is snacking. Eating five small meals rather than three large ones can be soothing to a nauseous stomach, while at the same time giving you the calories you need.

# 242 days to go...

### YOUR BABY TODAY

A front view of the embryo: the head region is bent downward so that the central nervous system can be seen. The tubelike structure in the head region is the developing spinal cord. The tail of the embryo is curving upward.

## Morning sickness is one of the most common and least welcome symptoms of pregnancy.

### Ease the nausea

**Unfortunately there is no definitive cure-all** for morning sickness, though you could try the following natural remedies:

■ **Eat little and often**—having low blood-sugar levels may make the nausea worse so even if you feel sick, eating small snacks may help.

■ **Try eating a plain cookie or cracker** first thing in the morning before you get out of bed.

■ **Stick to bland foods** such as cereal or toast and avoid eating fatty and oily foods.

■ **Try having foods and drinks that contain ginger** (see right) such as gingersnaps or ginger tea.

■ **Drink plenty** if you are vomiting, to avoid becoming dehydrated. Put a bottle of water in the fridge and sip it gradually throughout the day. If you feel you are getting dehydrated, for example if your urine is getting very concentrated, you may need to see a doctor.

If the nausea or vomiting is too much to bear, then consult your doctor, who will be able to prescribe anti-nausea medications.

**Feeling sick and vomiting** are common symptoms of early pregnancy. There are various theories to explain why morning sickness occurs; one is that it's due to the rising levels of hCG (human chorionic gonadotrophin) hormone during the first trimester. Morning sickness, unfortunately, doesn't only happen before breakfast; in fact it can happen at any time of day and more than once in 24 hours.

One of the greatest challenges of early pregnancy is keeping it a secret from colleagues. If you have to keep rushing to the bathroom to vomit, people are likely to become suspicious.

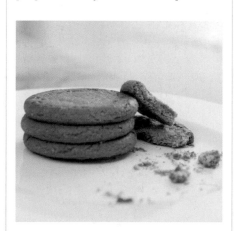

**Ginger contains properties that help to ease nausea.** Put a plate of cookies on your bedside table, and nibble them before you get out of bed.

They may also notice that you look unwell or are more tired than usual. To help you handle this, you may want to tell one or two colleagues or your boss. You could ask them to keep it a secret for the time being. It's a good idea to keep some face wipes, toothpaste, and a toothbrush in your drawer, together with any snacks that you have found help to ease your nausea.

If you're finding it difficult to handle your vomiting, or are worried you are vomiting too much, seek advice from your doctor. Rarely, the sickness can become more serious and require medical treatment (see p.111).

### AS A MATTER OF FACT

**Ginger** has been shown in studies to help with pregnancy-induced nausea.

One study found that the decrease in nausea happened four days after including ginger in the diet daily; so don't give up if you don't get relief right away. Try crystallized ginger chews or tasty ginger cookies; drink soothing ginger tea; and try cooking with fresh ginger. Be aware that most ginger ale does not contain real ginger, so is unlikely to ease nausea.

# A changing world

The family is an ever-changing unit and has undergone some major shifts in the past two decades. Although times have changed, your role as a parent is the same as ever: to give your child consistent love, loyalty, and care.

## THE STATISTICS

### Changing family life

The statistics below reveal how family life has changed over decades.

■ **In the US, 64 percent of moms with children under the age of six work;** in the UK, 55 percent of mothers of children under five work (compared with around 25 percent in 1975).

■ **About 25 percent of children under five** with working moms are cared for full-time by dad and 30 percent of working parents share child care.

■ **About 25 percent of married moms** stays at home full time with the children.

■ **Today, around 25 percent of children live in** one-parent families, of which about 9 percent have a single dad at the helm.

■ **Around 25 percent of babies in the UK are** born to immigrant moms, and in some parts of the country up to a third of all babies are born to ethnic minority families—a figure that is similar in New Zealand and Australia. In the US, about a third of all children are minorities.

■ **More than 41 percent of babies in the UK** are born to unmarried women; in the US, 37 percent of babies are born out of wedlock. This trend is echoed throughout the West, and the numbers are steadily rising.

■ **One in every 100 babies** grows up in a household with same-sex parents.

## The family today

Today, there are many varieties of family life. Although studies report on the problems of modern childhood, children are familiar with and tolerant of different cultures, and living and working practices.

**Mature moms** The number of births to women in the US between 35–39 has risen 52 percent since 1990; the birth rate in women 40–44 has risen 65 percent since 1990 and is at an all-time high. Benefits are that older women are more likely to be settled, financially stable, and mature.

**Single parenting** Single moms in the US have risen from 1 percent in 1971, to 12.5 percent in 2007. There's no doubt that children in single-parent families can be disadvantaged, but it's thought that much of this is due to financial constraints, and that those who have adequate socioeconomic resources do well.

**Stepfamilies** Stepfamilies are the fastest-growing family type. It's thought that at least 1 in 3 children will have a stepfamily situation within their lifetime. Siblings may be of wildly different ages, or of the same age; these are unique and beneficial relationships for all children.

### Modern dads

Dads today are more involved in family life. Some 93 percent attend the birth (compared to 5 percent in 1965), and over 70 percent take time off after the birth. In the 1970s, dads of children under five devoted less than 15 minutes a day to child-related activities, compared to over two hours by the 1990s. Research shows that children whose dads spend

## THE GENDER GAP

### Boys versus girls

**Historically, about 106 boys have been born for every 100 girls**—a phenomenon believed to be nature's way of compensating for the fact that males are more likely to be killed through conflicts. But ratios are changing with girls outnumbering boys. One factor may be increased stress (women under stress produce more girls than boys). However, the most important contributor is now thought to be the number of gender-bending chemicals in our environment, such as synthetic estrogens, PCBs (polychlorinated biphenyls), and pesticides.

considerable time with them do well educationally and at work.

### Child care

This is a necessity in most families. Studies show that good care outside the family has a positive impact on social skills, intellect, and language. Grandparents care for about 30 percent of US babies. A good grandparent relationship provides stability, family values, and is thought to improve cognitive development.

### Multiple cultures

Your baby will live in a multicultural society. This affects educational experience and friendships, and there's a strong chance a child will be cared for by someone from another culture at some point in her childhood.

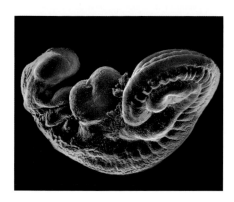

# 241 days to go...

## YOUR BABY TODAY

This image shows just how curled up the embryo is at this stage. The head end of the embryo is on the left. The embryo now has 22 pairs of somites (building blocks of the musculoskeletal system) running along the back.

## This is a crucial time for your developing baby as the neural tube, which will become the brain and spinal cord, is forming.

---

### TIME TO THINK ABOUT

## Whether to tell

You're excited to be pregnant, but should you tell people yet?

■ **Most parents-to-be** wait to share their exciting news until after week 12 when the risk of miscarriage falls. You, may, however, decide you want to confide in family and close friends. If they are people whom you would tell if you miscarried, then there is no harm in sharing your news.

■ **Most women don't tell** their employers yet, unless severe morning sickness interferes with their ability to keep up with work responsibilities. Most wait until after the first trimester or when they start to show. If you want time off for prenatal appointments before this, you'll need to explain why.

■ **Similarly, if your job** involves anything that could be a health and safety risk (for example, heavy lifting or working with chemicals), you should inform your employer early so your role can be adapted. It's also sensible to tell your boss the good news before office gossip about your expanding girth snowballs.

**This week your baby begins to grow rapidly** and will become much more recognizable as a baby over the next five weeks. There are three types of cell, each committed to a separate function. The first will form the skin and nervous system; the second forms blood vessels, muscles, and bones; the third forms the entire digestive system.

At this stage, it is the cells responsible for the spine and nervous system that are at work. Changing shape from a flat

**Not telling many people, if anyone,** in the first few weeks will give you both time to come to terms with the news.

disk, the embryo starts to curl up. The edges of the groove that has already partially formed along the back gradually start to meet, closing and fusing to form a tube, which will become the brain and spinal cord. The last parts of the tube to close are at the very top of the head and then the base of the spine, two days later.

Being careful to get an adequate intake of folic acid (see p.35) in early pregnancy is essential to ensure the neural tube closes completely, with no gaps.

---

### FOCUS ON... DADS

## Keeping quiet

**Your first reaction to finding out that your partner is pregnant** might be to tell the world. After all, you may be excited or nervous and may want to confide in people who you can trust. Think twice before telling lots of people (see box, left) and don't do so without talking to your partner. Of course your partner may find it hard to hide some aspects of pregnancy, such as morning sickness.

Most importantly, make sure that you are both in agreement that it is the right time to tell others.

# 240 days to go...

## YOUR BABY TODAY

This is a view of the right side of an embryo with the fronds of the chorionic villi in the background. The curled shape of the embryo is clearly demonstrated. The umbilical cord attachment to the early placenta can just be seen.

Are you feeling up one minute and down the next? Be reassured that this is a perfectly normal response to pregnancy hormones.

**It may not happen quite yet,** but be forewarned that you may become very emotional or irrational during pregnancy and suffer from mood swings. You may cry at things that had previously not affected you. This is due to a combination of your rapidly fluctuating hormones and the fact that pregnancy is a major life change.

Mood swings can be difficult for both you and your partner—try to keep communicating with each other and explain how you are feeling, no matter how irrational it may seem.

### MORE VEGGIES PLEASE!

**Be creative to stimulate your appetite** and get essential nutrients:
- **Try raw veggies** with a dip.
- **Throw in a few vegetables** when you make your morning smoothie (see p.135)—cucumber, celery, peppers, and carrots are mild in flavor, but deliciously nutritious.
- **Try grating** zucchini or carrots into soups, pasta sauces, and stews, or throwing a handful of squash, frozen peas, broccoli, asparagus, or green beans into a risotto.
- **Add vegetables** to a cheese sauce. If you cook them in the sauce, it will absorb all of the nutrients that would normally make their way into the cooking water.
- **Make your own pizza** topped with crunchy and colorful vegetables.
- **Choose vegetarian** dishes when you get takeout.

### FOCUS ON...YOUR HEALTH

## Tackling fatigue

**Fatigue is a common pregnancy complaint** and you might find you have a sudden loss of energy in the early stages as your body adapts to the changes caused by pregnancy. This often lasts throughout the first trimester, but after about week 13 you should start to feel more energized. When you're not resting, try to stay active.

Another cause of fatigue is anemia. When you see your doctor you will be offered a blood test to check your iron levels, and if these are found to be low you will be offered supplements. To avoid anemia, eat iron-rich foods, such as dark green leafy vegetables, red meat, whole-grain cereals, and legumes, and drink prune juice. Vitamin C helps your body absorb iron so try drinking fresh orange juice with meals. Limit caffeine intake (see p.66) since it inhibits iron absorption.

**The embryo is developing rapidly,** although still only 4 mm long. The spinal column is in place and the eyes have formed. The yellow yolk sac on the left is larger than the embryo which it is nourishing.

# 239 days to go...

**YOUR BABY TODAY**

Development in the upper body usually precedes that in the lower body—this image shows the bulge containing the heart and liver, and the very earliest sign of development of the upper limb buds, but as yet there is no sign of the lower limb buds.

## You may notice a marked increase in your breast size, even at this early stage of pregnancy.

**The first part of your body to change shape** is likely to be your chest. Your breasts may increase in size quite rapidly, looking bigger and feeling heavier. They may become quite tender to touch.

The nipples will change, the areola (the darker skin around the nipple) may become darker in color and your nipples may tingle. As your breasts get bigger, you might notice blue veins appearing. All these breast changes are due to the hormone estrogen.

### AS A MATTER OF FACT

**Each breast will increase,** on average, by 2 in (5 cm) and 3 lb (1.4 kg) during pregnancy.

That is why it is important to wear the right bra, even in the early stages of pregnancy.

**Read the labels on cleaning products** carefully to make sure they are not toxic, and always wear rubber gloves. Pregnancy can be a good time to ask your partner to clean the bathroom!

### ASK A... DOCTOR

**How can I ease the soreness in my breasts?** Wearing a supportive bra can help with both the feelings of heaviness and soreness in your breasts, which are common in pregnancy. If your breasts are very tender at night, try wearing your bra at night while you sleep which may help. Try to avoid sleeping on your front if this causes discomfort. You may find that rubbing in a cream containing aloe vera is soothing.

### FOCUS ON... SAFETY

## Detox yourself

**Once you know you're pregnant,** it's only natural to want to keep your baby safe, so...

**Be careful when you're cleaning.** Studies suggest there may be a link between pregnant women using bleach and spray air fresheners, and babies developing asthma. Plus, commercial oven cleaners contain toxic chemicals that experts believe could damage unborn babies.
- Don't use "toxic" products.
- Keep rooms well ventilated.
- Steer clear of fumes.
- Wear gloves.
- Make your home sparkle with a solution made of bicarbonate of soda, distilled white vinegar, lemon juice, and essential oils.

**Get someone else to clean your cat's litter box** (or if that's not possible, wear rubber gloves and wash your hands afterward). Cat feces may contain parasites that can cause toxoplasmosis (see p.101), an infection that could harm your unborn baby.

YOU ARE 6 WEEKS EXACTLY

# 238 days to go...

## YOUR BABY TODAY

Here the back of the embryo can be seen lying over the yolk sac. The opening overlying the developing brain has now closed (left side of image) and this will be followed two days later by closure of the opening at the base of the spine (out of view).

By the end of this sixth week, one of your baby's major organs—the heart—is rapidly developing and circulating blood.

**Your developing embryo may still be tiny,** but is undergoing rapid and complex development.

The heartbeat is now more easily recognized on an ultrasound scan. The heart continues to form from a simple smooth tube which, as it becomes more muscular, loops, folds, and divides to form four chambers. On the left side the upper chamber (left atrium) takes in blood from the lungs. From here blood passes through a one-way valve (the mitral valve) into the main left pumping chamber (the left ventricle). This then pumps blood out of the heart to the body along the main artery (the aorta). On the right-hand side of the heart, the upper chamber (right atrium) collects blood returning from the body and passes it through a one-way valve (tricuspid valve) into the right main pumping chamber (right ventricle). This pumps blood to the lungs and the cycle continues.

At this stage of development, the circulation is very basic with the heart tube simply sending blood around the length of your baby. No blood travels from your baby's circulation to the placenta (see p.127).

It's at an early stage of development, but the developing heart can be seen here as the dark red area. It lies just above the larger, slightly paler red area, which is the liver. Below the liver is the umbilical cord.

### TYPES OF MISCARRIAGE

**At this early stage,** a common concern is that the pregnancy will miscarry. A miscarriage is the spontaneous loss of a pregnancy at any time up until the 20th week. After 20 weeks the loss is referred to as a stillbirth. The signs of a miscarriage are vaginal bleeding and periodlike cramps.

Unfortunately, there is nothing that you can do to prevent a miscarriage. In around 60 percent of cases, it is caused by a one-time genetic problem. Bleeding does not always mean that the pregnancy is being miscarried.

Since not all miscarriages follow the same pattern, there are various terms to describe what happens:

■ **A threatened miscarriage** occurs when the pregnant woman experiences bleeding and possibly pain, but the baby survives.

■ **An inevitable miscarriage** occurs when there is bleeding and pain due to the pregnant woman's uterus contracting. The cervix opens, and the fetus is expelled.

■ **A missed miscarriage** is when the fetus dies but is not expelled. Surgery may be needed to remove it.

### ACTUAL SIZE OF YOUR BABY

**At 6 weeks**, your baby's crown to rump length is 0.15 in (4 mm).

5 weeks          6 weeks

Your 6th week

87

# Your 7th week

**SET YOURSELF SOME FITNESS STANDARDS TO SEE YOU THROUGH YOUR PREGNANCY**

Getting in shape now will stand you in good stead as your pregnancy continues. Keeping active is important, so work up a daily exercise routine to strengthen your muscles and reduce fatigue—but listen to your body and don't exhaust yourself. This week your baby's vital organs, including the lungs and gut, start to develop. Your baby's head already looks too big for his body as the brain rapidly enlarges.

**The embryo measures** 0.31 in (8 mm) crown to rump.

**The heart** is now providing your baby with a simple circulation.

**The yolk sac** has shrunk but is still supplying nutrients to the embryo.

**A prominent forehead** bulges out as the brain develops.

**Nostrils** appear as shallow pits.

**The placenta** is becoming well established, although it is not yet ready to function as a supply line.

EMBRYO AT 7 WEEKS

**The liver** is starting to make blood cells.

**The arm and leg buds** are lenghthening.

# 237 days to go...

## YOUR BABY TODAY

In this side view of the embryo the spinal cord is clearly curved as it begins to develop. The pale-yellow ridgelike structures along the back are somites—your baby's developing muscular system.

You may be spending a lot of time in front of the mirror trying to spot your "bump," but it could be weeks yet before you show.

**Like most newly pregnant women,** you're probably on the lookout for a rounded belly, but it's unlikely to make an appearance just yet. On average, the fourth month marks the greatest period of growth, with your pregnancy most definitely appearing as a rounded abdomen.

If it's not your first pregnancy, you might show earlier, possibly as early as eight to 10 weeks, since your abdominal muscles will be more relaxed. Conversely, women who have firm abdominal muscles may show later. If you are expecting twins or triplets, you can expect to show even earlier.

### ASK A... DOCTOR

**Can having sex in pregnancy harm the baby?** Unless you have been told by your doctor to avoid sex because of specific problems, such as a history of miscarriage or unexplained bleeding, then sex is safe at any stage. Enjoying intimacy with your partner is beneficial to your relationship.

Your baby is cushioned in fluid in the amniotic sac inside your uterus and protected by a plug of mucus at the cervix. Even deep penetration isn't harmful.

### STRENGTHEN YOUR ABDOMINALS

**It's safe to do abdominal exercises lying on your back** during your first trimester. Toward the end of the first trimester, or when you start "showing" (see left), you should stop doing abdominal exercises on your back (see p.250 for other exercises you can do at this point).

When you are doing abdominal exercises, it's important to breathe correctly: remember to inhale to start and exhale on each effort.

The purpose of abdominal exercises is to strengthen core muscles. The deeper transverse abdominis muscle that runs horizontally across your body is vital for core stability and strength as your baby develops. The rectus abdominis muscle that runs vertically down your body is the muscle that will stretch during pregnancy and weaken, so it's vital to keep the transverse muscle strong to help your posture and support your spine.

The sooner you begin to strengthen the transverse abdominis, the better. In the first trimester, one of the exercises you can do to strengthen this muscle is shown below.

Knees bent

Feet flat on the floor

Feel your abdominal muscles tightening

**Lie on your back,** feet flat on the floor and arms at your sides. Inhale to begin and as you slowly exhale, push your lower back flat on to the floor. Hold this position for 3–5 seconds and repeat.

# Strengthening and toning exercises

Exercises that strengthen your muscles will help you deal with the additional demands of pregnancy and to manage better during labor and birth.

The exercises shown are sometimes called "functional movement enhancers" because they increase the strength of the muscles that you use for everyday functions such as walking, carrying, lifting, sitting, and standing. The workout can be used alongside walking, swimming, or other cardiovascular exercises and can be done around 2–3 times a week.

**Warm up** Walk in place, swinging your arms back and forth. Continue for 3–5 minutes until your muscles are warm.

**Biceps curl** The biceps is an important muscle for carrying and lifting. You can use 3–5 lb (1–2 kg) weights for this sequence if you're a regular exerciser. Stand with feet hip-width apart, knees slightly bent, back straight, and arms at your sides. Breathe in, then exhale as you bend one elbow, raising your hand to shoulder level. Alternate arms until you've done 20 curls each side (40 in total). If you find this easy, try doing a total of 60 curls.

**Side lunges** (left) These (and the foward lunges, right) strengthen the abdominal and thigh muscles. Start with hands on hips, legs hip-width apart. Step one leg out to the side, bending the knee. Keep the other leg straight. Step back to the starting position, keeping the tummy pulled in and torso straight. Do 10 lunges on each leg. **Forward lunges** (right) Start with hands on hips, feet hip-width apart. Step one leg forward; bend the opposite knee toward the floor, allowing the heel to lift off the floor. Return to the starting position. Do 10 lunges on each leg.

**The bridge** This exercise works your bottom, hamstrings, and inner thighs, and builds strength in your lower body to support your growing belly. Lie on your back with your feet flat on the floor and knees slightly apart. Raise your hips (this relieves pressure on your back and is safe in the second and third trimesters). Keep your hands on the floor next to you, arms straight. Slowly bring your knees together while clenching your bottom; open and close your knees 10 times. Slowly lower your hips and roll onto your left side to end.

# 236 days to go...

## YOUR BABY TODAY

The first recognizable facial feature to be formed is the eye, visible as a black dot in the center of this image. The gray areas are the fluid-filled chambers of the underlying brain.

Try not to dwell on your lifestyle before you realized you were pregnant, but start making changes now.

**Have you only just discovered you're pregnant?** Not all women realize they are pregnant immediately, especially if it wasn't planned. If you've only just found out, it's natural to be concerned about things that you did before you knew, such as drinking alcohol or taking drugs. You may be worried that you've harmed your unborn baby. Use your pregnancy as an opportunity to assess your lifestyle and improve your health.

Because of how pregnancy is dated (see p.35), your baby is still only a little over four weeks old. If you have not been taking folic acid (see p.35), start taking supplements starting today.

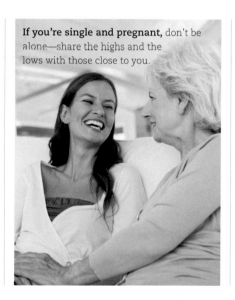

If you're single and pregnant, don't be alone—share the highs and the lows with those close to you.

## TIME TO THINK ABOUT

### Prenatal care

**The options for prenatal care in the US** are outlined on p.102, but they do vary from area to area. Whatever your type of prenatal care, any ultrasound scans, tests, and investigations may also take place at a hospital. Your options are likely to be:

- Group medical practice
- Solo medical practice
- Combination practice
- Maternity Center-based practice

## GOING SOLO

**The prospect of being pregnant and single,** especially if it wasn't your choice, can be tough. Make sure you:
- **Take care of yourself:** plan a healthy diet, and an exercise routine. Get as much rest and restful sleep as you can. Ask a friend to spur you on or get online and seek support from other single pregnant women in your area—you will have a ready-made support network after the birth.
- **Ask for help** from family and friends. You will probably find they

are delighted to be involved in your pregnancy and are willing to come to prenatal appointments and classes with you: you may want to consider asking one of these people to be your birth partner.
- **Discuss support and access** with your baby's father (if appropriate), and if you can't agree, seek legal advice. You and your baby will benefit if an amicable arrangement is reached, and the sooner you start talking, the easier it will be after the birth.

- **Arrange support** for after the birth. A survey found that grandparents who are actively involved in their grandchildren's lives contribute positively to their well-being. If you don't have family close by, try to build a network of other support that will see you through the early weeks.
- **Start thinking early** about your career options for after the birth. You don't have to make any decisions, but it helps to know some of the choices you may have to make later.

# 235 days to go...

**YOUR BABY TODAY**

The eyes begin life as shallow depressions, one on each side of the developing face. This image shows an early eye in the center right, together with the curve of the pale yellow somites of the developing musculoskeletal system.

Needing to urinate frequently is, unfortunately, one of the unwanted side effects of pregnancy.

## ASK A... DOCTOR

**Why do I have so much saliva in my mouth now that I'm pregnant?** Called pytalism, excess saliva is caused by increased hormone levels. Don't try to keep the saliva in your mouth; if you find yourself drooling, spit into a tissue or small cup. Place a towel on your pillow. Sucking lemon wedges or ice cubes may help. Pytalism usually subsides in later pregnancy.

**Are you spending a lot of time in the bathroom?** In addition to dealing with symptoms such as nausea and vomiting (see p.81), if you're like the majority of pregnant women, you'll need to urinate more frequently. It means you're unlikely to want to be too far away from the nearest bathroom.

It can feel as though your bladder cannot hold much urine so you may feel the need to go to the bathroom not long after you've just been, during the day and at night. This is because there is more blood being pumped through the kidneys so you produce more urine. As your uterus grows, it puts pressure on your bladder so it cannot expand as much as normal and will feel uncomfortably full earlier than usual. This can last throughout pregnancy, though you're most likely to experience it in the first and third trimesters.

If, however, you're concerned about the amount of urine you're passing, and/or develop pain or stinging while passing urine, you may have developed a urinary tract infection and should see your doctor immediately.

## FOCUS ON... NUTRITION

## Get carb loading

**Make carbohydrates part of your balanced diet,** but make sure you choose the right ones. Refined carbohydrates, such as white bread and white rice, are very quickly broken down, releasing a large amount of glucose into the bloodstream. This is quickly used up and then glucose levels fall rapidly. This fluctuation in glucose levels has been associated with diabetes, obesity, and heart disease, and recent data suggests it is not the optimal environment for adult or fetal health.

Unrefined carbohydrates, such as whole-wheat bread and brown rice, break down more slowly, releasing glucose steadily leaving you fuller. This can prevent the hunger signals that follow a rapidly digested meal and help with weight control. Your baby is constantly drawing glucose from your bloodstream, so a steady release of glucose leaves you both with plenty of fuel on an ongoing basis. New research has found that babies exposed to a diet based upon unrefined carbs may have more lean body mass and less body fat, though still a healthy birthweight. This will make them less likely to be overweight later in life.

# 234 days to go...

## YOUR BABY TODAY

The early limb bud that will form your baby's arm can be seen here (white area). The upper limb buds appear before the lower limb buds. At this early stage, the hands and fingers are not yet developed.

## Your baby's lungs won't be fully developed until late in pregnancy, but the foundations are being laid down right now.

### ECTOPIC PREGNANCY

Pregnancy sac with embryo    Fallopian tube

**In an ectopic pregnancy,** the embryo develops outside the uterus, usually in a fallopian tube.

**An ectopic pregnancy** can cause abdominal pain on one side and irregular vaginal bleeding. Some women get shoulder-tip pain, thought to be caused by internal bleeding. An ectopic pregnancy can rupture the fallopian tube causing severe pain. Emergency medical attention is essential.

If an ectopic pregnancy is suspected, you will be given a scan. Sometimes the pregnancy will naturally regress; if not medication or surgery will be necessary.

**In this 7th week of pregnancy,** your baby's lungs are starting to develop. This begins with a small lung bud branching out from the upper part of the tube (esophagus) between your baby's mouth and stomach. This lung bud forms the main windpipe or "trachea," which then divides into two main branches (bronchi) that will eventually form your baby's right and left lungs. These bronchi continue to branch into smaller tubes, a process that will be repeated many times.

Your baby's gut is also starting to develop, from the mouth downward. At the beginning of this week, his future digestive system consisted of a simple tube that lay along the length of the embryo; this tube was closed at each end. The tube remains closed but the esophagus has now started to separate from the trachea and connect to the stomach. The swelling that will become your baby's stomach forms around the center of his body, but undergoes a 90-degree rotation to lie more on the left-hand side.

Buds arise from the duodenum (the first part of the bowel that leaves the stomach) that will form the pancreas and bile duct to the gall bladder.

In just a couple of weeks, your baby will have all its major organs and body systems.

**The embryo is safely cocooned** in the fluid-filled amniotic sac. The yolk sac can be seen in the bottom left-hand corner, attached by what is now a very fine thread; its function is gradually replaced by the placenta.

### AS A MATTER OF FACT

**Music therapy** is a highly effective way to reduce stress.

A study found that pregnant women who listened to music that mimicked the human heartbeat had reduced stress levels compared to those who did not receive the treatment.

# Miscarriage

Miscarriage is the spontaneous loss of a pregnancy before the fetus is mature enough to survive outside the uterus. Miscarriage is common, affecting 15–20 percent of pregnancies, with the majority occurring in the first 12 weeks. Late miscarriage, after the first trimester, occurs in about 1 percent of pregnancies.

---

**DIAGNOSIS**

## Types of miscarriage

Different terms are used to describe miscarriage, depending on what is found during an ultrasound scan or an internal examination.

■ **Threatened miscarriage** is the term given to bleeding early in pregnancy, but in which the cervix remains closed. In this case, the bleeding stops after a few days, and the pregnancy is likely to continue.

■ **Inevitable miscarriage** occurs when there is bleeding and the cervix is open, meaning that the fetus will be lost. If the pregnancy is less than eight weeks, the bleeding may be like a heavy, painful period. After eight weeks, the bleeding may be considerably heavier.

■ **Incomplete miscarriage** occurs when there is bleeding and the cervix opens, but the uterus doesn't expel its entire contents and some pregnancy tissue is left behind.

■ **Complete miscarriage** is when there is bleeding, the cervix opens, and the uterus expels all the pregnancy tissues.

■ **Missed miscarriage** is less usual. There may be no miscarriage symptoms, but the pregnancy stops developing and the miscarriage isn't diagnosed until the routine scan at around 12 weeks.

## Why miscarriage happens

An early miscarriage is usually due to a problem such as a chromosomal or structural abnormality in the fetus. It may also be caused by a fibroid (a non-cancerous growth in the uterus), an infection, or an immune system disorder. Miscarriage occurs more commonly in older women, in smokers, and in multiple pregnancies.

If you miscarry, it's important to know that it wasn't linked to anything you did, such as exercise, sex, or travel. Also, there is no evidence that rest reduces the risk of a threatened miscarriage going on to become inevitable (see box, left).

## What will be done

If you bleed in early pregnancy, contact your doctor immediately who will arrange for you to have a pelvic exam and/or ultrasound scan. If a scan shows a healthy fetal heart, the chance of miscarriage is reduced. If there is no heartbeat, or no developing baby, the doctor will assess if you've had a complete or incomplete miscarriage (see box, left). A complete miscarriage doesn't require treatment. If it is incomplete, you may be offered medication to hasten the miscarriage, or a procedure to scrape the uterus, although your doctor may recommend expectant management—monitoring the situation while letting your uterus expel its contents. Expectant management means that you avoid risks such as infection from an invasive medical procedure, but its disadvantage is that you may bleed longer. Discuss the options with your doctor.

If you have two or more miscarriages in a row, known as "repeated miscarriage," your doctor may arrange tests to see if there is a cause. About half the time, no cause will be found but sometimes testing will find fetal chromosomal problems, uncommon uterine problems, or blood disorders or other medical conditions.

## After a miscarriage

Your period may be delayed by 6–12 weeks. Once the bleeding stops, there is no medical reason to not try to get pregnant again. The only problem is that you may not know if your period is late since your cycle is readjusting after the miscarriage, or whether you are pregnant again. It's wise to wait until you both feel mentally ready to try again. Talking to a close friend, family member, or a counselor, can help you come to terms with your loss.

---

**LATE MISCARRIAGE**

## Pregnancy loss after the first trimester

**Losing a pregnancy after the first trimester is much more unusual than an early miscarriage.** After 20 weeks, a pregnancy loss is referred to as a stillbirth. There are several reasons why late pregnancy loss may occur, including infection; uterine abnormalities or abnormalities in the baby; and a weak cervix. If you have a late miscarriage, your doctor will discuss the possible causes with you and, if a cause is identified, whether anything needs to be done in a future pregnancy.

# 233 days to go...

### YOUR BABY TODAY

This 3D ultrasound scan shows the embryo and its yolk sac, attached to the wall of the uterus. The yolk sac provides nourishment for the embryo until the placenta is fully functional, and produces blood cells until the liver can take over this role.

By this stage, you may have experienced bouts of dizziness. It's all part of your body and brain adjusting to the pregnancy.

### THE LOWDOWN

## Being a teetotaler

Your baby's health is the most important consideration, so before you've announced your pregnancy, you may need to take steps to discreetly avoid drinking alcohol.

■ **Buy the first round** and get yourself a carbonated mixer and ice and a slice without the alcohol. Once everyone else has had one drink, they're less likely to notice that you're on the wagon. For the next round, say you're pacing yourself and ask for a mixer.
■ **Claim you're detoxing** or hungover and order a juice or a Virgin Mary.
■ **Discreetly swap your full glass** with your partner's empty one.

### AS A MATTER OF FACT

**Exercising regularly** can help you sleep more deeply.

Insomnia is common in pregnancy, due to anxiety or difficulty in getting comfortable. Exercise is a destresser and will tire you out, increasing your chance of a good night's sleep.

**If you feel lightheaded,** especially when you get up from lying down, be extra careful. Dizzy spells are common, especially as your pregnancy progresses and you get bigger, since your heart has to work harder against the forces of gravity to get blood to the brain.

Try to stand up very gradually, in stages, from lying to sitting to standing. Dizziness can also occur if you have been standing for a long period of time, since blood may collect in your legs.

Keep moving to encourage the blood to be pumped back to your heart.

Alternatively, you may feel dizzy due to low blood-sugar levels. Other symptoms of low blood sugar include feeling sweaty, shaky, and hungry. Even if you're feeling or being sick, try to eat little and often to ensure that your blood-sugar levels remain stable.

If you regularly feel dizzy, speak to your doctor, who will carry out some basic health checks.

### KEEP ON MOVING

**The last thing you may feel like doing is exercising,** but it can play a significant role in alleviating and preventing pregnancy symptoms. Although a run through the park or a walk downtown may not sound as inviting as a cozy nap on the sofa, exercise is invigorating and the effects will last. Try to think of it as being active, rather than "exercising."

If after completing a physical activity you feel even more fatigued, decrease how hard and long you exercise. Always listen to your body. As you become more fit and your pregnancy progresses, these feelings of fatigue should diminish, usually by weeks 12–14.

# 232 days to go...

**YOUR BABY TODAY**

At this stage of your baby's development, the heart is a tubular structure, visible in the center of this image. It is, however, already providing your baby with a very simple circulation.

## What will become your baby's tiny arms and legs are beginning to develop during this seventh week of pregnancy.

**It's still some weeks before your baby**—still an embryo—will become recognizable as a human fetus. At the end of this seventh week, however, there are four simple limb buds, each slightly flattened at the end where, over the next two weeks, a hand or foot will form.

With the exception of muscle tone, which comes much later on, all stages of your baby's upper limb development precede any developments in his lower limbs.

The eyes are the first recognizable landmarks to form on the face. At this stage, the eyes consist of two simple surface indentations, which then develop a second indentation within the first; the inner one will become the lens and the outer the eyeball. Your baby's eyes are wide apart at this stage and his ears and nose have yet to form.

**At this stage of an unborn baby's** development, the circulatory system is at a very primitive stage. The upper dark bulge shown here is the heart and beneath it lies the liver, where blood cells are starting to be made.

### ASK A... DOCTOR

**Can exercising increase the risk of miscarriage?** There is no evidence to suggest that, as long as you're healthy and have been given the all-clear from your doctor, exercise will put you at a greater risk of having a miscarriage. In fact, the benefits of getting regular moderate exercise while you're pregnant far outweigh the risks to you and your baby.

The most important factors at this stage of your pregnancy are to exercise at the same level you did prior to being pregnant. Do not attempt any new high-impact and strenuous activity or take up a new sport. Follow the guidelines that are set out on page 18.

### FOCUS ON... NUTRITION

## Know your fish

**Fish is packed with essential nutrients** that are good for your baby's development, so try to eat at least two portions a week.

You do, however, need to be careful of consuming high levels of mercury, present in trace amounts in nearly all fish and shellfish, since it can harm an unborn baby's nervous system. The FDA and the EPA recommend the following for pregnant women:

- **Don't eat fish** that are highest in mercury, including shark and swordfish.
- **Eat up to** 12 ounces per week of lower-mercury seafood like shrimp, salmon, pollock, catfish, and canned light tuna.
- **For fish caught locally** check local advisories regarding mercury content. If no guidance is available, eat up to 6 ounces and consume no other fish that week.

# 231 days to go...

## YOUR BABY TODAY

This early vaginal ultrasound scan shows the first signs of pregnancy: the black central area is the fluid-filled cavity in which your baby (not visible) is developing. Within this is a small circular area, which is the yolk sac.

As your baby's body continues to develop, it won't be long before some very general movements will be visible on a scan.

**While you're dealing with early pregnancy symptoms,** your tiny embryo is tightly curled in your uterus. There is a short portion at the lower end of the spine that in other species goes on to develop into a tail. This portion now starts to disappear as more recognizably human features appear.

The ends of your baby's limb buds flatten, like paddles, and begin to form short digits that will become your baby's tiny fingers and toes. At first these are fused together—then, like the remainder of the skeleton, the digits grow around a soft framework of cartilage that will gradually harden into bone. As the upper limb buds lengthen, your baby's elbows begin to form.

Your baby's eyes continue to develop but won't be fully formed until around week 20; his nostrils now appear as two shallow nasal pits.

---

### ASK A... DOCTOR

**Help! I'm pregnant again and my little boy is only 12 months old. How will I cope?** Pregnancy can be exhausting, particularly in the first trimester, when your body is adjusting to the new demands placed upon it. Having a toddler to contend with at this time makes it even harder.

Find quiet activities to enjoy with your toddler and leave the rough and tumble play to someone else. Take time to nurture yourself, sleeping when your toddler naps, or just settling down on the sofa while he watches a DVD. Don't feel guilty about putting your feet up: it's important to take a step back at this stage and remember that your most important job right now is "growing" your baby.

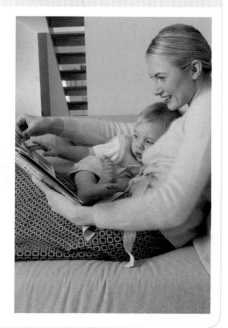

---

### THE LOWDOWN

## Good friends

Keeping your pregnancy quiet in these early weeks is difficult. Whether you want to tell people you're expecting is a matter of personal choice, but there's a good reason to keep it quiet for the time being (see p.83).

You may, however, need to talk to someone (other than your partner), so confide in a friend. Choose someone who will indulge your need to discuss everything—from pregnancy symptoms to birth fears and baby names. The ideal candidate will find your food cravings and 4 am trips to the bathroom riveting... and provide bowls of ice cream and pickles, and advice around the clock.

---

### ACTUAL SIZE OF YOUR BABY

**At 7 weeks,** your baby's crown to rump length is 0.31 in (8 mm).

5 weeks    6 weeks    7 weeks

# Your 8th week

**YOUR MOOD MAY SWING FROM HIGH TO LOW AS HORMONES AND EMOTIONS TAKE HOLD**

You're probably beginning to feel different, even though you don't look pregnant. You may feel a bit low and irritable at times; this is largely due to the changing levels of hormones in your body. You may sometimes have mixed feelings about being pregnant, however much you long for a baby. If the idea of going on vacation appeals to you, opt for short trips and a safe climate, and take extra care of yourself.

**The yolk sac** continues to shrink as the placenta now starts to take over nourishment of the embryo.

**The baby's head** is large relative to the trunk.

**The eyes** are getting larger and darkening with pigment.

**The umbilical cord** contains blood vessels that are beginning to transport nutrients to the embryo and remove waste products.

**Digits** begin to form on the hands and feet, although they are still fused together.

**Your uterus** is starting to enlarge, but you won't notice any changes in your shape yet.

**The ears** are just starting to develop; the small swelllings will form part of the outer ear.

**The embryo measures** 0.51 in (13 mm) from crown to rump.

**Elbows** are now visible.

**EMBRYO AT 8 WEEKS**

**The baby's spine** is straightening up, although the large head still topples forward.

# 230 days to go...

## YOUR BABY TODAY

The fronds that will form the early placenta can be clearly seen on the right here. At the bottom and separate from the embryo is the yolk sac, which is becoming ever smaller as its role is taken over by the placenta.

As your body begins to change shape, you may begin to worry about gaining too much weight.

**You're supposed to put on weight** during pregnancy and while this is not a time to overeat, neither is it a time for fad or restrictive diets. By eating sensibly and exercising moderately, you should gain a healthy amount of weight during pregnancy.

How much weight you should gain depends on your starting weight. If you are underweight when you become pregnant, you should put on more weight than someone who's overweight.

This starting weight is calculated by working out your BMI (see p.17), which is a measure of weight in relation to height. It's a useful tool to figure out approximately how much weight you should gain during your pregnancy.

If your BMI falls within the normal range, then your recommended pregnancy weight gain is 25–35 lb (11–14.5 kg). If your BMI is in the underweight category, you should gain 28–40 lb (12.5–18 kg). If you're overweight, your pregnancy weight gain should be 15–25 lb (7–11 kg). Women in the obese category should gain at least 15 lb (7 kg). Women carrying twins should plan to gain about 35–45 lb (16–20 kg).

As a rough guide, an ideal weight gain is no more than 5 lb (2.2 kg) in the first trimester; no more than 12–19 lb (5.5–9 kg) in the second trimester; and no more than 8–11 lb (3.5–5 kg) in the third trimester. Remember not all of this weight gain is fat (see box, below).

### HOW MUCH WEIGHT WILL YOU GAIN?

**Over the 40 weeks of pregnancy,** you are likely to gain very little weight in the first trimester and then experience a steady weight gain of around 1½–2 lb a week.

In the final few weeks of pregnancy, it's normal to gain a few more pounds. Remember that all figures given are averages and the amount you gain will depend on many individual factors;

where weight is gained can also differ from woman to woman. Always consult your doctor if you're concerned about any aspect of your weight gain or diet.

**Weight gain chart**

**Components of weight gain**

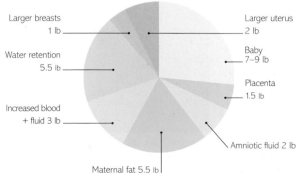

Larger breasts 1 lb
Water retention 5.5 lb
Increased blood + fluid 3 lb
Maternal fat 5.5 lb
Amniotic fluid 2 lb
Larger uterus 2 lb
Baby 7–9 lb
Placenta 1.5 lb

**The weight you'll gain during pregnancy** is a combination of your baby and her support system, the increased size of your breasts and uterus, essential fat reserves, and additional bodily fluids and blood.

YOU ARE 7 WEEKS AND 2 DAYS

# 229 days to go...

## YOUR BABY TODAY

Your baby won't look recognizably human yet, but the lower lip and jaw are formed; the upper lip is not yet complete, and the mouth appears very wide. The external ears are developing low down at the jaw line and the eyes are wide apart.

## Although your baby's brain is still very simply formed, it's undergoing some remarkable changes.

**This is a really important stage of development for your baby.** At this time, her brain is a hollow structure, which is joined to the spinal cord, but it's now starting to fold and form five distinct areas.

The lowest part, or hindbrain, is the first part to grow rapidly and will become structures known as the pons, medulla, and cerebellum. These structures are the most primitive areas of the brain and determine many basic actions that we do without conscious effort, such as breathing and keeping our balance.

Above this is the midbrain that conveys signals from the hindbrain, peripheral nerves, and spinal cord to the forebrain. This part of the brain consists of the thalamus—involved with emotions and sensory perception—and the two cerebral hemispheres, both

quite smooth at this point. Each hemisphere contains a fluid-filled chamber and within that the cerebrospinal fluid is produced.

At the 11–14 week scan (see p.139), brain development checkups will be done to confirm that the baby has normal early cerebral development.

**The dots that will form the eyes** are clearly visible now. At the side of the head, the deep cleft can be seen between the front and back of the brain; this is normal at this stage.

### AS A MATTER OF FACT

**Fish** really is brain food!

Research found that six-month-olds whose mothers had consumed high amounts of fish during pregnancy scored better in mental development tests. But only varieties low in mercury should be eaten (see p.96).

### ASK A... DOCTOR

**I'm eight weeks pregnant and have had some bleeding. Should I be concerned?** Bleeding in early pregnancy is common. If the bleeding is light, and not accompanied by abdominal cramping or pain, then it's unlikely that there is anything wrong. However, always consult your doctor if you have bleeding at any stage of pregnancy to rule out any complications.

Bleeding in early pregnancy can sometimes be due to a cervical ectropian, which is when the surface of the cervix becomes "raw." This results from hormonal changes and is not harmful to the baby. Sexual intercourse can aggravate a cervical ectropian, causing bleeding.

Bleeding in late pregnancy may be more serious since it can be due to the placenta partially, or totally, detaching from the wall of the uterus, known as placental abruption, or to a low-lying placenta (see p.212). If you have a mucus discharge tinged with blood in late pregnancy, this may be a "bloody show" (see p.391).

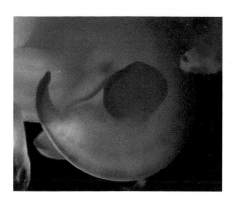

# 228 days to go...

## YOUR BABY TODAY

At this stage, the embryo's "tail," shown curving up on the left, is starting to disappear. The somites of this area of the musculoskeletal system will eventually form the four fused bones of your baby's coccyx—the lowest part of the spine.

Even if you're happy about having a baby, it's natural to have mixed emotions at times.

**Your emotions may fluctuate—** one minute you're laughing and the next you're irritable and yelling, or crying. You might be confused that at a time when you should be happy, you often feel tense and tearful. Be reassured that this is a normal and temporary part of pregnancy.

Don't be too hard on yourself since these changing moods are caused mainly by pregnancy hormones, which is something out of your control. They are the same hormones that cause the symptoms of PMS—rapid mood swings, crying, and irritability—that you might have experienced before.

Be kind to yourself during these down times and do what works best for you, whether it's taking time out to be alone or sharing your feelings with others.

### FOCUS ON... SAFETY

## Protect yourself

**Toxoplasmosis is a disorder caused by a parasite** that can harm a developing fetus. The symptoms may resemble those of mononucleosis with a fever and/or swollen glands in the neck.

It can be spread through cat feces. However, it can also be spread from undercooked meat. Thus, in addition to avoiding changing cat litter, use some caution in the kitchen. Beef, pork, and lamb need to be cooked well. Avoid cross-contamination in the kitchen when preparing foods. Be certain to clean chopping boards and utensils well with hot soapy water after preparing meat.

**When you're having a down day,** remember that these negative feelings will pass; mood swings are a normal part of pregnancy.

### AS A MATTER OF FACT

**Up to 70 percent** of pregnant women sometimes have symptoms of depression.

While one woman hardly has any mood swings, another could suffer for weeks, especially in the first trimester.

### ASK A... DOCTOR

**I'm struggling to deal with my wife's mood swings. Are these normal?** Yes, your partner will be emotional and all you can do is be as supportive, patient, and understanding as you can.

At this early stage of pregnancy, her changing hormone levels may cause mood swings and unexpected emotional responses. Sometimes things that have never been a problem, such as hearing a particular piece of music, might make her cry, or she may snap at you over something trivial. With her emotions out of kilter, she's likely to be as frustrated and confused by this behavior as you are. Until it passes, just bide your time, bite your tongue, and give her a hug.

# Prenatal care options

Throughout your pregnancy, you may be cared for by a family-practice doctor, obstetrician, or a combination of the two. The goal of your prenatal care is to monitor you and your baby so that problems can be identified and managed.

## Your care during pregnancy

Early in pregnancy, you will need to think about who you would like to care for you during pregnancy, labor, and the postpartum period. You will also need to consider where you want to give birth since this will have an influence on your choice of care provider. The main options are set out below, although these may vary depending on where you live. When you attend your first prenatal appointment at 8–12 weeks (see pp.122–3), you will be given information about the prenatal services you can access in your area. The medical checkups that are done during this appointment will also

### YOUR OPTIONS

## Informed choice

**Being able to choose the type of care you receive** is one of the most important aspects of pregnancy and childbirth. Make sure that you have the most up-to-date, evidence-based information available so that you can make informed decisions. The care you receive should take into account any special needs you have, such as a disability, or cultural or religious beliefs. You should be able to discuss the options with your doctor and feel free to ask her whatever you want, change your mind, and know that your preferences, regardless of the recommendations made by the doctor, will be supported.

help establish the best choice for your prenatal care.

## Types of prenatal care

The majority of your care will usually be provided by an ob/gyn. At your first appointment, she will outline the prenatal services you will receive.

**Group medical practice** With this type of care, you will see two or more doctors (typically ob/gyns and/or family practitioners) throughout your pregnancy on a rotating basis. One of these doctors will be present at the hospital when you deliver.

**Solo medical practice** You'll only have one doctor, and you will see her at every prenatal visit. She will attend your birth at the hospital, unless she's unavailable and arranges for another doctor who covers for her to be present for your delivery.

**Combination practice** With this type of care, you'll get to see both doctors and midwives. At least one ob/gyn and one nurse-midwife sees patients on a rotating basis. Depending on the practice, a midwife may or may not be able to assist in delivery at the hospital. Expect a doctor to be present.

**Maternity center-based practice** If your pregnancy is low-risk, you can see certified nurse-midwives for most of your appointments throughout pregnancy. Ob/gyns are available for consultations as required. If you choose this option, you'll deliver your baby at the maternity or birthing center that is

associated with the practice, unless complications arise, in which case your care would be transferred to the affiliated hospital.

**Independent certified nurse-midwife practice** Some states permit midwives to practice without a doctor in the office. If this type of care is available in your area and you have a low-risk pregnancy, you can see midwives for all of your appointments, and a midwife would be present at your delivery in a hospital, birthing center, or at home. The midwives generally have arrangements with doctors, who are available for consultations as needed.

## Where you give birth

This important decision doesn't have to be made at your initial appointment, but your midwife or doctor may discuss the options at this time. It's wise to be aware of the risks, benefits, and consequences of your choice. If you have a preexisting problem, or one that develops during pregnancy, this must be factored into your decision on where you will give birth.

**In the hospital** Some women prefer to give birth in a hospital with doctors and medical equipment close by. Also, some women need specialized care and input from obstetricians because of existing conditions or problems that develop in labor. In this case, the obstetrician and the midwife will work closely together. Other specialists may also need to be involved during labor, for example if a woman has diabetes or a heart condition.

**In a birthing center** These units provide a homelike setting. They are led by midwives with no obstetric input and have facilities such as birthing tubs and pools. The goal at a birthing center is to make labor and birth more natural, with less monitoring and fewer routine medical procedures and interventions. Some pain medication may be available, but epidurals are not. Some birthing centers are next to or affiliated with hospitals so that, if necessary, you can be transferred quickly. Birthing centers are an option that is recommended for low-risk pregnancies.

**At home** A home birth is an option for women who want to give birth in familiar surroundings. However, a home birth is only advised for women who have low-risk pregnancies and for those with no preexisting medical problems. In the US, home births are considered controversial because complications can develop during the labor or the delivery, even in women with low-risk pregnancies. The American College of Obstetricians and Gynecologists and the American Medical Association oppose home births because of the potential for complications.

## Your care providers

**Several different health-care professionals will care for you during pregnancy and labor, and in the postpartum period:**

**Ob/gyns** provide the vast majority of care for women in pregnancy, labor, and the postpartum period. They're specially trained to handle all phases of pregnancy and postpartum recovery. If you have a preexisting condition that could complicate your pregnancy, like diabetes or high blood pressure, or if you're pregnant with twins, you should see an ob/gyn. Special doctors known as high-risk obstetricians, or maternal-fetal medicine specialists, may see you for some appointments if you have a very high-risk pregnancy, such as a baby diagnosed with a serious medical condition or a history of pregnancy complications or repeated loss.

**General practitioners (GPs)** may alternate appointments with ob/gyns.

**Midwives** can provide care for women with low-risk pregnancies throughout all phases of pregnancy and the postpartum period. Certified-nurse midwives often work in a practice with ob/gyns but sometimes can practice on their own. They are registered nurses with extra education and training who are certified by the American College of Nurse-Midwives.

**Pediatricians** are doctors with special training in the health of babies and children. All babies born in a hospital have a newborn checkup by a pediatrician before being discharged.

**Neonatologists** specialize in the care of newborns with problems.

**Hospitals** have clinics where you may go for routine scans; (top). **Midwives** provide care at doctors' offices, maternity centers, or their own practices (bottom left). **Ob/gyns** see patients in their offices and may share care with midwives..

# 227 days to go...

## YOUR BABY TODAY

The upper and lower limb buds that will form the legs and arms are clearly visible by now. The baby's head is still curled over the chest, but the beginnings of ears can just be detected as raised areas at the base of the head.

Your baby's facial features are beginning to develop and over the next few weeks will become much more defined.

### AS A MATTER OF FACT

**According to one study,** eating apples during pregnancy could reduce the risk of your child developing asthma.

Following a Mediterranean diet may have the same effect. Researchers found that the babies of mothers who ate plenty of fish, olive oil, fruit, and vegetables were up to 30 percent less likely to wheeze as well as 50 percent less likely to develop skin allergies.

**Your baby has ears!** Low down, near the jaw line, the ears form, each arising from six small mounds, fusing together to give your baby his unique and individual ear shape. As the face and jaw forms and your baby's neck extends moving away from the chest wall, the ears migrate upward; they will come to lie at the same level as his eyes by 11 weeks.

The lips and nose are now beginning to take shape. To form the upper lip, two separate ridges of tissue grow from each side of your baby's face to fuse with the small piece of tissue in the midline extending downward beneath the nose (the grooved part of the upper lip).

At around this stage, your baby's small and large bowel lengthen. Because they have insufficient room to expand inside the still very curled-up embryo, the intestines appear as a bulge on the surface of the abdominal wall. This bulge is covered by a membrane, into which the umbilical cord becomes attached. The bowel will continue to grow in this embryonic sac until 11–12 weeks when it will be reabsorbed into the abdominal cavity, leaving just the surface attachment of the cord.

### FOCUS ON... SAFETY

## Cooking with care

**Scrupulous food hygiene is important in pregnancy** for a number of reasons. Firstly, your immune system is under extra pressure during pregnancy, making you more susceptible to food poisoning. Secondly, there's a risk that food-borne illnesses can affect the health of your baby, so it pays to be cautious. Do the following:
- **Wash your hands carefully** and regularly, with hot water and soap. Make sure they are completely dry before preparing food, since bacteria spread more easily on damp skin.
- **Keep food in your fridge** until you plan to prepare it, and cook it thoroughly before serving.
- **Serve food piping hot,** since germs can multiply in lukewarm conditions.
- **Refrigerate leftovers** immediately, and reheat them well, only once.
- **Thoroughly clean your hands,** implements, and work surfaces.
- **Set the correct temperature** on your fridge and freezer.

**Make time for preparation** and take the precaution of washing all fruit and vegetables. Keep raw foods away from cooked foods.

# 226 days to go...

## YOUR BABY TODAY

This ultrasound scan of the baby in side view shows that the head (at top) is relatively large compared to the rest of the body. The lighter, elongated area at the center of the baby's darker body is an upper arm bud.

Life goes on even though you're pregnant, but make sure you seek the right help if you're becoming overly tired.

### ASK A... DOCTOR

**I'm going on an overseas, pre-paid vacation to a tropical climate. Can I have vaccinations now that I'm pregnant?** In principle, it's a good idea to avoid traveling to parts of the world where there is a high risk of disease unless you really need to. Local health care might not be adequate and food and water may be contaminated, which poses dangerous risks.

If it isn't possible to change your destination or postpone your vacation, be aware of the following:
■ **Oral vaccines** to protect against yellow fever, typhoid, polio, and anthrax, for example, are contraindicated during pregnancy, although your doctor may decide that if you need to travel, the risk of having the vaccine is lower than the risks associated with contracting the disease.
■ **Some vaccines** (polio and typhoid) are safe when given by injection. Mefloquine tablets, taken to prevent malaria, are considered safe after week 16.
■ **It's safe to have a tetanus** vaccination if you're pregnant; check whether yours is up-to-date.

**You may find work a strain at times.** If you have symptoms, such as fatigue, and still haven't told colleagues you're pregnant, it can make for a stressful and day. If you've told some colleagues, or your boss, you're expecting it may be easier but you might feel you have to prove you can still do your job as efficiently as before.

Traveling can be tiring so explore the possibility of doing more flexible hours, so that you can commute when it's less busy. Be reassured that even though you aren't feeling your best, your unborn baby is unlikely to be affected. Do, however, take care of yourself.

If you find that you're struggling to deal with your workload, consider speaking to your boss (you can ask him or her to keep your pregnancy a secret until you are ready to tell), or someone in the human resources department, to give yourself a little breathing space. If you have colleagues who are close friends, lean on them for support in these early weeks.

### ARE YOU NESTING ALREADY?

**There's nothing like a new arrival** to inspire you to get all those do-it-yourself (DIY) jobs done around the home. For most women, the nesting bug occurs in the later weeks of pregnancy, but if you're itching to get your house in order before then, make sure you exercise a little caution.

First of all, avoid putting yourself and your baby at risk: don't stand on tall ladders, and don't bend and crouch for long periods since this may affect your circulation. Avoid contact with oil-based paints, polyurethane (used for flooring), spray paints, turpentine, and other paint removers, and avoid inhaling plaster dust.

# 225 days to go...

### YOUR BABY TODAY

The yolk sac can be seen floating like a balloon in the amniotic cavity on its fine stalk. As the embryo has drawn nutrition from the yolk sac it has gradually reduced in both size and importance. Meanwhile the placenta (on the right) is becoming established.

## If you're planning a vacation, take into account that you may not feel up to a long trip.

### BREATHE EASY

**Exercise can help keep breathlessness at bay,** and increase the efficiency of your heart and lungs (cardiovascular system), helping you to deal with the physical demands of pregnancy now and in later months.

A cardiovascular workout involves increasing your heart rate for at least 20–30 minutes. However, pregnancy is not a time to start training for a marathon; stick to moderate-intensity workouts. A way to test if you are exercising at the right level is to talk while you are working out (see p.161)—if you can't, lower the intensity.

Try doing interval training, which involves alternating five minutes of cardiovascular workouts with five minutes of toning for the upper body (see p.196). Breathe out as you lift the weights, and in as you relax.

Breathing deeply allows oxygen to travel to your vital organs and helps the cardiovascular system to function effectively. During pregnancy, it's important to avoid taking short, shallow breaths and to focus on expanding your rib cage and filling your lungs with air.

**You may have planned a vacation** before you found out you were pregnant, or just feel like getting away. If you're feeling tired and have morning sickness, however, you may not feel up to traveling too far.

One advantage of going away is being able to spend quality time with your partner and fully embrace the fact that you're going to be parents.

When going on vacation, check with travel insurance companies to see if you can get coverage during pregnancy and check the medical facilities at your destination. If you have prenatal records, take them with you. Some airlines may not accept pregnant women on flights after 36 weeks without a doctor's lettter written within 72 hours of the flight confirming your due date and your fitness to fly.

**Relax and take the opportunity** for a snooze on the plane trip, but make sure you get up regularly to stretch your legs. It's even more important to keep the blood circulating when you're pregnant.

# 224 days to go...

**YOUR BABY TODAY**

The head is disproportionately large at this stage. In the center of this image, the underlying structures of the brain can be seen: the forebrain has divided into two and these two halves will become the two cerebral hemispheres of your baby's brain.

You're probably already wondering if you're carrying a boy or a girl, but the physical signs of gender aren't apparent yet.

**Although the sex of your baby** was determined at the moment of fertilization, it will not yet be apparent whether the embryo is male or female.

At this stage of development, the external genitalia have exactly the same appearance (almost nonexistent). In a girl, no uterus or tubes have formed internally. The ovary in a female embryo and testes in a male embryo are currently just ridges of tissue, without any of the characteristics of either reproductive organ.

Incredibly, your baby's heart has already developed, with four chambers beating at about 160 beats per minute. The common tube leaving the heart has divided into the two main blood vessels: the aorta takes your baby's oxygen-carrying blood to his body and the pulmonary trunk takes his blood to the lungs. Valves within the heart ensure that the blood only travels one way and all of the major blood vessels are now established.

Your baby's eyes appear open because the eyelids have just started to appear and have yet to fuse. In reality, they won't properly open until week 26. Pigment is just starting to accumulate within the retina of the eye. The developing lens is supplied by a single blood vessel in the optic nerve, which will later disappear.

**Your baby is all curled up** at this stage of development, with her chin on her chest. Her head is quite large due to rapid underlying brain expansion giving the impression of an overhanging forehead.

---

**ASK A... DOCTOR**

**I'm eight weeks pregnant and have an ear and throat infection. Will I be allowed to take antibiotics?** You may be prescribed antibiotics by your doctor since there are some that can be taken during pregnancy. Penicillin-based antibiotics are usually prescribed, or if you are allergic to these your doctor will be able to offer other safe alternatives.

Never take antibiotics that have not been prescribed for you specifically. The following antibiotics should not be taken during pregnancy:

■ **Tetracylines** taken during pregnancy can adversely affect the development of an unborn baby's bones, and may cause some discoloration of the enamel on the baby's teeth.

■ **Streptomycin** can cause damage to the ears of the developing baby and result in hearing loss.

■ **Sulphonamides** can cause jaundice in the baby.

---

**ACTUAL SIZE OF YOUR BABY**

**At 8 weeks**, your baby's crown to rump length is 0.51 in (13 mm).

6 weeks    7 weeks    8 weeks

# Your 9th week

**YOUR BABY HAS HANDS AND FEET, AND HIS BONES ARE GROWING**

During this week, your baby starts to make tiny movements. You won't be aware of this, but it's exciting to think about. On the downside, you could be in the throes of nausea and sickness. However, many women find that the nausea starts to lessen from now on. There are various self-help measures you can take to relieve the sickness, but if it's making life miserable, talk to your doctor.

**The yolk sac** shrinks further and soon will not be needed.

**The baby's head** is still bowed over the bulge of his stomach.

**Chorionic villi** continue to branch as the placenta matures and so that it can fulfill all your baby's needs.

**Individual fingers** are distinct, but are still not totally separate.

**The major organs** of the baby's digestive system have all started to develop but are not ready to carry out any digestive functions.

**Your uterus** is growing to accommodate the baby and now starts to tilt upward.

**The toes** are less advanced than the fingers and still appear budlike.

**The eyes**, which until now have been on the side of the baby's head, have migrated around to the front.

**The embryo** now measures 0.70 in (18 mm) from crown to rump.

**The outer ears** are starting to take shape.

**Elbows** are now able to move.

EMBRYO AT 9 WEEKS

# 223 days to go...

**YOUR BABY TODAY**

At this early stage in the pregnancy the placenta is much larger than the fetus. The fetus can just be seen within the amniotic sac. The fronds (white area) on the surface of the sac make up the placenta and at this stage surround nearly all of the amniotic sac.

Not all pregnant women have cravings, but many women do experience a change in their food preferences.

**When it comes to being pregnant,** it seems your body instinctively knows what you like to eat. Experts are not sure how this can happen but it seems your body has natural protective mechanisms; certain foods are not good for the developing baby so your body turns you away from them; or your body is deficient in certain nutrients, so craves foods that will provide them.

Suddenly you can't stand the thought of food and drinks that you have always loved and find yourself craving things you never previously liked, or you long for bizarre combinations of foods. Aversions and cravings are often associated with nausea. It's common to be turned off by fatty foods since the smell alone can make you feel sick. You may start to dislike the taste or the smell of coffee or tea, cigarettes, and alcohol.

It is common to crave strong-tasting foods such as pickles, which may be due to the fact your taste buds change during pregnancy. What's termed "pica" is an unhealthy craving for bizzare items (see p.121).

You should try to eat healthily, but there are a few foods which should be avoided (see p.17). Otherwise eat whatever combinations you desire—and don't worry about the strange looks you might get in the sandwich shop!

(see p.121).
(see p.17).

**ASK A... NUTRITIONIST**

**Should I stop adding salt to my food?** There is no need to limit salt intake but don't have in excess of the recommended 0.2 oz (6 g) a day.

During pregnancy, your blood and other bodily fluids expand almost 50 percent, an expansion that requires extra water and salt. The majority of salt in the diet comes from processed foods, not from the salt shaker or the salt you add in cooking. To manage your intake, eat whole foods you cook yourself and add your own salt to taste.

**FOCUS ON... DADS**

## Satisfy her cravings

**If it's a mom-to-be's responsibility** to play host to baby for nine months, it most definitely falls within a your dad-to-be's job description to see that your partner gets everything she needs. A word of warning: cravings usually occur the minute the local store has closed, or in the evening when you're relaxing. Forget the pickles and ice cream you've been told to expect. Instead, be prepared for a last-minute dash to the local pizza place, a trek to a 24-hour supermarket that carries organic sour cream-flavored potato chips, beets, or a chocolate doughnut.

You can help by preparing meals and snacks some of the time: if your partner is presented with healthy food lovingly prepared by you, she may be less likely to reach for any unhealthy food she craves.

**If an ice cream craving strikes,** try to have one spoonful, not the whole container. Pair it with fresh fruit for a healthy combination.

# 222 days to go...

**YOUR BABY TODAY**

The baby's hands (seen here) and feet are gradually developing and they are formed of cartilage, not bone at this early stage. In the center left, the fused rays of the hand plate that will become the fingers can be seen. The ribs are in the background.

## Who will your baby look like? His unique facial features are beginning to take shape this week.

**If you were to have an ultrasound scan this week,** it would be possible to recognize several of your baby's facial features.

His eyelids fuse and will remain closed until around the 26th week. The lips have already formed and with the surrounding skin will have the greatest concentration of nerves. The muscular tongue arises from the base of your baby's mouth, but it will be two weeks before the first taste buds appear. The hard palate that forms the roof of the mouth arises from two "shelves" that start to grow, one each side, beneath the tongue; these shelves will lift upward to connect horizontally, allowing the tongue to drop down in to the mouth. Once they have joined together, the septum of the nose grows downward to meet them.

Your baby's tiny tooth buds are in place and this is critical to adequate jaw development. One branch of tooth buds will form the first milk teeth and a separate branch will eventually form the permanent teeth. The milk teeth develop slowly and it will not be until the six month of pregnancy that they acquire their hard enamel coating.

The embryo is still very curled up, with the head resting on the chest. Over the next two weeks as the jaw and neck grow, the head will gradually lift.

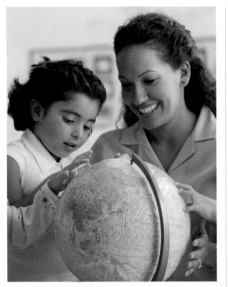

**If you are in regular contact** with young children while you're pregnant, it's even more important that you check your immunity to childhood illnesses.

### CHILDHOOD ILLNESSES

**Having immunity against common infectious illnesses** will protect your unborn baby. You may have natural immunity from having conditions such as chicken pox and fifth disease as a child. You will almost certainly have been vaccinated against mumps and measles, so your unborn baby will be protected from these.

If you are unsure about your immunity or medical history, or think you may have been in contact with any of these infections, contact your doctor immediately for further advice. He or she will be able to do a checkup and provide reassurance.

### ASK A... DOCTOR

**I work for a dry cleaner. Could the chemicals harm my unborn baby?**
Concerns about dry-cleaning chemicals stem from research showing that women who operated dry-cleaning machines had a higher risk of miscarriage. If touched or inhaled, some organic (carbon-containing) solvents used in dry-cleaning machines can pass through the placenta and some are thought to increase the risk of miscarriage or birth defects.

Talk to your employer to find out how your duties can be changed for the duration of your pregnancy to limit your contact with organic solvents and industrial chemicals.

# 221 days to go...

## YOUR BABY TODAY

In a matter of days, your baby's eyes have developed from slight ridges to clear depressions, on each side of the face. The face is developing rapidly at this stage, and your baby's heartbeat would be seen on an ultrasound scan.

It's a few weeks before the hormone responsible for morning sickness subsides, but the nausea will pass soon.

**You may be wondering when you'll wake up and no longer feel sick.** HCG (human chorionic gonadotrophin) levels, which may be responsible for feelings of nausea will begin to fall in about three weeks' time and most women begin to feel better then. For some women the sickness may continue beyond this time.

You may have just started to feel nauseous or your sickness may have begun weeks ago and now be worse, but by around week 12 you should be over the worst. Nausea that happens daily, especially if it is associated with fatigue, can be very wearing so try to remember that it's temporary.

It's normal to have some morning sickness and you should be able to keep some foods and fluids down. However, for a small minority of pregnant women—about 1 percent—the vomiting is severe, occurring regularly and lasting over a period of weeks. This more serious form of morning sickness is called hyperemesis gravidarum and can lead to dehydration. Hospital treatment with intravenous fluids and anti-nausea drugs may be required to rehydrate you.

Seek advice from your doctor if you're concerned about the amount of times you're vomiting or if you're struggling to keep fluids and food down.

### Fit—not sick

**If you're feeling particularly nauseous,** try going for a brisk walk in the fresh air while concentrating on your breathing and posture. Sometimes frequent sips of water help these feelings, and will allow you to exercise longer. Regular exercisers may find that nausea is absent during exercise, although it may resume after the session.

Extreme nausea and vomiting can be a sign of overexercising. Always drink water before, during, and after any physical activity.

## ACUPRESSURE WRISTBANDS

**A simple solution to help relieve feelings of nausea** is to wear acupressure wristbands. Available from pharmacists, these bands have been clinically tested in the treatment of pregnancy-induced nausea. Unlike anti-nausea drugs, they don't have any side effects and are easy to use.

The elastic bands, one worn on each arm, work by applying pressure on the Nei Kuan acupressure point (known as P6). They can be washed and reused as necessary.

**About 70–80 percent** of pregnant women suffer from morning sickness.

If you are one of the 20–30 percent who don't be thankful. You may get anxious if you're not feeling sick because it is such a common symptom, but don't worry and just count yourself lucky.

# Your baby's life support system

The placenta links your baby's blood supply to your own and carries out all the functions that your baby can't perform for himself. The placenta is rooted to the lining of your uterus and linked to the baby by the umbilical cord.

## HOW SUBSTANCES ARE EXCHANGED IN THE PLACENTA

### Inside the placenta

**The placenta contains a huge network of** tiny projections called chorionic villi that branch out from a thin membrane, the chorion, and contain fetal blood vessels. The chorionic villi are bathed in maternal blood within the intervillous space. Each villus is only one or two cells thick, which allows the transfer of gases and nutrients between the mother and the baby, while ensuring that the two circulations never come into direct contact. Through the process of diffusion, oxygen and nutrients such as glucose, your baby's primary source of energy, from the mother pass into the fetal circulation, and waste products from the baby are picked up and carried away in the mother's bloodstream. The chorionic membrane also acts as a protective barrier, preventing many harmful substances and infections from reaching the baby.

Uterine muscle

Maternal blood vessels

Fetal blood vessels in chorionic villus

Maternal blood in intervillous space

Chorion

Umbilical cord

Direction of blood flow to and from the fetus

Umbilical cord

**The vast network** of villi in the placenta facilitates the transfer of gases, nutrients, and waste products to and from your baby.

## How the placenta develops

The placenta forms from cells in the embryo shortly after the egg implants in the lining of the uterus. Early placental growth is rapid, and at the beginning of the first trimester, the placenta is larger than the baby. However, the baby's growth catches up by 16 weeks, and by the end of pregnancy the baby is almost six times heavier. The final weight of the placenta is between 12 oz (350 g) and 1 lb 5 oz (600 g). Once its structure is complete at the end of the first trimester, it takes on many important functions for the rest of the pregnancy (see opposite).

**Growth after the first trimester** The placenta grows throughout the second trimester. By the third trimester, growth slows, but placental efficiency continually improves as extra villi (through which substances are exchanged; see left) grow and increase the available surface area of the placenta by nearly fourfold. Cell layers also become thinner so that substances can be exchanged efficiently.

Placental blood flow is massive and many of the changes in your circulation are designed to meet its needs. By term, a tenfold increase in placental blood supply results in a fifth of your circulation supplying the placenta with up to half a liter of blood (almost a pint) each minute.

**The aging placenta** The placenta ages towards the end of pregnancy, especially after 40 weeks. However, at least 60–80 percent of its function would need to be lost before there were any signs of problems with blood flow in the umbilical cord.

## The role of the placenta

The placenta fulfills many essential roles that help sustain your pregnancy and enable your baby to grow and develop.

**The exchange of substances**. The placenta transports substances to and from your baby, acting as your baby's lungs, kidneys, and digestive system.

To obtain oxygen, the baby's blood cells grab oxygen molecules from your own hemoglobin (the oxygen-carrying subtance in blood). Fetal hemoglobin has a modified structure that makes it bind readily to oxygen. Your baby requires twice as much oxygen weight for weight as your own needs so the transfer of oxygen needs to be efficient. The placenta's enhanced blood supply, large surface area, and the characteristics of fetal hemoglobin all ensure the efficient transfer of oxygen from mother to baby.

As your hemoglobin gives up oxygen, it accepts carbon dioxide molecules. Your lungs breathe out air rich with the baby's carbon dioxide as well as your own and the cycle begins again.

To grow and develop your baby also needs amino acids, the building blocks for proteins, and minerals like calcium and iron and these all pass from your own circulation via the placenta to the baby.

**Protecting your baby** The placenta protects your baby from infections and harmful substances. Since your baby hasn't encountered any external threats he doesn't yet make protective antibodies known as immunoglobulins that can identify threats, such as viruses or bacteria. Instead he is reliant on the transfer of immunoglobulins from your circulation via the placenta and into his circulation. This means that you are able to protect your baby in the uterus from illnesses such as chickenpox. After your baby is born, the immunglobulins he acquired from you will eventually be lost, which means that later as a child he becomes susceptible to chickenpox.

**Hormone production** The placenta produces hormones, such as estrogen and progesterone, that are vital to your baby's well-being and lead to many of the changes in your body during pregnancy.

**Heat transfer** A baby's high metabolic rate generates heat. The placenta's big surface area and high blood flow disperses heat, controlling the baby's temperature.

# The umbilical cord

**The umbilical cord, which connects your baby to the placenta,** contains three vessels: two arteries, which carry blood from the baby to the placenta, and one vein, which carries blood back to the baby. The blood in the arteries contains waste products, such as carbon dioxide, from the baby's metabolism. Carbon dioxide is transferred across the placenta to your bloodstream and then to your lungs, where it's breathed out. Oxygen is transported from red bloods cells in your circulation, across the placenta to the baby in the umbilical vein. In addition to oxygen, the umbilical vein transports nutrients from the placenta to your baby.

The vessels in the umbilical cord have a protective coating called Wharton's jelly, and the cord is coiled like a spring so that the baby is free to move around. The coiling pattern of the cord has usually established itself by week nine and is usually in a counterclockwise direction. However, the cord can coil later, and sometimes isn't established until 20 weeks. The baby's movements seem to encourage the cord to coil.

The cord is usually attached to the center of the placenta, although sometimes it's attached near the edge. Very occasionally, it divides into its separate vessels before finally entering the placenta. The cord is usually under 1 in (1–2 cm) in diameter and 23 in (60 cm) long, which is twice the length needed to ensure that there are no problems at delivery.

After delivery, the cord vessels close by themselves. The arteries close first, helped by their thicker muscular walls. This prevents blood loss to the placenta from your baby. The umbilical vein closes slightly later (starting at 15 seconds, but only completed by 3 or 4 minutes). This allows blood to continue to return to your baby during the first few minutes of life. As a result, many feel that a slight delay before clamping the cord can be beneficial to the baby. There are no nerves within the cord, so cutting the cord after delivery is a painless procedure for your baby.

**This Doppler scan** shows the blood vessels in the umbilical cord. Blood flows through a single vein (blue) and two arteries (red).

**Some harmful substances** can cross the placenta

For this reason, it's important that you protect your baby by taking medical advice before you use any type of medication during pregnancy.

Your baby's life support system

113

# 220 days to go...

## YOUR BABY TODAY

In the upper limb bud, the flat expansion that will form the hand can be identified. The fingers are becoming more distinct and there will now be the first signs of movement at the elbows.

Your baby's bones are beginning to develop—and they will continue to lengthen from now until his teenage years.

---

### FOCUS ON... NUTRITION

## Good mood foods

**If being pregnant** gets you down at times, try a dietary boost. Happy, relaxed people tend to have high levels of serotonin, a brain chemical that is produced when you consume protein-rich foods. So eat meat (especially turkey), fish (see p.96), legumes, and well-cooked eggs (see p.17).

Eating foods that are rich in vitamin B, such as bananas and avocados, can also help increase your serotonin levels.

**You won't be aware of your developing baby's activities** inside the uterus for some months yet, but the fact that his elbows are forming allows him to make some small movements; the wrists do not yet move.

Your baby is looking more human by the day. His vertebrae and ribs are now in place, and his fingers are gradually lengthening. His body is less curled up than it was a few weeks ago.

The skeleton will gradually calcify and harden. With the exception of the cranial skull bones, all your baby's bones have a soft cartilage core that will later be reabsorbed as it is converted into hard bone. This process of hardening, known as ossification, starts in so-called primary ossification centers during the next five weeks of your pregnancy. Within these primary centers, specialized cells form spongy then hard bone as calcium salts are laid down. Within the hard bone is red bone marrow, which in later weeks will become the main producer of the baby's red blood cells.

Secondary ossification centers develop in the second trimester at the ends of each of your baby's bones.

The portion of bone between the hardening primary and secondary centers is known as the growth plate. This plate is responsible for the continued lengthening of your unborn baby's bones.

---

### MORE CHEESE PLEASE

**Tired of being told what you can't eat?** It is a common myth that eating cheese harms the unborn baby. Only unpasteurized cheeses are potentially dangerous because they increase the risk of listeria (a rare bacterium that can attack the baby). These products may be produced at local cheese stores or dairy farms.

All other types of cheeses pose no danger and are regarded as a good source of calcium.

So, while there are some cheeses you should avoid eating, you can enjoy all of the following, if they're pasteurized:
- Hard cheese, such as Cheddar and Parmesan
- Feta
- Ricotta
- Mascarpone
- Cream cheese
- Mozzarella
- Cottage cheese
- Processed cheese, such as spreads.

# 219 days to go...

### YOUR BABY TODAY

The development of the baby's lower limbs always lags slightly behind that of the upper limbs. At this stage, the toes are not distinct and the legs are not yet bending at the knee.

## It's understandable that your pregnancy will be on your mind. Try to find ways to communicate this to your partner.

**At a time when you want to feel close to your partner,** you may find that your relationship is changing, and it may be quite fraught with issues. Often men say that their pregnant partners are more sensitive or now react to things differently and that this can be difficult for them to handle.

Your relationship will inevitably change—going through pregnancy together is momentous—but as long as you keep communicating, you will be able to support each other. Being united now will stand you in good stead for the first year of parenting.

During the early stages of pregnancy, your partner may find it hard to relate to the fact that you're expecting a baby; the physical changes to your body won't be that visible at this stage and he is yet to see his baby on a scan. Conversely, you will be very aware of the pregnancy and undergoing many physical and emotional changes.

Your partner may need more time than you to adjust to the idea of becoming a parent. He may be concerned about practical issues, such as the changes to your lifestyle and the financial implications of having a baby. Talking openly to each other can help ease anxieties for you both. Remember, that although many changes are happening to your body, your partner

does have feelings and this is a big life change for him too. If you've told your family and close friends about the pregnancy, all the attention may be on you. Your partner may be feeling left out and this is something that often gets worse as the pregnancy progresses and after the baby arrives.

Take time to find out your partner's concerns and look for ways to involve him more in the pregnancy, if that's what he wants. If you have a good support network of friends, encourage him to spend time with male friends who have been through the expectant dad experience.

**Support each other** as you both go through the different emotions attached to becoming parents. Don't lose sight of your relationship and be understanding of each other's needs.

### ASK A... MOM

**I'm worried we won't have space in our small apartment, but is a house move inadvisable while I'm pregnant?** We started the process but thankfully it fell through since it was proving quite stressful, and it's not advisable to deal with those kinds of pressures while you're pregnant. We stayed in our apartment until our baby was one and it was fine. Remember that small babies have very few needs, other than being fed, loved, changed, and stimulated, and much of the paraphernalia that you think you need is unnecessary. If you have room for a crib, a stroller, a drawer for your baby's clothes, and a corner for toys, you'll be fine in a small space for the time being.

115

# 218 days to go...

## YOUR BABY TODAY

This 3D ultrasound scan shows a baby lying on its back, in exactly the same orientation as the image opposite. It is just possible to pick out the limb buds on an ultrasound scan taken at this stage.

## It's not long until you have your first prenatal appointment and will see your doctor.

**In a couple of weeks' time,** you will have your initial appointment (see p.129) with the doctor. If you haven't made an appointment for this yet, contact your doctor now to arrange it. You may or may not have a choice of hospitals. If you do have options, talk to women you know locally who have had their babies at those hospitals to find out about their experience. For example, some hospitals may have a birth center attached, and have a less medically managed approach to childbirth.

Start thinking now about the kind of questions you want to ask your doctor. It's a good idea to write these down. Also make a note, in advance, of the key details of your medical history and any pregnancy symptoms.

### TACKLING COLDS

**Cold medicines contain a variety of ingredients,** including antihistamines, that are best avoided in pregnancy. Check the label and talk to your doctor or pharmacist before taking any medications.

Try natural remedies, such as steam inhalations or saline nasal sprays before resorting to medication.

### ASK A... PANEL ABOUT HOME BIRTH

## It's my first pregnancy. Can I have a home birth?

**Midwife:** if you're in good health with no complications, giving birth at home is an option. Many women enjoy the experience of giving birth at home, because they may feel more comfortable with familiar surroundings and people. Some women find labor easier when they get into water, either a familiar bathtub at home or a birthing pool that has been purchased or rented.

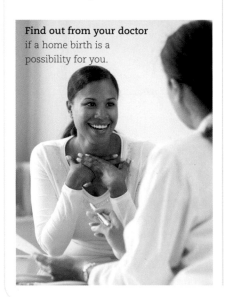

**Find out from your doctor** if a home birth is a possibility for you.

**Obstetrician:** there is no problem with this in general, but take advice from your doctor. You should avoid taking risks. If there is a history of long or complicated labors in your family, your baby is breech or very small, there are issues about the location of the cord or the placenta, you are very overweight or unhealthy, or you suffer from conditions such as diabetes, it might be worth erring on the side of caution. If you have your baby in a hospital, quick and early intervention can take place if needed. You may want to have a home birth; however, it is sensible to listen to the experts. Delivery of a healthy baby is the most important thing.

**Mom:** I had my first baby at home, and it was wonderful. I was nervous about what might go wrong, but my midwife reassured me that she would be monitoring me, and would get me to the hospital if there was a problem. She also explained I could change my mind if I didn't think things were going well, and go to the hospital for the birth (and some pain relief!).

# 217 days to go...

**YOUR BABY TODAY**

The baby's hands can be clearly seen here but the fingers are still fused at this stage. The fingers will be completely separate in just one week's time and wrist movement is just about to begin.

By the end of this ninth week, your baby's digestive system is rapidly developing but won't function properly for some time.

**Your baby is developing quickly** inside the uterus. The simple tube forming along his gut has undergone most changes at the upper end. Now the lower part dilates as the single tube then divides into what will become the rectum at the back and then the bladder and urethra at the front.

Although the mouth is open to the amniotic fluid, there is still a membrane in place, which will disappear in one to two weeks' time. The lower bowel is not yet mature and does not move material along its length.

The remainder of the large bowel and small bowel is still lengthening. The duodenum is the first part of the small bowel and it is still a solid tube. The pancreas, gall bladder, and liver have all formed buds leading off from the upper small bowel, but none are yet contributing any digestive function.

**Looking at a computer screen** for long periods of time can make headaches—a common side effect of pregnancy—even worse. Take regular breaks and drink plenty of water since being dehydrated can exacerbate headaches.

**ASK A... DOCTOR**

**Since I've been pregnant, I've had terrible headaches. Could computer work be the cause?**
Tension headaches and migraines are common in pregnancy, probably due to fluctuating hormones, and it is not uncommon to have severe headaches with prolonged computer use. This could be due to eye strain and the fact that you are immobile, which can cause tension.

Take even more breaks from your computer screen now that you're pregnant. You'll probably find you need more bathroom breaks anyway. If this doesn't help, ask if you can do tasks that don't require computer use for a short time. Headaches are often worse in the first trimester.

**ACTUAL SIZE OF YOUR BABY**

**At 9 weeks** your baby's crown to rump length is 0.70 in (18 mm).

7 weeks

8 weeks

9 weeks

Your 9th week

117

# Your 10th week

**NO LONGER AN EMBRYO, YOUR UNBORN BABY ENTERS A NEW PHASE**

This is your baby's last week as an embryo; next week she'll be known as a fetus. Her major organs are in place, although by no means in full working order. There's a long way to go yet and her body systems will continue to mature for the rest of pregnancy, and beyond. The most noticeable difference to your body will be in your breasts. You may well have gone up a cup size—or more.

**The baby's head** has lifted slightly off the chest.

**The nose** protrudes from the face and has a definite shape.

**The mouth and lips** are now nearly fully developed.

**The yolk sac** is not needed anymore and is shrinking away.

**The placenta** is now fully functioning. It will be the baby's lifeline until the end of your pregnancy.

**The umbilical cord** takes blood between the baby and the placenta.

**The bulge at the base** of the umbilical cord contains the developing intestines.

**The uterus** continues to enlarge and lift upward.

**The embryo** measures 1.18 in (3 cm) crown to rump.

**The outer ear** is fully formed but not yet in its final position, which will be higher up.

EMBRYO AT 10 WEEKS

**The wrist** has formed and is able to bend.

**The fingers and toes** have lengthened and separated.

# 216 days to go...

## YOUR BABY TODAY

At about seven weeks, the human embryo measures about 1.2 in (3 cm). Most of the primitive organ systems are formed: the arms and legs have budded; the retina of the eye, and the nose, can be seen. The large dark mass is the enlarged liver.

Your baby's welfare will be your main concern, but be reassured that, however you're feeling, she'll be getting sustenance.

**You may be very conscious of your health** and well-being at this time but be reassured that even if you've felt unwell during this first trimester, your baby will have been taking what she needs from you: you have internal reserves of various minerals and substances, such as iron, and will still be absorbing some nutrients from what you eat. However, if you're concerned about the amount of vitamins and minerals you're consuming through your diet, for the sake of your own health you could take a prenatal vitamin supplement. Remember, you should still be taking folic acid supplements and eating folate-rich foods (see p.35).

There is no cause for concern if you do not put on any weight in the first trimester, or even if you lose a bit of weight. The majority of weight gain takes place in the second and third trimesters (see p.99).

If you're vomiting a lot and struggling to keep food down (see p.111), don't hesitate to see your ob/gyn.

---

**FOCUS ON... YOUR BODY**

## Your changing breasts

**The changes to your breasts you will be noticing** are caused by both an increased blood supply and a rise in pregnancy hormones, particularly in the first 12 weeks.

Before your pregnancy was confirmed you may have felt tingling sensations (especially in the nipple area) as the blood supply increased.

- **As early as 6–8 weeks,** your breasts will have become larger and more tender and may have begun to look different on the surface, with threadlike veins starting to appear.
- **At around 8–12 weeks,** the nipples darken and can become more erect.
- **As early as the 16th week** of pregnancy, colostrum, the first milk, may leak from your breasts.

---

**THE LOWDOWN**

## He's "pregnant" too

**Can your partner ever really understand what you're going through?** According to a recent study, some dads don't need a fake pregnancy belly to empathize. Known as Couvade syndrome, symptoms experienced by expectant fathers ranged from morning sickness to backaches, mood swings, and food cravings. Although, interestingly, often it was the woman claiming her partner had these symptoms.

Couvade is thought to happen because men are so deeply involved in the pregnancy. While others believe it could be jealousy (you're getting all the attention) or guilt that he's responsible for your condition and therefore your symptoms.

# 215 days to go...

**YOUR BABY TODAY**

The baby now begins to bend her wrists. The natural position is for the limbs to be slightly bent at all joints, especially in the early stages. There is a more distinct neck area as the baby's head is now slightly lifted off the chest.

## The muscular diaphragm that will eventually enable your baby to breathe—and hiccup—is developing now.

**As your baby's lungs develop in the chest,** there is nothing to separate them from the stomach, liver, and bowel in what will later become her abdominal cavity.

In adults, the chest is separated from the abdomen by the muscular diaphragm. When we breathe, the diaphragm moves downward and the ribs expand outward. This process allows air to enter the lungs.

Your baby's diaphragm forms from four in-folds of tissue. First seen at around this week of pregnancy, these folds gradually expand inward, fusing together and closing the space by the end of this week.

In the center of the diaphragm there are openings for the esophagus to the stomach, main artery to the body—the aorta, and main vein returning blood from the lower body, the inferior vena cava. As your pregnancy progresses, muscle fibers gradually strengthen your baby's diaphragm, which later allows her to make breathing movements.

**The nuchal translucency screening** is a scan. It measures the width of the skin behind the baby's neck to assess if excess fluid has collected there—if a high level is found, it may indicate a greater risk of Down syndrome. Nuchal translucency is the most accurate way to screen for Down syndrome.

Red area shows the fluid under the skin at the back of the baby's neck.

### FOCUS ON... TWINS

## Twin tests

**If you're expecting twins or more,** blood-based screening tests for Down syndrome can mislead, since they rely on measuring the amounts of circulating AFP (alfa-fetoprotein) and other markers, which are present in much higher levels when there's more than one baby. That's why your best bet for screening is the nuchal translucency test from 11–14 weeks (see right).

### TIME TO THINK ABOUT

## Screening and diagnostic tests

It's useful to be aware of the screening tests (see pp.142–3) and diagnostic tests (see pp.152–3) that will be available in the weeks to come. Your doctor will talk through the pros and cons of having each test. Some abnormalities may be detected at the 18–22 week scan.

■ **Screening tests:** these tests identify the "risk factor" for a particular condition, but do not confirm that your baby definitely has a condition. For example, a screening test for Down syndrome may give your baby a risk factor of 1:200. This means that your baby has a 1 in 200 chance of being affected by Down syndrome, but it does not mean that he actually has the condition.

■ **Diagnostic tests:** if screening tests reveal your baby has a high risk factor for a chromosomal abnormality, you will be offered a diagnostic test, such as amniocentesis or chorionic villus sampling (see pp.152–3), which gives a definite result as to whether or not a condition is present.

# 212 days to go...

### YOUR BABY TODAY

The lower limbs are now held flexed at the hip and knee joints, leading to a slightly crossed-legs position. The separate toes can be distinguished. Further growth of the thigh and shin bones will bring the foot length into proportion with the rest of the leg.

## One of the downsides of pregnancy is being at greater risk of urinary tract infections, so you need to be aware of the signs.

**It's important to be on the lookout** for any signs of a urinary tract infection while you're pregnant. While it's not very serious, and can be easily treated, it's a complication you can do without.

An infection may cause you to urinate more frequently, but this is also a symptom of early pregnancy so can be hard to spot. If, however, you also have stinging or discomfort when you actually urinate, lower abdominal pain, or even blood in the urine you may have

developed a urinary tract infection. These infections are very common in women in general, because the urethra (tube which carries urine from the bladder to the outside) is very close to the anus and so bacteria do not have far to travel to create an infection.

In pregnancy, there are high levels of the hormone progesterone; this relaxes the tubes of the urinary system making it even easier for bacteria to enter and infect the bladder or even the kidneys. It is very important that if you have the

symptoms of a urinary tract infection that your doctor tests your urine. In general, urinary tract infections are easily treatable in pregnancy. If there is an infection, you will be prescribed antibiotics that are safe to take in pregnancy. The infection must be treated because, if left, it may cause damage to your kidneys.

### STAYING IN SHAPE

**If you were a regular exerciser prior to becoming pregnant,** it is important to continue with some form of exercise. Stopping entirely, just because you're pregnant, would be a shock to your fit body.

There are some contraindications to exercising (see p.18), but if you have clearance from your doctor, take the following steps to ensure that you are continuing to exercise safely and effectively, and getting all the benefits from your program without putting you or your baby at risk.

■ **Continue with activities,** such as jogging, and swimming, as long as you feel comfortable.

■ **Listen to your body** very carefully—look for signs that you should slow down or take a break.
■ **Get adequate rest** between workouts, and drink water before, during, and after all forms of exercise.
■ **Exercise at a moderate level—** you should be able to do the talk test (see page 161).
■ **Keep to low-impact** and low-risk activities (avoid sports that involve contact and the risk of falling).
■ **Wear the right clothing:** cotton will enable your body to dissipate heat, and a supportive sports bra is vital for your growing breasts, especially if you're jogging.

**If you're used to bicycling,** switch to a stationary bike at the gym during pregnancy. It's best to avoid activities that can lead to falls, such as biking outside.

# 211 days to go...

## YOUR BABY TODAY

The umbilical cord widens where it enters the baby's abdomen. This bulge is necessary to accommodate the bowel that is forming underneath at this stage of development. The bones of the head are not yet fully formed.

## Your baby's organ systems are now present, in a basic form, so at this point she changes from being an embryo to a fetus.

**The early embryonic period** is complete at the end of this week, and it is the start of the fetal period. The development of the embryo was characterized by the three cell lines each developing into their own types of tissues and organs, as it grew from a flat disk of cells into a human shape. Many of the changes took place concurrently, but it was the heart, circulation, and nervous systems that developed initially with the gut, limbs, and face development following.

During next week (your 11th week), your baby's kidneys and genital system will undergo their most rapid development. All your baby's organs need to mature fully, and many of them, such as the brain, lungs, and kidneys, will continue to mature throughout pregnancy and after birth.

During this ninth week, your baby's facial features are becoming more recognizable. The ears will take on their final shape, although they are still positioned low.

**The eyes** which started on the side of the face start to move more centrally, the nose is visible, and the head achieves a more rounded contour.

### FOCUS ON... NUTRITION

## Vegetarian mom-to-be

**A vegetarian diet can be safe and healthy in pregnancy.** Lacto-ovo vegetarians, those who consume dairy products, usually have no trouble getting enough nutrients, though they should be careful to eat a varied diet rich in whole grains, beans, legumes, fruit, and vegetables, in order to obtain the proper mix of amino acids, vitamins, and minerals.

Vegetarians also need to obtain enough, as well as complete, protein since vegetarian sources tend to be lower than animal proteins. An intake of 2 oz (60 g) of protein is needed daily

in pregnancy, which for vegetarians usually means that a protein source be included in all three meals, as well as a protein-containing snack.

In addition, vegetarians need to obtain all 23 essential amino acids, since vegetarian proteins don't usually have all of these in any one source. To obtain all 23 amino acids, eating a variety of protein types at several meals will usually do the trick. It is not necessary for each meal to contain all 23, since the body can store them over several meals. If you're vegan, see p.121.

### AS A MATTER OF FACT

**A new noninvasive test** to detect chromosomal disorders could soon be available.

This could require simply a sample of blood from the pregnant woman, unlike current tests that require a needle to be inserted into the uterus.

YOU ARE 10 WEEKS EXACTLY

# 210 days to go...

## YOUR BABY TODAY

The bones of the front of the skull are starting to grow over the baby's forehead and harden from cartilage to bone. The forehead is still very prominent and the top of the head still very flexible to accommodate the baby's rapidly developing brain.

The placenta is rapidly developing and once it's fully formed, will supply all your baby's needs.

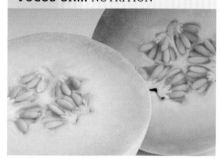

### FOCUS ON... NUTRITION

## Refreshing melons

**Staying hydrated is essential throughout pregnancy.** A good tip is to eat fruit that is high in water. Water contained in fruit is easily absorbed into the body, because fruit contains natural sugars that draw water into the bloodstream. Melons—watermelon, cantaloupe, and honeydew—are naturally high in water. In addition, their mellow and less acidic nature make them well tolerated in pregnancy.

In addition to staying hydrated, by eating melons you will get some extra folate, as well as other vitamins and nutrients. Try combining melons with cottage cheese or yogurt, sprinkled with granola, for a light meal, or blend them into a nutritious smoothie.

**A milestone in your baby's development**—the placenta takes over from the yolk sac to provide your baby with nutrients. Just like your baby, the placenta has needed to grow and develop a circulation to support the ever-increasing demands that are being placed on it.

One week into the pregnancy, the placenta formed a distinct inner and outer layer of cells that gradually

### ASK A... DOCTOR

**What is meant by Rhesus negative?** Red blood carries a positive or negative Rhesus factor (Rh-factor). Problems arise if a Rh-negative woman carries a Rh-positive baby who has inherited the Rh-positive status from the father. If the mother's blood comes into contact with the baby's during delivery, she may produce antibodies against it.

This may cause problems in subsequent pregnancies when a mother's antibodies attack the cells of another Rh-positive baby, which can lead to severe anemia and heart failure in the baby after the birth. You will be given Rh immune-globulin to combat this.

penetrated the lining of the uterus, with fingerlike fronds. You may have noticed a very slight bleed at this implantation stage (see pp.67). More and more fronds spread out into the lining of the uterus, which itself undergoes a transformation process that enables each frond or villus to be bathed by small pools of maternal blood, enabling oxygen and nutrient transfer to take place.

Up until now, this blood flow has been limited by plugs of tissue, but at this stage of pregnancy these plugs begin to disappear. This means the placenta is sufficiently developed to withstand the pressure of maternal blood on each delicate villous. Villi will continue to branch out until around 30 weeks of pregnancy.

### ACTUAL SIZE OF YOUR BABY

**After 10 weeks** your baby's crown to rump length is 1.2 in (3 cm).

9 weeks

10 weeks

Your 10th week

127

# Your 11th week

**YOU'LL NOW BE SETTING UP THE HEALTH CARE THAT WILL SUPPORT YOU OVER THE COMING MONTHS**

Your baby is now unmistakeably human and is undergoing many sophisticated changes, such as development of the sense organs. To mark his new status, he's now called a fetus. If pregnancy hasn't seemed quite real to you so far, it soon will. It's time to get down to such practicalities as your first prenatal checkup. Procedures such as ultrasound scans and blood tests are about to become part of your normal pregnancy routine.

**The eyelids** are sealed shut and will remain this way until the 26th week.

**Within the amniotic sac**, the baby is becoming very active, kicking and squirming. You cannot feel any movements yet.

**The placenta** will get larger as pregnancy progresses. In addition to allowing food and wastes to circulate, the placenta helps prevent harmful microorganisms and substances from reaching the baby.

**The diaphragm** is complete, and your baby can make breathing movements.

**Your growing uterus** may begin to cause discomfort as ligaments and muscles stretch to make room.

**The fetus** measures 2 in (5 cm) from crown to rump.

**The ear** has started to move into its final position.

**The neck** has lengthened, allowing the baby to nod and shake his head from side to side.

FETUS AT 11 WEEKS

**The ovaries or testes** are beginning to develop.

# 209 days to go...

## YOUR BABY TODAY

In this side view of a fetus, the right ear and eye are just visible and the right hand and leg can be seen in characteristically bent positions. The reddish, tubelike structure, to the right of the image, is the umbilical cord.

Your prenatal care begins with your first appointment, where you will get to talk with your ob/gyn about your pregnancy care.

**You should have your first prenatal appointment around now.** The exact timing of it will vary depending on when your doctor sees pregnant patients for the first time. This is the first time you will see your ob/gyn during pregnancy. Unless your doctor has a solo practice (see p.91), your prenatal team is likely to consist of several doctors who will take care of you throughout your pregnancy.

The purpose of this appointment is for a doctor to obtain your medical history, provide information, and plan your care for pregnancy and the birth. It's also an opportunity for you to ask any questions you may have and discuss the schedule for appointments, blood tests, scans, and prenatal classes. You will be given booklets, information leaflets, and important contact telephone numbers.

### AS A MATTER OF FACT

**Midwife comes from the anglo-saxon word "mit wif,"** meaning "with woman."

A midwife's role is to respect the ability of a woman to give birth independently, and to only intervene when it is essential to do so.

The doctor will ask you about your medical history; your family's medical history; your partner and your partner's family's medical history; about any previous pregnancies you have had; and how this pregnancy has been so far.

Your answers will help the doctor identify factors that may affect your pregnancy, for example if there is a family history of preeclampsia (see p.474). The doctor will also do some health tests, such as urine tests, at this and other prenatal appointments.

**At your prenatal appointments** you will have routine checks, including taking your blood pressure. It's the doctor's job to take care of your health throughout pregnancy.

### ASK A... DOCTOR

**How should I decide which tests I want?** Your doctor will give you lots of information regarding tests and it is up to you to decide whether you want them. There are two different types: screening tests (see pp.142–3) and diagnostic tests (see pp.152–3). The goal of screening tests is to figure out the risk of there being a problem—based on the result, you may be advised to have a follow-up diagnostic test.

Most women opt to have the screening tests, but it's worth considering how far you would continue with the process. For example, if you had a high-risk result from the screening test, would you opt to have a diagnostic test? If you did, and the results of that were positive, would you want to continue with the pregnancy?

Such considerations are difficult but important. For example, if you know that, no matter what, you and your partner would want to continue with the pregnancy then you may decide not to have a test, or decide to have the test so that you can prepare yourself for a baby with potential problems.

Your 11th week

# 208 days to go...

### YOUR BABY TODAY

The baby's head is just under half the length of his body. His limbs are still relatively short but the hands and feet can look quite big. Early basic trunk and limb movements are taking place but it's too early to feel them at this stage.

## Will it be a boy or a girl? Significant changes are taking place that enable your baby's sexual organs to develop.

**Hormones are influencing your unborn baby's development** and the ovaries or testes now begin to form. The testes will gradually descend but there structural development won't be complete until your child hits puberty. The ovary will produce eggs (see p.226) but these will remain in the early stages of development.

A minute genital tube forms the external genitalia but each sex appears the same at this stage. This is not entirely surprising since the phallus is only 0.09 in (2.5 mm) long.

Your baby's bladder and rectum have now separated. The kidneys will take some time to fully develop: two buds grow up from the bladder to the tissue that will become the kidneys, one on each side. These so-called uteric buds form the ureters—the tubes that transport urine from the kidney to the bladder. The ureteric bud must successfully fuse with the kidney tissue in the pelvis. As the ureteric buds expands upward, the early kidneys developing in the pelvis will move upward to lie in the abdomen.

### ASK A... DOCTOR

**I have hay fever. Can I take antihistamines?** The potential effects of taking antihistamines in pregnancy aren't known, so it's best to err on the side of caution and not take them. However, if your symptoms are very severe, see your doctor since there is one antihistamine available by prescription that can be taken during pregnancy.

### FOCUS ON... TWINS

## A shared support system

**Nonidentical twins are always in separate amniotic sacs** with a placenta each. If your babies are identical (from one fertilized egg) they may share the same placenta and/or amniotic sac, with a single membrane called the chorion surrounding them. These are known as monochorionic twins and will require greater monitoring. The arrangement of the placenta and amniotic sacs can be analyzed on an ultrasound scan.

When twins share a placenta, a blood vessel directly connects them.

This can cause one twin to receive too much blood, which can cause heart problems; the other twin will get too little blood and not grow at the correct rate. This is called twin-to-twin transfusion and happens in about 10–15 percent of monochorionic pregnancies. The imbalance can sometimes be corrected by draining amniotic fluid from around the twin with the greater blood supply, or by using laser treatment to seal off some blood vessels in the placenta. An early delivery may be necessary.

Shared placenta

One baby is bigger than the other

Amniotic sac

# 207 days to go...

## YOUR BABY TODAY

This color 2D ultrasound scan shows a baby lying on its back with its head to the right. This is the ideal position when measuring the crown (head) to rump (bottom) length to accurately date the pregnancy: it simply measures in a straight line.

You may begin to notice some discomfort around your pelvic as your body begins to accommodate your growing uterus.

### ASK A... NUTRITIONIST

**I'm allergic to dairy products. What can I eat to make sure my baby gets the nutrients these provide?** Dairy products are an excellent source of protein, calcium (which is required for the development of your baby's teeth and bones), some B vitamins, and a little iron. And milk contains vitamins A and D. Eat foods that provide the same nutrients:

■ **For calcium:** leafy green vegetables, particularly broccoli and kale; fish (see p.96) with soft, edible bones, such as salmon (canned is fine), whitebait, and sardines; calcium-fortified soy milk.

■ **For vitamin A:** brightly colored vegetables, meats, eggs, and liver. Although most nutritionists do not recommend liver during pregnancy, if you aren't getting much vitamin A in your diet, a little will not harm.

■ **For vitamin D:** eggs. Vitamin D is also found in most fish (see p.96).

■ **For vitamin E:** eggs, canned salmon, fortified orange juice and cereals, and fatty fish. As long as you're getting plenty of other sources of these key nutrients, your baby's health will not be adversely affected.

**Having a few minor aches and pains during pregnancy** is nothing to be concerned about. They occur because the ligaments and muscles of your pelvis are stretching to fit your ever-growing uterus. This can cause some discomfort but should be manageable.

### FOCUS ON... SAFETY

## Bon voyage

**Whether you're going on vacation or on a business trip,** it's important to be prepared:

■ **Check you're healthy enough to travel**—speak to your doctor.

■ **Find out whether you need any vaccinations** and discuss these with your doctor (see p.105). It's advisable to avoid traveling to areas where there is a high risk of disease while you're pregnant if at all possible.

■ **Get travel insurance** and make sure it covers you during pregnancy.

■ **Carry your prenatal records** with you at all times and stay within reach of medical help.

■ **Don't stay seated** for long periods in transit and stay hydrated. Wear support socks to reduce the risk of DVT (see p.186).

If the pain you're experiencing does become crampy, like period pain, and there is any bleeding, or if the pain becomes very severe and constant, then you should go to the doctor or the hospital to be checked. You will be examined to rule out a miscarriage (see p.94) or ectopic pregnancy (see p.93).

■ **Wear adequate sun protection** if you're going to a hot climate.

■ **Be careful** about what you eat and drink bottled water.

Your 11th week

131

# 206 days to go...

**YOUR BABY TODAY**

The umbilical cord gradually becomes more coiled as the pregnancy progresses—as seen here on the left of the image. This coiling is thought to occur because of the many movements the embryo makes.

Your baby's limbs are more developed now, enabling him to move, and his hands and fingers can be clearly seen on a scan.

**Your baby takes on a more human form** as his neck lengthens and his head is seen as separate from his body. The head is still about half the total length of your baby. The length of your baby can be measured on an ultrasound by measuring the distance between your baby's head (crown) and his bottom (rump). This is noted as the CRL (crown-rump length) measurement. The head is also measured: this is the biparietal diameter (BPD), which is the distance between the two parietal bones on each side of the baby's head.

Now that the neck is more developed and all the limb joints have formed, your baby can begin to make several movements. The completed diaphragm allows for breathing movements. In the gut, your baby's duodenum now opens up along its length, the small bowel starts to rotate and prepares to re-enter the abdominal cavity.

Within your baby's mouth, the hard palate has formed; the relatively large tongue makes it easier for your baby to move amniotic fluid through the nostrils rather than through his mouth with each breath.

**This endoscopic image,** obtained by passing a fine light-emitting tube into the uterus, shows the hands obscuring the fetus's face.

**TIME TO THINK ABOUT**

## Nuchal fold screening

At around 11 weeks of pregnancy, you may be offered a nuchal translucency screening. This test assesses the risk of Down syndrome by measuring the width of the fold of skin behind your baby's neck to see if any excess fluid has collected there.

■ **The nuchal fold scan** is considered to be 80 percent accurate. If your doctor offers you a blood test (PAPP-A—see p.142) with the scan, it becomes 85–90 percent accurate. When the nasal bone is measured, the accuracy rises to 95 percent.
■ **If the results** show a high risk, another test (see pp.152–3) is offered.

**FOCUS ON... TWINS**

## Double the trouble

**Since your body is growing two or more babies,** there will be physical effects. But there is a positive side: Since your growing size and hormones are the cause, these symptoms are often worse if the babies are doing well.
■ **In the first three months,** your heart has to work harder to pump more fluid around your body, which can lead to a greater feeling of fatigue.
■ **Morning sickness** can be more severe because you have higher amounts of pregnancy hormones.

Mention severe symptoms if you're suffering, but remember these symptoms are not serious. You may be seen earlier if you suspect you're having twins, and will go on to have more prenatal appointments and ultrasound scans. You may be asked to limit activities like travel and exercise as your pregnancy progresses.

# 202 days to go...

**YOUR BABY TODAY**

Although on a scan it might look as though the baby is resting on her back, the fluid in the amniotic sac means that she is floating in a near weightless environment and can easily move into any position within the uterus.

In this final week of your first trimester, you'll probably have your first ultrasound scan and see your baby for the first time.

**You and your partner have reached an exciting milestone.**
You'll have your first ultrasound around now and see your baby; this may help you feel closer to her. For many men, seeing the baby on the scan may be the first time the pregnancy becomes a reality.

At this scan, your baby's length will be measured (see p.139) and this will be used to figure out her age. Up until about 12 weeks of pregnancy, all babies grow at around the same rate so irrespective of whether you and your partner are tall or short, at this time your baby will be the same size as others at this stage of development.

Figuring out your due date (see p.74) using the first day of your period, isn't always accurate, especially if your menstrual cycle is long or irregular. The dating scan can give a more accurate expected date of delivery, but it by no means tells you for certain—very few babies arrive on their actual due date.

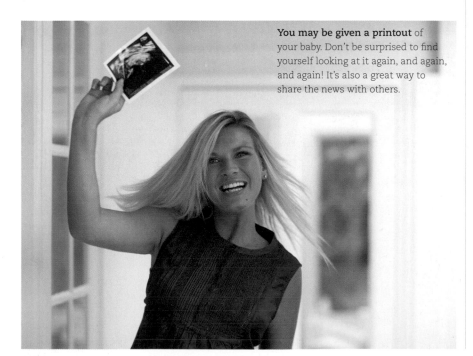

**You may be given a printout** of your baby. Don't be surprised to find yourself looking at it again, and again, and again! It's also a great way to share the news with others.

## It's really happening!

**As a dad-to-be, going to your first scan** will be a time of great excitement, but you may be anxious too. It's normal for you and your partner to wonder if your baby is okay and be desperate to hear that all is well.

The first scan may seem quite technical since it is used to detect your baby's heartbeat and take some measurements, but it's also very emotional. In reality, the first scan gives you the first look at this new life. It lets you see your baby moving around, with legs kicking and arms flailing, even though your partner can't feel these movements yet.

Perhaps, as a man, the biggest shock of the scan is the fact that it confronts you for the first time with the physical evidence that your baby really exists. Your partner is likely to be more used to the idea of pregnancy, because she's carrying the baby, but the scan will make the pregnancy much more real to you, and you may be surprised at how emotional you feel.

Your 12th week

137

# First ultrasound scan

Your first scan at 8–14 weeks can pinpoint the length of your pregnancy to within a five to seven day window. Such accurate dating helps to estimate your due date and determine the right time to perform tests later in pregnancy.

## Your first scan

This ultrasound helps to accurately establish your baby's gestational age. This is particularly useful if you are not sure when your last menstrual period was, if you have irregular periods, or you became pregnant immediately after you stopped using contraception such as the pill. At this stage of pregnancy, your baby can be measured from crown to rump (from the top of the baby's head to its bottom). In addition to establishing your due date and the timing of other screening and diagnostic tests, accurate dating of your pregnancy is important since it helps avoid misdiagnosis of problems such as poor fetal growth (see p.284). Your due date will usually be changed at this scan if there is more than a five to seven day difference between your menstrual dates and the dates based on the crown–rump length.

A scan may be given before 10 weeks if you have bleeding or pain to rule out the possibility of a miscarriage or ectopic pregnancy (see p.93).

**How the scan is done** During an ultrasound scan, high-frequency sound waves are emitted through the abdomen via a handheld device called a transducer. As the sound waves hit solid tissue, they translate into an image that is viewed on a computer screen and interpreted by the sonographer.

At this scan, you will need to drink plenty of water to raise the uterus and provide a clearer image. The sonographer will put some cold gel on your abdomen to maximize contact with the skin and will then move the transducer gently over the area.

**By 12 weeks** the fetus has taken on a human appearance. The forehead, eye sockets, and small button nose are all visible in profile.

**Measuring the diameter** of your baby's head (the biparietal diameter) helps assess your baby's growth and date your pregnancy.

### WHAT THE SCAN SHOWS

## What can be seen on a first scan?

In addition to confirming your dates, your first scan may reveal some other useful information.

■ **This scan usually confirms whether** you have a single or multiple pregnancy (twins, triplets, or more).

■ **Uterine anomalies** can be seen, such as a double uterus, although this is rare. Uterine fibroids (benign tumors) will also be identified.

■ **The scan may reveal an ovarian cyst** (corpus luteum) on the ovary that produced the egg. These are common and can persist in the first trimester.

■ **Major anomalies** may be seen, but most are diagnosed at the 20-week scan when the organs are seen (see p.214).

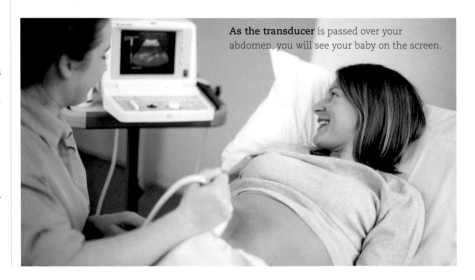

**As the transducer** is passed over your abdomen, you will see your baby on the screen.

# 201 days to go...

## YOUR BABY TODAY

This image shows the yolk sac at the 12 o'clock position with the placenta seen as a thickening to the lining of the uterus on the left. The baby is in the lower part of the uterus and is positioned lying on her back.

## The dating scan is reassuring because it's an opportunity for your baby's progress and development to be thoroughly checked.

**At your ultrasound scan, the pregnancy is dated** according to your baby's length from crown (head) to rump (bottom) because he is—and will remain—quite curled up. This is known as the CRL (crown–rump length).

Since your baby can flex his spine and stretch his neck, this measurement needs to be taken with your baby in a specific position so it can take some time to achieve. The measurement is used to estimate your baby's date of delivery and this may be different than the EDD you calculated (see p.74)

This first ultrasound scan should be able to recognize all four limbs, your baby's hands and feet, the spine, some aspects of brain development, the fluid-filled stomach, and the bladder. From now on your baby's kidneys will be producing small amounts of very dilute urine and the bladder will start to fill.

### AS A MATTER OF FACT

**Dating scans are only an estimate.** The chance of delivering on your due date is only around 5 percent.

So keep the estimated due date in mind but don't expect your baby to abide by it!

### ASK A... DOCTOR

**I've had quite a few pregnancy symptoms and don't feel as though my body is my own. How can I relax and enjoy being pregnant?**
Not all women adapt well to pregnancy and for some dealing with the symptoms and worrying about issues such as weight gain, makes them feel out of control. The best way to cope with these feelings is to embrace the changes and remain in touch with your body by exercising and taking time to focus on what is happening inside you. We spend most of our lives listening to all the things that happen on the outside, but very little time focusing on the inside.

Take a few minutes each day to practice deep breathing and relaxation and consider learning some pregnancy yoga and meditation techniques (see right).

The dramatic changes happening to your body may be mirrored in the wide swings of emotions and feelings you experience throughout your pregnancy. Some days you may feel excited and elated at the prospect of becoming a parent, and on others you may feel overwhelmed and anxious.

Perhaps the nine months' gestation period is nature's way of giving us time to get used to the idea of becoming a parent, and allowing us time to deal with our emotions and prepare for the birth. So try to relax but if you're feeling really anxious, speak to your doctor.

**This simple yoga pose** allows you to fully relax your body and mind. Consider joining a pregnancy yoga class since it's a great way to learn techniques and also an opportunity meet other moms-to-be.

# 200 days to go...

## YOUR BABY TODAY

As the baby floats in the amniotic fluid, her limbs are now more fully developed, allowing her to make many movements. The lips and fingers—which are now completely separated—stimulate sensory feelings.

Does your face resemble the pimply complexion of your teenage years? Don't worry, it's those hormones again and it will pass.

**Your skin is likely to change during pregnancy.** Some women find that they develop pimples or acne, due to the high levels of progesterone. Conversely, you may get dry skin, also due to pregnancy hormones. The dryness may become worse over your abdomen as your belly grows and the skin is stretched.

Freckles and moles may get darker. You may also notice tiny red lines on your chest or legs: these are called spider nevi (see p.134) and are due to the increased blood supply to the skin which makes the vessels dilate and become more visible.

Other women find that the high levels of estrogen mean that their skin is in a better condition than before they were pregnant. The "glow" of pregnancy is due to the increased blood supply that occurs in pregnancy, which gives you a rosy healthy looking complexion.

**Your skin may become dry and flaky,** on your face, as well as elsewhere on your body. Using a good moisturizer should help.

### ASK A... DOCTOR

**Since going to the scan my partner is very overprotective. Is this normal?**
Your partner is now realizing his responsibilities and affection for the baby, and is showing these feelings by taking care of you. If you're finding that his pampering of you is a little too much, you might want to discuss other ways he can feel involved in the pregnancy and prepare for the baby. Try to embrace his involvement and enthusiasm—it's a great way for you to strengthen your relationship and prepare for parenthood together.

### TIME TO THINK ABOUT

## Telling your employer

As soon as your employer knows you're pregnant, you should be protected by the Pregnancy Discrimination Act, which says that pregnant employees must be treated the same as other employees with disabilities or limitations. Most parents-to-be wait until 12 weeks when the risk of miscarriage is lower. Some wait longer.

■ **Each company has its own policy** on maternity leave. Some offer paid or unpaid leave for a set period. Others let employees use sick leave or vacation days. Meet with a human resources representative to learn your options.

■ **You can discuss** when your maternity leave will start. If your baby is born early or your maternity leave starts earlier than planned due to illness, the arrangements can be altered at short notice.

■ **Your employer** should respect your right to confidentiality. If you want the news of your pregnancy to remain under wraps until a certain date, make this known.

# 199 days to go...

## YOUR BABY TODAY

The fetus can be seen inside the uterus on this color ultrasound scan. At this stage of development, the fetus measures approximately 2.4 in (6 cm) crown to rump and weighs around 0.3 oz (10 g).

**At around 12 weeks, the doctor might be able to hear your baby's heartbeat with a handheld monitor.**

**At this stage your baby's heart beats** at approximately 140 beats per minute, so at least twice as fast as your own. The heart and its internal electrical conducting system are structurally complete but its external nerve supply is still quite immature. The nerves to the heart influence its rhythm, gradually slowing the rate as the pregnancy advances.

The heart is tiny and to maintain an adequate output the heart is unable to increase the amount of blood it pumps with each beat (as we can), but instead increases the number of times it beats each minute.

The abdominal cavity is large enough to hold the intestines. Whereas before they were bulging outside of your baby's body, they now fit into her abdominal cavity. Having started to rotate while outside the body, the bowel completes its final rotation in the abdominal cavity. Once inside, the bowel position remains fixed, and its diameter increases as the loops of bowel become hollow.

### SMOKING: THE FACTS

**If you've only cut down, rather than quitting, read on.** Many smokers inhale more deeply when smoking less and their intake of damaging toxins increases. Here's how smoking affects your baby:

■ **The carbon monoxide,** nicotine, and other substances that you inhale pass from your lungs, into your bloodstream, and cross the placenta.
■ **Nicotine** makes your baby's heart beat faster as she struggles for oxygen, which can affect her growth rate.
■ **Smoking increases the risk** of miscarriage, premature birth, and low birth weight, and exposure to tobacco chemicals makes your baby more likely to suffer from conditions such as asthma and chest infections after the birth, which may be bad enough to warrant a hospital stay.
■ **There is also a higher risk** of crib death if you or your partner smokes. Your partner should stop too.
■ **If you live with a smoker,** you will be inhaling thousands of toxic carcinogenic chemicals that are released into the air around you from the burning end of the cigarette and the exhaled smoke.
■ **Several studies** have confirmed that passive smoking can damage the baby's health and increase the risk of miscarriage and premature birth.

### FOCUS ON... TWINS

## Feeding two?

**If you're carrying twins,** you're likely to have put on some weight by now, perhaps around 11 lb (5 kg). Early weight gain is usually a good thing, especially in your case, since this is a vital time for the formation and development for your babies organs. As a rough guide, a good recommended weight gain is:

■ **For twins,** total weight gain of 35–45 lb (16–20 kg), preferably 24 lb (11 kg) by week 24, then a gradual increase until the birth.
■ **For triplets,** a total weight gain of 50–60 lb (23–27 kg), preferably 35 lb (16 kg) by week 24, then a gradual increase until the birth.
■ **For quads,** total weight gain of 65–80 lb (31–36 kg), ideally 50 pounds of it by week 24.

# Screening tests

Optional routine screening tests in the first trimester assess the risk of your baby having a chromosomal disorder such as Down syndrome. If your risk is high, you will be offered a diagnostic test (see pp.152–3) for a definite result.

**Your doctor will discuss** in advance the available screening tests so you are fully informed before agreeing to a test.

## What is screened for

In addition to Down syndrome, screening tests also assess the risk of another chromosomal abnormality called trisomy 18. Babies with this condition have more severe mental and physical abnormalities than babies with Down syndrome and seldom survive beyond a year. The condition is rare, with each year around 1 in 6000 babies born with trisomy 18, compared to 1 in 800 babies born with Down. Screening can also detect neural tube defects like spina bifida and anencephaly, which occur in about 1 in 1000 pregnancies.

## The "combined" test

The recommended screening test, and the one most commonly offered, for Down is the "nuchal translucency screening," performed between 11 and 14 weeks. This test has a high accuracy rate and the results are produced quickly.

The test uses a combination of a maternal blood test and an ultrasound of your baby. The ultrasound measures the thickness of the skin at the back of your baby's neck, called the nuchal fold (see box, opposite). The blood test looks at the levels of two chemicals: pregnancy associated plasma protein A (PAPP-A) and one of the pregnancy hormones, human chorionic gonadotrophin (hCG). The results of the blood test is combined with your age, and the measurement of the nuchal fold. A mathematical formula is then used to calculate your baby's risk of Down syndrome.

If you have your blood test before your ultrasound, you will usually receive your results immediately following your ultrasound. If you have your blood drawn at the time of the ultrasound you will receive your results a few days later. Your risk based on the combined test may be higher than your risk based on your age alone, lower, or stay the same.

## The integrated test

This test is done in two stages using results from a range of screening tests done in the first and second trimesters. Your age will also be taken into account when calculating your risk. In the first trimester, a blood test at 12 weeks measures the PAPP-A and hCG. You will also have a nuchal translucency screening. At between 15 and 22 weeks, another blood test measures the levels of hCG, AFP, inhibin A, and estriol. The integrated test is the most sensitive screening test, but it has the disadvantage that the results are not available until later in pregnancy. It is not available everywhere.

---

**UNDERSTANDING TESTS**

## Accuracy of screening tests

**As more screening tests have become available,** the detection rate for Down syndrome, which used to be assessed on maternal age alone, has significantly increased. The aim of screening tests is to provide a high detection rate for Down syndrome and a low "false positive" rate. A false positive means the screening test indicated a high risk of Down syndrome, but subsequent diagnostic tests gave the all clear, which means the mother would exposed to unnecessary testing.

| Tests | Timing (weeks) | Detection rate | False positive rate |
|---|---|---|---|
| Combined test | 11–14 | 85% | 5% |
| Integrated test | 11–13/15–22 | 85% | 1% |
| Quadruple test | 15–20 | 76% | 5% |
| Triple test | 15–20 | 69% | 5% |

## Triple and quadruple tests

These screening tests are done in the second trimester, usually between 15 and 20 weeks gestation, and assess your baby's risk of Down syndrome from blood tests alone. The triple test measures levels of the hormones hCG, AFP and estriol. The quadruple test measures levels of inhibin-A in addition to these three hormones. If your doctor or hospital doesn't offer a nuchal translucency screening, then a triple or quadruple test will be offered instead.

## A positive screen

It's important to remember that a positive result does not mean your baby has Down syndrome. For example, if you have a 1 in 100 risk of Down syndrome, your test will be positive. However, the chance that your baby has Down syndrome is low since your baby will be normal 99 times out of 100. Talking to your doctor or a genetic counselor can help you understand your actual risk and decide if you want to have a diagnostic test such as amniocentesis (see p.153) for a definite result. Since diagnostic tests carry a risk of miscarriage, you need to weigh the risks before deciding to go ahead.

Some research suggests that women are more likely to enjoy their pregnancy and birth and come to terms with the diagnosis if they know in advance that their baby has Down syndrome. So don't assume therefore that you should only have a diagnostic test to decide whether or not to continue your pregnancy.

If you have a positive screening test for another more severe chromosomal disorder, such as trisomy 18, your doctor will talk to you about the outlook for babies with these conditions—the majority of whom die early in life, sometimes within the first week—to help you decide what to do. In some cases these disorders are associated with abnormalities detected during the dating scan (see p.138), and the presence of these abnormalities

HOW THE TEST IS DONE

## Nuchal translucency screening

**An ultrasound scan, known as the nuchal translucency screening, is done between 11 and 14 weeks** of pregnancy and is used to help assess your baby's risk of Down syndrome. During this test, the sonographer measures the depth of fluid under the skin at the back of the baby's neck, known as the nuchal fold. If this measurement is high, it indicates that excess fluid is present, which means that the baby has a higher risk of Down syndrome. The measurement is then combined with the results of blood tests and the average risk based on your age to give your baby's individual risk for Down syndrome. If your risk is higher than 1 in 250, you will be counseled and offered a diagnostic test, such as amniocentesis or chorionic villus sampling, to give a definitive result (see p.152).

The small depth of fluid seen in the neck's nuchal fold in this scan means that the fetus has a low risk of developing Down syndrome.

The thicker nuchal fold seen here indicates an increased risk of Down syndrome in this fetus and a diagnostic test will be recommended.

combined with a positive test may confirm the diagnosis. Nevertheless, many women opt to have a diagnostic test before deciding whether or not to terminate their pregnancy.

**Further screening** Another option is to have a specialized ultrasound scan to look for Down syndrome markers between 17 and 22 weeks. If the ultrasound doesn't show any signs of Down syndrome, the risk of your baby being affected is reduced. However, a second trimester ultrasound is not such an accurate test for Down syndrome as other screening tests and so you should only consider this path if you are strongly against having a diagnostic test such as amniocentesis and feel that you don't need a definite diagnosis.

CHECK LIST

## Should I have a diagnostic test?

Deciding on whether or not to go ahead with genetic or diagnostic testing (see pp.152–3) is a personal choice. Factors that may affect your decision–making process include:

■ **Your anxiety level** without knowing for sure, and how this will affect your enjoyment of pregnancy.

■ **Your fears about** pregnancy loss.

■ **What you would do if** you found out your baby had Down syndrome or another condition such as Trisomy 18.

# 198 days to go...

## YOUR BABY TODAY

At this stage the eye—not yet in its final position—still dominates the appearance of the face. The eye is not yet responsive to light and remains well protected behind the covering eyelid.

Having your first scan this week and knowing your risk of miscarriage is reduced now, should mean you can start to relax.

**This can be a very positive time for you,** especially if you've been anxious from day one of your pregnancy. The risk of miscarriage falls as your pregnancy progresses and by the end of this 12th week, it's no more than 1 percent.

As you enter the second trimester, you should begin to feel better (see opposite), and this, combined with the knowledge that you have passed the most risky time, may help you relax. If you've been keeping your pregnancy a secret, you can also enjoy telling others.

---

**FOCUS ON... SAFETY**

## Safe scans

**Ultrasound has been used for years** and is thought to be safe. Children who've been exposed to prenatal ultrasound do not have differences in speech, hearing, vision, or school performance, or an increased risk of cancer. However, ultrasound should only be done when necessary.

---

**AS A MATTER OF FACT**

**Medical ultrasound** has been used since the early 1960s.

However, the first discovery of high-frequency echo-sounding techniques, on which ultrasound is based, was as long ago as 1880 in Paris. In the early 20th century, ultrasound was used as a therapy tool and it was not until the 1940s that research began into its use as a diagnostic tool.

---

**ASK A... NUTRITIONIST**

**I have a really sweet tooth. Is it okay to indulge this while I'm pregnancy?** While occasional treats of cookies or chocolate are fine, processed foods usually contain hidden fats and sugars and provide few nutrients, so it's best to try to find healthier sweet alternatives to snack on, such as fresh fruit.

Always read food labels and look for alternative foods containing less fat and less added sugars. Just as you would consider carefully how you feed your child, you should take care of yourself in the same way while you're pregnant.

One of the best ways to curb your sweet tooth is to eat regular meals. This helps to steady your blood-sugar level and reduce sweet cravings. Try not to go longer than three hours without eating and, if you're hungry, have a healthy snack between meals, such as a chicken sandwich, a low-fat yogurt, or fruit, which can be fresh, canned, or dried, such as raisins or apricots.

Try to drink about two quarts of water a day, since perceived hunger is often really dehydration. Drinking a glass or two of water may stop you from reaching for the cookie jar.

**It's possible to satisfy sweet cravings** with refreshing fruit. You may find that you feel better after eating a fruit salad than if you eat a bar of chocolate.

# 197 days to go...

**YOUR BABY TODAY**

The bones of the front of the skull have continued to expand and cover the head, protecting the delicate brain structures beneath. The soft spot in between the skull bones (center) remains through pregnancy and into babyhood.

If you're finding you're out of breath when you get to the top of the stairs, accept this as a normal side effect of pregnancy.

**By the end of the first trimester** it's normal to begin feeling a little breathless. This is because your heart and lungs are having to work much harder to supply your body with oxygen due to all the changes that are taking place to allow the baby to grow.

The amount of oxygen you need in pregnancy is about 20 percent more than normal; some of this goes to the placenta (see p.127) and baby and the rest to your other organs. To get this increased amount of oxygen you breathe faster and deeper, almost hyperventilating so you feel short of breath, especially when you exercise.

As your pregnancy continues, you may find that this shortness of breath or feeling that you are not breathing very deeply continues, or worsens. As the baby grows, your uterus will expand upward and your other abdominal organs will rearrange themselves to create more room. Your organs and uterus push up against your diaphragm so it becomes more difficult to take a deep breath, so in order to get all the oxygen you need, you then have to breathe much faster. The hormone progesterone may also affect the rate at which you breathe.

If you have any concerns about breathlessness, don't hesitate to speak to your doctor.

---

**FOCUS ON... HEALTH**

## Feeling better?

**By the end of this trimester,** many of the early pregnancy symptoms are likely to have passed.

■ **Nausea** may have begun to lessen and it can be a complete relief to wake up in the morning without feeling sick. Your loss of appetite will return, and you can stop worrying about whether your baby is being properly nourished, which is often a common concern for women who suffer from morning sickness.

■ **You won't need to urinate** quite so often, which will be good news if you've spent an inordinate amount of time in the bathroom. This is because your uterus is now moving up the abdominal cavity and therefore is placing less pressure on your bladder.

■ **The fatigue** that you may have felt in these early months is likely to have lifted by now, and you may be sleeping more deeply now that you're relaxing into your pregnancy.

If your sickness hasn't passed yet, don't worry—for some women, it does last longer (see p.159).

---

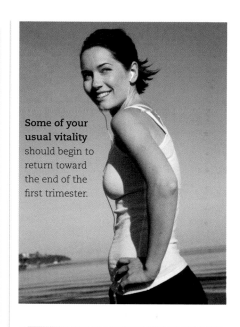

**Some of your usual vitality** should begin to return toward the end of the first trimester.

---

**ASK A... DOCTOR**

**I've gone from an A cup to D cup. Will this increase in size last forever?** The majority of women who have had babies do report a permanent increase in breast size but it's unlikely to be to this extent! The effects of estrogen cause fat to be deposited in the breasts and when your milk comes in after the birth your breasts will get bigger, but reduce again once you have stopped breast-feeding.

# 196 days to go...

**YOUR BABY TODAY**

Here the legs are crossed and the arms outstretched. The umbilical cord is short and thick at this stage, but will lengthen as the baby grows, and become much thinner with many coils.

You've reached the end of the first trimester and in this time your baby has developed from a ball of cells to an active fetus.

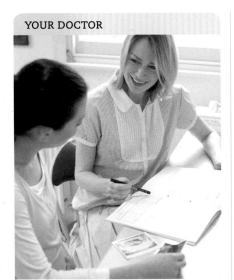

**YOUR DOCTOR**

**Most women develop a good relationship with their doctor,** who can be a fountain of fantastic information, and a wonderful source of comfort and reassurance.

It's important that you are as honest as you can be with your doctor. Like many women, you may be reluctant to reveal concerns, or to admit to unhealthy habits for fear of being embarrassed or scolded. It's very likely that your doctor will have heard it all before, and will be able to help and advise—with a few tried-and-tested tricks up her sleeve.

**Your amazing baby can do so many things already,** including being able to open his mouth and yawn, hiccup, and swallow. Swallowing develops earlier than sucking. Your baby will be swallowing the amniotic fluid regularly but the more complex sucking movements cannot be identified until 18–20 weeks. Swallowing will encourage gut development. The amniotic fluid enters into the stomach not the lungs, which are protected now by the vocal cords and the higher pressure of the lung's own fluid. The amniotic fluid will later be excreted as urine when the fetal kidneys start to function.

After the stomach, the amniotic fluid will enter the small bowel. The intestinal walls are developing muscular layers but these do not yet contract in a coordinated way to move the fluid along the digestive tract. It will be 20 weeks before the structural organization of the gut is finally complete. Many digestive enzymes are starting to be released into the gut but these currently act as a stimulus to development rather than for the absorption of nutrients.

Your baby is reliant on a steady stream of glucose, which is stored as glycogen in the liver. This continues throughout pregnancy and at birth your baby will, for her size, have significantly larger glycogen reserves than adults do.

The correct level of glucose is controlled by insulin secreted by the pancreas. The placenta, however, has little control over the amount it takes from your bloodstream and passes on. For this reason if your glucose level is very high, for example in poorly controlled diabetes, the baby will be presented with high levels of glucose. He will maintain a normal glucose level but the insulin released leads to increased fat deposition and weight gain.

**ACTUAL SIZE OF YOUR BABY**

**At 12 weeks** your baby's crown to rump length is 2.4 in (6.1 cm).

9 weeks

12 weeks

**All your baby's organs**, limbs, and facial features are in place, but her head is still disproportionately large. She can open and close her mouth, and her eyes are developing behind closed lids.

# Welcome to your second trimester

**Spreading the word** Safely past the first trimester, you will probably want to tell people your good news.

**Visibly pregnant** As your belly expands and your waistline disappears, you'll start to look as well as feel pregnant.

**At 16 weeks** your baby has taken on a definite human form. The body and limbs have grown substantially and a translucent layer of skin reveals underlying blood vessels.

**By 17 weeks** the arms and hands are well developed; the fingers now move freely and start to grasp.

**At three months** your pregnancy becomes noticeable. By five months, there's no mistaking it.

**Second trimester** As your pregnancy starts to show, you may feel renewed energy as the fatigue and nausea of early pregnancy fade.
**Looking good** By the end of this trimester, you'll look clearly pregnant as your baby steadily grows.

**Feeling energized** Regular exercise throughout pregnancy will positively benefit you and your baby in the months ahead and help prepare your body for labor.

**Time for a vacation** The second trimester is the ideal time to get away from it all as your hormones settle down, energy levels lift, and labor is still a safe distance away.

**Facts and figures** Even in the uterus, rhythmic movements such as walking send your baby to sleep.

# Now your pregnancy starts to feel "real" as your body changes rapidly and you feel your baby move.

| 19 | 20 | 21 | 22 | 23 | 24 | 25 |
|---|---|---|---|---|---|---|

**The 20-week ultrasound** Your baby's major organs are now clearly visible and will be studied in detail to ensure they're developing normally.

**By 23 weeks** your baby's facial features are distinct, with eyebrows and eyelashes visible. On the hands, fingernails start to grow.

**Facts and figures** At 21 weeks, your baby measures about 10 in (25 cm) from crown to heel.

**Loud and clear** By 24 weeks, your baby is able to hear sounds from the outside world and becomes familiar with your voice.

**Exercise classes** Prenatal exercise classes are tailored to meet your requirements in pregnancy and are also a great way to get acquainted with other moms-to-be.

**First flutters** As your baby's movements increase and strengthen, your partner can begin to share in your pregnancy experience.

**Nutritious bites** A varied diet with plenty of vegetables benefits your own and your baby's health.

**Your active baby** Surrounded and cushioned by amniotic fluid, your baby is free to move around in the uterus without risk of being bumped or hurt.

# Your 13th week

For most women, any discomforts of early pregnancy start to disappear this trimester. The high levels of pregnancy hormones, which are thought to contribute to sickness, are subsiding, and fatigue should begin to diminish. Meanwhile, your baby floats peacefully in the amniotic sac. As he goes on growing, so the sac will expand to give him plenty of room to kick and stretch. His brain is developing at a rapid rate.

**Arms and legs** are lengthening rapidly and muscle control is developing.

**The eyes** have moved more toward the front of the face but they are still tightly closed.

**At 13 weeks** the average crown to rump length is 1.6 in (4.1 cm) and the average weight is 0.25 oz (7 g).

**The ankle joints** have matured and the toes have separated.

**In the amniotic sac,** there is room to move freely and your baby is very active. Amniotic fluid cushions the kicks and wiggles, so you won't feel anything.

**The baby's body** has no underlying fat, and the bones look prominent beneath the delicate skin.

Your second trimester

150

# 195 days to go...

## YOUR BABY TODAY

This 3D ultrasound scan clearly demonstrates that the baby's arms and legs are now fully formed and much more in proportion with the trunk. All of the baby's joints are now formed, enabling a full range of movement.

This is a good time to start telling the important people in your life your exciting news—before they guess for themselves.

**Now that you're in your second trimester** and have had your dating scan (see p.138), you may want to start telling a wider circle of people that you're pregnant. You can feel confident doing this, knowing that the risk of miscarriage is reduced to no more than 1 percent after the 12th week. Besides this, your belly will begin to show in a few weeks, if it hasn't already, so hiding the pregnancy will become difficult.

If you and your partner have been keeping the pregnancy a secret for the past three months, announcing it will be a huge release and it can be a positive experience to share the news with others. However, be prepared for an onslaught of advice and people's tales of their pregnancy and birth experiences!

Sometimes letting others know that you're pregnant can be difficult. Be sensitive to other people's feelings: friends who also want to be parents, but are having difficulty conceiving, may find it difficult to share your happiness right away. It's preferable to tell these people face to face rather than them hearing it through the grapevine. Even if they don't react positively, and don't want to talk about your pregnancy all the time, give them time to come to terms with it at their own pace. Remember they can be sad for themselves while being happy for you.

### TIME TO THINK ABOUT

## Second trimester tests

If you haven't had a nuchal translucency scan (see p.143), blood tests will be offered this trimester to screen for Down (see pp.142–3).

■ **The triple test** is done at 16–18 weeks. It measures levels of the hormones hCG, AFP, and estriol.
■ **The quadruple test** is done at 15–22 weeks. It measures levels of inhibin A in addition to the hormones measured in the triple test.

### FOCUS ON... YOUR BODY

## Become a clothes cheat!

**Although your clothes may be feeling a little tight by this stage,** you probably aren't ready to wear voluminous maternity clothing just yet, so it's time to get creative! Simply bridge the gap between your button and button-hole with an rubber band (see right) or by sewing in an elastic panel. Assuming he's bigger than you, try raiding your partner's wardrobe—his T-shirts, shirts, and sweaters can be ruched in with a low-slung belt.

Check what's in your wardrobe already: empire-cut dresses will see you through most of your pregnancy; looser smock tops can be layered over tight-fitting T-shirts; low-slung pants can sit neatly under your belly, topped with an oversized shirt. The one item you might want to purchase is a pair of maternity pants—something stretchy with an adjustable waist.

# Diagnostic tests

If you've had a positive screening test for Down syndrome or another genetic abnormality, you will be offered a diagnostic test, which gives a definitive answer as to whether or not your baby has an abnormality.

### What are diagnostic tests?

Diagnostic tests are tests that involve taking a sample of either the placenta, the amniotic fluid, or fetal blood. The samples are then sent away and examined in a laboratory for chromosomal or genetic abnormalities. The two main diagnostic tests are amniocentesis and chorionic villus sampling, or CVS. Since both of these tests carry a small risk of miscarriage (see right), you will need to carefully consider the advantages and disadvantages of the tests before going ahead with either of them.

### Chorionic villus sampling (CVS)

Chorionic villi are fragments of placental tissue. Because the placenta originates from the fertilized egg, the chromosomes in the cells that make up the placenta are representative of your baby's chromosomes. During CVS, a small amount of tissue from your placenta is removed and tested in a laboratory to reveal if your baby has a chromosomal disorder such as Down syndrome or another trisomy disorder, such as trisomy 18. CVS is done between 10 and 12½ weeks' gestation and the results are usually available within 7 to 10 days. The procedure can also definitely identify your baby's sex, if you want to know. If you don't want to have this information, make your wishes clear before the test. In rare cases, the doctor will be unable to perform CVS due to the placenta's position. In this case, you may be asked to return for an amniocentesis at 15 weeks.

**Amniocentesis** This is the most common diagnostic test, done at around 15 to 19 weeks of pregnancy. The amniotic fluid around your baby mainly consists of your baby's urine and contains cells from your baby's skin and urinary tract. During amniocentesis, a number of cells are collected from the amniotic fluid. They are then sent to a laboratory and grown in a cell culture, until there is a sufficient number of cells to examine your baby's chromosomes and identify whether your baby has a chromosomal abnormality such as Down syndrome. Amniotic fluid can also be tested for high levels of the substance alpha-fetoprotein (AFP), which could mean that your baby has a neural tube defect such as spina bifida or anencephaly. Other DNA testing can also be done during amniocentesis to check for congenital conditions that may run in either parent's family. (see p.431).

---

### HOW THE TEST IS DONE

## Chorionic villus sampling

**There are two ways of doing chorionic villus sampling.** In the transabdominal method, a fine needle is placed through the abdomen to collect placental fragments. In the transcervical procedure, a thin tube (catheter) is inserted into the cervix. The method used depends on the position of the placenta and the doctor's training and expertise. During the procedure, ultrasound guidance is used so that the doctor can see the placenta's position.

CVS can also be done in a multiple pregnancy; in this case both the transabdominal and transcervical methods of collection may be used.

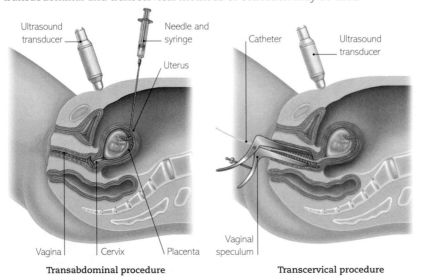

Transabdominal procedure labels: Ultrasound transducer, Needle and syringe, Uterus, Vagina, Cervix, Placenta

Transcervical procedure labels: Catheter, Ultrasound transducer, Vaginal speculum

**Transabdominal procedure**　　　　**Transcervical procedure**

## WHEN TO WORRY

**If, following the procedure, you experience severe abdominal pain,** fever greater than 100.5° F (38° C), vaginal bleeding, or a large gush of clear fluid from your vagina you should call your doctor immediately.

## How you might feel

You may be concerned about the idea of a needle going through your abdomen, or a catheter into your cervix; however, the majority of women find that these procedures are not particularly painful. If you are having a transabdominal procedure, the needle usually doesn't hurt any more than it does when you are having a blood test. Some doctors use a small amount of local anesthetic before the transabdominal procedure to numb the area, although the anesthetic itself can occasionally sting. Although afterward it's common to experience uterine cramps, similar to the cramps you feel during menstruation, rest assured that these cramps alone do not mean that you have an increased risk of miscarriage.

If your blood type is Rh negative (see p.127) you should receive an injection of anti-Rh after the procedure to prevent complications from occurring during this and future pregnancies.

## After the procedure

It's generally thought that being active after CVS or amniocentesis does not increase your risk of miscarriage. However, you may feel better if you don't exercise heavily right away; it's not necessary to remain in bed. In most cases, you should be physically able to return to work within a day or so after a diagnostic procedure, although some women may feel emotionally fragile and may not feel up to returning to work right away.

## Getting the results

Usually, chromosomal results from diagnostic tests take around 1–2 weeks to return, and sometimes may take as long as three weeks. If you have had your AFP level tested with amniocentesis (see left), the results for this are usually available fairly quickly, after around 1–3 days. If you are considering terminating your pregnancy based on the results of a diagnostic test, opt for testing earlier in the time frame during which it is offered, rather than later, to reduce risks of complications.

## RISKS AND BENEFITS

# Comparison of CVS and amniocentesis

Before deciding on a diagnostic test, you may want to weigh their pros and cons. Consider too that the risks may be reduced with a doctor who has expertise in a particular test.

### CVS: the pros

■ CVS can be done up to five weeks earlier than amniocentesis, so if an abnormality is found and you decide to terminate, this can be done in a safer, less traumatic way.
■ Since more genetic material is collected, the results may arrive sooner, decreasing the anxious wait.
■ If you're nervous about a needle going into the abdomen, transcervical CVS means that you can avoid this but still have a prenatal diagnosis.

### CVS: the cons

■ The risk of miscarriage after CVS is similar to amniocentesis, at around 1 in 400. The miscarriage rate is the same whether it's done transabdominally or transvaginally.
■ In the past, some women had CVS then had babies with limb abnormalities. It's now thought that most of these cases occurred when CVS was done before 10 weeks when the limbs were starting to form.

### Amniocentesis: the pros

■ Amniocentesis is highly accurate and has the lowest risk of miscarriage at around 1 in 400.

### Amniocentesis: the cons

■ Since this is done later than CVS and the results take longer, if you terminate you may be offered an induction for vaginal delivery, but most doctors can perform D&E until 20 to 24 weeks depending on the state.

## HOW THE TEST IS DONE

# Amniocentesis

**During amniocentesis, the doctor uses ultrasound to locate** an open pocket of amniotic fluid. Under continued ultrasound guidance, a thin needle is placed through the skin of the abdomen and then through the uterus and into the amniotic fluid. A small amount of the fluid is drawn up into the needle and an attached syringe. A local anesthetic may be applied to your abdomen before the procedure to ease any discomfort.

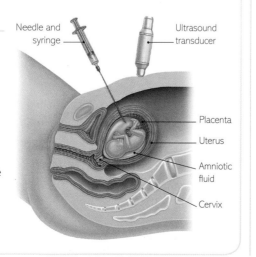

Needle and syringe
Ultrasound transducer
Placenta
Uterus
Amniotic fluid
Cervix

# 194 days to go...

**YOUR BABY TODAY**

In this ultrasound scan, the baby is seen floating in amniotic fluid, which provides plenty of space for him to move around in. Later in pregnancy, your baby will excrete waste products into the fluid, but his bladder is still tiny and kidney function not yet established.

## The bag of amniotic fluid is your baby's home—it will keep him safe and free from infection until he is ready to be born.

**Your baby is safely cushioned in the amniotic fluid.** This surrounds him, gives him space to move and grow, and helps him maintain a constant temperature.

The volume of fluid is only 1 ml at seven weeks but is 25 ml by this stage of your pregnancy. In about six weeks' time there will be around 60 ml, with plenty of room for your baby to do lots of somersaults.

The amniotic fluid increases steadily until around 32 weeks of pregnancy, then stays constant until 37 weeks. It begins to reduce slightly thereafter by about 8 percent per week.

Further on in the pregnancy, waste products excreted in your baby's urine will be absorbed from the fluid back into your bloodstream. At 37 weeks, your baby will urinate an astonishing one quarter to one third of his body weight every day. Compare this with your own production of 2–3 percent body weight as urine.

Your temperature directly influences your baby's temperature. Temperature control is not an important requirement until later in pregnancy when your baby's high metabolic rate means that he needs to transfer heat to you in order to cool himself down.

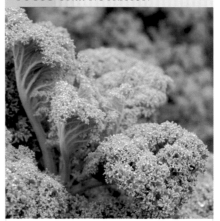

**FOCUS ON...** NUTRITION

### Iron-rich foods

**If you're suffering from pregnancy fatigue,** try boosting your intake of foods that are rich in iron. Eat plenty of:
- Dark leafy green vegetables
- Red meat
- Whole-grain cereals
- Legumes
- Prune juice.

Vitamin C helps your body absorb more iron from your diet, so try drinking fresh orange juice with meals, and limit your intake of coffee and other caffeinated drinks: caffeine inhibits your body's ability to absorb iron.

---

**ASK A...** NUTRITIONIST

**My appetite has come back, but how many calories should I be eating at this stage of my pregnancy?** Like many women, you're finding that the second trimester has brought relief from the discomforts of early pregnancy. As a result, you may have noticed you're less nauseous and have more of an appetite.

Caloric needs in the second trimester are approximately 2,100–2,500 calories per day, depending upon your level of physical activity. You shouldn't eat unlimited snacks, and when you do snack, opt for foods with nutritional value. For example, one banana has about 100 calories, and a handful (1 oz) of nuts about 170 calories. For a light 200-calorie snack, you can eat two pieces of whole-wheat toast spread with a small amount of butter and jam; a small bowl of cereal with skim milk; or a small can of soup with a slice of bread and butter.

If you're exercising regularly, you can of course increase your calorie intake without gaining excess weight.

# 193 days to go...

**YOUR BABY TODAY**

The toes are now separate and are all the same length. The ankle joints are now mature enough to be working, although it will still be many weeks before you are likely to be conscious of any kicks.

## As your uterus grows to accommodate your baby, you may begin to notice a few twinges around your pelvis.

**There's a strong band of** connective tissue in your pelvis, supporting your uterus. Known as the round ligament, this band has to stretch as your uterus expands, which can cause some discomfort. The pain is generally felt in the groin or lower abdomen and can be on either side. Although the pain starts in the pelvis, it may travel up to your hips. You may feel a short, sharp stabbing pain or a more prolonged, dull ache.

You will soon adapt and find sitting and lying positions that cause you the least discomfort and which may relieve discomfort. Also, try other common methods of pain relief, too, such as taking a warm bath or resting comfortably with your feet up.

Round ligament pain is common in pregnancy and isn't a cause for concern. See your doctor, however, if you have sharp abdominal or pelvic pains don't resolve quickly or if your pain becomes crampy; if there is any bleeding; if there is a burning sensation when you urinate; or if you're feverish. If you're in any doubt, always seek medical advice.

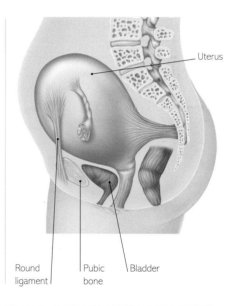

**The round ligaments,** which help support the uterus, stretch as the uterus enlarges and pull on nearby nerve fibers and sensitive structures, causing discomfort.

Uterus

Round ligament | Pubic bone | Bladder

---

**AS A MATTER OF FACT**

**Fertility treatment has had** a huge impact on the number of multiple pregnancies.

In 1977, the year before the world's first "test tube baby" was born, the natural occurrence of multiples in live births in the US was: twins 1 in 53; triplets and other multiple births, 1 in 3,092.

Today, with the increased use of fertility treatments, those numbers are 1 in 618 for triplets and other multiple births.

---

**FOCUS ON... TWINS**

## Carrying twins

**If you're expecting twins,** or more, it's good to know that most multiple pregnancies are straightforward and without complications. However, being pregnant with multiple babies is going to be more challenging for your body to handle than if you were carrying just one baby.

It's wise to know about the slightly higher risk of certain conditions that can occur. These include:

- Placenta previa (see p.212)
- Polyhydramnios (see p.473)
- Poor growth of one or more babies, which may be caused by twin-to-twin transfusion syndrome (see p.130)
- Premature labor (see p.431).

The fact that any of these conditions can develop is the reason why you'll have more prenatal checkups to preempt problems and minimize their effects.

# 192 days to go...

## YOUR BABY TODAY

By now the fetus's forehead is high and bulging, with visible joins in the plates of bone that comprise the skull. The eyes have migrated from the sides of the head at this stage of development.

Complex brain development is gradually enabling your unborn baby to become more responsive and mobile.

**Your baby's brain is undergoing rapid development.** The right and left cerebral hemispheres begin to connect. Each hemisphere controls the opposite side of the body, so the right side of the brain controls muscles on the left side of the body and the left side controls muscles on the right side of the body.

Motor fibers (those that control movement) mature first, so your baby can make increasingly complex limb movements. Sensory nerves (those that control feeding) mature later and are first present on your baby's hands and in his mouth. The brain matures quickly over the next three weeks and will be complete in around 10 weeks' time, as the rest of the upper and lower limbs and trunk achieve adult levels of sensitivity to stimuli. All your baby's nerves are very immature at this stage and he doesn't have any perception of position, pain, temperature, or touch.

**As your baby's brain develops,** he is able to make larger movements with his arms and legs, but this activity won't be well coordinated at this stage.

### FOCUS ON... NUTRITION

## Yummy yogurt

**For a calcium-packed snack,** stock up on yogurt. Those with so-called friendly bacteria are okay to eat during pregnancy and may help your digestion. Just make sure that the milk ingredients in your yogurts have been pasteurized to reduce the risk of infection with listeria (see p.17).

### ASK A... DOCTOR

**I've been diagnosed with diabetes. How will this affect my pregnancy?** Whether you develop diabetes in pregnancy (known as gestational diabetes), or have pre-existing diabetes, you will require special care from a diabetic health-care team and a obstetrician. This is because diabetes poses risks in pregnancy, particularly if there is poor control of blood-glucose levels.

All this can be managed with close prenatal care: your blood glucose needs to be well controlled since your insulin requirements will increase during pregnancy. You will also need to adapt your diet and may need insulin injections.

Pregnant women who are diabetic are at a greater risk of high blood pressure, blood clots, and preeclampsia (see p.474). If you have diabetic kidney disease, and diabetic retinopathy, a condition that affects the retina in the eye, there's a chance it will worsen during pregnancy. For your baby, there is an increased risk of congenital abnormalities and growth may be too fast or too slow.

YOU ARE 12 WEEKS AND 5 DAYS

# 191 days to go...

## YOUR BABY TODAY

This image is a close-up of your baby's umbilical cord. The umbilical arteries can be seen as they carry blood from the baby to the placenta. Since there are no nerve fibers in the cord, your baby is unaware that this is happening—or even that the cord is there.

## You and your partner will be developing your own special relationship with your baby.

At this point in your pregnancy, you won't be able to feel your baby move but it is still possible to interact and bond with him. Some women feel comfortable talking to their babies, while others don't; do what feels natural for you, whether that is talking out loud or in your head.

Very soon, your baby will be able to hear (see. p.171) and recognize your voice and that of your partner, and hear other sounds, such as music.

You might want to think of an interim name for your baby. This might be "the bump" or "the bun" or an in-joke between you and your partner. It can be helpful to give your baby an identity because it's difficult to talk about him or her at this relatively early stage, and when you don't know the gender.

If you're still keeping the pregnancy a secret in some quarters, using a code phrase to refer to the pregnancy may be useful in some circumstances.

(see. p.171)

### AS A MATTER OF FACT

**At this stage, your baby may squirm** if your abdomen is pressed.

He will gradually develop more reflexes: his eye muscles will clench if his eyelids are touched; touching the soles of his feet makes his toes curl; his fingers curl if you touch his palm.

## ACTIVITIES TO AVOID IN THE SECOND TRIMESTER

**The second trimester is generally when fatigue lifts,** and you begin to feel more energetic. This is a great time to continue your exercise program, making good use of your increased energy levels before you are too big and too uncomfortable to move and enjoy being fully active.

While you're encouraged to continue to exercise during the second trimester, there are some high-risk exercises that should be avoided. You should avoid any activity that potentially could cause you to fall, activities that involve a high degree of balance and agility, and specifically exercises that require lying on your back for extended

periods, or twisting of the upper body. Changes in your center of gravity can increase the chances of stumbling and falling, risking injury to you and your baby.

The following activities are best avoided during your second (and third) trimesters:
- Vigorous exercise at a high altitude (unless you are used to it)
- Diving and scuba diving
- Road or mountain bicycling
- Rock climbing
- Skiing, snow boarding, and waterskiing
- Ice skating/ice hockey
- Horse riding
- Bungee-jumping!

**Racquet sports** You should curtail activities such as tennis and badminton since your changing balance can be affected by quick movements and turns, increasing your risk of falling.

# 190 days to go...

**YOUR BABY TODAY**

The developing eyes are now facing forward and the baby's right ear can also be seen here. Your baby spends most of the time in a curled position, often with legs crossed, and hands close to the face.

It's never too early to start planning what you'll need to buy for your baby, even if you don't want to start shopping just yet.

**Now that you're in your safer second trimester,** you may be tempted to start buying a few baby items, unless you're superstitious and would prefer to wait. A good reason to start shopping in this trimester is that your energy levels should be at their pregnancy peak. In later months, you will find it too tiring to carry your belly, as well as your bags, around the stores and a shopping trip may not be your favorite pastime.

Even if you're not shopping yet, start planning. Ask friends to recommend their favorite strollers, cribs, slings, and car seats, then check prices so you can plan your budget. You might also find that family and friends offer used goods you can buy or borrow.

If you purchase new baby clothes, leave the tags on and check the store's return policy in case you have a baby who's too big for the newborn clothes or you decide against the items you've bought.

**ASK A... DOCTOR**

**I've just told my parents I'm pregnant but they reacted very negatively because they don't approve of my partner. What can I do?** First, give them time to come to terms with the news. Creating a baby with someone is the ultimate commitment, and marks an important life-changing event. For your parents, it is a signal that your partner isn't going anywhere, however much they might disapprove of him.

Once things have calmed down, suggest that your parents take the pregnancy as an opportunity to reestablish their relationship with your partner and wipe the slate clean. Reassure them that you and your partner very much want them to be a part of their grandchild's life, and that you'd rather clear the air now, so that there aren't any negative feelings and tension once your baby is born.

Remember that all is likely to be forgotten when your parents hold a much-loved grandchild in their arms, and since part of that baby will be your partner's that should help them to feel warmer toward him.

**FOCUS ON... YOUR BODY**

## Managing hair growth

**Changing hormones can play havoc with hair growth.** To deal with any new unwanted hair:
- **Shave larger areas** and pluck out the odd stray hair.
- **Depilatory creams and hair-lightening bleaches** may be absorbed through the skin so shaving and tweezing are safer. If you feel you must use depilatory creams and bleaches, do a patch test first and keep the room well ventilated to avoid fumes.
- **If you're waxing**, be aware that your skin may be more sensitive during pregnancy.

# 189 days to go...

**YOUR BABY TODAY**

This 2D black-and-white ultrasound scan is similar to the scan you may see and may be given. The baby is the white area, and the amniotic fluid is black. This type of scan is the best way to measure your baby's length at this stage.

Your hormones have done all the hard work to establish your pregnancy and as they settle down, so should your nausea.

**AS A MATTER OF FACT**

**Your immune system weakens during pregnancy** to stop your body from rejecting your developing baby.

This, unfortunately, makes you more prone to colds and bugs. As an added burden, pregnancy hormones can worsen a stuffed nose and nausea.

**Morning sickness usually subsides** around the start of the second trimester. It's believed that the rapid hormonal changes required to establish and maintain the pregnancy in the early stages may cause the sickness. By this stage your pregnancy is well established and your baby's major internal organs and support system are fully formed, so these hormone levels start to stabilize. This may be why the nausea passes.

Furthermore, there is a theory that nausea is the body's way of protecting your baby from harmful substances in the early crucial stages of development, so you become naturally adverse to alcohol and junk food, for example.

If your nausea and sickness hasn't begun to subside by this stage don't worry since for some women it does continue into the second trimester. See your doctor if you are concerned about your level of sickness.

**There doesn't have to be a loss of intimacy,** even if you and your partner are having less sex. Take the time to be affectionate and show your partner you want to be physically close.

**ASK A... MOM**

**My partner hasn't wanted sex at all since I've become pregnant. Will he ever desire me again?** Yes! Although it's difficult, try not to take his reluctance to have sex personally. When I was pregnant, my husband didn't want to have penetrative sex, and most of his fears centered around harming the baby or me. This was made worse by the fact that I'd taken a long time to get pregnant, and was also having a difficult pregnancy, with lots of nausea and sickness.

We spoke to our doctor and she was able to reassure my partner that he couldn't harm the baby in any way by having penetrative sex. She also told us that it wasn't uncommon for either partner to experience a reduced sexual desire in pregnancy for a variety of reasons. Although many women experience an increased libido at this stage of pregnancy, the same may not be true for their partner.

It's important that you talk to your partner to find out his fears and explain your own thoughts and feelings. Don't let this issue cause an argument between you. Each couple is different and you will need to talk to each other to find your way through this problem.

You may also find it helpful to talk to someone who isn't so closely involved, such as your doctor or a trusted friend.

Your 13th week

159

# Your 14th week

**THERE ARE SUBTLE CHANGES HAPPENING TO YOUR SHAPE THAT ONLY YOU WILL NOTICE**

Your baby isn't big enough to give you an obvious pregnancy belly, but you'll definitely notice your waistline become thicker. At this stage of pregnancy, many women feel re-energized and have a strong sense of well-being. Healthy eating is very important, so be clued in about the best food choices. In particular, your body needs plenty of protein; and your baby needs it, too, to sustain her rapid growth.

**Facial features** are becoming more clearly defined. The eyes and ears have reached their final positions.

**The brain** is developing rapidly, and your baby's head accounts for about half her total length.

**At 14 weeks** the average crown to rump length is 2.1 in (5.4 cm) and the average weight is 0.5 oz (14 g).

**The fundus**, the top of the uterus, can now be felt in your abdomen.

**The ears** have already developed their helical pattern, although your baby cannot hear yet.

**The first hairs** of the baby's scalp and eyebrows often appear at this stage.

YOU ARE 13 WEEKS AND 1 DAY

# 188 days to go...

### YOUR BABY TODAY

It's easy to see where your baby's bones are on an ultrasound as they show up as brighter areas. Other features may be harder to see. If you have a scan and are unsure what you are looking at, ask your doctor to interpret it for you.

## Relief, excitement, apprehension... it's normal to feel all this and more at this stage of your pregnancy.

**While you're undoubtedly feeling better physically,** and probably have lots more energy, you may still be up and down emotionally. This is completely normal.

This stage of pregnancy can be a very emotional time: reaching the second trimester is a pregnancy milestone and coincides with seeing your baby on the scan (see p.138). You know that, with the chances of miscarrying now being so minimal, you're really going to have

a baby. However, like many pregnant women, you may find that the feeling of relief at reaching this stage is followed by occasional anxieties.

One good outlet for all this emotional energy is exercising, which you may find easier now that you're over the first trimester fatigue. Exercise releases endorphins, the feel-good hormones, and so can improve your emotional as well as physical well-being, but always exercise safely (see box, below).

### AS A MATTER OF FACT

**Exercising** may reduce the time you are in labor.

Research has shown that women who exercise at a moderate to high intensity can cut their time in labor by up to three hours, and they tend to have less complicated deliveries than those who don't exercise.

### LISTENING TO YOUR BODY

**Check with your doctor** whether there's any reason why you shouldn't be exercising; there are certain pregnancy conditions, such as placenta previa (see p.212) and the risk of premature labor, that may preclude you from exercising.

When exercising during pregnancy, always use your common sense and look out for symptoms that may indicate you are exercising too hard. Aerobic exercise is often tracked by measuring the heart rate, but this is difficult during pregnancy since there is a natural increase in your heart rate, even at rest. So the most effective way to keep your exercise at a safe level is the talk test: you should

be able to carry on a conversation while exercising. This will indicate that you are not exercising to exhaustion and potentially restricting the oxygen flow to your baby.

There are other symptoms that indicate you're exercising too hard or should not be exercising at all:
- Vaginal bleeding
- Dizziness and headaches
- Chest pain
- Extreme and sudden muscle weakness
- Calf pain and leg swelling
- Leakage of amniotic fluid.

If you suffer from any of the above symptoms, even momentarily, stop exercising and seek medical advice.

**Rather than taking a gentle stroll,** try walking at a brisk pace, but make sure you can still talk. This will ensure you're exercising at a moderate aerobic level.

# 187 days to go...

**YOUR BABY TODAY**

This scan shows a cross section of your baby's brain, with the two hemispheres clearly seen. From this point on, your baby's brain measurement from one side to the other, taken just above the ear, is used as a reliable indicator of her growth and development.

## Even at this early stage of development, your baby has started to urinate, although in very small quantities.

**Your baby's bladder** now fills and empties every 30 minutes; she swallows the amniotic fluid, filters it through her kidneys, and then passes it as urine. The bladder volume is tiny at this stage, and even by 32 weeks it will only be 10 ml, reaching 40 ml by 40 weeks. Your baby produces very dilute urine, having only a limited capacity to reabsorb water in the kidney to concentrate the urine. However, the placenta performs most of the kidney functions until birth.

Your baby's blood system can now make and break down blood clots. The placenta has been able to form clots for some time, reducing the risk of bleeding.

A small number of white blood cells are now being produced by your baby but she is still relying on yours to fight infection. Her red blood cells contain hemoglobin that transfers oxygen to all the cells of the body. Before birth she has several forms of hemoglobin that differ from yours. These are more stable at a lower acidity and bind more easily to oxygen. This allows your baby's body to extract the oxygen in your hemoglobin for her own use.

**The toes are now fully formed** and separated, and their individual bones can be clearly discerned on an ultrasound.

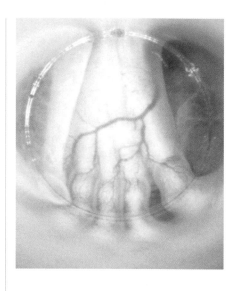

---

**ASK A... DOCTOR**

**I'm expecting triplets. How will my prenatal care differ?** All the usual risks of pregnancy are increased for women having more than one baby. This is partly because hormone levels are higher when there is more than one baby, and, in your case, it will be hard work for your body to carry and nourish three fetuses.

You can expect to be referred to an obstetrician, who will plan your prenatal care with you. You'll have more frequent checkups and scans to check the health and progress of your babies. Although many of the risks are outside your control, if you go to all your appointments and take care of your health, it is likely that you will have three healthy babies.

With triplets, you will probably need to give birth by cesarean section. The average pregnancy length for triplets is 34 weeks.

For more information about multiple pregnancy and details of local support groups, visit nomotc.org, the National Organization of Mothers of Twins Clubs' website (see p.481).

**TIME TO THINK ABOUT**

## Amniocentesis

This involves testing the amniotic fluid and is normally done at 16–18 weeks (see pp.152–3) It may be offered:

■ **When there's** a family or pregnancy history of a genetic problem.
■ **To older women** who are more at risk of having a baby with a chromosomal abnormality.
■ **When a screening test** (see pp. 142–3) has shown there is a high risk of a chromosomal abnormality.

# 186 days to go...

**YOUR BABY TODAY**

It is surprising how much detail is already present in your baby's body. This closeup of an ear shows that its helical pattern of folds is nearly fully developed, although it is still too soon for your baby to hear anything.

## Your waistline will be increasing and your body shape changing but your belly is unlikely to be very prominent for several weeks.

**By week 14,** if you stand in your underwear in front of the mirror, you will see a change in your body shape, but to the outside world you may not look very different. Women who have previously been pregnant tend to show earlier than those who are pregnant for the first time, because their stomach muscles have already been stretched once and so stretch much more quickly.

Women often say that this is the time when they look as though they have put on weight and feel fat, not pregnant! But it won't be long before your belly will be visible for the world to see.

If you're feeling uncomfortable and heavy, make sure you choose the right clothes. See page 151 for some tips on how to adapt your wardrobe without having to spend any money yet.

### SLEEP PROBLEMS

**Now that you're in the second trimester,** you may be sleeping better, since the urge to go to the bathroom frequently may have subsided, allowing you to stay in bed all night long once again. Or maybe not, since sleep-related problems can affect women during the entire pregnancy. Here are some common problems and solutions:

■ **Heartburn** Lying down soon after a big meal can cause acid reflux, known as heartburn, which can make it uncomfortable for you to sleep. To lessen the possibility of disrupted sleep due to heartburn, avoid eating big meals 2–3 hours before bed. If your heartburn is severe, discuss over-the-counter medication options with your doctor.

■ **Restless leg syndrome** This condition, which makes you feel the need to move your legs around to relieve a creepy-crawly feeling while you're lying in bed, is fairly common in pregnancy. It's a good idea to mention it to your doctor, since it can sometimes be caused by a deficiency (like anemia) that can be treated by taking supplements.

■ **Napping** If pregnancy makes you tired, you may want to grab 40 winks in the afternoon. But for some pregnant women, this extra shut-eye makes it more difficult to fall asleep at night. If this happens to you, skip the afternoon nap and go to bed at night a little earlier than you usually do.

### ASK A... DOCTOR

**Is it safe to use complementary therapies?** Check with your doctor before opting for complementary and alternative medicine. This umbrella term covers medical practices and products that are not considered part of conventional medicine, and studies of their effects on pregnancy may not have been done. "Natural" doesn't mean "safe."

**Reflexology** is a complementary therapy that involves applying pressure to reflexes on the hands and feet. It's believed to help with morning sickness, backaches, fluid retention, and swelling during pregnancy.

Your 14th week

# 185 days to go...

## YOUR BABY TODAY

Whether your baby's legs are crossed or uncrossed, it is very difficult to tell from an ultrasound at this stage whether your baby is a boy or girl: male and female look too similar to reliably tell them apart.

Your baby's central nervous system, including the brain and the spine, now has all its basic components.

**The core development of your baby's central nervous system** has taken place, and it will now progress further using four overlapping processes. The number of nerve cells increases and their positions alter during migration—a process by which cells move to their final locations and develop specific functions. The connections between individual nerve cells become more organized, and the fibers become insulated.

The growth of the nervous system now enters its most active phase. Reflecting this, the head accounts for half of the entire length of the baby. Both the nerves and their supporting cells increase in number. Although most of the nerve cells are produced during pregnancy, the supporting cells continue to increase in number during your baby's first year. The supporting cells assist in the migration process, which is largely completed by 22 weeks.

### ASK A... DOCTOR

**Can I continue jogging?** There's no reason why not if you were a regular runner before you became pregnant, but take it easy—now is not the time to run a marathon!

You need to avoid becoming overheated so don't run on hot days and drink plenty of water, regardless of the temperature. Wear a good sports bra to support your growing breasts. Whenever you can, run on soft surfaces, such as grass, to reduce the stress on your joints, especially your knees.

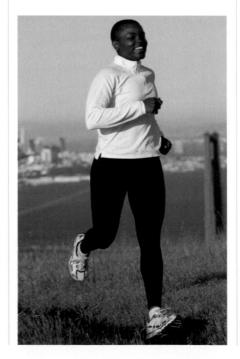

**Jogging is a good aerobic activity** during pregnancy in the early months, but is only advised if you're used to jogging. Don't take it up as a new activity in pregnancy.

### FOCUS ON... NUTRITION

## Perfect pork

**Pork is an excellent source of protein,** vitamin B6, and zinc—which are all essential nutrients for pregnancy. Pork has a reputation as a fatty meat, but this is not deserved; it is probably due to the fact that some cuts can be fatty, such as spare ribs, bacon, and ham, but many cuts of pork have less saturated fat than beef.

The key to eating healthily is to look for the leanest cuts. These usually have the word "loin" in the name, such as tenderloin or top loin chop. A serving of pork should be approximately 3 oz (85 g).

Pork is healthy and delicious, and quick and easy to prepare. Sprinkle some salt on lean pork chops, grill, and serve with some apple sauce on the side; your craving for something both salty and sweet can be met in a healthy way. Always make sure that the pork is prepared on a separate cutting board than other foods and thoroughly cooked to reduce your chances of getting a food-borne illness (see p.104).

# 184 days to go...

## YOUR BABY TODAY

At this stage the head, although still large, has a much more rounded shape than before and, as the jaw and neck lengthen, the chin moves away from the neck. An ultrasound now will show the thumb as distinct from the fingers.

## It's only a minor pregnancy symptom, but nasal congestion can happen most days—and make you a snorer at night!

**Is your partner nudging you in the night because you're keeping him awake?** It's common for pregnant women to snore. This is largely due to increased swelling of the nasal passages, but it can also be caused by increased weight and the fact that you may roll over onto your back during the night.

Your stuffy nose is due to the increased volume of blood in your body while you're pregnant. This can cause congestion and make your ears feel blocked, too. Nosebleeds are also very common in pregnancy; some women find that every time they blow their nose they have a small amount of bleeding. This is because the blood vessels in the nose are very fragile, and with the increased volume of blood flowing through them, they tend to bleed more easily. However, the bleeding should be very light.

To treat a nosebleed, tip your head forward and pinch the middle of your nose (in the soft part) hard. It should stop quickly. If it doesn't, try an icepack on the nose to help the blood vessels constrict. In the rare situation of heavy bleeding, go to the hospital. Seek medical advice if you are getting heavy bleeding regularly.

### ASK A... NUTRITIONIST

**Is it safe to eat peanuts or foods containing them during pregnancy?** Some experts feel that if a child is at a particular risk of developing a peanut allergy, the problem may have started to develop before birth. Due to the mother's diet, a sensitivity to peanuts may have begun when the baby was exposed to them in the uterus.

However, recent studies have suggested that avoiding peanuts during pregnancy may be increasing the incidence of allergies, pinpointing countries where peanuts are a staple food and allergies relatively rare. Although studies have been inconclusive, your baby may be at risk of developing a peanut allergy if you, or your partner, or your baby's siblings suffer from asthma, eczema, hay fever, or other allergies. If any of these apply to you, ask your doctor whether you should eat peanuts during your pregnancy or while you are breast-feeding.

There is no need for you to avoid eating peanuts if your baby is not at risk of peanut allergy.

### FOCUS ON... DADS

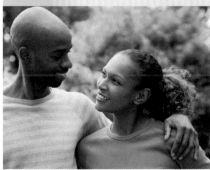

## Looking forward

**During the first trimester,** you probably anxiously awaited developments in the pregnancy and supported your partner when the going got tough. Now that her early pregnancy symptoms, such as nausea and sickness and fatigue, are likely to have passed, and the risk of miscarriage is reduced, you may begin to feel differently about the pregnancy and your future.

As your partner starts to show increasing strength and vigor, and as you begin to notice her changing body shape and small belly, you may find that the reality of the pregnancy hits you and your sense of trepidation is replaced by optimism as you both look forward.

# 183 days to go...

**YOUR BABY TODAY**

In this color ultrasound image the baby is red and the placenta green. It is just possible to see the two crosses that measure the depth of fluid in the nuchal fold at the back of the neck (see p.143). Now is the last opportunity to measure this reliably.

Your baby is growing and getting stronger every day, and it's all thanks to her life support system—the placenta.

**Your baby's rapid growth** continues and she'll nearly double in size from 2.25 in (5.5 cm) to 4 in (10 cm) during the next three weeks. Muscle and bone growth advances, but, although all joints are present, it will be three weeks before the skeleton begins to harden.

Your baby is now totally dependent on the placenta for her nourishment. Environmental factors have almost no influence on your baby's size at this stage; all babies up until around 20 weeks' gestation are the same size.

The placenta is larger than your baby and supplies all the nutrients she needs. To aid her growth, the placenta extracts amino acids from your circulation, giving her high levels. Amino acids are the building blocks of protein, from which muscles and organs develop.

**FOCUS ON... NUTRITION**

## Protein plus

**Protein is required** for the development of the baby and placenta, as well as to fuel changes taking place in your body (see p.14). The protein requirement for pregnancy is 6 or 6.5 oz daily, instead of the usual 5 or 5.5 oz. Include a source in all three meals daily. Protein sources include meat, poultry, fish, milk, cheese, beans, nuts, and seeds.

The best protein foods are those that are lower in saturated fat and cholesterol. Trim the fat off meat and eat one or two servings of fish (see p.96) or seafood. When choosing dairy products, pick skim milk and low-fat cheeses. These retain all the protein benefits of the whole milk versions. Nuts and seeds are rich in heart-healthy oils. Vegetarians need to eat a wide range of plant proteins to ensure they are getting adequate amino acids (see p.126).

**The umbilical cord** can be seen connecting this 13-week-old fetus with the placenta, which nourishes your baby. The incredible blood vessels of the placenta are clearly visible in the background.

# 182 days to go...

**YOUR BABY TODAY**

This 2D ultrasound shows the profile of the baby particularly well. The nasal bone can just be seen at the bridge of the nose, as can bright echoes from the lower and upper jaws; the umbilical cord is rising from the center of the abdomen.

## It can be difficult to avoid information overload—everyone, it seems, will have advice to share with you.

### ASK A... DOCTOR

**Why are varicose veins common in pregnancy and what can I do to avoid getting them?** Your blood volume increases up to 30 percent during pregnancy, due to the added needs of your baby and your expanding body. In addition, the hormone relaxin (which is produced to soften ligaments and joints) also softens the walls of your blood vessels. The blood vessels relax and the increased blood and extra weight of the baby make you susceptible to varicose veins.

To reduce the likelihood of getting varicose veins:

■ **Avoid sitting or standing in one position** for prolonged periods: walk around regularly, moving your arms as you do so to increase the blood flow in your body.

■ **Exercise daily:** most forms of cardiovascular exercise will help increase blood flow. Water aerobics is a good choice since the pressure of the water helps increase blood circulation.

■ **Sleep with your legs slightly elevated** by placing a pillow under your bottom sheet at the end of your bed.

**One side effect of pregnancy** all women have to deal with is conflicting information and advice. One article says to do something, while a friend says the exact opposite. It can be confusing and irritating. While you can choose to stop reading a newspaper or turn to a different television channel, it's more difficult to avoid the unwanted advice of other women. Even more difficult is the advice from close relatives, such as your mother and mother-in-law. You'll need the support of your family and friends,

**The second trimester is a great time** to pamper yourself with a new haircut and color. Your new hairstyle will complement your glowing skin.

so won't want to alienate them, but don't feel pressured to act in a certain way. Also don't reject everything immediately—some of the advice may in fact be useful and accurate.

If someone is persistently advising you explain that you're overwhelmed by information and would rather not talk about the pregnancy at this time. Or listen to the person's advice, smile politely, and then do what you want. You could subtly hint that you will ask for advice as and when you need it.

### FOCUS ON... YOUR BODY

## Style challenge

**Give yourself a hair makeover.**

■ **There is no evidence** that the chemicals in hair dyes are harmful for your baby although only a limited amount of research has been done on pregnant women. If you're cautious, skip the chemicals and get a new cut.

■ **If you're worried** stick to highlights, which don't expose the whole scalp to dye and make sure the room is well ventilated.

■ **When coloring your own hair,** do so in a well-ventilated space and always wear the gloves provided.

# Your 15th week

**START TALKING TO YOUR BABY—HE CAN HEAR YOUR VOICE**

Like many pregnant women in the second trimester, you may now be reaping the benefits of the pregnancy "glow," as hormones improve the appearance of your skin and hair. Enjoy this time and the attention that often comes with it. Amazingly, your baby's ears have formed enough for him to hear you speaking. He'll recognize your voice—and your partner's—when he comes out into the world.

**The arms** have grown long enough to allow the baby to place his hands together in front of his face.

**The placenta** undergoes a new wave of development to meet all your baby's needs.

**At 15 weeks** the average crown to rump length is 2.9 in (7.4 cm) and the average weight is 0.8 oz (23 g).

**The inner ear bones** have developed sufficiently to pick up sounds, including your voice.

**The neck** is lengthening and the baby can raise his head further, lifting up his chin from his chest.

**The fully formed spinal cord** now extends the entire length of the vertebral canal, with nerves leaving between every vertebra.

# 181 days to go...

**YOUR BABY TODAY**

At this stage, the fetus's forearms, wrists, hands, and fingers are all well differentiated. The eyes, which are visible as dark areas behind the sealed eyelids, have migrated inward from the sides of the head.

Now that some pregnancy discomforts have passed and while you await your belly "bump," you may feel strangely "normal."

**You may not feel as though you are pregnant** at the moment. The beginning of the second trimester is an interesting transition period: you know you're expecting a baby—you've seen the ultrasound scan—but you may not look or feel that pregnant, and you won't feel the baby move for several weeks yet (see p.213).

The physical reminders that were common in the first trimester—such as nausea and fatigue—may have greatly lessened or passed entirely.

Many women say they feel completely ordinary and find this strange because they think that they "should" be feeling something. Try to enjoy this time and keep looking at that scan picture if you need a reminder that your baby is there. You may long to feel normal once you hit the third trimester and some of that fatigue returns.

---

**THE POWER OF OMEGA 3**

**It's a fact that what you eat could make your baby's brain and nervous system work better.** Recent studies suggest that women who eat a diet enriched in omega-3 fatty acids during pregnancy and breast-feeding may enhance their baby's language development, IQ, and cognitive development. These essential fatty acids may also decrease allergies in children of mothers who eat them during pregnancy and breast-feeding, and decrease postpartum depression although more research is needed.

Omega-3 fatty acids are found in oily fish. In fact, only seafood contains two essential omega-3 fatty acids; essential because the body can't manufacture them.

Although fish is a main source of omega 3, you need to ensure you don't consume varieties that are high in mercury (see p.96). Salmon and anchovies are two oily fish that are low in mercury yet rich in omega-3 fatty acids. Wild salmon is a particularly rich, and delicious, source of these healthy fatty acids.

Other nonseafood sources of omega-3 fatty acids are canola oil, walnuts, flaxseed, and omega-3 enriched eggs. These sources contain only one essential omega-3 fatty acid, but it is still worth eating them. Note that flaxseed, which is also a great source of fiber, must be ground for the body to absorb it. Sprinkle it on cereal or yogurt.

---

**FOCUS ON... DADS**

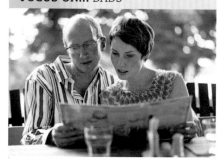

## The two of you

**Make the effort to set aside time** for you and your partner to be alone together while she's pregnant. Whether it's an evening out once a week, or that weekend away you've been promising yourselves for ages, do it now! Remember, the second trimester is also a good time to go on vacation (see p.185).

It's common for there to be fundamental changes to a relationship when a baby arrives; some new fathers feel a bit pushed out, especially in the early weeks. By spending time together now, you will build a greater bond for when the baby is born and feel satisfied that you enjoyed lots of pleasurable time together during the pregnancy.

Your 15th week

YOU ARE 14 WEEKS AND 2 DAYS

# 180 days to go...

### YOUR BABY TODAY

In this 3D ultrasound scan, the baby is lying on his back. The arms and legs have lengthened and the baby is able to move them freely. His head is still relatively large compared to the trunk and the forehead bulges out.

## He's well-developed on the outside, but complex changes are taking place as your baby's internal organs continue to mature.

### WORKING DURING PREGNANCY

**The majority of employers are supportive when they find out an employee is pregnant,** and hopefully this will be the case for you. However, should a problem arise, there is employment law in place to protect pregnant women:

■ **You can't be fired** during pregnancy, unless you breach the terms of your agreement.

■ **You can't be laid off** because you're pregnant or on maternity leave. However, if the reason for the lay off is a legitimate one, unconnected with your pregnancy, it is allowed.

■ **Your employer** has extra responsibilities when you're pregnant, and these include ensuring that your workplace is safe. For example, you should be protected from handling or lifting heavy loads, standing for long periods of time, or handling toxic substances.

■ **If you need time off** for a pregnancy-related absence, your employer must hold your job for you the same length of time that jobs are held for employees on sick or disability leave.

**Your baby's neck is growing,** and he's now looking more and more like a human being. Internally, the thyroid gland first develops at the base of the tongue but gradually moves down to lie in the neck, overlying the trachea (windpipe). The thyroid gland is producing the hormone thyroxine, using iodine transported from your body across the placenta.

### ASK A... DOCTOR

**I've developed a dark vertical line down the middle of my belly. What is this?** This line is called the linea nigra, which occurs due to changes in

skin pigmentation. It's extremely common, affecting 90 percent of all pregnant women in some way or another, and is often more noticeable if you are darker skinned.

You may also notice a darkening of the skin around your nipples and a darkening of freckles, moles, or birthmarks. A few women may also experience brown patches on their face called chloasma or the "mask of pregnancy" (see pp.190 and 467). These changes are caused by the extra amounts of the hormone estrogen during pregnancy, which affects the melanin-producing cells of the skin—these cells produce the pigment that darkens the skin. These color changes are normal and will usually fade once the baby is born.

The baby's kidneys are starting to function. The nephrons in the kidneys are lengthening and maturing: these essential units enable the kidney to function by filtering the blood and eliminating waste from the body.

New nephrons will be produced up until the 37th week and the kidneys continue to lengthen by around 1 mm a week during the entire pregnancy.

Your second trimester

# 179 days to go...

**YOUR BABY TODAY**

The hands are well developed at this stage, but, as can be seen here, the skin is very thin and transparent, which means the developing bones of the fingers and the blood vessels can be seen.

Feel free to talk to your baby. His ears have now developed to the point where he can hear your voice.

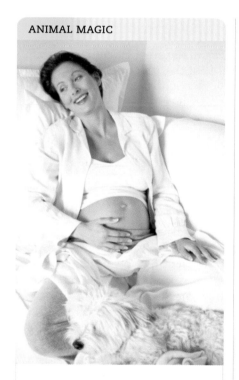

**ANIMAL MAGIC**

**Do you share your home with a pet?** Recent research shows that living with a cat or dog in early childhood may reduce the risk of your child developing asthmatic symptoms. The study found that children residing with cats were more likely to have allergy-related antibodies to felines. Never leave your baby alone with a dog or cat.

**Around this point in the second trimester,** the bones of your baby's inner ear have formed and he starts to hear. Previously, your baby would have been able to feel the vibrations created by noise, especially when you talked, even though he couldn't hear sounds. Research has found that when an unborn baby hears something, his heart rate might change or he might move. You may be able to feel your baby move in response to a certain noise or type of music.

Your baby can now hear you when you talk to him, or when your partner talks to him (in fact, babies are thought to be able to hear deeper male voices more clearly than female ones), and when you give birth he will already be familiar with the sound of your voices.

---

**ASK A... DOCTOR**

**How can I relieve my constipation?**
Constipation is a common symptom of pregnancy, mainly because the hormone progesterone slows down your bowel function, making everything more sluggish. Many women exercise less than usual during pregnancy, which can also cause things to become blocked. Finally, iron pills, which may be prescribed for anemia, are notorious for causing constipation.

There are, thankfully, many ways to relieve the problem:
■ **Eat more fiber:** ensure that you are getting plenty of fiber in your diet, in the form of fresh fruit and vegetables, and whole grains, and drink plenty of water to aid the passing of stools.

■ **Go natural:** Psyllium (or ispaghula), a common ingredient in some laxatives, appears to be safe during pregnancy, although studies in pregnant women have not been done.
■ **Exercise regularly:** Exercise during pregnancy helps to reduce constipation.
■ **Constipation during pregnancy can lead to itchy or painful hemorrhoids:** If this happens to you, ask your doctor what medicines you can use for soothing relief.
■ **Don't ignore the urge to go:** Ignoring the urge too often can lead to constipation. Take care of your needs, even if you think you're too busy to stop what you're doing or if it means that you'll have to use a public toilet.

# 178 days to go...

## YOUR BABY TODAY

In this image the placenta can be seen to the left of the baby. The placenta is still very much larger than your baby and is growing at a faster rate, preparing to meet the demands of your baby, who will later overtake it in size and weight.

## To function successfully, the placenta needs a good maternal blood supply to the arteries in the wall of the uterus.

**The placenta now starts a second wave of growth** that will take almost six weeks. The outer layer of cells in the placenta move into the coiled, or spiral, arteries in the uterus, destroying their muscular wall. This causes the arteries to dilate, resulting in a low resistance to blood flow. Only those arteries beneath the placenta (80–100 vessels) are invaded by the placental cells in this way. If these cells move too deeply, they can fuse too tightly with the muscle of the uterus and have difficulty separating after delivery. If the wave of invading cells is inadequate, however, the low resistance to blood flow doesn't develop. This can increase the risk of the mother developing preeclampsia (see p.474), and cause the baby growth problems.

### AS A MATTER OF FACT

**It is a native Hawaiian belief that the placenta** is part of the child.

It is a tradition to plant the placenta with a tree, which then grows alongside the child.

### ASK A... DOCTOR

**I'm trying to stay out of the sun but is it okay to use fake tanning lotions?** Sunless tanning lotions are safer than sunbathing or tanning beds but they have not been tested on pregnant women so their effects aren't known. It may be better to err on the side of caution and go without a tan while you're pregnant. Bear in mind that a fake tan does not protect your skin so, if you do wear it, you'll need to wear additional protection when you are in the sun.

No tanning pills of any kind have been approved by the Food and Drug Administration. They may contain canthaxanthin and can be toxic to your unborn baby, and also have been known to cause hepatitis and eye damage.

### SLEEP REMEDIES

**Even though you may not need to go to the bathroom** as much at night as you did in the first trimester, and may not yet be suffering from too many aches and pains, sleep may still escape you in the second trimester.

You may find that during this life-changing time you may be having especially vivid dreams, which can disrupt your sleep. Even if you're feeling well, it's essential to get adequate sleep: after all, your body is working hard to create another life. To get more sleep:

■ **Eat a late-night snack** containing the amino acid tryptophan (see p.177), which is sleep inducing.

■ **Don't watch TV in bed** for an easier time falling asleep.

■ **Cut down on caffeine** (see p.66) and make non-herbal fruit tea your bedtime drink instead.

■ **Take a bath before bedtime,** with soft music or candlelight (see below). Make sure the water isn't hot since because this can stimulate rather than relax.

# 177 days to go...

**YOUR BABY TODAY**

This 3D ultrasound shows the hands held up in front of the face. The knees seem "knobby" with every bone clearly seen on the scan. The soft spot on the baby's head can also be seen: this protects the brain while still allowing for its rapid growth.

## You might receive some compliments, because at this stage of pregnancy you're likely to look glowing with good health.

**The terms "blooming" or "glowing"** are often used to describe pregnant women, especially during the second trimester. The ideal image is a woman with thick shiny hair and perfect skin that has a healthy blush.

The improved condition of your skin is thanks to the hormone estrogen (pregnancy hormones can have positive effects, too!) and the increased blood supply to the skin; the many blood vessels just below the skin's surface give you a healthy glow, or at least stop you from looking pale and tired. The glands also secrete more oil, giving your skin a healthy-looking sheen.

Again due to hormonal changes, your hair may look thicker. Less hair than normal falls out during pregnancy and hair grows more quickly. After the birth you may find that your hair appears to be falling out more than normal as you lose the hair that's built up during the nine months. Normal hair loss is about 100–125 hairs a day; after the birth you might lose 500 hairs a day.

If you don't feel you match this picture of good health, it may just be that you can't see it yourself, especially if you're still adapting to your pregnancy. If you're looking pale and feeling tired, speak to your doctor because you may be anemic and need to boost your iron intake (see p.154).

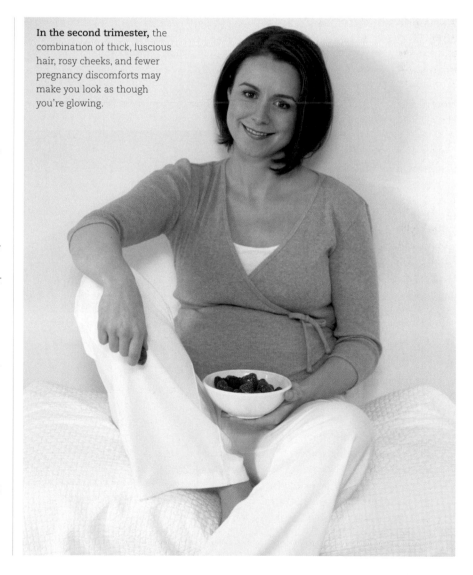

**In the second trimester,** the combination of thick, luscious hair, rosy cheeks, and fewer pregnancy discomforts may make you look as though you're glowing.

# 176 days to go...

## YOUR BABY TODAY

Your baby is starting to swallow amniotic fluid more regularly: this enters the stomach (seen here as a dark circle in the center of the abdomen). The tiny bladder is also visible as a black fluid-filled structure within the lower pelvis.

The neural tube, the basis of your baby's spinal cord, developed in the very early weeks; now the spinal cord is fully formed.

**Nerves from your baby's spinal cord** are linked to each set of vertebrae, but as your baby lengthens the spinal cord does not grow at the same rate, and the lower tip ends up lying at the mid-lumbar level, half way between the hips and lowest rib.

Below the mid-lumbar level, the nerves leaving the spinal cord have lengthened so that they still exit between the lowest vertebrae. In adult life, the cord will end slightly higher than in the newborn baby. Because the spinal cord does not extend the entire length of the vertebral canal, a fluid-filled space fills the lower portion.

By the end of this week, your baby is able to use fat as a source of energy. This isn't, however, an important source of energy because that need is met largely by glucose crossing the placenta from your bloodstream. Free fatty acids in your circulation easily cross the placenta to your baby and are used for organ growth, forming cell walls, making myelin sheaths around nerves to insulate them, and for many other functions.

Cholesterol is not only supplied to your unborn baby via the placenta, but he is also forming it within his own body. For this reason, your cholesterol level bears little relation to your baby's, which needs to be high for your baby to produce fat, especially in the first few months of pregnancy.

### AS A MATTER OF FACT

**Your baby could be tuning in** to your favorite TV show!

Research examined babies of mothers who watched the Australian show, *Neighbours*, while pregnant alongside women who didn't. After the birth those babies who had heard the music in the uterus became quiet and "paid attention" to the tune, while the other group of babies ignored it.

**In this computer-generated image**, the internal organs of the fetus can be seen. The skull, spine, and rib cage are also clearly visible. The lungs (pink) are protected by the rib cage; the kidneys (red) are below.

### ASK A... DOCTOR

**When can my baby first suck his thumb?** Ultrasound scans have shown unborn babies sucking their thumbs from as early as 12–14 weeks of pregnancy. However, this is likely to be a reflex at this stage as the brain does not have any conscious control over movement until the fetus is much more developed later on in pregnancy.

Some research has suggested that if an unborn baby shows a preference for sucking, for example, his right thumb, then he will prefer to lie with his head turned to the right after the birth. The same research suggested that this preference could be used to predict right- or left-handedness in the baby as he grows older.

# 175 days to go...

**YOUR BABY TODAY**

This profile view shows that the bridge of the nose is shallow and the eyes are still dominating the face. The jaw is lengthening and the chin held away from the chest. The hands (with outstretched fingers) are in a common position—close to the face.

It's worthwhile finding comfortable sleeping positions now; these will stand you in good stead throughout pregnancy.

**FOCUS ON... YOUR BABY**

## Quiet times

**Times when you can focus quietly** on your baby are precious bonding opportunities and a great way to relax. You may want to visualize your baby floating in the amniotic fluid.

Try this "butterfly" pose with the soles of your feet together. Place your hands on your abdomen and massage your baby using different strokes. Think of your baby and shed your preoccupations with each out-breath.

**Your belly will be getting bigger** by the day and, as a result, you may find it increasingly difficult to get comfortable when you're lying down, especially during the night.

You should avoid sleeping on your back in the second half of your pregnancy, so start practicing some new positions now. This is because the weight of your uterus will press on the major veins that return blood to your heart, which may result in dizziness, low blood pressure, and possibly a reduction in blood flow to the uterus.

Ideally, lie on your left side (although it will do you or your baby no harm to lie on your right side) since this is actually good for you and the baby. It improves blood flow to the placenta and helps your kidneys eliminate fluids and waste products. Don't worry if you wake to find you're lying on your back: just roll onto your side and support yourself with pillows if necessary.

It's fine to lie on your front if you prefer (your baby is safely cushioned in the amniotic fluid), but the bigger you get, the more difficult this will become.

**ASK A... DOCTOR**

**My doctor is great but she's always in a hurry. How can I get her to answer my questions?** This is a common problem. Doctors' practices are often very busy, with lots of women for the doctor to see. As a result, many doctors allow only a certain amount of time for each appointment—sometimes barely enough time to go through the basic physical checkup. However, it is important that your questions are addressed and it may be helpful to write them down so that you remember what you want to ask. If your doctor doesn't have time to discuss the issues during your appointment, ask her to arrange to talk to you at a mutually convenient time. This could be in the form of a phone call, or another appointment at her office. Or she may be able to direct you to other sources of information such as books, websites, or other health-care professionals.

It's a crucial part of your prenatal care that you feel comfortable with your caregivers and are given the opportunity to discuss any questions you have or issues that arise since they will be involved with your labor and delivery, which is a very important time for you.

# Your 16th week

**THE BELLY STARTS HERE, ANNOUNCING YOUR PREGNANCY TO THE WORLD**

Some days, you'll take huge pride in your emerging belly, on other days you may sigh for the loss of a trim figure. Enjoy your changing shape—you'll probably find that your partner loves it, too. For many couples, this can be a time of increased interest in sex. If you have any emotional or physical worries, there'll be an opportunity to discuss them with your doctor. Another prenatal checkup is likely to take place this week.

**Facial muscles** have developed enough for the baby to make faces, such as frowning, although she has no control over her expressions.

**In the brain**, nerve cells are forming and moving from the central to the outer areas. As yet, any neural activity is still very immature.

**Greater mobility** in the hands means that the baby is able to suck her thumb.

**The skin** is quite smooth and has a reddish tinge, since there is very little underlying fat.

**At 16 weeks** the average crown to rump length is 3.4 in (8.7 cm) and the average weight is 1.52 oz (43 g).

**The gut** is too immature to function properly but it can take in the tiny amounts of amniotic fluid that the baby swallows at infrequent intervals.

# 174 days to go...

## YOUR BABY TODAY

In this artificially colored ultrasound scan of the baby within the uterus, the spine shows up especially clearly. The two blue crosses, at the top of the baby's head and at his bottom, indicate where the rump to crown measurement is taken.

Your belly "bump" may be clearly visible by this 16th week of pregnancy, and you'll be amazed at how quickly it grows.

**At around this stage you may begin to "show,"** that is, instead of having a slightly bigger waist you develop a definite "bump" and start to look pregnant. You may begin to notice people's eyes are drawn toward your abdomen. If you'd rather keep the pregnancy quiet in some circles—for example, at work—wear baggy clothes.

While some women have neat little bellies positioned more to the front, others have bellies that are more spread out. The size and shape of yours will be individual to you, so try not to compare. There are old wives' tales that if you're carrying in front you're having a boy, and if you're carrying spread out over your hips you're carrying a girl, though this hasn't been proved.

If you haven't bought any maternity clothes, you may want to shop for some or adapt your clothes (see p.179).

(see p.179)

### AS A MATTER OF FACT

**Twin bonding occurs well before** the babies are born.

Advanced video technology has captured the special relationship between twins in the uterus. They have been seen to interact and even grasp each other's hands.

**Your belly may not be obvious** to others when you're wearing baggy clothes, but in tight-fitting ones it will be quite prominent. Although your shape changes gradually, some women find that their belly gets larger more quickly during some weeks than others.

### ASK A... NUTRITIONIST

**I keep waking up hungry at night—what should I do?** It is normal to get the nighttime munchies during pregnancy, but annoying, especially if you're already having difficulties sleeping. Try to preempt nighttime hunger by snacking on the right foods before you go to bed:

- **Eggs, milk** (and therefore cheese, and yogurt, too), and turkey are good sources of the amino acid tryptophan, which encourages the body to produce the B vitamin niacin. This helps the production of serotonin, a brain chemical that has a calming effect and aids sleep.
- **Eat slow-release carbohydrates,** such as whole-wheat bread or pasta. So, for example, half a cheese or turkey sandwich, a small amount of whole-wheat pasta with some cheese, or a bowl of good-quality whole-grain breakfast cereal with some warm milk and honey will fill you up, while also helping you sleep better.
- **A handful of nuts and seeds,** or some plain yogurt with honey and fruit, are high in protein and will stop your stomach from rumbling.

Your 16th week

# 173 days to go...

### YOUR BABY TODAY

The fingertips are prominent and the fingers still quite short. Each finger is separate and moves independently of the rest. This is the most comfortable position for the hand, with the thumb and fingers outstretched rather than curled into a fist.

## You're unlikely to feel her move yet, but your baby is becoming increasingly active inside your uterus.

**By now, your baby may be active for up to five minutes at a time.** In the next few weeks, you may begin to feel some slight fluttering movements, particularly if this is not your first pregnancy (see p.193). You'll only be aware of those movements that cause your baby to make contact with the inner muscular wall of your uterus.

The placenta itself can act like a cushion absorbing the impact of all but the strongest of the baby's movements. For this reason, women with an anterior placenta (one lying on the front wall of the uterus—that closest to the skin) often feel the movements at a much later stage than those with a posteriorly sited placenta (one that lies closer to the back).

Your baby's brain is continuing to develop. The nerve cells that will form the outer gray matter start centrally within the brain, and need to move outward to their final position. This process takes place in waves that occur from 8 to 16 weeks. The migration process is not complete until 25 weeks and electrical activity cannot be detected until 29 weeks. Even after this point, gray matter continues to mature and organize neural connections in the brain throughout the pregnancy. Your baby's body is now longer than her head for the first time.

**3D ultrasound scanning** uses computer technology to produce more detailed images than conventional 2D scans. This scan shows a 15-week-old fetus in the uterus. At this stage all of the organs are formed, as are the vocal cords.

### ASK A... DOCTOR

**Can using tanning beds and hot tubs harm my unborn baby?**
Tanning beds expose you to ultraviolet light which can prevent you from absorbing folic acid, which the baby needs for development. Also, it's been reported that a rise in the mother's temperature, which can happen on a tanning bed, in a hot tub or sauna, may increase the fetus's temperature. A temperature above 102° F (39° C) has been associated with spinal malformations in developing babies, and if a rise in temperature is maintained long enough, it may cause brain damage. The temperature of the amniotic fluid can also increase and it's thought that an extreme rise in your temperature can cause problems with the flow of blood to the baby. So avoid tanning beds and hot tubs while you're pregnant.

# 167 days to go...

## YOUR BABY TODAY

At this stage of development, your baby's lips and mouth are well formed, and she can open and close her mouth and swallow. Inside her mouth, her taste buds are now mature, but she cannot taste anything yet because nerve connections are immature.

## Since this is considered a safe stage of pregnancy, with no, or few, symptoms to contend with, it's a great time to go on vacation.

**At this time,** you're likely to be over the sickness and fatigue of the first trimester and not overburdened by, or uncomfortable from, a large belly yet. You can also rest easy knowing that your baby is developing well, with very little chance of a miscarriage occurring. Going on vacation is a great opportunity to spend quality time with your partner and pamper yourselves.

Relax and enjoy yourself, but be aware of the extra health precautions you need to take during pregnancy (see below and pp.28–9). If you've had any complications, check with your doctor that it is safe to go on vacation.

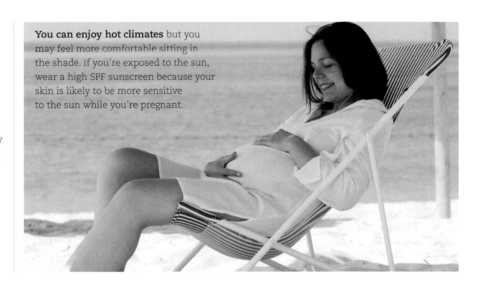

**You can enjoy hot climates** but you may feel more comfortable sitting in the shade. If you're exposed to the sun, wear a high SPF sunscreen because your skin is likely to be more sensitive to the sun while you're pregnant.

---

**FOCUS ON... SAFETY**

## Enjoy a healthy vacation

**If you go on vacation while you're pregnant,** there are a few additional factors to consider, not least the fact that you might not have as much energy as you had before:

■ **Give yourself plenty of time** when you're trying to finish all those pre-vacation preparations at home and at work; getting ready for a vacation can be stressful. Pack hand luggage for a flight sensibly so that you won't have to carry heavy bags with you.

■ **Plan a car trip carefully,** bearing in mind that you may need more bathroom stops or snack breaks than usual.

■ **Be aware that sightseeing** will be more tiring than usual, so pace yourself and allow yourself to spend time in a cafe, just watching the world go by.

■ **If you're abroad,** drink bottled water —lots of it, especially if you're in a hot climate. Avoid having ice in your drinks since this tends to be made using tap water.

■ **Peel fruit** or wash fruit and vegetables with bottled water.

■ **If you get diarrhea,** it's even more important than usual to drink plenty of water to replace the fluid you've lost. Don't take diarrhea medication and check with your doctor before taking any type of treatment for diarrhea. If your urine is very concentrated and you can't keep fluid down, see a doctor.

# 166 days to go...

**YOUR BABY TODAY**

In this color 2D ultrasound scan the baby is facing upward. The skull bones reflect the ultrasound beam most effectively and show as bright areas. The curved frontal bone of the forehead is seen just above the short nasal bone forming the bridge of the nose.

## Your baby is at his most mobile about now, and he may even be doing somersaults in your uterus.

Your second trimester

---

**ASK A... DOCTOR**

**What is DVT and am I at increased risk of it when I fly?**

DVT stands for deep vein thrombosis, a condition in which a blood clot forms in a deep leg vein. DVT partially or completely blocks the blood flow in the vein, causing pain and discomfort. The most serious form of DVT is a pulmonary embolism, when part of the clot breaks off and travels to the lungs, blocking a pulmonary artery. This can cause chest pain, shortness of breath, and blood-tinged phlegm to be coughed up. In severe cases, a pulmonary embolism can be fatal.

Pregnancy is considered to be a thrombotic condition, meaning it can lead to clots forming in blood vessels, so you are at increased risk of DVT even when you're not traveling by plane. Women who have previously had DVT or who are obese are more at risk of getting the condition.

Wearing support stockings (see p.225), drinking plenty of fluids, and moving around while flying can help prevent DVT. If you've had blood-clotting issues in the past, avoid flying at all during pregnancy.

---

**There are several ways in which your baby** can now move: he can curl and stretch his trunk, move his head up and down and from side to side, and move his arms and legs independently. Regular chest wall breathing movements occur, along with occasional hiccups. The mouth can open and shut, and your baby can yawn and swallow amniotic fluid. He'll bring his hands up to the face and prefer lying on his side rather than back. He has plenty of space in which to move.

Your baby's taste buds first appeared at 10 weeks and by now have an appearance very close to that of a mature taste bud. They also have their own nerve supply, connected to a branch of the facial nerve. Because these neural connections have not yet matured, it is too early for your baby to be able to taste anything.

---

**FOCUS ON... TWINS**

## How your babies interact

**By now, you may be starting to feel your twin babies move.** Contact between them probably began a few weeks ago, long before you knew

about it, and it becomes more complex as their brains develop. By this stage of pregnancy, a baby has the elementary brain circuits that help him feel the parts of his body and appreciate their position, so it's no wonder that your babies can now interact at a basic level.

Your babies will move around 50 times an hour and can touch each other, even though in all but a tiny percentage of cases they're in separate amniotic sacs so there's a membrane between them. Ultrasound studies show that twin babies make physical contact and sometimes react to each other's touch and pressure.

# 165 days to go...

**YOUR BABY TODAY**

This 3D scan is taken from a viewpoint above the baby's head and looking over the shoulder, but since the baby is curled up the face cannot be seen. The placenta is to the right of the image, with the umbilical cord over the baby's arm.

While you're pregnant, it's even more important to find ways to relieve stress and keep any worries in perspective.

## RELIEVING STRESS

**Learn to recognize the signs that you're stressed:** you may feel your heart racing or a rise in your body temperature. When you know you're stressed, take action.

■ **Identify the cause** and try to keep it in perspective. Let go of the stress by breathing deeply and relaxing your muscles. Imagine blowing the stress away as you exhale.

■ **Stay busy**—sometimes having too much time to think can make you more stressed.

■ **Go swimming:** it's a great stress reliever and a fantastic way to stay in shape, too.

■ **Take time to relax,** especially if you have a lot on your mind or are juggling lots of things. Put your feet up, watch TV, read a book, or think about your growing baby.

■ **Talk through your problems** with your partner or a close friend. If you're worrying about any aspect of your health or how your baby is developing, seek reassurance from your doctor.

■ **If work is an issue,** be honest with your boss or the human resources department and they may be able to help. Your most important job right now is to nurture your baby.

**You may be pregnant and happy,** but life goes on: you might still be working full time, as well as running a home, and you're bound to have stressful days and times when you feel you can't cope. And, of course, you're still contending with those challenging pregnancy hormones that can cause some emotional ups and downs.

Like many women, you may become stressed about the big changes that are going to happen, and worry about factors such as finances, whether you'll be a good mother, and how your relationship will change. It's important to keep worries in perspective and maintain an emotional balance because being stressed isn't good for your health or that of your baby.

Find ways to destress (see left), as well as talking to others—your partner, friends, and doctor—about any concerns.

### AS A MATTER OF FACT

**A mother's stress** can be transmitted to the fetus.

The level of the stress hormone cortisol in the amniotic fluid matches that in the mother's blood. Cortisol is thought to adversely affect fetal development.

# 164 days to go...

**YOUR BABY TODAY**

In this 2D ultrasound, the baby's head is to the left, with the arms not visible, although the knee and lower leg can be seen. At this stage, details of the brain developing under the skull are becoming much more apparent.

## Until you feel your baby move, hearing his heartbeat is the next best way for you to bond with him.

188

---

**ASK A PANEL ABOUT...** MONITORING YOUR BABY'S HEARTBEAT AT HOME

### My partner is eager to rent a handheld Doppler so we can listen to our baby's heartbeat. Do you think this is a good idea?

**Doctor:** Handheld ultrasound Doppler devices, which allow parents-to-be to listen to the fetal heartbeat at home, are currently sold over the counter in the US. Parents are told they can listen to their baby "in complete safety as early as 10 weeks of pregnancy" and "any time they want," implying there is no limit on frequency of exposure.

However, there has been no research into the effects of frequent scanning, which would be more than the baby receives during prenatal care. A Doppler is not a toy and using it in this way is an unnecessary risk.

**Midwife:** Using your own Doppler may help reassure you if you are very anxious about your baby's well-being, but it is just as likely to have the opposite effect if you can't pick up the heartbeat. Identifying different sounds takes practice and if you have difficulty finding the heartbeat (this happens to midwives, too!), it could be distressing. If you're worried about your baby for any reason, help and advice is only a phone call away.

**Mom:** I used a Doppler because I am a worrier and it really gave me peace of mind. I didn't use it very often and only when there was a good reason to. For example, at one stage of my pregnancy, I had an episode of bleeding and clots. After this, I was very worried about my baby's health and hearing his heartbeat really helped to calm me down, so it had benefits for the baby, too. I don't think a Doppler is a substitute for medical advice but it's a useful addition.

---

**At this stage of pregnancy,** your doctor may be able to hear your baby's heartbeat using a handheld Doppler ultrasound machine. Because ultrasound waves do not travel well in air, gel is applied to the end of the probe or "transducer" as it is placed on your abdomen. This then detects the heartbeat and converts it into a sound that we can hear.

It's quite easy to distinguish your baby's heartbeat from your own since it beats almost twice as fast. However, your baby's heart rate peaked around five weeks ago and, since then, has slowed down as the nerves controlling the heart's rhythm have matured.

During the second half of pregnancy, the range of the heartbeat is between 120 and 160 beats per minute and will be responsive to many stimuli, as well as to your baby's activity.

**AS A MATTER OF FACT**

**The baby's heart rate is** not an indication of gender.

A study in the mid-1990s, using over 10,000 measurements, dispelled the theory that the speed of a baby's heartbeat predicted whether it would be a boy or a girl.

# 163 days to go...

### YOUR BABY TODAY

The baby's face is partially obscured by the hand in this 3D image. Babies at this stage are small enough to fit onto the ultrasound screen, but beyond 20 weeks it is increasingly only possible to see a smaller part of the baby at any one time.

## Ensuring you drink enough fluids is essential to good health in pregnancy, so carry your bottle of water everywhere.

**Staying hydrated in pregnancy can be a challenge.** Because of the hormonal changes taking place, some of the fluid you take in leaks into your body tissues, rather than staying within the bloodstream.

It's difficult to recommend an exact amount of fluid that should be drunk to keep you hydrated, since this depends on many factors, such as the foods you eat (some naturally contain water), your size, the amount you exercise, and the heat and humidity in the environment. Therefore, you need to listen to your own body to determine if you're adequately hydrated. One of the best

ways to do this is to look at your urine. If it's clear to light yellow, you're adequately hydrated. If it's bright yellow or orange, you're likely to be dehydrated.

Drinking plenty of water is important. Sometimes, though, if you are nauseous, or just plain tired of drinking water, you may want to try other options for hydration, such as drinking juice or eating more fruit (see box, below). Remember that caffeinated beverages, such as coffee, are not hydrating;

caffeine has a diuretic effect, which means that you will want to urinate more often.

In the second and third trimester, dehydration in pregnancy can lead to premature contractions. This is because an anti-diuretic hormone is produced to help your body hold on to water. This hormone acts a lot like oxytocin, the hormone that triggers labor, causing contractions. Staying hydrated will prevent this from happening.

---

### FOCUS ON... NUTRITION

## Fabulous fruit

**One great way to stay hydrated** is to eat fruit. Many fruits are very high in water, especially melons, grapes, and strawberries. The water in fruit is very well absorbed in your body, because it comes partnered with sugar, which helps the water stay in your bloodstream.

In addition, fruit is highly nutritious and contains many of the vitamins and electrolytes that your body needs to stay in balance.

---

### ASK A... DOCTOR

**Should I stop picking up my toddler while I'm pregnant?** You may be experiencing some back pain and discomfort as your hormones begin to soften your ligaments. This means that your joints are less stable than usual, and injury is more likely.

Lifting your toddler will not harm your baby, but it may cause you discomfort, and you may be more likely to lose your balance. Ask your toddler to climb onto a chair so that you don't need to lift from bending position. To lift from floor level, squat down and use your legs to bear the weight. Avoid bending, which strains your back. Encourage your toddler to get onto your lap for a hug.

Your 17th week

189

# 162 days to go...

**YOUR BABY TODAY**

Your baby often brings his hands to his face and sometimes sucks his thumb at this stage; however, the sucking action is not well coordinated and the thumb is more likely to enter the mouth by luck than design. The arms are now in proportion with the rest of the body.

## Your baby is practicing his breathing movements, which are vital to develop his chest muscles and enable his lungs to grow.

**While he's in the uterus,** your baby is practicing his breathing movements and this also aids his lung development. When he breathes in, the diaphragm moves downward and the chest wall moves inward.

Each "breath" the baby takes lasts less than a second. Breathing might only happen occasionally at this stage and when it does it can be either regular or irregular.

Your baby might also open his jaw and swallow at the same time as making a breathing movement.

A single breathing movement with a large movement of the diaphragm may resemble a sigh.

For the chest wall movements to be effective, there must be adequate amniotic fluid (see p.182). This is especially true for the critical time of lung development, from 16–26 weeks.

By the 24th week of pregnancy, your baby will spend approximately three hours in a 24-hour period practicing breathing movements, and around eight hours in a 24-hour period in the last eight weeks of pregnancy.

**AS A MATTER OF FACT**

**When a pregnant woman smokes,** it reduces the number of times her baby practices breathing movements.

In a *British Medical Journal* research study, the proportion of time that the baby practiced breathing movements was found to fall within five minutes of the mother beginning to smoke her cigarette.

---

**FOCUS ON... TWINS**

### Growth rate

**While most unborn twins grow at much the same pace,** from now on some don't.

Your babies are almost certainly developing all the right organs at the right time, even when there's a size discrepancy. If, however, a scan detects a growth difference between your twins, you'll have additional scans to monitor growth. Lesser degrees aren't usually a problem. Doctors aren't usually concerned unless there's a growth difference of more than 15 percent.

**ASK A... DOCTOR**

**Why am I beginning to get brown patches on my face?** As many as 70 percent of pregnant women find the color of their skin changes. You may notice brown patches appearing on your forehead, cheeks, and neck, known as chloasma or the "mask of pregnancy." Darker-skinned women may develop lighter-colored patches.

Chloasma is caused by an increase in the production of melanin, the pigment that gives the skin and hair its natural color. It will gradually fade after the birth. To minimize the patches, stay out of the sun as much as possible, use a high protection

sunscreen, and wear a hat outdoors. Try covering larger patches with a tinted moisturizer or foundation and use concealer on smaller patches.

Your second trimester

190

# 161 days to go...

## YOUR BABY TODAY

Every part of your baby has an enhanced blood supply bringing nutrients for growth. Blood vessels are easy to see on scans because the skin is still quite transparent, with little fat yet deposited beneath the skin.

While your energy levels are at a peak, make the most of eating out but choose your meals wisely.

### STRONGER NAILS

**Your nails are likely to be stronger and healthier than ever,** due to the hormonal changes that occur during pregnancy.

Since your nails are in good condition, you can simply file them and they'll look nice even without nail polish. If you do decide to have a manicure, make sure it takes place in a well-ventilated room. Avoid using nail polishes that contain dibutyl phthalate (DBP), an ingredient that is linked to birth defects in animals.

**Being pregnant doesn't have to cramp your lifestyle,** and it's perfectly possible to eat out safely. You may, however, have to ask what's in particular dishes to avoid eating foods that aren't recommended during pregnancy, such as soft cheeses, shellfish, and raw eggs (see p.17).

Don't be afraid to ask questions about what exactly is in a dish and always request that your meat and fish are cooked to well done, to avoid any possible contamination. Check that all cheese and milk products, including yogurts, included in recipes, have been pasteurized.

You may find that fatty foods upset your stomach and cause heartburn (see p.194), and, if so, stick with foods that have been grilled or steamed, rather than fried. Beware of accompaniments such as pickles and chutneys that may not be entirely fresh. Pâtés and terrines should also be avoided.

### ASK A... NUTRITIONIST

**I'm a vegetarian but keep craving meat. Is this normal?** When you're pregnant, it's common for your body to crave things that might be missing from your diet. You may be craving meat because you are low in iron or protein, for example, both of which are required in higher quantities during pregnancy.

When you're pregnant, it's particularly important to ensure that you're getting the nutrients you need. If you don't eat meat, you can get iron from whole-grain cereals and flours, leafy green vegetables, molasses, legumes, such as lentils and kidney beans, and dried fruit, such as raisins, and apricots.

It helps to have a glass of orange juice, or another drink or food high in vitamin C, such as peppers and other citrus fruit, with your meals, since this encourages the absorption of iron.

Protein is also crucial to your baby's development. Legumes, whole grains, nuts, seeds, eggs, and dairy produce all contain good quantities of protein. Try adding some quinoa—a protein-packed grain—to your diet. Quinoa is a great alternative to rice and is one of the few plant sources of protein that contains all the essential amino acids. It's also high in omega oils, which will encourage the development of your baby's nervous system and brain.

# Your 18th week

**YOU'LL FIND YOU'RE GAINING WEIGHT WEEK BY WEEK, WHICH IS PERFECTLY NORMAL**

Not all the weight you're gaining is your baby. In fact, most of the increase is because parts of your body, such as your breasts, are getting bigger and your blood volume is increasing. You might want to think about signing up for prenatal classes now because they fill up quickly. They are a great source of information, as well as a good way to make friends and compare notes with other pregnant women.

**Your uterus** is likely to be large enough to give you a noticeably rounded belly.

**The baby's movements** are getting more vigorous and you may now be able to feel them.

**The placenta** is still growing, although not as fast as in earlier weeks. It continues to be a vital supply line for the baby.

**The sex organs** are developing well, both externally and internally. In baby girls, follicles containing immature eggs are already forming in the ovaries.

**At 18 weeks** the average crown to rump length is 4.6 in (11.6 cm) and the average weight is 3.5 oz (100 g).

**Your baby** is now bigger than the placenta for the first time, and will continue to outgrow it.

# 160 days to go...

## YOUR BABY TODAY

Your baby's jaw continues to grow throughout the pregnancy, but at this time it can still appear to be quite short. The early tooth buds are hardening within both jaws and, just as with the other bones, calcium is being laid down to strengthen their structure.

Around this time, you may become aware of your baby moving, although for some women first movements are felt much later.

**Although your baby is very active,** she's not big enough for you to feel any but the strongest kicks on the walls of your uterus. "Quickening" is the term used to describe these first movements, which feel like tiny flutterings or bubbles in your lower abdomen. You may not notice them or not realize that they are the baby at first, since they feel similar to having gas.

If you've been pregnant before, you will be more familiar with the sensation and able to recognize it. First-time moms generally don't feel movements until a bit later, at about 18 to 20 weeks (see p.213), so don't worry if you haven't felt anything yet. The flutterings become more persistent and definite over time, and there will eventually be recognizable kicks and nudges.

Once you can feel the activity, you will become very conscious of them and may become aware of a pattern to them.

**At around this time,** you may begin to feel some slight sensations when your baby moves around.

### THE LOWDOWN

## That funny feeling

**Was it gas, or did your baby move?** The first time you notice your baby moving marks the start of a new chapter in the bonding process, and it seems it has always been the case, even in ancient times.

In many cultures, until the advent of pregnancy tests, "quickening" was the first conclusive evidence of pregnancy, and was viewed as the point at which human life began.

According to ancient Egyptian, Greek, American, and Indian beliefs, the first movement marked the moment when the soul entered the fetus. Aboriginals regard the location where the first quickening is felt as highly significant for the baby.

### FOCUS ON... DADS

## Being patient

**It will be exciting when your partner tells you** she can feel the baby move and a great milestone of the pregnancy, but when you touch your partner's belly, you won't feel anything at all. Just be a little patient since there will be plenty of opportunities later on in the pregnancy to feel the movements. Meanwhile, keep talking to your baby—she can hear you!

### AS A MATTER OF FACT

**Babies are rocked to sleep** by their mother's movements.

This is why you're less likely to feel your baby move when you're active. You're also likely to be distracted yourself and miss some movement.

YOU ARE 17 WEEKS AND 2 DAYS

# 159 days to go...

## YOUR BABY TODAY

Here, the baby's legs are in the typical crossed-legs position. The right arm is on the right side of the image. The limbs and umbilical cord appear to be in a tangle, but the umbilical cord is filled with a jellylike fluid and does not become compressed.

## The tiny embryo was once dwarfed by the placenta but now your baby has outgrown it and will continue to do so.

**In the early stages of pregnancy, the placenta grew** at a far greater rate than your baby. Your baby has now caught up and from now on will be larger than the placenta.

The structure of the placenta will change over the course of the next few weeks as the second wave of cells move into the spiral arteries in the uterus

(see p.172). The placenta is currently at its thickest but as it continues to grow, albeit at a slower rate for a time, it thins out.

Your baby's more rapid growth means that at 2.5 oz (70 g) she is now heavier than the placenta and by the time she is full term she will be six or seven times its weight. Nutrients supplied across the

placenta provide your baby with energy for growth, but growth is in part regulated by her own insulin production and insulin-like growth factors.

Although your baby has relatively high concentrations of growth hormone, which is responsible for growth after birth, this does not seem to play an important role in her growth during pregnancy.

FOCUS ON... HEALTH

## Tackling heartburn

**If you're battling with the burning sensation** and sour taste of heartburn, try these solutions:
■ Eat smaller meals, and ensure you chew your food well
■ Avoid foods that aggravate your symptoms, such as spicy, rich, and fatty dishes
■ Don't smoke or drink alcohol
■ Drink milk
■ Wear loose-fitting clothing
■ Chew gum after eating, except for mint varieties
■ Remain upright after meals; bending can increase discomfort
■ Don't eat 2 to 3 hours before going to bed
■ Raise the head of your bed by 6 in and lie on your left side.

**The baby is in a typical position**, curled with feet and elbows bent. The well-developed ear is still a little low on the side of the head at this point, and the baby's blood vessels show up well.

# 155 days to go...

## YOUR BABY TODAY

In this image the whole baby is seen in one view. The legs, held straight, will now be kicking more strongly and, especially if you have had a baby before, you will be increasingly aware of these movements over the next few weeks.

## You might want to think about signing up for prenatal classes now since in many areas they get filled up well in advance.

**Prenatal classes help to prepare you** for the birth of your baby. They usually start in the sixth or seventh month. You'll learn about the signs that you're in labor; breathing and relaxation techniques; pain-relief options; and medical interventions. You'll also be given practical advice on caring for your newborn baby, which can be invaluable if you're a first-time parent.

Depending on where you live, there are various types of classes. These range from classes run by a nurse or other certified instructor at the hospital or classes run by organizations like Lamaze International (lamaze.org) or the Bradley Method (bradleybirth.com). Classes are a great way to meet other expectant parents, and by doing so you'll gain an invaluable mutual support system through the rest of your pregnancy and the early weeks of parenting.

By attending prenatal classes with you, your partner can help to prepare for the labor and early weeks of parenting. Classes are also a good way for your partner to meet other dads-to-be. The significant role fathers can play during labor and in the early weeks of parenting is widely acknowledged, and as a result prenatal classes have become much more father-friendly.

**By going to classes,** you and your partner can practice and feel more confident about the techniques you'll use in labor.

### FOCUS ON... TWINS

## Classes for two

**Since twins are likely to arrive** ahead of schedule, you should definitely look into signing up for prenatal classes now so that you can start them early. Besides, your belly could be very large toward the end, and you may feel less mobile and inclined to go. Because twins sometimes need special care, you should arrange a tour of the Neonatal Intensive Care Unit too.

In some areas, there are special prenatal sessions for those having twins or more, often in the evenings. If your hospital doesn't provide these, a neighboring hospital might. Ask your doctor.

### FIND A CLASSMATE

**If you're single, you don't have to go it alone.** There's no reason why you can't go to a class with a friend or relative—preferably the person who will be attending the birth. If you'd prefer not to do this, you could find out if there are any classes in your area for single expectant moms. You may feel more comfortable in this environment and you will get the opportunity to meet other women who are in the same position as you.

Don't skip classes just because you're single: they're an invaluable way of learning about pregnancy, labor, and parenting.

Your 18th week

# 154 days to go...

## YOUR BABY TODAY

Like your own ear, your baby's ear is made of soft and flexible cartilage. Although the outer ear is well developed at this stage, inner ear structures will not be mature enough to enable your baby to hear for about another five weeks.

Is it a boy or a girl? You and your partner may want to start thinking about whether you would like to find out.

**The sex of your baby should now be apparent** on an ultrasound scan, but you may not have this for a couple of weeks yet (see p.211).

Whether your baby develops into a boy or a girl depends on the presence or absence of a Y chromosome. Males are

**Some pregnant women** will want to delay buying a complete set of clothes for the baby until they know the sex, but not everyone wants to settle for either pink or blue.

XY and the Y chromosome instructs the reproductive glands (gonads) to become testes. These then produce testosterone and other hormones that inhibit the development of the female organs and in turn stimulate the normal development of the external male genitalia.

If there is no Y chromosome, the gonad becomes an ovary and the internal genitals are female by default; it's not the ovary that dictates that the female reproductive organs will develop but the lack of testosterone. In the female the uterus is formed first and the vagina lengthens upward to meet it.

### THINK ABOUT: GENDER

**Many women** have a strong opinion about whether or not they want to find out the sex of their baby at the 20-week ultrasound, but others are ambivalent. If your partner has strong feelings one way or the other, you can choose to follow his lead. Otherwise, try to figure out your feelings by deciding if you want to choose two names (boy and girl) and get mostly yellow and green baby clothing at your shower, or if identifying with the baby's gender will make these upcoming baby tasks more enjoyable for you.

### ASK A... MOM

**Our 20-week scan is fast approaching. I want to know the baby's sex but my husband doesn't. What should we do?**
When one person in a relationship wants something that is at odds with what his or her partner wants, tensions can arise.

Like you, I wanted to find out the sex of my baby but my partner didn't. We both explained our reasons: I felt that knowing the sex would better help me prepare for the birth, both emotionally and practically; my partner said he wanted the surprise element of discovering the sex of the baby at the actual birth.

Talk to each other openly and hopefully you'll be able to reach an agreement. Try not to let the issue get out of hand and consider backing down if necessary. It's important that you feel united at this special time.

You may find either one of you doesn't feel as strongly once you start talking. You could agree to find out but not tell anyone else. If you do find out, don't forget the result is not 100 percent accurate.

**The umbilical cord** is growing thicker and stronger as it continues to transport blood and nutrients to your growing baby. Your baby is now bigger and heavier than the placenta.

# Your 19th week

**YOU'LL PROBABLY FIND YOU'RE BECOMING MORE ATTACHED TO YOUR BABY EACH DAY**

It's easier now to think of your baby as a real person, especially if you see him on another scan around this time. He's almost fully formed and the function of his organs is well advanced. You'll be taking your maternal responsibilities very seriously, but don't let anxieties build up. Talk over any worries you may have with your partner and your doctor; many pregnant women also seek comfort and advice from their own mothers.

**The top of your uterus** is now level with your belly button.

**On the pads of the fingers** the ridged pattern of the baby's fingerprints, his personal badge of identity, is becoming apparent.

**A little fat** has started to cover the baby's body but he still looks very skinny and his head appears too large for his fragile neck.

**The eyes** make random movements under the still-closed lids.

**At 19 weeks** the average crown to rump length is 5.1 in (13 cm) and the average weight is 4.9 oz (140 g).

**The ears** have moved up from the jaw line to their final position on the side of the head; the eyes too are now in their final position, and face forward.

# 153 days to go...

**YOUR BABY TODAY**

Anchored to the placenta by the umbilical cord, your baby floats in amniotic fluid. Your uterus provides a warm, protective environment for your baby with lots of room to move in near weightless conditions.

As you approach the halfway mark of your pregnancy, you'll continue to be astounded that there's a baby growing inside you!

**The further along the path of pregnancy you are,** the more attached and protective you're likely to feel toward your baby. What was once a tiny bundle of cells now looks like an almost fully formed baby—and you will continue to be amazed that you and your partner have made that baby and that this incredible process is happening inside your body.

Once you feel your baby move (see p.213) within the next few weeks, the attachment to him is likely to grow even stronger. While you may have some anxieties at times, try to relax and enjoy your pregnancy—it will be over before you know it.

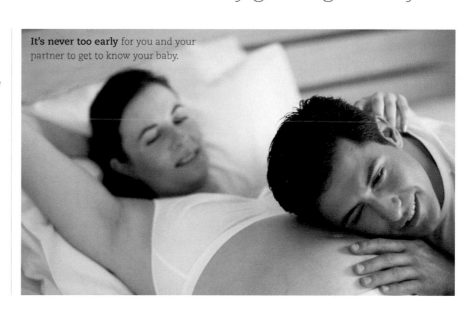

It's never too early for you and your partner to get to know your baby.

---

**ASK A... DOCTOR**

I have a high-powered career and have hardly had any time to think about the baby since I've been pregnant. Will this stop us from bonding? Even if you work full time while you're pregnant, this doesn't have to have a negative effect on your relationship with your baby. As your baby grows, you will probably find that you start to develop a relationship with your "belly" as you anticipate your baby's movements and perhaps talk to him. Make sure you plan enough maternity leave before your due date since this gives you time for practical and emotional preparations, as well as time to rest.

There's some evidence to suggest that too much stress in a mother can affect her unborn baby's brain development (see p.187). This highlights the importance of ensuring you have regular opportunities to relax during pregnancy and so, if your work is stressful, maybe this would be a good time to look at your priorities.

---

**FOCUS ON... HEALTH**

## It's all a blur

**Water retention in pregnancy** can affect the eyes. Both the lens and cornea can become thicker, and there can be an increase in fluid in the eyeball, causing pressure and blurred vision. This usually resolves itself after the birth. Exercising to keep the fluid moving, and avoiding wearing contact lenses can help. Notify your doctor if you have vision problems.

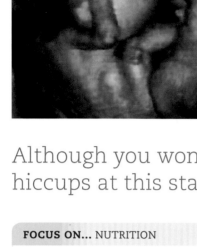

# 152 days to go...

**YOUR BABY TODAY**

The sound of your baby's rapidly moving heart muscle can be detected using a simple handheld listening device—the frequency change it produces is converted into a sound that is easy for you and your doctor to hear.

Although you won't feel it yet, your baby may start to have hiccups at this stage of his development.

**FOCUS ON... NUTRITION**

## Not all fat is bad

**Many fats are healthy, and should be consumed** as part of a heart-healthy diet. The key is to choose healthy fat. For example unsaturated fats, such as those found in olive oil, canola oil, and in nuts and avocados, are good for you and your baby.

Saturated fats, such as those found in butter and whole milk, and trans fats (chemically altered vegetable oils) found in many processed foods, should be kept to a minimum. Substitute good fats for bad fats in your diet:

■ **When making a salad dressing** or in cooking, choose olive oil or canola oil. Store-bought salad dressings are often high in saturated fat.

■ **Eat nuts and avocados,** which are full of healthy fats.

■ **Eat white meat** since it is lower in saturated fat than red meat.

**At around this time,** your baby may start to hiccup. Just like your own, his hiccup is a short, powerful, jerky contraction of his diaphragm, which will last for less than a second.

Hiccups frequently follow each other in rapid succession and are often followed by gentle limb-stretching movements. No one is certain why babies hiccup. Perhaps it's due to the immaturity of the nerves supplying the diaphragm, or else to your baby's small stomach quickly becoming overdistended.

Your baby's ears and eyes are now in their final position on his face. The ears have moved up from the jaw line and the eyes have moved from the side of the head to lie closer together, looking forward. The eyes move beneath the lids but not yet in a coordinated way. He will open them at around 26 weeks.

**Your baby is looking more human and fully formed** every day, with well-developed facial features and limbs—and he may even get the hiccups.

# 151 days to go...

## YOUR BABY TODAY

Coiling is now well established in the umbilical cord. This coiling protects the cord from kinking and from pressing on the umbilical arteries and vein. The coils help ensure that there is a continuous flow of blood both to the placenta and also back to the baby.

Wanting to protect your baby is a natural maternal instinct and it's likely to have started already.

**It's understandable that you want your baby** to have the best start in life, but this may lead you to unnecessary anxiety about his health and well-being.

You may find yourself worried about things that previously did not bother you. For example, you may use a computer regularly and only now become concerned about the radiation it might produce (see box, right).

Try to relax and keep concerns in perspective; remember that your baby is very resilient and well-protected inside the uterus. If you have concerns about lifestyle issues or how your baby is developing, your doctor can provide information and reassurance.

Meanwhile, you can take good care of yourself by eating well, exercising regularly, and attending all your prenatal appointments.

### AS A MATTER OF FACT

**There is no significant radiation** from a computer that can affect an unborn baby.

Many studies have been done to examine the low-level radiation that computers and laptops emit, but they've found computers to be safe.

### ASK A... DOCTOR

**What are the risks if I gain too much weight?** Pregnant women who overeat tend to have larger babies, which can make the delivery more difficult (the baby is more likely to get stuck during the birth) and increase the likelihood of having a cesarean section.

Pregnant women who are overweight are also more likely to experience health complications, such as gestational diabetes (see p.473) and preeclampsia (see p.474). Their children may be at greater risk of becoming diabetic and being obese in later life.

Most of the research seems to focus on pregnant women who have gained more than 40 lb (18 kg).

**Taking care of your baby** will become your main concern and there's unlikely to be a day that goes by where you don't consider your baby's well-being.

YOU ARE 18 WEEKS AND 4 DAYS

# 150 days to go...

## YOUR BABY TODAY

This is a side view ultrasound scan with the baby's head in the top left. Your baby appears completely human with all fingers and toes fully developed. The skin is now covered with lanugo, fine protective hair.

There's no harm in encouraging your baby to move to increase the likelihood of you feeling his wiggles.

**If you're waiting to feel your baby's first movements,** be patient. Although it's reassuring to feel him wiggling around, becoming stressed about it won't be good for either of you. Remember, many pregnant women—first-time moms especially—don't feel those first flutterings until 18 to 20 weeks or later. Also remember that while you're awake, your baby spends a lot of time sleeping.

There are a few ways you can try to stimulate your baby into action—the more he moves, the more chance there is that you'll feel it. First of all, stop and relax. If you've been busy all day, you may have been distracted and not felt your baby's movements. Keeping still may also waken him, since he isn't being "rocked" within your uterus.

Try playing loud music to him, which will not only wake him, but also encourage him to respond. Some women report that their unborn babies "kicked" to a rhythm!

It may also help to lie down on your side, with your belly supported. Doing this may stimulate your baby to move, as he changes his position to accommodate yours. If all else fails, have a sweet, icy cold drink, which may do the trick.

### ASK A... DOCTOR

**My baby seems to "jump" when he hears loud noises—is this likely or am I imagining it?**
Yes, this is common. Research has shown that a baby can react to sounds in the uterus from as early as nine weeks' gestation.

Premature babies react to sounds with a "startle reflex," so this provides strong evidence that babies in the uterus will hear and react to loud sounds, too, possibly with sudden movements.

**You will probably not be able** to feel your baby move yet, but he is incredibly active inside your uterus. Somersaults and stretches

are part of his daily routine, as are thumb and toe sucking. Your baby moves when awake and asleep: he has no control over his

movements at this stage. Ultrasound scans reveal a huge range of movement in between inactive periods.

Your second trimester

# 149 days to go...

**YOUR BABY TODAY**

Your baby's hands—and feet—look quite large at this stage in pregnancy: it is as if your baby needs time to grow into them. The past few weeks have seen rapid changes in the hands and feet and it's now time for the limbs to catch up.

## Your baby's fingers and toes are fully developed and their unique prints are beginning to form.

**Your baby will be a unique individual** and his fingerprints will be proof of this. The ridge patterns in the dermis that will eventually form fingerprints (and "toeprints") are fully developed by this stage of pregnancy. These skin ridges are genetically determined and, as with most developments, are seen about a week earlier in the hands than the feet.

Your baby's sweat glands appeared in his skin in the eighth week, and will continue to increase up to 28 weeks; but they do not function until after birth. The color of your baby's skin is due to melanin, a pigment produced by "melanocytes," specialized skin cells that have now migrated into the skin. Different skin tones are not due to differing numbers of these cells but due to the amount and shade of pigment that each cell produces. Melanin protects the skin from ultraviolet light which damages DNA.

Although unborn babies produce melanin pigment, they do not achieve their final amount of skin pigment until well into childhood. For this reason it follows that all newborn babies are particularly vulnerable to sunburn. Dark-skinned babies are likely to have a light skin tone when they're born.

---

**AS A MATTER OF FACT**

**Eating plenty of foods that are rich in vitamin E** could reduce the risk of your baby developing allergies, including asthma.

Researchers believe that low levels of vitamin E during pregnancy could adversely affect your baby's lung development or immune system. To boost your intake, improve your diet rather than taking supplements. If you eat more than you need, vitamin E is stored in the body for future use.

---

**ACUPUNCTURE**

**In acupuncture, certain points on the body** associated with energy channels or meridians are stimulated by the insertion of fine needles. The belief is that these conduct vital energy or "qi" around the body. Illness or symptoms are associated with an imbalance of this vital energy.

Acupuncture has been widely and successfully used in pregnancy and regular treatments can help to treat a number of health problems:
■ Pain and nausea—a recent study has shown it to be effective in relieving nausea and vomiting or the potentially more dangerous hyperemesis gravidarum (see p.111).
■ Heartburn (see p.194)
■ Hemorrhoids (see p.468)
■ Stress (see p.187)
■ Headaches and backaches
■ Carpal tunnel syndrome (see p.471).

Acupuncture may be effective in "turning" breech babies (see p.433), and can also be used during labor to boost energy and relieve pain.

Use a registered practitioner with experience treating pregnant women.

**Boost your intake of vitamin E** by eating salad greens, green leafy vegetables, nuts, avocados, eggs, and wheatgerm.

# 148 days to go...

### YOUR BABY TODAY

Your baby appears to be quite thin on early scans. Fat reserves are not yet laid down underneath the skin, which can seem quite thin and almost transparent. An ultrasound image also highlights the underlying bony skeleton, enhancing this effect.

## At around this time you'll have another scan, and your baby will get a thorough health checkup.

**From 18–20 weeks most doctors' offices or hospitals** offer a detailed ultrasound scan, which is termed an "anatomy" scan. The scan is used to check the baby's overall development and examine his organs and body systems (see pp.214–5) to check for signs of problems. For most women and their partners, this scan will reassure them that all is progressing well with the baby's development.

The scan can take some time to perform because of the detailed measurements and investigations taking place. The sonographer can only do the checks when the baby is in the correct position—this can be a challenge, given that the baby is likely to be moving around a lot. If the position of your baby makes it difficult to do all the checks, you may be asked to walk around for a little while and then return, or even to come back in a week or two for another attempt.

### EXERCISING IN WATER

**Water is a great environment to work out in during pregnancy:** the added support for your belly and extra resistance will enable you to maintain your fitness.

When standing, the water should be just above your waist—too deep and you will not be stable enough and too shallow and you won't get enough support from the water.

You are likely to find pregnancy water aerobics classes at your local gym, but here are a few simple exercises you can do yourself:

■ **Running in place:** bring your knees up and push your arms forward and back in a pumping motion. Run for 3–4 minutes, if possible, but always stop if you feel tired. This exercise has cardiovascular benefits, and will help tone your legs and arms.

■ **Bicycle exercise:** stand in the water and place a float under each arm. Once you're comfortable, lean back slightly and move your legs in front of you as if you are rotating the pedals on a bicycle. Continue the cycling motion for 3–4 minutes, if possible, but always stop if you feel tired. This exercise will help you maintain your fitness and help tone your legs. It's also a good way to strengthen your back and arms.

■ **Arm exercises:** stand with your feet apart and knees slightly bent, then crouch to submerge your shoulders in the water. Lift your arms from your sides to the height of your shoulders and back down again. Pull your arms down in the water toward you and push up as hard as you can (see right). This exercise will help tone and strengthen the muscles in your arms, back, and abdomen.

Your second trimester

# 147 days to go...

**YOUR BABY TODAY**

Your baby has highly flexible joints, enabling her to raise her arms high. This is because her bones are first made of cartilage, which is soft and flexible. Gradually, the cartilage is being replaced by calcium-containing bone.

You'll be getting advice from all quarters, but there's one person you might want to listen to—your mother.

## FOCUS ON... YOUR BODY

### Taking the strain

**There are a number of changes in your body during pregnancy** that impact how you can exercise and how your body moves:

■ **The increased weight** of your baby, placenta, extra blood, enlarged uterus, and breast tissue can cause stress on your body, and most notably on your skeleton.

■ **Postural changes** due to changes in the center of gravity can increase your chances of developing hip, back, and knee problems.

■ **Relaxin** (see p.197), a pregnancy-related hormone that affects the ligaments, can increase flexibility and result in improper alignment of the spine and pelvis.

Effective and safe exercises are the most efficient way of maintaining and improving your posture and minimizing the stress on your body (see p.196 for a great second trimester workout).

Regular exercise (especially weight bearing exercise such as walking, and using weights—see p.196) generally improves the bone density of your skeleton.

**Whether or not you're already close to your mother,** being pregnant is likely to affect your relationship with each other. Many women feel naturally closer to their mothers as they go through this significant life event, turning to them for help and reassurance during the course of pregnancy and wanting them to be there in the days and weeks following the birth of the baby.

It's normal for a mother to respond to her daughter being pregnant by being very protective, so expect a few more phone calls than usual. Your mother is bound to offer lots of advice. Whether or not you take it all in, listen—you may just find some of it useful.

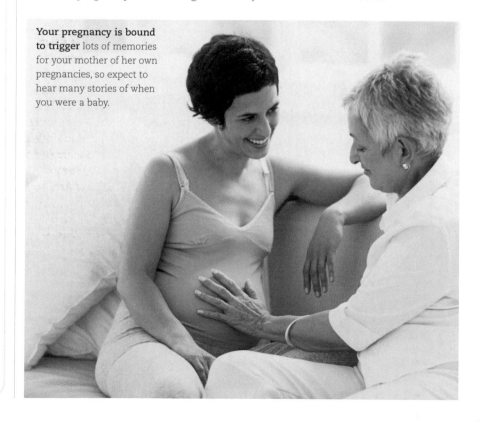

**Your pregnancy is bound to trigger** lots of memories for your mother of her own pregnancies, so expect to hear many stories of when you were a baby.

# Your 20th week

**THOSE BUTTERFLIES IN YOUR STOMACH MAY BE MORE THAN JUST GAS**

In the next few days, you might feel your baby's movements for the first time. The little flutter can be such a tiny sensation that many women write it off as gas. But what a wonderful moment when you realize the truth! If you want to find out the sex of your baby, it could be revealed on the ultrasound scan you have this week.

**Tooth buds**, for both the milk teeth and the underlying permanent teeth, are now in place under the gums.

**Abdominal organs**, including the stomach, intestines, and liver, are fully enclosed within the abdominal cavity.

**At 20 weeks** the average crown to heel length is 8.7 in (22 cm) and the average weight is 6.7 oz (190 g).

**The eyebrows** have thickened and are clearly visible.

**The baby's body** has a covering of fine hair, called lanugo hair. Most of this hair disappears before birth, although it may still be present in very premature babies.

**The spine** is now quite straight. Your 20-week scan will reveal each vertebra.

YOU ARE 19 WEEKS AND 1 DAY

# 146 days to go...

**YOUR BABY TODAY**

This image shows the entire baby lying within the amniotic sac. Every finger and toe, and even the lower ribs in the chest, can be seen. Although the head is still quite large, the limbs are much more in proportion with the body.

If you want to know whether you're having a boy or a girl, this is the week you might be able to find out.

**You'll have a scan this week**
and may be given the opportunity to find out the sex of your baby. Identifying the gender is dependent on a number of factors, including the expertise of the sonographer, the quality of the equipment being used, the position of the baby and, specifically, of the legs, which could obstruct the genitals. Even if all of these factors are favorable and the genitals can be seen, there is an error factor, so the information given is never 100 percent accurate. You may be able

to identify the genitals yourself as you're watching the screen, so if you don't want to know, it's advisable to look away.

If you have an amniocentesis test (see pp.152–3) and want to know the sex of your baby, it can be identified with close to 100 percent accuracy.

**This 2D scan** is a close-up of the baby's profile, showing the bright frontal bone of the forehead, the nose, lips, and chin. The nasal bone appears as a bright area at the top of the bridge of the nose.

**TIME TO THINK ABOUT**

## Finding out the sex of your baby

Is it a good idea to find out the sex of your baby before he (or she) is born?

**Yes...**
■ **Being able to call your baby** "he" or "she" rather than "it" or "the baby" may help you and your partner to bond with him or her.
■ **Knowing the sex** means you can choose a name before the big day, although bear in mind that it's not guaranteed to suit him or her.
■ **Decorating the nursery** and buying baby clothes may be simpler.

**No...**
■ **Not knowing is a huge motivator** during labor and birth for many women, and the excitement of finding out right at the end can help keep you focused through all the stages of labor and delivery.
■ **Remember that unless you had** an amniocentesis test or CVS test (see pp.152–3), there's no way of knowing your baby's sex for certain. Sonographers can (and do) get it wrong, so don't get too attached just yet to the name you've chosen.

Your 20th week

211

YOU ARE 19 WEEKS AND 2 DAYS

# 145 days to go...

**YOUR BABY TODAY**

Your baby is increasingly using her hands and feet to explore her surroundings. All limbs have a full and unobstructed range of movements and the fingertips especially are extremely sensitive. Most of her movements are reflex responses at this stage.

Comfortably floating in her fluid-filled amniotic sac, your baby is made up almost completely of water.

**Pregnant women used to believe** that not drinking enough water would make the baby dirty!

While it is important to stay hydrated during pregnancy, the amniotic fluid is not affected by what you drink.

**Because water can travel through the skin** and the baby is floating in amniotic fluid, her water content is really high, nearly 90 percent. As your baby's skin thickens and becomes less permeable, and her kidneys better regulate the amount of water lost in the urine, her proportion of water will reduce to 70 percent at delivery and again to about 60 percent

by the age of 10 as kidney function continues to improve.

Fluids conduct sound waves but the inner ear is still immature and it will be three weeks before a startle response to sounds can be reliably seen on a scan. As both the uterine wall and the ear drums become thinner, she will gradually respond to higher frequencies and quieter sounds.

**FOCUS ON... YOUR BABY**

## Low-lying placenta

**Placenta previa is when the placenta** is either partially covering (minor) or completely covering (major) the cervix. In major placenta previa, the baby cannot be born vaginally. Major/complete placenta previa poses a high risk of heavy bleeding, either in the later stages of pregnancy or during the actual labor, which is treated as an emergency.

If a low-lying placenta is detected at your 20-week scan, you may be offered another scan at about 34 weeks; the placenta may "move up" as the uterus grows, and by about 34 weeks no longer be low. With major placenta previa, you may be admitted to the hospital for bed rest in late pregnancy.

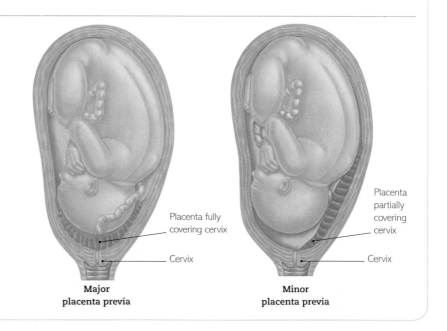

Placenta fully covering cervix

Cervix

Placenta partially covering cervix

Cervix

**Major placenta previa**

**Minor placenta previa**

# 144 days to go...

### YOUR BABY TODAY

The toes will wiggle and stretch just as much as the hands and fingers. Your baby is extremely flexible at this time and as likely to bring one or both feet up to her mouth as she is her hands in order to explore them with her sensitive mouth and lips.

Are you feeling your baby kicking? She's letting you know she's definitely in there—a wonderful pregnancy milestone.

**At around this time, you're likely to feel that awe-inspiring first kick**. While your baby has been moving in your uterus since around the sixth week of gestation, it's only at this stage that she'll make her movements so definitely felt (although some women do feel movements from around 15 to 16 weeks). When exactly you feel that movement can be affected by your body weight, your baby's position, the location of your placenta, and whether it's your first pregnancy.

Experiencing the first sensation of movement, whether it's a feeling of bubbles, butterflies, flipping goldfish, or even a resounding kick, is likely to be an emotionally charged moment. After all, this is the first time your baby has communicated with you, even though she's not aware of what she's doing.

Once you've felt your baby move, you may want her to do it again—just to make sure you didn't imagine it. You may, however, not feel another movement for a few days. Your partner may want to rest his hand on your belly when your baby is most active (usually when you're resting so that your baby isn't being rocked to sleep by movement) to experience those first thumps himself. It won't hurt your baby to play with her, so gently press on your abdomen when she kicks.

---

### MATERNITY SWIMWEAR

**Swimming is fantastic exercise** during pregnancy, but you may need to invest in new swimwear as your breasts and abdomen grow.

■ **Comfort and support:** maternity swimsuits have additional support. These swimsuits are designed to be higher at the back and have more support in the cups. Maternity swimwear is made with stretchy fabric that is comfortable and will give as you grow.

■ **Try a tankini:** this is a two-piece swimsuit that has a tank-style, rather than bra, top. It will flash your belly without revealing too much.

■ **If you're self-conscious** about your belly, wear a sarong. If you prefer to bare your belly to females only, go to women's sessions at your local pool.

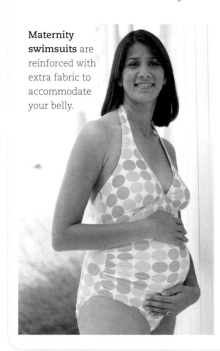

**Maternity swimsuits** are reinforced with extra fabric to accommodate your belly.

**Maternity bikinis** are designed with a generous cup size, and the bottoms fit neatly under your belly.

# Your 20-week scan

This second-trimester ultrasound, typically done between 18–22 weeks, looks in detail at how your baby's major organs and body systems have developed, as well as checking the placenta and the volume of the amniotic fluid.

## YOUR BABY'S CHECKUPS

### What the ultrasound looks at

During this scan, your baby's organs are examined in detail and therefore it can take a little longer to perform than previous scans. For most, the scan provides reassurance that their baby is developing normally. The following areas will be checked.

■ **The brain**, including the fluid-filled spaces inside the brain and the shape of the back of your baby's brain (cerebellum).

■ **The spine**, to check for spina bifida or other problems.

■ **The upper lip**, to check for cleft lip (see p.476).

■ **The heart**, to rule out any major heart malformations. The heartbeat will be checked too.

■ **The stomach** and diaphragm.

■ **The kidneys and bladder**, making sure that both kidneys are present and there are no blockages or malformations.

■ **The abdominal wall**, to look for a defect, known as gastroschisis.

■ **Your baby's limbs**, to make sure there are no hand or feet malformations, such as club foot.

■ **The umbilical cord**, to check that this has a normal number of blood vessels.

## What the scan reveals

By 20 weeks, your baby's organs and body systems are well developed and can be seen clearly on an ultrasound scan. The sonographer performing the scan will look closely at how your baby's major organs and body systems have formed and whether there are any indications of a problem (see box, left). In the majority of cases, the scan will reassure women that their baby is developing normally.

If your baby is found to have a problem, the sonographer will refer you to a maternal medicine expert who will confirm the findings and offer follow-up scans throughout the rest of your pregnancy. He or she will also talk to a pediatrician to ensure that they have enough information to take care of your baby at birth.

**A picture of your 20-week scan** shows the incredible detail visible on an ultrasound at this stage of your pregnancy.

## Your due date

If you had a scan in the first trimester, your dates are unlikely to be changed after a second trimester scan. This is because dating is most accurate in early pregnancy when all babies essentially grow at the same rate. Later on, individual differences in growth start to appear, making it harder to tell if your baby is just big for dates or if you are further along than thought.

However, if you didn't have a first trimester scan, the sonographer may change your dates if your baby is 10–14 days smaller or larger than expected. If your dates have been confirmed by a first trimester scan, a substantial lag may be a sign of a growth problem in your baby (see p.284), although this is rare.

**Measuring your baby** Because your whole baby no longer fits on the screen, the crown–rump length won't be measured. Instead, your baby's size will be calculated by combining a series of measurements in a mathematical formula. The sonographer will measure the width (biparietal diameter) and circumference of your baby's head, the circumference of your baby's tummy (abdominal circumference), and the length of your baby's upper leg bone (femur length). These measurements help estimate the size of your baby and check that this is within the normal range for this stage of pregnancy.

## Placenta and amniotic fluid

The placenta will be examined to ensure that it appears normal and isn't blocking the baby's exit route (the cervix). It's quite common in early

## HOW THE SCAN IS INTERPRETED

**During your ultrasound, a picture of your baby is produced** when high-frequency sound waves bounce off your baby and translate into an image on screen. In this image, solid matter, such as bones, are white, while softer tissue appears gray. Areas that contain fluid, such as blood vessels or the stomach, as well as the amniotic fluid, do not respond to the sound waves and therefore appear as black areas on the scan. The sonographer will study these details to assess how your baby is developing in the uterus.

The skull is well developed by now, and features such as the ears are clearly seen.

The leg bones are measured to assess how your baby is growing.

The four chambers of the heart can be identified and certain defects spotted.

Each vertebra in your baby's spine will be counted to check for spina bifida.

for example, because you are over 35 years of age, or were given a high risk from a previous screening test. Common markers include a bright spot in your baby's heart, seen in about 1–2 percent of normal babies; extra fluid in your baby's kidneys; short leg or arm bones; thickened neck skin (nuchal fold); and bright (echogenic) fetal intestines.

Some specific abnormalities are linked with a far higher risk of Down syndrome or other chromosomal abnormalities. These include certain kinds of heart defects and other major malformations, such as abnormalities in the spleen.

**What happens next** If the sonographer detects soft markers, he or she will discuss the findings and may suggest a diagnostic test (see p.152), especially if you already have an increased risk of Down syndrome. However, an earlier all-clear from a diagnostic test means that you can be confident your baby's chromosomes are normal. If an obvious abnormality is seen, and you haven't had a diagnostic test, this will probably be strongly advised. Having information from the scan will help you decide whether you want to proceed with a test. Whatever your decision, any associated abnormalities will be monitored throughout your pregnancy.

---

pregnancy for the placenta to be low-lying and to cover the cervix, but in 95 percent of cases, the placenta moves up and out of the way by the third trimester as the uterus grows. If your placenta is low lying, your doctor will arrange a follow-up scan later in pregnancy to check that the placenta has moved up out of the way. If a later scan shows that it has failed to move up, a condition known as placenta previa (see p.473), you will be monitored until the birth.

The amniotic fluid is assessed to check that there isn't too little or too much. If there is too much fluid, it may be possible to drain some using

amniocentesis (see p.152) to decrease the risk of later complications such as premature labor (see p.431). Too little fluid can indicate a problem with fetal growth or your baby's renal tract and your baby may need to be monitored.

## Markers for Down syndrome

Although ultrasound at this stage is not a reliable way to detect Down syndrome, it can pick up certain signs known as "soft markers" that may suggest that your baby has an increased risk of Down syndrome. However, many markers are very common and are not usually a cause for alarm unless you already have an increased risk for Down syndrome,

**BOY OR GIRL?**

**Unless your baby is curled up or the legs** are closed tight, the sonographer will have a pretty good idea of whether you're going to have a boy or a girl. If you don't want to know the sex, tell the sonographer at the start of the scan. If you do, consider asking the sonographer to point out the baby's genitalia onscreen. If you are told which sex your baby is, resist the urge to go out and spend money on all-blue or all-pink decor since sonographers have been known to get it wrong!

Your 20-week scan

# 143 days to go...

## YOUR BABY TODAY

The appearance of your baby's head is still dominated by a prominent forehead due to the rapidly growing brain. The jaw can seem small but as the toothbuds grow and expand within the jaw, it lengthens and changes proportion.

## The foundations are already laid for your baby's teeth—both the milk teeth and the permanent ones that will follow.

**Although it's very rare for any teeth** to have come through by birth (only a 1 in 3,000 chance), your baby's tooth buds that will form her teeth are already in place within the jawbone.

All of your baby's teeth—both her "milk" teeth and her underlying permanent teeth—start their development beneath the gums while she is developing in your uterus. The milk teeth buds began to develop at eight weeks of pregnancy and by this week all of the buds are formed.

The first milk teeth to harden, as calcium builds up, are the central incisor teeth and the last are the back molars, at around 19 weeks. The crown of each milk tooth does not complete development until after birth and root completion takes until your child is more than three years old.

Buds for the permanent teeth begin to form between the 14th and 20th weeks. These lie deeper than those for the milk teeth and closer to the inner edge of the jaw and gum. They remain dormant until it is time for the milk teeth to be lost.

Your baby's milk teeth will start coming through at around six to eight months and she'll have a complete set of milk teeth by the age of 2½.

### AS A MATTER OF FACT

**Fetal alcohol syndrome leads** to serious oral and dental problems in the baby.

Smaller teeth that have weak enamel is just one of the many unfortunate consequences of this condition.

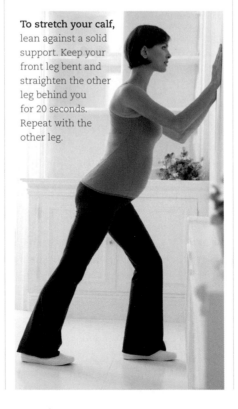

**To stretch your calf,** lean against a solid support. Keep your front leg bent and straighten the other leg behind you for 20 seconds. Repeat with the other leg.

### FEELING FLEXIBLE

**Stretching and flexibility exercises** should be a regular part of your fitness program at all times, but especially during pregnancy. Being flexible enables your muscles to work more efficiently, alleviates tightness, helps prevent cramping, and leads to improved balance and posture. Stretching can also help you feel confident and calm, especially if the exercises are combined with deep breathing.

Flexibility can be maintained or improved during pregnancy by doing a series of exercises that stretch your muscles in a safe and effective way.

■ **Do not stretch further** than feels comfortable or you risk injuring the ligaments and stressing your joints.

■ **Ensure that you're stretching** when the muscles are warm, at the end of a workout or after a warm bath.

During the second and third trimester you should avoid any exercises—stretching or otherwise—that require you to lie on your back for extended periods.

# 142 days to go...

## YOUR BABY TODAY

Your baby often rests against the placenta. This has no effect on the placenta since its surface is protected by the amniotic sac and its composition and blood flow maintain its circulation at all times, leaving your baby free to explore her environment.

As the weeks go by, you'll find that you'll need to rest more and limit the amount of time you are on your feet.

**By this stage, you may find it tiring** to be on your feet for long periods of time. For one thing, the growing weight of your baby and uterus will lead to discomfort, and potentially to muscle strain. Because your center of gravity is shifting, too, you may find that you stand awkwardly, putting pressure on your ligaments, which are, themselves, softened due to hormonal changes (see p.197). What's more, prolonged standing can cause blood and other fluids to pool in your legs, which can cause pain and dizziness.

If possible, take short, frequent breaks, so that you can put your feet up. If you do have to stand for long periods, you may find that resting one foot on a stool or box from time to time can help. Make sure your shoes offer good support (see p.257), and consider wearing maternity hose (see p.225).

It's important not to stand for more than three hours at a time, so if your work involves standing make sure you are given adequate breaks.

### ASK A... DOCTOR

**The bigger I get, the more difficult it's becoming to have sex. What should we do?** As your pregnancy continues, you will have no choice but to try new sexual positions that will more easily accommodate your growing belly.

You can still use the missionary position but your partner may have to support his weight on his hands instead of lying on you; that way he won't press on your belly. However, you'll find that positioning yourself on top is a better alternative, and as your belly gets bigger you can squat or kneel over your partner. Side-by-side or rear-entry positions are also comfortable during pregnancy. Have fun experimenting to find out what's right for you.

### FOCUS ON... YOUR BABY

## That's tasty!

**The flavors from the foods you eat** will be transferred to the amniotic fluid, which is swallowed by your baby in the uterus. Therefore the types of food you eat can influence your baby before her first exposure to solid foods.

Studies show that prenatal and postpartum (through breast milk) exposure to a flavor enhances a baby's enjoyment of it in solid foods. These early flavor experiences may provide the foundation for healthy choices, as well as explain the cultural and ethnic differences in cuisine. So get your baby started on the road to good food choices by making healthy selections now.

**Being out and about** will make you tired. When you're going out for the day, plan lots of breaks so you can sit and rest.

# 141 days to go...

## YOUR BABY TODAY

You will become much more aware of your baby moving as her size and strength increase. You will not be aware of the more gentle movements, or those movements that do not hit the side of the uterus.

You're likely to experience some backaches as your baby grows in size and your body continually adapts to accommodate her.

**The increasing weight of your developing baby,** and the fact that your joints and ligaments soften in pregnancy, can cause backaches, but thankfully you don't just have to put up with this pain. There are many simple ways in which you can ease a backache or even prevent it (see below).

See your doctor to make sure that the problem and its exact location is properly diagnosed. This way you'll have more chance of stopping it from becoming worse. A common problem, often in later pregnancy, is sciatica (see p.470)—a sharp pain that travels down the back and leg.

### BANISH BACKACHES

**To nip backaches in the bud,** try the following:
- **Take a warm bath** or use a hot-water bottle on the painful area.
- **Ask your partner** to give you a nice back rub, or get yourself a massage with an experienced prenatal practitioner.
- **Go to yoga or Pilates classes** to strengthen your back muscles.
- **Watch your posture** (see p.249), and raise your legs when seated.
- **Ensure your car seat** is properly positioned to support your back.

### FOCUS ON... YOUR HEALTH

## Fibroids during pregnancy

**In the second trimester,** fibroids—a benign mass of muscle fiber within the uterine wall, or occasionally attached to it—can become problematic. Increased levels of the hormones estrogen and progesterone during pregnancy encourage them to grow along with the uterus.

In some circumstances, the rapid growth of the fibroid causes feelings of pressure, discomfort, or pain. Fibroids may increase a woman's risk of miscarriage, preterm birth, or having a baby in the breech position which usually resolves the problem. Fibroids that do not cause discomfort do not require treatment.

The fibroid will not usually affect the developing baby, but if a large fibroid is positioned low down in the uterus or near to the cervix it can prevent the baby from descending into the pelvis, and a cesarean delivery will be necessary.

Once the baby is born and the uterus shrinks, the fibroids will also usually shrink to their pre-pregnancy size.

**Potential sites of fibroids**

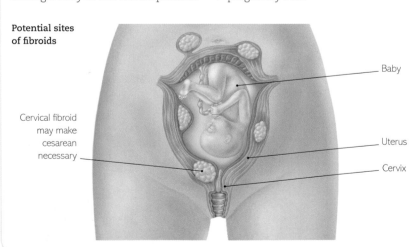

Baby

Cervical fibroid may make cesarean necessary

Uterus

Cervix

# 140 days to go...

## YOUR BABY TODAY

Although your baby may be sucking her thumb, this is a very complex action that is not fully developed at this stage. For this reason, your baby is as likely to put her fingers or toes in her mouth as her thumb.

Congratulations—you're now halfway through your pregnancy. In around 20 weeks' time, you'll be a mom.

**Does it seem like a lifetime, or has it flown by?** At least from now on, you really will be counting down. Hopefully, at this halfway point you are feeling fine physically. You're not yet encumbered by a large belly and probably have a reasonable amount of energy. Psychologically, you may still be very emotional, although you will no doubt have gotten used to any mood swings by now (as will your partner).

At this stage you will continue going to prenatal appointments around every four weeks. Remember, your doctor is there to monitor your health and your baby's progress, but also to help, so get her advice on how to deal with some of the discomforts you might experience as you grow bigger.

### AS A MATTER OF FACT

**The gestation period for an elephant is an incredible 22 months**, making it the longest of any land animal.

In addition to this, the common birth weight for elephants is 260 lb (120 kg). So, if your pregnancy is already starting to feel long, and your baby a tad heavy, spare a thought for our large-eared friends!

### ASK A... DOCTOR

**I haven't felt my baby move yet. Should I be worried?** While you understandably want to feel your baby's movements, there is no cause for concern yet since your recent scan should have shown you that all is well with your baby.

If it's your first baby, you may not notice the early movements since you won't know what to expect. Also, if you're an active person, these slight flutters may be missed. Women with a placenta lying at the front of the uterus may feel movements later, as may larger women since the movement may not be detected through the flesh.

Once you do feel movements, don't become too focused on every one. It's not until around 28 weeks that it becomes important to monitor the pattern. From this stage, the amount your baby moves, as well as the type of movement and when it happens, are relevant since these indicate that the placenta is sustaining the pregnancy and your baby's muscles are developing.

If you're concerned about lack of movement from your baby at any stage, speak to your doctor.

### SITTING CORRECTLY

**Sit upright on a chair** with your legs wide apart and your feet firmly on the floor to align your spine. Make sure your lower back is resting against the chair.

**Good posture can help to minimize** pregnancy discomforts, including backaches (see opposite page). When seated, make sure your lower back is supported by the back of the chair and keep your feet flat on the floor (see above).

Yoga is a great way to learn to hold your body correctly, including how to keep your spine aligned and your lower back supported.

# Your 21st week

**YOU'RE HALFWAY THROUGH YOUR PREGNANCY ALREADY—IT'S ALL HAPPENING SO FAST**

Not all women happily accept their changing body shape, even though they're overjoyed to be pregnant. But a belly "bump" doesn't have to mean frump. You've got a good excuse to treat yourself to a few attractive maternity clothes or to indulge in some pampering, perhaps by having a gentle massage. Keep up your exercise routine, because you'll feel energized and all the better for it.

**The developing brain** is picking up electrical signals from the baby's body about sensations such as pressure and temperature. At this stage, a baby's nervous reactions are not conscious but simply reflexes.

**The baby** is regularly swallowing the amniotic fluid in increasing amounts.

**Fingernails** are beginning to grow. There's no danger of the baby scratching himself, since his skin is covered in vernix, a protective waxy coating.

**At 21 weeks** the average crown to heel length is 9.7 in (24.5 cm) and the average weight is 8.8 oz (240 g).

**In girl babies** the ovaries have descended from the abdomen into the pelvis.

# 139 days to go...

**YOUR BABY TODAY**

Your baby's movements are still based on a set of reflex actions but this is now beginning to change. As the nerve pathways develop, expand, and mature, your baby gains greater and greater control of his actions.

You're in the second half of your pregnancy and in the months that follow you'll have more regular contact with your doctor.

**Your prenatal appointments will become more frequent** in the second half of your pregnancy. Even if you are in good health, and your baby has been thoroughly assessed at the 20-week ultrasound scan (see pp.214–5), it can be reassuring to have these regular checkups with the doctor.

The number of appointments you have will differ depending on whether you've had any complications, or whether you are having a high-risk pregnancy for another reason, such as a preexisting medical condition like diabetes. If it's a low-risk pregnancy, you can expect around 14 appointments unless there are complications. As a general rule you can expect to have prenatal appointments from now on: every 4 weeks until you reach 30 weeks' gestation, then appointments at 2-week intervals until you reach 36 weeks' gestation. From then on, you'll have appointments weekly. And if you pass your due date (see p.139), you'll need to see your doctor once or twice weekly

However, you can contact your doctor if you have any concerns.

If you're expecting twins, appointments will be more frequent and will depend on the type of twins you're having: non-identical or identical. If identical, care will depend on whether they share any of their support system (see p.130).

**The wide range of maternity clothes** that is now available means you can still look good at work. Look for items that you can also wear after the birth.

---

**FOCUS ON... YOUR BODY**

## Dressing well

**With your usual office clothing straining at the seams,** you might have to rethink your work wardrobe. The good news is that, unlike in years gone by, there is now a wealth of beautiful maternity clothing available and much at affordable everyday prices. These are often designed as coordinated sets, which makes putting them together easy.

Remember that you'll be wearing maternity clothing for a few months, and it's easy to become bored by the same items. If possible, designate a little of your wardrobe budget to buy yourself one or two items every month. If you're tired of your black elastic pants, sleeveless top, and smock dress, buy a pretty new shirt or jacket to jazz them up; you can wear them unbuttoned if necessary.

Don't hesitate to accept hand-me-downs; even if they are not right for your office dress code, wearing them at home will enable you to spend a little more on work clothing. And don't forget your shoes; if you were a stiletto girl before becoming pregnant, you'll need to rethink (see p.257).

# 138 days to go...

**YOUR BABY TODAY**

This close-up of the fingertips shows that the nail beds have formed and the nails are starting to grow. The nails have not yet hardened: this prevents your baby from scratching himself accidentally while he has no control over hand movements.

## Twin babies have been sharing a home in the uterus for a while now, but how are they relating to each other?

**At 21 weeks, a baby's eyes are still closed,** but he'll still be aware of light and dark. Because of this, twins can probably make out their sibling changing position and they're increasingly becoming aware of each other. It's thought that because memory starts developing around now, twin babies may begin to bond at this stage.

As ultrasound scanning has proven, there's plenty of contact between twin babies in the uterus, especially as the amount of space decreases. They have been seen to touch often, kick, and try to grab. Each twin reacts to the other's movements.

They may not act in the same way, with one twin favoring different movements than the other one. For instance, one baby may prefer sucking his thumb, while the other likes clutching his cord. Nor do they necessarily have the same body clock, so they may be active at different times. This proves that, even in the uterus, twin babies are already individuals.

**ASK A... DOCTOR**

**Can my baby feel anything when we have sex?** He may be aware of some movements when you have sex and of a change in your heart rate, but he won't be harmed by either. You may find that your baby responds to these sensations by moving a lot while you're having sex, or just afterward. Some women find this inhibiting, but remember that it doesn't mean the baby is uncomfortable and, of course, he doesn't understand what you're doing! If you have an orgasm, your uterus will feel tight and you may have Braxton-Hicks contractions (see p.410) but, again, this is not harmful to your baby.

Be reassured that your baby is well protected by the pool of amniotic fluid. Also, the cervix is closed by a plug of mucus during pregnancy so no semen can enter the uterus; this helps to guard against infection.

**As the pregnancy progresses,** contact between your twin babies will increase. Because you'll have more ultrasound scans in a twin pregnancy, you'll have plenty of opportunities to see them interacting with each other.

# 137 days to go...

**YOUR BABY TODAY**

The eyelids are still fused shut to protect your baby's developing eyes from prying fingers and toes. Deep within the brain, connections are starting to form to link the senses to those areas within the brain that are able to process information.

Part of the fun of not knowing your baby's sex is anticipating what it might be, but be prepared for others to do the same.

**If you and your partner decided** against finding out the sex of your baby at the 20-week scan, the guessing games will begin and you won't be short of people telling you what they think you're having.

Perhaps your own instinct is the best of all: in one study that asked women to guess the sex of their baby, 71 percent of the expectant moms surveyed guessed correctly.

### THE LOWDOWN

## It's definitely a...

If you like testing a few old wives' tales on gender, consider these:

■ Ask someone to tie a gold ring on to a piece of string and dangle it over your belly to "dowse" for the sex. If it swings from side to side or back and forth, it's a boy; if it spins around in a circular motion, you're having a girl.
■ Hairier than usual? Apparently, according to the "old wives," you're more likely to be carrying a boy.
■ If your baby's heart rate is faster than 140 beats per minute, you're having a girl (but see p.188!).
■ Craving sugar, spice, and all things sweet: girl. Sour or salty foods: boy.

### ASK A... MOM

**I've found out at the 20-week scan that I'm having my third girl, but I so wanted a boy. How can I feel better about this?** It can be enormously disappointing to find out that your baby's sex is different than what you wanted, and perhaps even expected. I felt that I'd let my husband down in some way, especially since I knew he wanted a son.

The good news is that by the time our daughter was born, we were both over the disappointment, and were able to focus on being parents. We always said that if we'd waited until the birth to find out, it would have been hard to come to terms with it at the same time as trying to bond with our newborn baby.

Remember that you haven't met your new daughter yet, and it may be difficult to imagine loving another daughter, but you will do, in time. Try to focus on the fact that she is healthy and that you're having a beautiful baby.

**Although you may prefer** to have a child of a different gender, you might find that your children are delighted to be having another same-sex playmate.

# 136 days to go...

### YOUR BABY TODAY

Shown here is a Doppler ultrasound scan. Your doctor may use a handheld Doppler ultrasound machine to identify your baby's heartbeat; Doppler scanning can also pick up sudden movements and the whoosh of blood through the placenta.

There are few better ways to relieve those pregnancy aches and pains, and to wind down, than to have a soothing massage.

**When you book a massage, make sure** you do so with a therapist who is experienced in prenatal massage. Although it's unlikely to occur at this stage, massaging the wrong areas or certain acupressure points can trigger uterine contractions (this can actually make a massage beneficial during labor when you want to speed things up).

Before making an appointment for a massage, check with your doctor that it's okay to have one. Massage may not be recommended if you've had complications such as high blood pressure or diabetes.

Comfort is crucial and most therapists will position you lying on your side with your head supported by a pillow (see right). Don't hesitate to tell the therapist if you're uncomfortable or if any aspect of the massage hurts. An experienced therapist should check that you're comfortable throughout the massage and stop if you're not.

If you don't want to book a professional massage, you can always call on your partner or a willing friend. It is, however, important that the person who is massaging you is careful and does not attempt to work on the abdominal area.

In addition to making a world of difference to those aches and pains and helping you to relax, a massage from your partner is a good way to be intimate with him at times when you might not feel like having sex.

If you don't feel up to having a full massage, a foot, hand, or head massage can be very soothing.

**Having a professional massage** during pregnancy can be a real treat. Besides feeling blissful, research shows that it eases aches and pains, helps you sleep, and can reduce stress.

---

### ASK A... DOCTOR

**I can't look in the mirror because I'm feeling so down about my size. Will things get better?** You're not alone in battling with your self-image in pregnancy. For some women, their changing body shape can create negative feelings. Eating a healthy diet and getting some exercise helps prevent excessive weight gain, and exercising will also lift your spirits and improve your sense of well-being.

There's no set emotional response to pregnancy, but in addition to coming to terms with a momentous life and body change, you are also under the influence of fluctuating hormones, all of which affects your mood and can add to feelings of negativity.

Mild depression in pregnancy is often helped by reassurance and support from your partner, family, or friends. Talking over your fears and concerns may help relieve your anxieties—you'll probably find that other pregnant women are experiencing the same feelings.

If you are feeling very low and desperate, don't hesitate to consult your doctor.

# 135 days to go...

## YOUR BABY TODAY

The skin is less translucent now as your baby is starting to lay down fat reserves, which after the birth will help with temperature control and provide an energy reservoir for your baby to call upon when necessary.

Your developing baby is becoming more responsive and aware every day as his nervous system begins to work more effectively.

**By this stage, your baby can use his senses** and recognize the sensations of light, pressure, pain, and temperature. Sound is thought to be the first sense to develop, although taste buds are at least present on the tongue from as early as 10 weeks. Nerves carrying the sensations of pain, temperature, and light touch from your baby's body reach his spinal cord and then travel to the hypothalamus, which lies in the center of the brain. This then sends signals to another part of your baby's brain so that the stimuli can be recognized and also evoke an emotional response. Many, but not all, of these nerves require insulation around them to conduct signals effectively. Known as myelin sheaths, these do not develop until much later, after 29 weeks in the spine and 37 weeks in the brain.

Painful stimuli result in a reflex action (such as pulling your hand away from a hot object). Reflexes don't have to involve the brain and for these sensations to be recognized at a conscious level, rather than as a simple reflex, the nerves need to connect the hypothalamus to the gray matter in the brain. These connections are thought to function after 26 weeks of pregnancy, but it may be 34 weeks before their electrical activity can be clearly seen on an electroencephalogram (EEG).

### ASK A... MOM

**This is my second baby—does it make sense to go to prenatal classes again?** I think so. There were three years between my pregnancies and it helped to have a refresher course; I even found that some of the advice had changed in that time. My partner found it helpful, too.

One reason to go is to meet some pregnant moms again; it's always useful to share the experience with others and, as with your first pregnancy, you'll probably find you make some great friends.

### WEARING MATERNITY HOSE

**You probably can't imagine wearing maternity hose,** but they have their uses. They work by promoting circulation and the return of blood back to the heart and may be recommended to prevent vein-related problems, particularly if you suffer from varicose veins (see p.167) or spider veins (see p.134).

They also help to relieve aching feet, mild swelling in the feet, ankles, and legs, as well as fluid retention. They may be particularly helpful if your work means that you must be on your feet for long periods of time.

Thankfully, an element of fashion has been introduced and many brands are sheer and pretty. There is a variety available: some are thigh- or knee-high (see right) and others cover the whole leg. There are also some that provide support for your baby and uterus, taking the pressure off your back. You'll find lighter stockings for summer wear, when the hot weather can lead to further swelling.

YOU ARE 20 WEEKS AND 6 DAYS

# 134 days to go...

## YOUR BABY TODAY

Your baby is now developing periods of movement and activity and periods of rest and quiet. Soon these periods will become definite cycles of activity, providing something of a daily (and nightly) routine to his movement.

## Your baby's reproductive organs are gradually developing and the differences in the genitals are increasingly obvious.

**In the absence of high levels** of testosterone in a female baby, the reproductive glands become ovaries, which contain 6–8 million follicles at this stage, of which about 1–2 million will remain at birth. The ovaries have now descended from the abdomen into the pelvis. The testes also undergo a similar descent, but have not yet reached the

scrotum. Under the influence of the hormone estrogen you produce, your baby of either sex may develop breast buds, although these will disappear after birth. Whether your baby is a boy or a girl has very little impact on the pregnancy. Later in pregnancy, there is a slight weight difference, with boys being slightly heavier than girls on average.

> ### ASK A... DOCTOR
>
> **I fell recently. Could I have harmed my baby?** Falling during pregnancy is extremely common, as your increasingly protruding abdomen, softening ligaments and joints, and changing center of gravity can cause you to lose your balance. The good news is that your baby is safely cocooned in amniotic fluid, which protects and cushions him when you fall. Your injuries would have to be quite severe to cause any harm to your baby.
>
> The best thing you can do is to monitor your baby's movements after a fall. If he's moving as much as normal all should be fine, but if you want reassurance, pay a visit to your doctor. If you do experience any discomfort, or unusual discharge or bleeding from your vagina, seek medical help. If you pass water, this is likely to be urine caused by stress incontinence (see opposite), not amniotic fluid.

**The amniotic sac** is sometimes referred to as a "bubble" because of its appearance. It may be transparent, but it's tough and extremely difficult to pierce, so your baby is very well protected in this safe environment.

Your second trimester

226

# 133 days to go...

**YOUR BABY TODAY**

This image shows just how large the developing eyes are underneath the lids. At birth, your baby's eyes will be large and blue. There are no eyebrows or eyelashes yet, but this will be the first adult type of hair to grow.

Try to find ways to fit in small amounts of energizing exercise every day—you'll feel much better for it.

**I seem to have a lot of vaginal discharge. Is this normal?** Yes, in the second trimester you may find that you have more discharge than normal. This is usually clear, stringy, or full of mucus and shouldn't smell offensive. If the discharge changes, becoming thick, white, and causes itching, you may have developed a yeast infection, which is common in pregnancy and easily treated (see p.133).

You should see your doctor immediately if the vaginal discharge becomes yellow or greener, or offensive in smell; see your doctor too if you have burning when you urinate, or your external genitals become sore. This may be a sign that you have an infection that must be treated. Don't ignore any abnormal discharge since, although it won't directly affect your developing baby, an infection can increase the risk of you going in to premature labor.

You may find that you leak urine, especially when you cough, laugh, or run. This is called stress incontinence (see p.471).

**Maintaining your exercise routine** while you're still working can be challenging. The last thing you may feel like doing is exercising after a day at work, especially as your pregnancy progresses. There are ways of exercising without a visit to the gym; it will just take some thought and planning. For example, every now and then, take the stairs, carefully, instead of the elevator, or get off the bus or train at a different stop, so that you walk some of the way.

If there's a pool close to work, try to fit in an invigorating lunchtime swim. You'll feel much better in the afternoon.

Walk wherever you can, but be prepared: wear comfortable sneakers and take your work shoes in a bag with you. Remember to take some water with you when exercising, and keep hydrated throughout the day.

At night before you go to bed, try to fit in some abdominal exercises (see p.250) to strengthen those muscles.

**OFFICE WORKOUT**

**If your job involves sitting down all day,** it's even more important to find ways to keep on the move.
- **Get up from your desk** at least once every hour. Walk to speak to your colleagues instead of phoning or emailing them. Volunteer to get coffee for people—this will also make you very popular!
- **Try this exercise while seated:** straighten your leg out in front of you (see right), keeping your thigh parallel to the floor. Then repeatedly bend and straighten your leg to help your circulation. Follow with flexing and pointing your foot from the ankle. Do each of these exercises at least 10 times with each leg.

# Your 22nd week

**DECIDING ON A NAME FOR YOUR BABY CAN BE TRICKY, SO START MAKING THAT LIST**

You may not know the sex of your baby but you and your partner can still have fun choosing names. This is a discussion that can run on and on. Some couples don't make up their minds until the baby is born. With such matters to preoccupy you, it's probably hard to stay focused at work. Try to pace yourself without letting standards slip. Eating little and often, and drinking lots of water, will help you stay alert.

**Your uterus** may now reach above your belly button, but there is a wide variation in belly size among women at the same week of pregnancy.

**The hands** move constantly, reaching out to touch the face or clutch at the umbilical cord.

**Every bone** in your baby's body now contains bone marrow capable of producing blood cells.

**Beneath the skin**, layers of body fat are being stored. Fats are essential because they contribute to the full development of the nervous system.

**At 22 weeks** the average crown to heel length is 10.1 in (25.6 cm), and the average weight is 10.6 oz (300 g).

**In boy babies**, the testes are still hidden within the pelvic cavity.

# 128 days to go...

## YOUR BABY TODAY

There is still plenty of room for your baby to move around. Your baby is able to perform complete somersaults and change position several times a day or even several times in a few minutes.

## Bellies come in all shapes and sizes and your doctor will keep track of how your baby is growing.

**If, like some pregnant women, you are feeling big for this halfway stage,** it doesn't necessarily mean that you'll have a big baby. Being large doesn't mean that all your weight is in your belly and from your baby; you may have put on weight on the rest of your body that doesn't affect your baby's size. Women who are carrying twins or triplets do, of course, show earlier and have much larger bellies than those expecting one baby.

The size of your belly is, however, a good indicator of your baby's growth, so it will be measured by your doctor (see pp.284–5). She will measure from a point on your pubic bone in your pelvis to the top, or fundus, of the uterus. This measurement should correlate with the number of weeks you're pregnant, with an accuracy of within ¾ in (2 cm). So, if you're 28 weeks pregnant your belly should measure 10¼–11¾ in (26–30 cm). This symphysis fundal height (SFH) will be written in your notes.

If your belly is found to be significantly larger or smaller than it should be for your dates, you're likely

**While it's good to spend time** with women who are at the same stage of pregnancy as you, try not to make comparisons. Your belly may be bigger than your friend's, but you may end up having a smaller baby.

to be referred for an ultrasound scan since this can give a much more accurate measurement of your baby's size.

Remember, though, what you think of as huge and what your doctor feels is too large can be two very different things! You are used to your body being a certain size and shape and you are much bigger than you used to be, even though to doctors you are a normal and healthy size. This can feel particularly the case if you're someone who has always been slim.

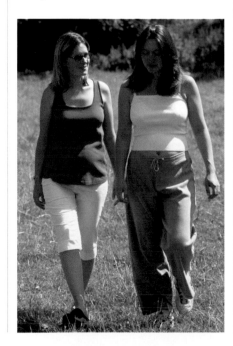

### ASK A... NUTRITIONIST

**I've been told to rest but will I gain too much weight?** It's important that you follow this advice, even though it can be frustrating. Ask your doctor if you're allowed to do gentle walking or swimming because this will help keep you fit and burn some calories.

If you're eating a healthy, nutritious diet that includes plenty of fresh fruits and vegetables, complex carbohydrates, and lean protein, you shouldn't gain too much weight.

Never be tempted to diet, or go hungry just because you're less active at the moment. Regular meals and snacks are important. Listen to your body; if you're hungry, it needs fuel.

If full bed rest has been prescribed, light exercise will be out of the question, but make sure you establish at the outset what is and isn't allowed. If you aren't active you are likely to gain some weight, but the goal of bed rest is to ensure that you deliver a healthy baby at full-term, and that's worth a few extra pounds.

Your 22nd week

233

# 127 days to go...

## YOUR BABY TODAY

This is a close-up of the baby's skin just behind the ear. Every part of the skin's surface has small ridges and hollows in a unique pattern. During this week the dermal ridges—the deeper layers of skin—start to mature, giving rise to finger- and toeprints.

## Your baby has been filtering amniotic fluid and storing the waste as a substance called meconium.

**At the end of this week,** your baby's anal sphincter muscle is fully functional. This should prevent any small particles of meconium from being passed into the amniotic fluid. Meconium is first produced at 12 weeks. It is the somewhat greenish/black first poop that nine out of 10 newborn babies pass in the first 24 hours.

Meconium is formed mainly from cells discarded from the lining of the gut as it lengthens and expands, and the waste of any nutrients which have been absorbed from the swallowed amniotic fluid. It is continuously produced, slowly moving down the gut to enter the large bowel (colon) by 16 weeks. Meconium is sterile since there are no organisms inside the gut and no bowel gas is produced.

### AS A MATTER OF FACT

**The unborn baby will move her hand to her mouth** and even suck her thumb.

Research has shown that the baby may even open her mouth in anticipation. Anything that the hands encounter is firmly grasped and this grip is strong enough to support all of the baby's body weight.

### KEEP TONED

**Effective strength training during pregnancy,** using free weights (see right) or a machine at your gym, will help your body deal with the demands of pregnancy. Being stronger will help you carry the increase in body weight and also help you recover after the baby is born. Having more toned limbs will help you look and feel better, too.

Like all aspects of exercise during pregnancy, there are guidelines that should be followed:

■ **If you've been doing regular weight training,** continue with your program, but do not increase the weight loads or repetitions.

■ **If you're new to using weights,** begin with very light ones and few repetitions and build up slowly. Do not increase the weight load until you are confident that you are able to manage the increase.

■ **Take a deep breath** to start and breathe out as you lift the weight.

■ **Free weights,** rather than machines, are safer to use during pregnancy. If you're using a machine, make sure a trainer has shown you how to use it correctly.

■ **If you find standing up while doing strength training too tiring,** sit on a chair to lift your weights (see below).

**If you're sitting and using weights,** keep your back straight and relax your shoulders. When standing, make sure that you have your legs hip-width apart and your knees slightly bent.

# 126 days to go...

**YOUR BABY TODAY**

The vertebrae that make up your baby's spinal column encircle and protect the spinal cord. The vertebrae are seen here on an ultrasound scan, forming a long chain (white areas) that narrows at the base of the spine and ends with a slight outward curve.

## Maintaining a professional manner at work will set the standard for how colleagues treat you during pregnancy.

**Chances are that everyone in your office** will be aware that you are expecting a baby by this stage, even if you haven't told them personally. Good news does have a habit of traveling fast, and you may have that pregnancy "glow" that makes your condition pretty clear—as well as a fairly prominent belly.

If word of your pregnancy is getting around the office, it might be best to tell your boss now. It's always better and more professional if your boss hears this news before other people in your company.

You may need to adapt your working day a little, but play it carefully. Try to keep up with your work, and act professionally. Your colleagues are, hopefully, thrilled that you're pregnant, but try not to expect special favors or extra attention.

While being pregnant isn't an illness, do take adequate breaks to recharge your batteries, or work flexible hours, if that's an option, so that you can avoid traveling at the busiest times.

Try to go for a short walk on your lunch hour for fresh air and to get some gentle exercise. Drink plenty of water to keep you hydrated and alert, and eat little and often to keep your energy levels high.

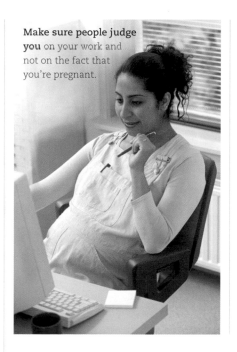

Make sure people judge **you** on your work and not on the fact that you're pregnant.

**FOCUS ON... HEALTH**

## Vaginal bleeding

**If you have any vaginal bleeding,** always see your doctor. Growths on your cervix, or some inflammation, can produce light bleeding from time to time.

Heavy bleeding in the second trimester may suggest a problem with your placenta, such as placenta previa (see p.212). Similarly, the placenta may pull away from the wall of the uterus, causing some bleeding, or, very rarely, uterine rupture can occur, usually only in women who have had a cesarean section in the past.

**ASK A... DOCTOR**

**My manager said I can't have time off to go to my prenatal doctor appointments. What should I do?**
You'll be spending a lot of time at the doctor's office for prenatal care during the next several months— every 4 weeks now, but as frequently as once a week at the end of your pregnancy. If you also work full-time, it's a good idea to to schedule your prenatal appointments for the early morning, before you begin work, or during your lunch hour. If your appointments tend to run long or your doctor's office is far from work and your boss isn't understanding, ask if you should use your sick leave or your vacation time for the hours that you'll be away from the office.

# Your 23rd week

**YOU COULD BE FEELING A LITTLE OFF-BALANCE, BOTH PHYSICALLY AND EMOTIONALLY**

Being pregnant can have all kinds of unexpected effects. There will probably be days when you just don't feel in control of your emotions and they get the better of you, making you cry for no reason. Or your body feels clumsy and uncoordinated, and you keep walking into the furniture. Just talk to some other moms-to-be and you'll find that these side effects are all a normal part of the pregnancy experience!

**As your abdominal organs** become ever more compressed, you may suffer from frequent digestive disturbances, such as heartburn or trapped gas.

**The umbilical cord** may be held in your baby's hands as he floats in the amniotic cavity.

**Kicks are becoming** quite strong and there's no mistaking your baby's movements.

**At 23 weeks** the average crown to heel length is 10.5 in (26.7 cm) and the average weight is 12.7 oz (360 g).

**The inner ear organs** have matured enough to send nerve signals to the brain. Soon, the baby will start responding to many more sounds.

# 125 days to go...

**YOUR BABY TODAY**

This is a landmark week for your baby's senses: hearing and balance, both controlled by the inner ear, start to mature now. As this image shows, the ears are still not in their final position at the side of the head.

If your emotions are all over the place, try having a good cry, preferably on someone's shoulder. You'll feel a whole lot better.

**It's normal to feel a bit up and down emotionally.** The best way to manage is to give yourself some time out and the low points will soon pass. If you find yourself crying at a commerical yet again, try to see the funny side! Sharing this fact with someone else may also help, especially a pregnant friend or new mom—she more than anyone else will be able to relate to how you're feeling and reassure you.

The good news is you don't need to worry about your baby—he won't be affected by your occasional mood swings. However, it might not be good for him if you get too stressed since this causes your body to produce more cortisol, a hormone which can have adverse effects on your baby (see p.187). So, when you're feeling stressed, make adequate time to relax and take care of yourself, for your baby's sake.

**FOCUS ON... TWINS**

## Maternity matters

**If you're having twins,** now is the time to discuss your maternity leave with your employers. Some women start their leave toward the end of their pregnancy, while others wait for their babies to be born. Ask your doctor for advice.

You may also want to take off as much time as possible after the babies are born, and your partner will want to take the maximum amount of leave he's eligible for (see p.349). Aside from help from family and friends, which will be essential, consider what you can afford in terms of additional child care.

**ASK A... DOCTOR**

**I think I may have food poisoning. Will this harm my baby?** Some food-borne illnesses, such as salmonella, campylobacter, and E. coli will not directly harm your baby but can make you very ill, causing profuse vomiting and diarrhea that could lead to extreme dehydration. It's important to keep your fluid intake up both to flush out the offending pathogens, and to ensure you're sufficiently hydrated. If the vomiting is so serious that you can't keep any fluid down, ask for an emergency appointment with your doctor.

Infection with listeria bacteria is the most serious since it can infect the baby and may cause a miscarriage or premature labor. It is, therefore, essential that you contact your doctor if you believe that you've eaten a contaminated food (see p.17), so that the relevant checkup can be done and treatment given, if necessary.

Always be especially careful when choosing food and follow hygiene rules when preparing it. Avoid eating foods commonly associated with food poisoning (see p.17).

# 124 days to go...

## YOUR BABY TODAY

The hands and fingers are clearly visible and the nail beds have been laid down. The baby's fingers will close if the palm of his hand is touched. The tips of the two bones in the forearm, the radius and the ulna, can just be seen in the lower part of this image.

Now that your baby's ears are sufficiently well developed to process sounds, his hearing will gradually improve.

**Your baby's external ears have been developed** for some time but for him to hear, the internal ear structures also need to mature. In the middle ear, three bones—the malleus ("hammer"), incus ("anvil"), and stapes ("stirrup")—conduct sound into the inner ear. These bones are formed initially from soft cartilage and embedded within connective tissue. The bones begin to harden and the connective tissue gradually dissolves. This allows the ear drum to vibrate onto the hammer, which passes the movement on to the anvil, and then the stirrup. The vibrations are then passed to the cochlea, a cavity of the inner ear, where they are translated into nerve impulses to be sent to the brain.

At 22 weeks, your baby's inner ear has matured adequately for sound to be processed into neural signals to the brain. The first part of the cochlea to develop is responsible for receiving lower-sound frequencies. As your baby develops, he will gradually be able to recognize and respond to higher sound frequencies. Over the next three weeks, your baby's responsiveness to sounds will gradually increase. At first the responses are slow and sluggish, but by 25 weeks he will react to a range of sounds by moving around.

In addition to being responsible for your baby's hearing, the inner ear also controls his balance. Small fibers within three semicircular canals of the inner ear are able to sense acceleration in any direction, providing the sense of motion and balance. Floating in the amniotic fluid is similar to weightlessness and, although your baby is very active, he has no sense yet of moving up and down.

## AS A MATTER OF FACT

**Men are faster than women** at changing diapers.

Research shows that the average time a woman takes is 2 minutes and 5 seconds, whereas the average man takes 1 minute and 36 seconds! So that's a job for him, then.

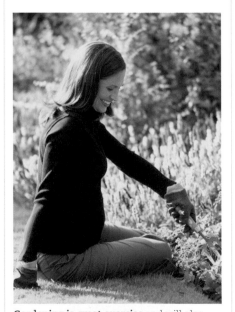

**Gardening is great exercise** and will also ensure you get some fresh air. Make sure you wear gloves because the soil may contain toxoplasmosis parasites (see pp.25 and 86).

## RARING TO GO

**If, like many pregnant women at this stage,** you feel incredibly energized, make the most of it. Here are some ways to direct that energy:
- **Get some exercise,** including doing some gardening (see left).
- **Organize your paperwork** and get your finances in order.
- **Clear out any clothes** that you know you won't wear again.
- **Learn to knit** or, if you already can, get going on some baby clothes.
- **Make time to see all the friends** you haven't been in touch with for a while—you may not feel up to socializing in later months.

However good you're feeling, always make time to relax and recharge your batteries.

# 123 days to go...

**YOUR BABY TODAY**

The baby's mouth and nose are well developed. The nervous and muscular systems are now mature enough for the baby to suck in amniotic fluid, which the kidneys slowly process. Waste is eliminated via the placenta.

During your pregnancy you'll probably make some new friends, but you may find that some old friendships are affected.

**One thing you may not have anticipated** before you were pregnant is how your friendships might change. It's normal to be drawn to other women who are pregnant or who have recently had a baby, and common to make friends at prenatal classes (see p.199). It's natural to want to surround yourself with people who are going through or who have been through the same experience as you, not least because you will have so many questions they can answer. You might also feel closer to female relatives, especially your mother (see p.209).

You may find that friends who are not pregnant or who don't have children may not be as interested in all the details of your pregnancy. It may be difficult for them to comprehend how all-encompassing pregnancy and then having a child is; it may be literally all you can think about. If these are friendships you value, make an effort to have some "nonpregnancy" chats. It will be good for you not to be 100 percent focused on the pregnancy.

If you find you drift apart from these friends for a while, don't worry. Good friends will always remain just that, whether or not your lives temporarily go in different directions.

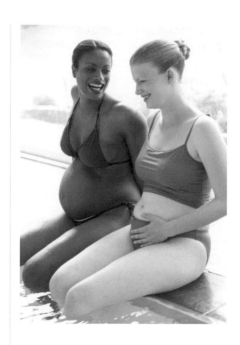

**By spending time with women** who are also expecting a baby, you can share the ups and downs of your pregnancy experiences. It can also be fun to do activities together, such as going swimming or to water aerobics classes.

---

**ASK A... DOCTOR**

**My fingers are tingling and I've been told I have carpal tunnel syndrome. What is it?** This condition occurs when swollen tissues in the wrist compress the nerves and cause pins and needles and numbness in your fingers. There may also be difficulty grasping and a weakness in the hands. In pregnancy, it's caused by an increase in blood volume and fluid, especially in the second and third trimesters. There are ways to reduce the symptoms, such as circling and stretching exercises to improve circulation and increase wrist mobility. Your doctor will be able to demonstrate these exercises. Wearing wrist splints and elevating your hands on a pillow at night can also help.

Carpal tunnel syndrome disappears after the birth, once there is no longer excess fluid.

---

**AS A MATTER OF FACT**

**The number of women over 40 becoming pregnant** is at its highest level ever.

According to the National Center for Health Statistics, the birth rate for women 40–44 more than doubled since 1981 and rose 65 percent since 1990. Birth rates for women 45–49 and 50 and over have also risen. The mean age for first-time moms giving birth is 25.2.

# 122 days to go...

**YOUR BABY TODAY**

Seeing your baby on a 3D or 4D scan gives you a better view, but most of the information that enables doctors to plan your care comes from looking inside your baby using 2D ultrasound, which provides the clearest images of internal structures.

## Now that he can hear, your amazing baby is starting to develop the ability to remember things, too.

**As your baby's nervous system develops,** and especially once his sense of hearing evolves, he has the opportunity to learn and remember from experience. How this process develops is not fully understood, but experts believe that the first signs of learning coincide with the unborn baby's ability to hear, at around this mid-stage of pregnancy.

In later months, more sound will reach your baby as the walls of the uterus become thinner. Although babies have been seen to be startled by a noise at this stage, they seem to learn not to react to the sound if it is repeated again and again, gradually adapting to it as it's repeated over time, and eventually ignoring it.

This simple test demonstrates that a fetus can adapt to a repeated stimulus. If, however, the sound pattern is not repeated for some time, your baby will have forgotten it and become startled by it if it occurs again.

Retaining a memory for events is a much more complex function and relies on pathways in the gray matter of the brain. It will be weeks before learning and memory are linked in the last stages of your pregnancy.

**3D scans enable you to see** your baby's face and features, such as the hands, in incredible detail. As these images are so real, they often improve the feeling of bonding a mother has for her baby.

### AS A MATTER OF FACT

**Your baby is likely to be** increasingly more active and predictable in his movements.

At around this time you're likely to start feeling regular, more definite movements, and become accustomed to your baby's activities.

### UP CLOSE AND PERSONAL

**State-of-the-art technology means it's possible** to see what your baby will look like before you give birth. Some ultrasound scans enable parents to see their unborn baby close up either in 3D, as a still image, or 4D as a moving picture.

Clear scans of the facial features can be seen from around this week. However, the optimum time to have one of these scans is between 26 and 34 weeks, when your baby still has room to move around easily. You will be able to see an amazing level of detail that won't be visible on a standard prenatal scan. Remember to inform the sonographer if you don't want to discover the sex of your baby.

The US FDA cautions against keepsake ultrasound images, since the ultrasonography may be done by someone not well-trained, using higher levels of energy for a longer time which could be harmful.

Be aware that it's expensive to have these scans and if your baby is in the wrong position, you may not get a great result. The position of the placenta, amount of amniotic fluid, and your size can also affect the quality of the picture.

# 121 days to go...

**YOUR BABY TODAY**

Extremely fine hairs called lanugo hairs cover your baby's entire skin surface. These are constantly shed and replaced but, during the final few weeks of pregnancy, will be replaced by thicker, permanent hairs. Lanugo cells help insulate the skin.

## The occasional dizzy spell is common in pregnancy and not a sign that anything is wrong.

**As your body works hard** to nourish your baby, you may find yourself feeling dizzy from time to time. It's common to feel dizzy when you stand up suddenly; this is because, although your blood supply has increased during pregnancy, getting up quickly causes the blood to rush into your legs. This reduces the supply of blood to your brain, making you feel light-headed.

Dizziness can also be a symptom of anemia. Although you produce more red blood cells in pregnancy than before, your volume of blood also increases. This means that proportionally there are fewer red blood cells and your blood count will drop.

You may also become short of iron and, if this is the case, you will be prescribed iron supplements. In addition to dizziness, symptoms of anemia include fatigue and shortness of breath. Low blood-sugar levels (see p.92) can also cause dizziness and can be prevented by eating snacks regularly.

If you're feeling dizzy, although it's likely to be due to the physiological changes in pregnancy, inform your doctor so you can be examined and any relevant blood tests taken. If you feel dizzy when you're out and about, or if you need a seat on a bus or train, always tell someone—the majority of people will be understanding.

**AS A MATTER OF FACT**

**Not all pregnant women** toe the good health line.

Healthy-eating messages abound so pregnant women are well informed, especially about calcium-rich foods needed for strong bones among other things. A recent study found that pregnant women who rarely drank milk gave birth to smaller babies than those who drank the recommended three 8-oz glasses per day.

**If you can't face crowds,** see one friend at a time in a home environment. Be selective and prioritize those people who really matter to you, rather than trying to fit everyone in.

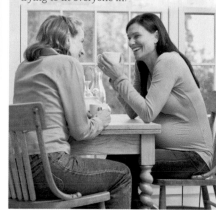

### ASK A... MOM

**I don't feel up to socializing but should I force myself to go out?**
I remember that feeling well! When you're pregnant, it's normal to feel like battening down the hatches sometimes because you're too tired to socialize. It's worth, however, trying to make the most of your leisure time before the baby arrives. You may not feel like getting out and about, but once you do you'll probably be glad you made the effort and it will help you maintain friendships.

I chose my activities carefully, opting for early evening or weekend get togethers, and went to cafés rather than bars. I also had friends over for lunch and dinner but asked everyone to bring a dish. I realized I might not get to the movies or theater for a while once the baby was born, so planned lots of great trips. You can always go to weekend matinées if you're too tired in the evening. When I was really too tired to go out, I'd catch up with a friend on the phone.

241

# 120 days to go...

**YOUR BABY TODAY**

Your baby's nervous system and muscular coordination are now much more developed. He has a grasping reflex—when his palm is touched his fingers will close—and he is able to suck his thumb purposefully, rather than through random movements.

## When clumsiness strikes, something as simple as walking in a straight line may prove difficult!

**If you find that you're often bumping into things** and tripping over, it sounds as though you've been hit by clumsiness, a common side effect of being pregnant.

Clumsiness in pregnancy has physical causes: the hormone relaxin causes your joints to loosen, your center of gravity changes as your abdomen expands, and your extra weight shifts you off balance. There are, however, also emotional reasons: if you're preoccupied by being pregnant, your concentration is bound to slip now and then, making you less likely to notice potential hazards in your path.

The good news is that your usual grace will return once you're no longer pregnant, but until that time it's important to avoid situations that might put you at risk of injury. So wear flat shoes rather than heels, avoid wet or slippery surfaces, and be careful on steep staircases. Tape down the edges of loose rugs, and keep the stairs and hallways clear of things that might trip you up. Be particularly careful when you're lifting something because it's very easy to lose your balance if you're leaning forward. Be careful also, getting into and out of the bath or shower, since these are notorious hotspots for pregnancy-related injuries.

It's worth noting that normal clumsiness in pregnancy is not accompanied by visual disturbances, headaches, or dizziness, so if you have any of these symptoms, you should see your doctor.

---

**TIME TO THINK ABOUT**

## Preparing your home

If your partner's nesting instinct has kicked in, make the most of it by figuring out what needs to be done around your home.

■ **Decorate the room** your baby will eventually sleep in once you move him out of your bedroom.
■ **Take the opportunity** to have a look around and take any unwanted clutter to the dump or charity shop.
■ **Make storage space** by putting up some extra shelves and cupboards where you can. Figure out where you'll store large items, such as the carriage.

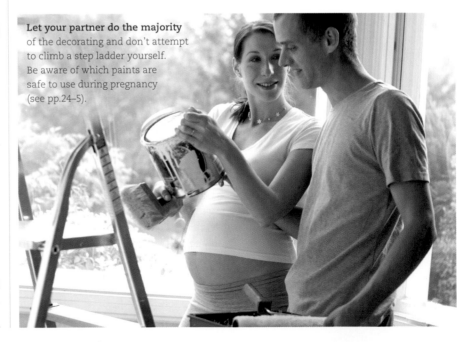

**Let your partner do the majority** of the decorating and don't attempt to climb a step ladder yourself. Be aware of which paints are safe to use during pregnancy (see pp.24–5).

# 119 days to go...

**YOUR BABY TODAY**

External appearances are deceptive: although your baby seems very well developed, it's still early in the pregnancy—the state of the cervix and progesterone produced by the placenta both play a part in ensuring that labor does not start for some months yet.

You may be surprised by the strength of feeling you have for your baby, and this maternal instinct will grow stronger each day.

**Do you feel as though you're a mom yet?** Whether or not you're a maternal person, you'll already have started, instinctively, the process of becoming a mother. You may be taking better care of yourself, eating better, and making lifestyle changes, not necessarily to benefit your own health but for your baby. You're likely to find yourself being very protective and nurturing toward your growing belly, wanting the best for your baby, and being worried about anything happening to him. It's nothing to worry about if you don't feel this bond: all women are different and it may not be until you're holding and caring for your baby that you experience strong maternal feelings.

Your partner may not have this strong parental instinct, but the more you involve him in the pregnancy, the greater the chance of him getting close to his unborn child. By reading books or on the internet about how the baby is developing at every stage, and attending some or all of the prenatal appointments with you, he will be able to picture the baby and follow his progress as closely as possible.

**You'll find that your baby** occupies your thoughts a lot of the time. Being pregnant makes most women act selflessly in the best interests of their baby.

---

**FOCUS ON... RELATIONSHIPS**

## What's that, Mom?

**If you have a toddler already, she will undoubtedly be curious** about why you have suddenly got so fat! Keep things simple, along the lines of "Mommy is growing you a baby sister or brother, but she/he won't be here just yet." Over the coming weeks, explain in more detail what having a new baby means.

There's no need to tell your toddler how the baby got there, or to keep reminding her about it. Just answer her questions when she asks, without showing too much preoccupation with the matter.

---

**ASK A... DOCTOR**

**I've got the flu. Will this harm my baby?** No, your baby should be fine but because your immune system is compromised during pregnancy, your symptoms might last longer than usual. Drink plenty of fluid to stay hydrated, and eat several small meals a day to maintain your energy levels. Call your doctor if you don't improve after 24–48 hours, or your temperature exceeds 101° F (38° C).

Very few pregnant women do experience complications, but if you feel very unwell, and, in particular, you experience problems breathing, see your doctor immediately. Ask the pharmacist's advice before taking any over-the-counter medication.

# Your 24th week

**YOUR BABY'S BODY SYSTEMS ARE BECOMING MORE AND MORE EFFICIENT**

A baby getting prepared for independent life needs all the help you can give her. Keep up your good habits by nourishing the two of you with healthy food; and make sure your own body is in peak physical condition to support your pregnancy. Some minor discomforts, such as feeling too hot, leg cramps, and hemorrhoids may be plaguing you. These annoying problems are only temporary and will disappear once your baby is born.

**The eyelids** are still closed. Beneath them, the eyes are protected by a thin membrane.

**The lungs** are not ready for the outside world but their function is rapidly improving.

**The baby's rapid heart rate** has slowed down a little. It is usually easy to detect the heart's beating during a scan.

**Fine, soft lanugo hairs** keep a layer of greasy vernix on the skin.

**At 24 weeks** the average crown to heel length is 10.9 in (27.8 cm) and the average weight is 15.2 oz (430 g).

**The skin** is starting to develop a protective outer layer of keratinized cells.

# 118 days to go...

**YOUR BABY TODAY**

There is no light in the uterus, but 3D ultrasound is designed to produce highlights and shadows to give the same effect as if you shone a flashlight into the uterus. Now your baby may be holding her hands flexed into a fist.

## From this point onward, your baby is considered "viable" and would receive life-saving treatment were she born early.

**Week 24 is considered the age of viability for your baby,** and therefore an important pregnancy milestone. Like many women, you may feel relieved to get past this point.

If you went into labor and delivered your baby before this week, she would be unlikely to survive and you would be considered to have had a miscarriage. After 24 weeks, the doctors will to do everything they can to save the baby, although babies delivered this early have an increased risk of long-term disability. The more advanced you are in your pregnancy before you deliver, the less likely it is that your baby will face the problems associated with being born prematurely.

**Incredible scientific and technological** advancements have meant a huge increase in the survival of premature babies.

### AS A MATTER OF FACT

**The world's youngest surviving premature baby** was born in Florida in October, 2006 at just 21 weeks and six days.

The baby weighed only 10 oz (283 g) and measured 9.5 in (24 cm). Her feet were the size of an adult's fingernail. It was the first time a baby born before 23 weeks had survived.

### NEONATAL INTENSIVE CARE UNITS

**Babies who are born prematurely,** or newborns who are sick, will receive specialized round-the-clock care in a neonatal intensive care unit (NICU) (see pp.452–3). The earlier the baby is born, the more chance there is of complications, such as infections, occurring. If your baby is born several weeks prematurely, she may need to be cared for in a level 3 NICU—this may not be in the hospital where your baby was born.

Your baby may be put in an incubator with monitors attached and receive oxygen through a special ventilator. Some of the equipment looks very frightening, but remember it is there to help your baby stay warm and nourished and improve her health.

The staff will readily explain what is going on, and they will be eager for you to be involved as closely as possible in your baby's care and encourage bonding.

YOU ARE 23 WEEKS AND 2 DAYS

# 117 days to go...

**YOUR BABY TODAY**

You will probably be aware of your baby's movements by now: the number of movements and their nature will vary during the day and night and you may notice that they start to form into a particular pattern or respond to your own activity.

## With a layer of fat and a tough layer of cells, your baby's skin is now becoming more resilient.

**Your baby's skin is continuing to develop** and has now started to "keratinize." Keratin is the substance that transforms the skin's outer layer into a protective layer of dead cells. Hair and nails also form from keratin.

The outer keratinized layer of skin cells, plus a layer of fat laid down between the skin cells, gives the skin a waterproof covering. This process of keratanization reduces the amount of water your baby loses into the amniotic fluid. Each new skin cell, made in the deepest part of the skin, matures as it gradually moves up toward the surface and, now keratinized, becomes part of the outer protective layer before it is eventually shed. The cycle takes approximately 30 days.

The thickest layers of keratinized cells are on the palms of the hands and the soles of the feet. The keratinizing process has only just begun. Since the fat layer is very thin at this stage, your baby's skin will still appear translucent, but less so than it did in earlier weeks.

At this stage of pregnancy, your baby still has plenty of room to maneuver inside the uterus, and although you're likely to be feeling lots of movements by now this will only be a fraction of the total. This is because the only movements you'll feel are those that cause your baby to kick or bump into the wall of your uterus. You will be unaware of many of the finer movements that are performed close to the baby's body since they won't make any contact with your uterus.

---

### COPING WITH LEG CRAMPS

**Getting painful spasms in the leg muscles** is common in pregnancy, particularly at night. You may find that you wake up due to the sudden and severe localized pain in your legs or feet. This is thought to be due to the pressure of the uterus on the pelvic nerves.

Some experts believe that cramps during pregnancy may be caused by a lack of calcium or salt or an excess of phosphorus, but these theories are as yet unproven.

When you get a spasm, relieve it by flexing your foot or leg (see far right), and gently massaging the affected area. The cramp should resolve itself once you are out of bed and using the muscle. However, if the pain doesn't recede and there is any reddening or swelling in the leg, you should seek medical advice immediately to eliminate the possibility of a clot (see p.186), since this can be dangerous.

To reduce the incidence of cramps or its severity, drink lots of water to prevent dehydration and regularly do leg stretches (see right) and ankle exercises, circling your heel and wiggling your toes.

Getting gentle exercise, such as walking or swimming, can also help, as can regularly massaging the calf muscle to improve circulation.

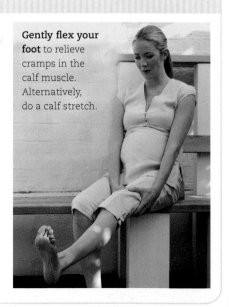

**Gently flex your foot** to relieve cramps in the calf muscle. Alternatively, do a calf stretch.

**Your baby's bones** are
hardening and her arms and
legs are beginning to flesh out.
She brings her hands to her
face often. Her skin is starting
to develop a protective outer
covering of vernix.

# 116 days to go...

**YOUR BABY TODAY**

Ultrasound uses sound waves of a very high frequency, well beyond the audible range of the human ear, so your baby's hearing will be completely unaffected by the sound waves transmitted during these scans that check her growth and development.

## Are you feeling hot? Being pregnant can sometimes feel as though you have your own personal radiator strapped to you.

**You may find that you're much hotter** and sweating more than normal during pregnancy. This is because you're carrying more weight than usual and you have more blood pumping around your body.

If you're pregnant during the summer, this can be difficult to bear, so find ways to stay cool (see p.324). If you're pregnant in the winter, you may find yourself walking down the street in a light sweater while other people are all bundled up in coats and scarves. You might get into debates with your partner if he wants the heat on and you want the windows open!

Make sure you drink enough fluid throughout the day. You might find that the increased sweat causes a rash in the creases under your breasts or in your groin, so wash frequently and make sure that you dry these areas well.

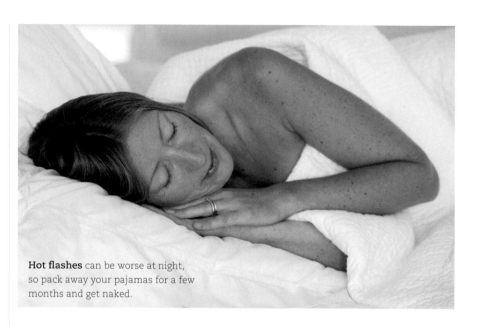

**Hot flashes** can be worse at night, so pack away your pajamas for a few months and get naked.

### AS A MATTER OF FACT

**It's common to dream that** you give birth to an older baby, who is born walking and talking!

This is thought to reflect a mother-to-be's insecurities about caring for a tiny, helpless baby. The older the baby, the more self-sufficient she appears.

### ASK A... DOCTOR

**I keep having really strange and vivid dreams. Is this normal in pregnancy?** Yes, when you're pregnant, it's common to dream more and to remember your dreams. Experts attribute the vividness of these dreams to all the emotional and physical changes a pregnant woman is going through.

The vivid dreams may be a way for your unconscious to deal with all the hopes and fears you may have about your unborn baby and impending motherhood.

The increase is also believed to be due to hormonal changes: increased levels of estrogen are thought to cause longer periods of REM (rapid eye movement) sleep—the phase of sleep in which we are most likely to dream.

If your dreams are disturbing, try writing them down to get them off your mind.

# 115 days to go...

**YOUR BABY TODAY**

The joints and bones of the hand are still very soft, although the cartilage skeleton is now gradually being replaced by bone. This image shows well the numerous capillaries supplying blood to the hands, right down to the fingertips.

Over the next few weeks, your baby will take on more of the appearance of a newborn.

**Your baby's eyelids and eyebrows are well developed** by this week of pregnancy, but the eyelids remain fused. The cells that are destined to become your baby's fingernails were present at 10 weeks, and the cells for the toenails were present four weeks later.

Now, at 23 weeks, the nails are just beginning to make an appearance at the base of the nail bed. The nails will grow continuously throughout life, but it will be several weeks before they have reached the tips of the fingers and then the toes.

Your baby's skin is developing quickly and often appears wrinkled at this stage; it is as if the baby has yet to grow into it. Your baby is now covered in extremely fine and short hairs, known as "lanugo." This layer of hair will be almost completely lost before birth. The hairs help trap vernix onto the surface of the skin; this is the white, greasy layer that you often see in patches on a baby's skin at birth. It collects in the skin folds and creases and helps protect the baby's skin not only from the water content of the amniotic fluid, but also the waste products within it.

As your pregnancy advances, your baby's kidney function is improving and the amniotic fluid produced becomes increasingly similar to urine in its composition.

---

**PREGNANCY POSTURE**

**Your posture will naturally change as a result of pregnancy;** this is due to the extra weight you're carrying and the softening of your joints.

Prior to pregnancy, your center of gravity was directly over your hips; during later pregnancy it shifts forward to your enlarged abdomen. This dramatic shift in your center of gravity increases the curve of your lower spine, and can result in lower back pain (see p.218). The weight you gain during pregnancy can also put strain on the back.

Exercises can help balance your body and alleviate the muscular aches associated with changes in your posture (see right for one example).

It's important to adapt to these postural changes in pregnancy:
- **Do abdominal exercises** (see p.250), to strengthen the core muscles, as well as back stretches. These help maintain good posture and avoid back pain later in pregnancy.
- **Be aware of** the way you're walking and standing: pull your shoulders down and back, do not arch your lower back and keep your pelvis in a neutral position.
- **Avoid balancing anything** on your hip, because this can affect your hip and back alignment.
- **Don't hold a phone between** your head and shoulder because this can result in neck pain.

**Your growing abdomen** affects the curvature of your spine. Practice tilting your pelvis to lengthen your spine.

Pull your shoulders back

Roll your pelvis under

Bend your knees slightly

Support your lower back

# Abdominal exercises

Strong abdominal muscles are beneficial during pregnancy because they will help you carry the weight of your baby and assist you during labor and birth.

Abdominal exercises done while lying on your back aren't recommended after the first trimester. The reason for this is that when you lie on your back, your enlarged uterus presses on one of your major blood vessels, reducing the amount of blood pumped around the body and to the baby. However, you can strengthen abdominal muscles without lying on your back by using gravity and your body to strengthen and tone the torso. In pregnancy, you can tone your abdomen with exercises where you adopt an all-fours position or an upright sitting position. Try to do the exercises below around 2–3 times a week.

**Benefits of abdominal exercises**
Strong abdominal muscles enable your body to work more efficiently in labor. They also help support the weight of the baby, which takes pressure off the spine, reducing the likelihood of backaches. In addition, keeping your abdominal muscles strong means that you may be less likely to get a condition called *diastasis recti*, in which the abdominal wall muscles separate, often following childbirth. making it harder to regain your figure.

**The sling** Get down on all fours with your hands on the floor, feet apart, and arms straight. Keep your back flat in a neutral position, being careful not to arch your back. Imagine your abdominal muscles as a sling holding your baby. Take a deep breath, then slowly pull your abdominal muscles (the sling) in toward your back, pulling the baby closer to you, and gently release, returning to the starting position. Repeat at least 20 times. Remember to breathe properly while doing this exercise, breathing in to start and breathing out as you pull in your belly.

**The superman pose** This exercise will strengthen your core muscles, keeping your abdomen and back strong, and helping prevent lower back pain. It also stretches your leg and arm muscles. Start from an all-fours position. Keeping your back in a neutral position, lift your left arm in front of you and your right leg up behind you. Be careful not to arch your back or lift your leg higher than the hips. Hold for a count of five and slowly lower. Then repeat with your right arm and left leg. Do around 10 repetitions for each arm and leg.

**The abdominal pull** This can be done anywhere and at any time. It's advisable to start by doing it sitting in an upright chair with your shoulders relaxed and back straight. Put your hands around your belly below your navel. Breathe in slowly and pull in your abdominal muscles for two seconds and then release; repeat 10 times. Take a short break, then start again. Once you've mastered this, move on to the next level. In the same position, pull in your muscles and release quickly, almost every second. Breathe properly and do not hold your breath.

# 114 days to go...

**YOUR BABY TODAY**

In this color 2D ultrasound scan the baby is lying face upward. it is now increasingly difficult to show the whole baby using this type of ultrasound because it only shows a thin slice at any one time. Here, only the upper part of the baby can be seen.

## Practicing yoga in pregnancy can be hugely beneficial, both physically and emotionally.

**In addition to strengthening and toning** muscles, yoga aims to bring about a greater awareness of your breathing. Learning to control your breathing is a great way to relax during pregnancy and an invaluable way to prepare to breathe through the contractions when you're in labor.

Standing poses in yoga focus on achieving core stability, thereby strengthening the back and abdominal muscles. This is beneficial during pregnancy when the additional weight you're carrying can affect your balance and cause unsteadiness. Calm sitting poses that concentrate on aligning your spine help you focus on steadying your breathing and centering yourself. If you feel unsteady doing yoga poses, you can simply lean against a wall.

Pilates is also a good exercise to do in pregnancy because it heightens your bodily awareness, giving you greater control of—and confidence in—your body. Pilates also incorporates Kegel exercises (see p.69).

Whatever classes you're doing, it's important to find an accredited instructor who is experienced in teaching pregnant women. There are now many specialized pregnancy yoga and Pilates classes.

**AS A MATTER OF FACT**

**Practicing prenatal yoga** under expert supervision can be safe and may reduce the risk of complications.

A recent study found that pregnant women who practiced yoga had a reduced risk of developing pregnancy-induced high blood pressure and of going into premature labor.

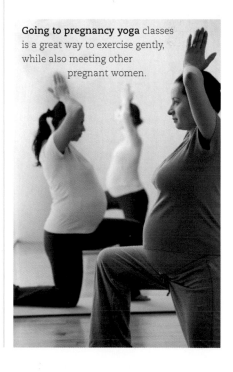

**Going to pregnancy yoga** classes is a great way to exercise gently, while also meeting other pregnant women.

---

**ASK A... DOCTOR**

**Why are hemorrhoids common in pregnancy?** Hemorrhoids are, like varicose veins (see p.167), dilated veins, but they occur around your anus. The weight of your baby pushes down on your back passage, restricting blood flow and causing the veins to dilate.

Hemorrhoids can be itchy and sore, and may cause a throbbing sensation. The discomfort can be relieved with cold packs and creams containing lubricants to help the passage of stools, and/or local anesthetics to relieve soreness. Hemorrhoids can bleed— you may notice bright red blood on the toilet paper after you pass a stool.

If you have hemorrhoids, it is important to try not to get constipated (see p.468) since this means you have to strain and push to pass stools, which increases the pressure on the hemorrhoids and makes them worse. Ensure that you drink lots of water and eat sufficient fiber.

If your hemorrhoids are becoming very problematic and uncomfortable, seek your doctor's advice.

Your 24th week

# 113 days to go...

**YOUR BABY TODAY**

Your baby is now making regular deep breathing movements. These have been present for some weeks, but not in a sustained and coordinated fashion. These breathing movements are critical for the development and expansion of your baby's lungs.

## Although the lungs are the last of your baby's organs to be fully functional, they are undergoing rapid development now.

### ASK A... DOCTOR

**Is it true that playing music to my unborn baby will enhance her development?** Some research into this claim finds that playing music to an unborn baby will lead to a shorter labor and easier birth, and to the newborn baby crying less, being more relaxed, and, overall, being in better health. At the moment, there doesn't seem to be any significant research to suggest that babies who listen to music in the uterus are more intelligent, or develop at a greater speed.

The jury is still out on these findings, but there is anecdotal evidence from pregnant women that their babies move to the rhythm of music. It makes sense that as you relax to gentle music or are invigorated by livelier music, your baby will respond in kind. Many moms say that music played frequently during pregnancy seems to be familiar to their newborns, and soothes them.

So whether your baby is simply experiencing the benefits of your happy state as you listen, or responding to the rhythm, playing music is a good idea.

**At this stage, your baby's lungs** are starting to mature, as the barrier between the bloodstream and what will become air-containing sacs gradually starts to thin. The thinner this barrier, the more easily oxygen and carbon dioxide will transfer into and out of the baby's bloodstream.

The lungs remain filled with fluid during your pregnancy and when your baby practices breathing, the fluid moves out of her lungs into the amniotic fluid.

At 23 weeks, cells begin to line the smallest branches within the lung and start to produce surfactant, a substance that greatly assists lung function. This substance enables the smallest air sacs to remain open when the newborn baby breathes in and out so that gas transfer can continually take place. Without it, the tiny air sacs would collapse after each breath and it would take much more effort to move air in and out of the lungs. The cells that produce surfactant are not, however, fully functional yet.

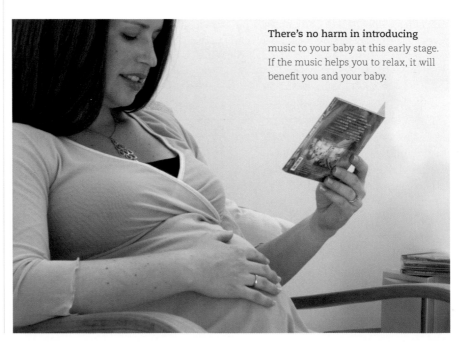

**There's no harm in introducing** music to your baby at this early stage. If the music helps you to relax, it will benefit you and your baby.

# 112 days to go...

**YOUR BABY TODAY**

As your pregnancy advances your baby's skeleton starts to harden, reflecting more of the ultrasound beam and casting black shadows. In this scan, the forehead casts a shadow, and it is no longer allowing the brain beneath to be easily seen.

Even though you're well settled into your pregnancy, ensure you maintain all those healthy lifestyle habits you've established.

**You've been pregnant for almost six months** and are, hopefully, feeling great in yourself. Don't, however, let this make you complacent. Even though your baby is well developed by this stage, it's important to maximize her health, and your own, by continuing to eat well and taking care of yourself. Changes, such as not smoking or drinking alcohol, will probably be part of your normal lifestyle now as opposed to something that you have to think about and work hard at.

If you have not managed to change your lifestyle to become more healthy, then it is never too late to start. Any changes you make now will benefit both you and your baby.

While you'll need to adapt your exercise routine, if you have one, in these later stages, ensure you continue to be active and, ideally, do something physical every day, even if it's just a 20-minute stroll. Also keep up your daily Kegel exercises (see p.69)—once the baby is born, you'll be thankful you did.

(see p.69)

---

**AS A MATTER OF FACT**

**A correctly worn seat belt reduces the risk of injury** to the unborn baby by 70 percent.

In recent research, over half of pregnant women did not wear their seat belt correctly, positioning it too high across the abdomen and putting the torso strap behind them rather than over the shoulder.

---

**FOCUS ON... DADS**

## Hello, it's Daddy

**Don't be afraid to talk to your baby.** To begin with, she will recognize lower-pitched sounds, such as deep male voices, more than higher-pitched sounds, like your partner's voice. This is good for you since it means that there is plenty of time for your baby to get to know your voice before she is born. After birth, your baby will recognize your voice and this will have a calming effect when she is distressed. So tell her about your day and even read to her—it helps create a bond.

**For maximum safety and comfort,** wear the seat belt positioned between your breasts and under your belly.

---

**HOW TO WEAR A SEAT BELT**

**It may feel cumbersome to wear a seat belt** while you're pregnant, but it is essential, and a legal requirement. The good news is it's possible to buckle up comfortably.
- **Fasten the belt** over your shoulder, as normal, and between your breasts (see left).
- **Position the lower part** of the belt below your belly, and flat over your hips (see left).

If an emergency stop is necessary, be reassured that your baby is very safely cushioned by the amniotic fluid that surrounds her and your strong uterine muscles.

# Your 25th week

**IT'S THE END OF THE SECOND TRIMESTER, SO YOU MIGHT WANT TO START LOOKING AHEAD**

The rest of your pregnancy will pass before you know it. Make sure you have all the practicalities in hand, such as deciding what date to stop work, and you might want to give some thought to the birth. Meanwhile, friends and family will no doubt be monitoring your growing belly with interest. Try to be patient if they bombard you with advice and don't listen to too many "tall tales" about pregnancy and childbirth.

**Your baby yawns** often, perhaps as a way to regulate the amount of fluid or blood in his lungs at any one time.

**Blood flow** through the umbilical cord and placenta regulates the baby's temperature, keeping it much the same as your own body temperature.

**At 25 weeks** the average crown to heel length is 11.7 in (28.9 cm) and the average weight is 1.1 lb (501 g).

**The baby's head** still seems too large for his body, but overall he's beginning to look more in proportion.

**Hearing is now acute** and loud noises may startle the baby into sudden movement.

**The limbs** appear more rounded as fat continues to be laid down.

# 111 days to go...

## YOUR BABY TODAY

From this week, brown fat is laid down in your baby's neck, chest, and back to be used after birth to produce heat and energy. At the moment he has no control over his temperature, which is efficiently maintained at a perfect level by the placenta.

This week, think about starting discussions with your employer about your upcoming maternity leave.

**Since you're more** than halfway through your pregnancy by now and are likely showing, you've probably already told your boss that you're pregnant. But just informing your company isn't enough—you need to know all the details that pertain to your upcoming maternity leave and what will happen if you decide to stop working before the baby is born.

Every company has different guidelines; some include paid maternity leave while others do not. Talk with a human resources representative to discuss your company's policies on maternity leave and time off. If paid time off isn't available, your company may allow you to use paid vacation days or sick leave, and you may be eligible for FMLA leave.

### FOCUS ON... YOUR BODY

## Stretchy skin

**You may have developed stretch marks** due to your skin stretching rapidly as you gain pregnancy weight. Initially, these marks are pinky/red and can be itchy. After pregnancy, stretch marks fade to a lighter, silvery color and become less obvious. They generally occur on the breasts, belly, hips, and thighs, and affect the majority of pregnant women.

Stretch marks can be genetic and are more likely to occur the older you are because older skin is less elastic. Moisturizing the skin won't prevent stretch marks but it may help to keep it smooth. A combination of exercising and eating healthily can minimize the rate at which you gain weight and "stretch."

### ASK A... DOCTOR

**My doctor measured me and said I seem small for dates. What does this mean?** It means your baby appears to be small for your stage of pregnancy, but it doesn't necessarily mean there's a problem. You'll be given a scan for an accurate measurement and so that your baby's development can be thoroughly checked.

Sometimes slow growth is due to a condition called intrauterine growth restriction or retardation (IUGR). It can be due to a problem with the placenta, multiple babies, or heart disease in the mother, affecting the nutrients reaching the baby. Preeclampsia (see p.474) can cause IUGR, as can smoking, alcohol, and recreational drugs.

### AS A MATTER OF FACT

**You may be eligible for Family and Medical Leave Act leave.**

You must have worked for an employer for at least 12 months (1,250 hours in the past 12 months), and within 75 miles of 50 or more company employees.

# 110 days to go...

**YOUR BABY TODAY**

In the uterus, your baby's ears not only have fluid around them but also inside. This is part of the reason that he can only hear certain lower sound frequencies. Yawning may be a way to unblock the ears, and from now on your baby spends a lot of time yawning.

## If you're feeling tired, you're not alone. Your developing baby has been yawning for some weeks now.

**All babies are known to yawn in the uterus,** although the reason why they do this remains unclear. Yawning is often accompanied by shrugging of the shoulders or stretching, exactly as you would do when tired. Unborn babies have even been seen to rub their eyes!

Your baby first started yawning at around 15 weeks and has gradually yawned more and more frequently. The precise function of yawning for the baby remains in doubt and there are several hypotheses. While it's difficult to imagine that an unborn baby is actually tired, it has been found that babies who are anemic yawn much more frequently than others. Another theory is that yawning may help the unborn baby to regulate the amount of fluid or blood flow he has within his lungs. Or yawning may simply be a primitive reflex, a remnant from an earlier evolutionary stage, with no current function.

Whatever the reason for yawning, the early stage at which this develops in the unborn baby, and the fact that all mammals are known to yawn in the uterus, does suggest that it plays an important, though unknown, role in fetal development.

### AS A MATTER OF FACT

**Women aged over 40 are more than twice as likely** to have left-handed babies.

This is according to a Canadian study and may be related to the fact that older women are more likely to experience complications in pregnancy and have more arduous deliveries. Several studies show a correlation between left-handedness and birth stress.

**Many unborn babies have been filmed** yawning on 4D scans, which give a very up close view of fetal behavior.

### FOCUS ON... YOUR BABY

## Listen to Mommy

**Your developing baby's ears are structurally complete,** and studies show that he can hear clearly now. Far from cushioning him against noise, the amniotic fluid that surrounds your baby has excellent sound-conducting properties. Your heartbeat and digestive system provide a constant background rhythm, but he's also aware of other sounds.

Talking to your baby will help you to bond: research indicates that newborns recognize—and turn toward—the sound of their mother's voice in preference to other female voices. To begin with he'll hear deeper voices more clearly, but later he'll register higher-pitched sounds. He will, of course, become more familiar with his mother's voice because this is what he will hear most often.

You may have noticed that sudden noises make your baby startle. In one study, ultrasound scans of fetuses showed that they had a "blink-startle" response to loud noises from around 26 weeks.

# 109 days to go...

## YOUR BABY TODAY

Here the baby is lying with an arm up to the face and the face lying on the placenta. The eyes are shut at this time and it will be a couple of weeks before they start to open. The hand is held in the most relaxed position, with the fingers slightly curled.

## Your body is working hard to grow your baby, so take care of it by enjoying some pampering.

**Think of your pregnancy** as a time to focus on yourself and your body; once your baby is born, the majority of your focus will be on baby care.

If you have the time and money, treat yourself to a day at a spa. Most spas will have special packages for pregnant women. Spending time at a spa, where you can go for a gentle swim, have some pampering treatments, and enjoy being in a tranquil environment, is a great way to relax and unwind. If a spa day is out of the question, create your own at home. Run a bath, add some relaxing music (for a background soundtrack), light some candles, and relax. If you don't want to be disturbed, let your partner know and turn off the phone.

Pregnancy massage (see p.224) either from a professional or your partner, can be very therapeutic, both physically and emotionally. Another great treatment to have at this stage is a pedicure; you'll increasingly be unable to see your toes, let alone reach them, so it's a treat for someone else to take care of them for you.

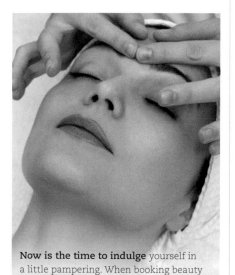

**Now is the time to indulge** yourself in a little pampering. When booking beauty treatments, always make it known that you're pregnant.

**ASK A... DOCTOR**

**I haven't felt my baby move for four hours. Should I be worried?** Contact your doctor and explain your baby's usual pattern of movements. She can examine you and provide reassurance.

If you're not familiar with your baby's movements, lie down—he is more likely to sleep when you're active. Try encouraging him to move around (see p.206).

**ON YOUR FEET**

**You may now find it more of a struggle** to be on your feet, especially for long periods of time. Weight gain, changes in your center of gravity (particularly during the second and third trimesters), and hormones can cause foot pain and swelling (see p.225 and p.466). The pregnancy hormones that relax your joints ready for childbirth can also work to loosen the ligaments in your feet and hips, which can cause some discomfort.

To minimize foot discomfort:
■ **Wear sports shoes** that have a good arch support to help reduce strain on your spine. They may also prevent a condition called *plantar fascitis*—this is where the large ligament that connects the heel to the ball of the foot becomes inflamed.
■ **Avoid wearing high-heeled shoes.** In addition to being uncomfortable, they may make you unsteady on your feet and cause you to fall.
■ **Ensure that your shoes fit** correctly and invest in new ones if not. Some pregnant women's feet expand by a size, and never return to their normal size after pregnancy.
■ **Get regular exercise,** and avoid standing for long periods. Take regular breaks if your job involves standing.

# 108 days to go...

**YOUR BABY TODAY**

This 3D scan shows the baby thumb sucking. The 3D technique uses several routine 2D images, linked together to give the 3D effect. In a 4D scan, a series of 3D images are shown in quick succession to give almost real-time movements: the 4th dimension is time.

## A natural temperature-regulating mechanism within the uterus means your baby never gets cold.

**The temperature inside the uterus** is between a third and half a degree higher than yours. Because your body temperature is so closely controlled, your baby never becomes cold so never needs to shiver. He has started to lay down a special form of brown fat, particularly around the neck, chest, and back. After birth, metabolism of this fat produces both energy and heat. In the uterus, however, the baby cannot use this fat to raise his temperature. Some temperature control occurs as heat is lost from the baby's skin into the amniotic fluid through the uterine wall and then into your body tissues. However, the regulation of temperature is predominantly achieved by means of the blood flow to the placenta. The large surface area of the placenta allows it to act as a heat exchange, keeping the temperature of the blood leaving the baby in the umbilical arteries constant with that of the oxygenated blood returning to the baby through the umbilical vein.

After birth, babies lose heat quickly. They are still unable to shiver and cannot maintain their temperature, cooling rapidly if they're not wrapped up warmly or held skin-to-skin shortly after the birth.

### SENSIBLE SNACKING

**In addition to eating three meals a day,** you may find you need to snack throughout the day, too. There's nothing wrong with that as long as you're choosing the right foods, and not reaching for the cookies and chips all the time. These tempting foods might satisfy a hunger pang, but the lack of nutrients and empty calories won't serve you any real purpose. Healthy snacking can be accomplished with a bit of planning before you go shopping:

■ **Dried fruits** should be a mainstay of your snacking, since they can easily be stored and carried. Enjoy a wide variety of dried fruits, since the more variety you consume, the more likely you are to obtain the nutrients you need. Try dried apricots, raisins, cranberries, cherries, and peaches.

■ **Lightly salted mixed nuts** will satisfy any salt craving you may have in a healthy way.

■ **Opt for pretzels, oatcakes,** or crackers, rather than potato chips.

■ **Fresh fruit** is a convenient and nutrient-rich snack; always carry one or two pieces with you when you're out and about, and make fruit salads that you can keep in the fridge. Keep frozen fruit on hand, and along with some vanilla yogurt, you can whip up a smoothie in no time at all.

■ **Frozen yogurt and low-fat ice cream** both make good snacks and desserts. Stock up on a variety of low-fat yogurt brands.

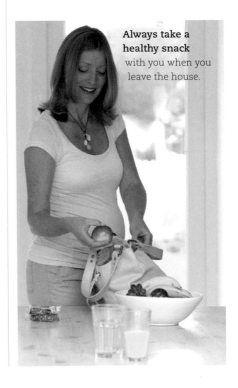

**Always take a healthy snack** with you when you leave the house.

# 107 days to go...

**YOUR BABY TODAY**

Here the skin looks almost loose around the neck as the baby has turned his head slightly. This is normal at this stage: the lack of fat beneath the skin and the need to grow rapidly can make your baby appear as if he needs time to "grow into" his own skin.

## Some meals may be followed by an uncomfortable bout of indigestion, but you can take steps to prevent and relieve this.

### THINK ABOUT GAS

**I seem to be gassier than usual lately. Is the pregnancy to blame?**
Yes, pregnancy slows down your digestive tract, which can lead to unpleasant burping, bloating, passing gas, and an uncomfortable feeling in the stomach. Symptoms can be worse after you eat a large meal. To minimize problems:

■ **Steer clear of foods that make you gassy.** For many women, this may include cabbage, beans, and other foods rich in fiber. Some women have trouble with large amounts of dairy products.

■ **Eat smaller meals more frequently** rather than a couple of large meals.

■ **Avoid swallowing air.** This means you shouldn't hurry when you eat, you should chew every mouthful thoroughly, and you should avoid drinking through straws. Also, skip carbonated beverages and chewing gum.

■ **Reduce your intake of fatty, fried foods** which can contribute to bloating and discomfort.

■ **Don't take any OTC indigestion remedies** without first checking with your doctor.

**While you may be enjoying your food,** you could be paying the price with indigestion. The pregnancy hormone progesterone relaxes the muscles in the entire digestive tract. This slows digestion and the sphincters,

or rings of muscles, at each end of the stomach become less effective. This can cause heartburn and indigestion as acidic juices from the stomach leak back into the esophagus. In addition, as your pregnancy progresses, your growing baby is squashing your stomach so that you have a smaller space to digest food.

To relieve indigestion, eat little and often, eat slowly, don't eat late at night, and cut down on fatty or spicy foods. Make sure to talk to your doctor about any natural remedies, including peppermint tea. Rather than lie flat, prop yourself up with pillows. Check with your pharmacist before taking over-the-counter medicine.

**Natural remedies** might seem harmless, but taking any herbal preparation, even peppermint tea, should be discussed with your doctor.

### FOCUS ON... DADS

## Arranging paternity leave

**Although it's much less common than paid maternity leave,** you may be entitled to paternity leave and pay (see p.349). Speak to your human resources department now to find out your rights and whether your company offers additional perks. To maximize the time you can take off once the baby is born, figure out how much vacation you have left and consider saving up days. You may also qualify for FMLA leave, but this is unpaid.

# 106 days to go...

**YOUR BABY TODAY**

The nose is well defined and in addition to regularly swallowing the amniotic fluid your baby is breathing it in and out through each nostril. Just as adults do, your baby will tend to favor breathing more through one nostril than the other.

From this point onward, babies grow at an individual rate, which is largely influenced by their genes.

**The proportions of your baby's body** are becoming much closer to those of a newborn baby. Up until the third month, his head accounted for almost half of his overall length. Now his head, trunk, and legs each account for a third. At birth your baby's head will still be large in proportion compared to an adult's, but it will be just a quarter of his overall length.

Still very skinny, your baby is now starting to fill out more as fat reserves continue to be laid down.

Up until this point most babies are approximately the same size and weight. Genetic and especially environmental forces increasingly come into play, influencing how quickly your baby can grow and whether his full growth potential is eventually reached.

Because different babies increasingly vary in size from this stage of pregnancy, ultrasound dating becomes less accurate at determining the number of weeks you are into your pregnancy. The best time to date the

pregnancy is between 11 and 14 weeks, simply measuring top to bottom (the crown rump length) (see p.138). The 20-week scan (see pp.214–15) also dates the pregnancy very accurately from the head and abdominal circumferences and the bone measurement in the leg.

If your first scan is at this late stage, it is only possible to estimate roughly the stage of pregnancy and age of the baby. It is never appropriate to change your due date if an earlier, more accurate scan has been performed.

---

**IT'S ALL IN THE BELLY**

**The general story goes that if you're carrying your baby low,** you're having a boy, if you're carrying high, then you're having a girl. The truth is, the way you carry is probably determined by the tone of your abdominal and uterine muscles as well as the position of your baby.

According to those "old wives," there are other physical clues: if you've gained weight on your face and it's round and full, you're having a girl. If your right breast is larger than your left, it's a boy—and if your partner gains weight, you're "definitely" having a girl!

**Small-framed woman carrying baby to the front**

**Medium-framed woman carrying baby low**

**Larger-framed woman carrying baby high**

# 105 days to go...

**YOUR BABY TODAY**

Here the baby's head is looking down toward the chest. The right arm is bent at the elbow to lie across the neck, the left arm is only just visible as it is partly in shadow, and finally the tip of a knee can be seen tucked up just below the right forearm.

## You can expect to be subjected to a few unwelcome birth stories, whether you want to hear them or not!

TIME TO THINK ABOUT

## Birth partners

The benefits of having a supportive birth partner are indisputable, so it's a good idea to think about it now.

■ **Research shows that** women who receive continuous emotional and physical encouragement during labor are less likely to need pain relief or medical intervention such as an epidural (see pp.404–5), assisted delivery (see pp.436–7), or cesarean (see pp.438–9), and should experience a shorter labor.

■ **Women who feel their birth partner** was supportive are more likely to view their birth in a positive light, and to take to motherhood and breast-feeding easily, and are less prone to postpartum depression.

■ **Your birth partner** doesn't have to be the baby's father (although he may be there as well); in fact, studies indicate that a woman may do the job better. A close female friend who's had her own children could be ideal; your mom is another option.

■ **You could consider** hiring a doula (see right).

**It appears to be a rite of passage** for some women to describe the birth of their babies in minute detail, literally giving an hour-by-hour account. For these women, it appears to be part of the recovery process and they like nothing better than a new audience, and, especially, a woman who is pregnant for the first time. So you'll no doubt find yourself on the receiving end of a few birth horror stories—sometimes from complete strangers!

These women may feel it's their duty to "warn" you about the "reality" of childbirth, and what you should and shouldn't do—for example, "definitely

**Having a close female friend** or relative with you during labor, even if it's only at home in the early stages, may prove to be a great help to you and your partner.

have an epidural, otherwise the pain is horrendous." Remember that every woman's experience is different and stay focused on your own birth plan. Childbirth is undoubtedly difficult for some women, while others have straightforward deliveries, without complications. Tell the story-teller you'd rather not hear the gory details but promise to book a date for a joint debrief once your baby is born!

MOTHER'S HELP

**The prospect of giving birth and then taking care of a newborn** can be daunting. For some moms, hiring a doula is the perfect way to ensure a gentle progression from pregnancy to motherhood.

Doulas are women who "mother the mother" by providing emotional and physical (but nonmedical) support before, during, and after childbirth. Widespread research shows that the presence of a doula can help you have a shorter, easier birth, making it less likely that you'll need pain relief or medical intervention (including an epidural or cesarean). To find out more about hiring a doula, visit dona.org/mothers/find_a_doula.php.

Your 25th week

261

# Welcome to your third trimester

**A new person emerges** Your baby is close to being a fully functioning individual. His major organs are almost ready to work in the outside world, but he would need medical help if he were born now.

**From weeks 26 to 40,** your baby will probably grow by about 5½ lb (2.5 kg) and 8 in (20 cm).

**Third trimester** Your growing baby pushes out your lower ribs and fills up most of the space in the uterus. **Ready for birth** Your belly is huge and you're tired and breathless, but excited too.

**Monitoring growth** By measuring your growing abdomen, your baby's rate of growth is assessed and any concerns addressed with further tests.

**A new brother or sister** Include older children as you prepare for your new baby. They can help you choose clothes and think about names.

**Sleeping comfortably** You need to take the weight off your belly, but relaxing is easier said than done. Use lots of pillows to cushion you when you rest in bed.

**Preparing for labor** Going to prenatal classes and exercise sessions will help you prepare both mentally and physically for the approaching labor and birth, and feel confident about how you'll manage.

# You're in the home stretch now and your thoughts turn increasingly to the birth of your baby.

| 33 | 34 | 35 | 36 | 37 | 38 | 39 | 40 |
|----|----|----|----|----|----|----|----|

**Fiber fit** An adequate fiber intake is especially important in late pregnancy when a sluggish digestion makes constipation more likely.

**Ready to go** Delivery date is on the horizon. Before you go to the hospital, pack your bags some time in advance. Start gathering essential items.

**Nearing the end** As you reach the end of your pregnancy, you'll marvel at the size of your belly.

**38 weeks** It's a tight fit now for your baby, so he doesn't have much room to turn and kick. You should still feel him moving, though—so it's important to be aware of any change in activity.

**Facts and figures** By week 38, the placenta's role is nearly over and it starts to age.

**Bringing on labor** If you've reached 40 weeks with no sign of labor, you may be starting to think about ways to trigger its onset—making love is one of several methods to try.

**Taking the weight** It's worthwhile to continue swimming as long as you feel able since the water supports all your additional weight, bringing welcome relief.

**Facts and figures** By 33 weeks, your baby is rapidly putting down fat deposits and is starting to look more like a newborn baby.

**Hello, baby** Here at last, and worth all the waiting. Immediate skin-to-skin contact has significant benefits for your baby.

# Your 26th week

**YOU'VE REACHED THE THIRD AND FINAL TRIMESTER AND WILL BE HEAVILY PREGNANT BY NOW**

You're in the last lap and, although your belly is probably big, you've still got a lot more expanding to do. Your baby will be moving around quite vigorously and may even respond to loud noises and music. Nerve cells in her brain are beginning to connect and her coordination is improving. Keep your own brain stimulated by going to prenatal classes for fun, company, and information.

**All the nerve cells** that make up the outer surface of the brain are in place. They will gradually branch out to form neural connections.

**The toes** are often grabbed by the baby's hand and may even be brought up to her mouth.

**Hand coordination** is improving and your baby often brings her hands to her face, and especially her mouth.

**At 26 weeks** the average crown to heel length is 11.8 in (30 cm) and the average weight is 1.3 lb (600 g).

**Your baby's body** is very flexible and she can double herself up with ease. As she gets bigger, her movements become stronger.

# 104 days to go...

**YOUR BABY TODAY**

Here the baby is looking directly upward. The profile is nicely detailed with the nose, lips, and chin clearly outlined. The neck is still quite short so, as this image shows, the head is still held quite close to the chest.

## Your prenatal classes will give you a chance to learn about labor, birth, and life with a newborn, and make new friends.

**If you arranged them earlier** in your pregnancy (see p.199), You may be starting prenatal classes, also called childbirth education classes, about now. The Lamaze Method and The Bradley Method are common classes. Ask your health-care provider, friends, and staff at the hospital where you're giving birth about where to find a class near you. In the class, you may be taught, for example, relaxation or breathing techniques, or be told about the different types of pain relief available. Some hospitals also offer newborn care classes, where you'll learn all the basics: How to diaper, dress, feed, carry, and generally take care of your baby when she is brought home from the hospital.

It's common to feel excited about the classes and eager to learn about what's going to happen and to meet other people going through the same experience. But prenatal classes are not just about gathering information, they're also about meeting others, which is difficult for some people. However, since you're all parents-to-be, you're likely to find things to talk about. Just talking with others about your symptoms or worries can help, especially if they're going through the same emotions as you. It can be reassuring to know that you're not the only person to feel a certain way.

If you do make friends in your prenatal class, this support group can also be very helpful after you all have your babies.

---

**FOCUS ON... YOUR BODY**

### Rib pain

**As the uterus expands,** the rib cage is pushed outward to make room for it, and this can lead to rib pain or discomfort. This is not inevitable, but it is more likely if you have a smaller than average body frame or you're carrying twins or more. It can be worse if your baby kicks a lot or if she spends a lot of time in the breech position since her head will push against your diaphragm and rib cage.

Sitting down may make the pain worse since being seated compresses your internal organs more. If you have a sedentary job, get up and move around as often as you can, and if you're forced to sit for long periods, keep adjusting your position until you find one that's comfortable.

Intestines | Liver | Rib | Stomach

Expanding uterus reduces space for stomach and intestines

---

**ASK A... DOCTOR**

**I think I have a vaginal infection. Will this harm my baby?** A vaginal infection is very unlikely to harm your baby since the mucus plug around the cervix stops infection from reaching her. The symptoms of an infection—itching, irritation, and a discharge with an unpleasant odor—are uncomfortable. Your doctor will prescribe medication to clear it up.

# 103 days to go...

### YOUR BABY TODAY

This image shows the baby in profile, this time in 3D. The coils of the umbilical cord are just seen in the background passing behind the baby's head. The eyelids can be seen, still firmly closed. Fat reserves are now giving the face a much more rounded contour.

## Two tiny glands control your baby's growth and development now, and give her the ability to face life's stresses later.

**Relative to body size,** your baby's adrenal glands are 20 times larger than your own. The adrenal glands are roughly triangular in shape, with their base wrapped over the top of each kidney. They have an outer layer, or cortex, which releases steroid hormones such as cortisol, and an inner layer, or medulla. Adrenaline and the related hormone noradrenaline are secreted from the medulla in response to stress.

Adrenaline prepares the body for a "fight or flight" response, increasing the availability of glucose, speeding up the heart rate, and maintaining or raising blood pressure. These are vital adaptive responses for your baby that will help to maintain a stable environment

within the uterus and prepare her for the stresses of life later on in the outside world.

It is the outer cortex, however, that needs to work hard, producing many hormones that help to coordinate your baby's growth and development. The cortex produces three types of hormones: mineralocorticoids that

regulate salt balance; glucocorticoids that help to control the availability of sugars, fat, and amino acids in the bloodstream; and androgens, male-type sex hormones, such as testosterone. It is the cortex that accounts for the large size of your baby's adrenal glands. After birth, in the first couple of weeks, the adrenal glands rapidly reduce in size.

---

### ASK A... DOCTOR

**I've noticed lumps in both my breasts. Should I be worried?**
Breast lumps can be normal in pregnancy, especially in the third trimester as the breasts get ready for breast-feeding. These lumps are generally soft and may move around; they may also be tender. However, breast lumps should never be ignored, so always see your doctor who will be able to confirm that they are pregnancy related.

---

### FOCUS ON... TWINS

## How identical are identical twins?

**Twins from the same egg** have the same DNA. In a way, they're natural clones, so you might expect them to

be identical in every way. They will certainly look very alike, and have the same hair color, eye color, and skin color. They will also have the same blood group and tissue type.

However, the environment isn't the same for each baby, even pre-birth. Small differences in blood flow, and in location in the uterus, can have far-reaching effects.
■ **There may be recognizable differences** in the weight, height, and head shape of identical twins.
■ **Each twin** has unique fingerprints and iris patterns.
■ **Identical twins** can have different personalities too, partly because of subtle dissimilarities in their very early environment.

# 102 days to go...

**YOUR BABY TODAY**

This baby has her hands held up in front of her face. In the top right-hand corner, the curved inner lining of the uterus can be seen. Shadows in the image give the impression of hair but ultrasound is not detailed enough to show hair—even if there was any to see at this stage.

## Going to prenatal classes together is a good way for your partner to stay closely involved with your pregnancy.

**Not all dads-to-be** are eager to go to prenatal classes. They might not feel the classes apply to them, and may fear that they will be asked to do exercises that they find embarrassing.

If your partner is reluctant, discuss it with him, pointing out what the classes are for and why you feel that you need his support. You could explain that you want him to be informed about labor so that he is not anxious in the delivery room. He might find it useful to talk to male friends who went to classes when they were expectant dads.

Classes may include some sessions with men and women together and others where the women go on their own, for example to practice breathing techniques, while the men have a separate session where they can share any concerns. If time off work is an issue for your partner, ask for a list of what topics will be covered each week and pick those sessions that you think are the most relevant for him. If your partner is well informed, he'll feel more involved in the pregnancy and more confident in helping you during labor and birth.

**What you learn at prenatal classes** may bring you closer. Try to stay in touch with each other at home, spending time relaxing together and feeling your baby moving.

---

**TIME TO THINK ABOUT**

## Family leave

Thanks to the Family and Medical Leave Act (FMLA), most companies must give employees (men and women) up to 12 weeks of unpaid family leave after your baby is born. The rules: If your company has fewer than 50 employees, they don't have to offer FMLA. Also, you must have worked for the company for at least one year. It's a good idea to ask your human resources department about your company's policy about leave and have your partner do the same.

---

**FOCUS ON... RELATIONSHIPS**

## Anticipating changes in your relationship

**It might seem obvious,** but once your baby is born your relationship won't just be about you and your partner any more. Suddenly there is a tiny new person around, who wakes during the night and who has her own needs. By necessity, after your baby is born you and your partner will pay less attention to each other. There

may also be less physical intimacy between the two of you, not least because you both will be very tired.

It's best to talk about, and acknowledge, these issues before the birth. This way, you and your partner will better accept that these factors are a normal part of making the life change from coupledom to being a family.

# 101 days to go...

### YOUR BABY TODAY

This 3D image shows the back of the baby, taken using a scanner setting that enhances the reflections from the skeleton. The back of the spine, ribs, and shoulder blades are clear: this technique has opened up many new possibilities for visualizing your baby's development.

## All the nerve cells are now on the surface of your baby's brain; what they need to do next is make connections with each other.

**Your baby's brain** is so complex that it needs the entire length of your pregnancy not only to grow, but also to mature. It is continually forming new connections and sensory pathways.

The nerves that make up the brain's gray matter started in the center of the brain on the outer surface of the lateral ventricles (there is one ventricle in each hemisphere of the brain). The lateral ventricles contain the part of the brain known as the choroid plexus, a loose, seaweedlike structure that produces the fluid that bathes your baby's brain and spinal cord. Constantly circulating around the brain, this fluid protects and buffers the brain from the harder structure of the bones of the surrounding skull.

The gradual, wavelike, outward movement of nerve cells in the gray matter, which started more than 12 weeks ago, is now complete. Coming to rest close to the brain's surface, these cells need to mature, branching out to make multiple connections, or "synapses," with other nerve cells.

The surface of your baby's brain is very smooth at this stage but as the cortex matures, beginning to form six clear layers, it takes on its familiar wrinkled appearance.

---

**FOCUS ON...** YOUR BELLY

## Your belly: to show or not to show?

**Whether you want to clothe your belly** in figure-hugging fabrics and proudly show it off, or choose looser styles that may fit you longer and obscure just how pregnant you are, is a personal choice.

■ **If you're fine showing your belly,** you may feel comfortable in stretchy fabrics that can expand as your belly does. The downside to wearing tight clothing is that your skin may be sensitive to anything snug-fitting. Tight tops will also bring attention to your breasts.

■ **If you feel more comfortable** not showing the profile of your belly, choose baggier clothes, such as tunics, smocks, and overshirts. These may be more comfortable and will cloak your belly longer.

■ **If you want to bare your belly,** do so when the weather is warm enough. One advantage is you may find you can wear some pre-pregnancy tops.

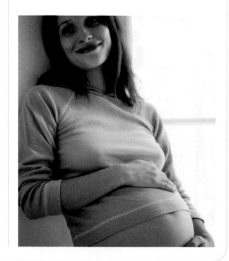

---

**ASK A...** DOCTOR

**I'm getting quite big—should I adapt my swimming style?**
You may find that in these final couple of months, you need to change your swimming style to one that is more comfortable; many women opt for breaststroke, which can also help to get the baby in to an optimum position (see p.329).

If you don't feel up to swimming laps, just relax in the pool instead. Being in the water will relieve pressure on your abdomen and help to ease lower back pain.

# 100 days to go...

## YOUR BABY TODAY

With fingers held up to the cheek, eyes closed, and the ear just visible in the background, this image shows a very peaceful baby. To the left, the umbilical cord is visible on its way to the placenta, seen further to the left.

**It will be some years before you'll know your child's personality, but even in the uterus she has some likes and dislikes.**

**As your baby continues** to grow you may find yourself wondering what she is going to be like: easy going or demanding? Funny or serious? Happy playing alone or social? Boisterous or quiet? You may believe that babies are born with their personalities already developed, or that they are born with a personality that is further shaped and developed as they grow. The nature versus nurture debate rages on and, in all likelihood, it's a combination of the two: some aspects of your child's personality may already be decided before birth, some may be developed later in childhood, or even adulthood.

You may already have noticed that your baby has certain likes or dislikes, for example she may kick or move in response to loud music or to a certain genre of music, though it's difficult to tell whether the increased movements mean your baby is enjoying it or not.

Your baby is very stimulated inside the uterus. By this third trimester, she can feel vibrations, and hear not just sounds from inside your body, such as your heartbeat, but also sounds from outside, such as people talking. Your baby is aware of when you're moving or are still and you may have noticed a pattern of movements from her, not least that she "communicates" more when you're resting.

As part of her activity, she will continue practicing for life after the birth, with breathing movements and swallowing—and she may even suck her thumb.

## BUYING FOR YOUR BABY

**Preparing for your baby's arrival** doesn't have to break the bank.
**What your baby needs:**
■ **Milk:** breast milk is free (and best for your baby). For bottle-feeding, you'll need bottles, nipples, formula, and a sterilizing system.
■ **Diapers:** you'll need to decide between disposables, reusables, or a combination of the two (see p.291). Whichever type you choose, you'll also need to use diaper wipes.
■ **Somewhere to sleep:** she can sleep in a crib from birth if you don't want to buy a bassinet. Even if you buy a used crib, you should always buy a new mattress.

■ **Lots of onesies:** don't buy too many newborn size.
■ **Transportation:** a stroller (with a lie-option until your baby can sit up), or a sling or frontpack to carry your baby.
■ **Car seat:** this is a legal requirement for car travel. Don't buy used.
**What your baby can live without:**
■ **Changing station:** a mat (or towel) on the floor is cheaper and safer.
■ **Bottle warmer:** heat in a jug instead.
■ **Designer wardrobe.**
■ **Pack-n-Play:** borrow one if necessary. Save money by shopping online. Scour second-hand shops and yard sales. Swap clothes and toys with friends, family members, and other parents.

**Babies soon outgrow onesies** and get little wear out of them so you may be offered some from friends. You can cut the feet off the onesies if they're too tight.

# 99 days to go...

**YOUR BABY TODAY**

A 3D scan can be colored in different ways: this image demonstrates that by this stage your baby's lip shape is clearly defined. The lips are the most sensitive part of the entire body and your baby's hands are often held up toward them.

## Your baby can make coordinated movements with her hands and feet, make a fist, and grab hold of her toes.

**Your baby's hand coordination** dramatically improves now and she constantly brings her hands up to her face, particularly her mouth. The face, and especially the lips, are extremely sensitive, and this heightened sensitivity provides strong positive feedback as your baby successfully coordinates smooth, purposeful movements between hand (and foot) and mouth.

There is still plenty of room in the uterus for all sorts of movements and your baby is extremely flexible. It is quite easy for her to adopt a doubled-up position, with her feet up by her mouth or even on top of her head, and to do full somersaults.

Your baby's bones are hardening from the center out so their outer edges are still formed of soft cartilage.

### ASK A... DOCTOR

**Why do I get so hot when I'm exercising?** During pregnancy, your core body temperature rises due to the effects of the hormone progesterone, your increased weight, and the greater demands on your body. Exercise generates heat and raises your core temperature even further, which is why you're likely to feel extra hot when you exercise during pregnancy.

You'll also sweat more easily while you are pregnant. This is because pregnancy-related hormones cause dilation of blood vessels and thus blood flow to your skin (this explains the rosy "glow" some women get), allowing your body to lose heat through the skin more readily. This means that, although you

get hotter while you're exercising, you'll cool down more quickly than usual. When you're exercising, always remember to:

■ **Drink water** before, during, and after a workout.
■ **Wear appropriate clothing** that will allow your skin to breathe.
■ **Avoid exercising** when conditions are hot and humid.

### FOCUS ON... YOUR BABY

## Birth weight

**A woman's weight gain** during pregnancy influences her baby's birth weight, which in turn influences the future health of the baby. Birth weights that are too high or too low have been associated with an increased chance of health problems in the baby's future. Thus, pregnancy is a balancing act, in which women need to take in enough, but not too many, calories and gain the right amount of weight (see p.99).

Health experts are increasingly concerned about the fact that fetal over-nutrition is resulting in high birth weight. Being overweight, or putting on excessive amounts of weight during pregnancy, increases the chances of gestational diabetes in the mother (see p.473), a cesarean delivery, complications during delivery, large newborns, and childhood obesity. If a child is obese, there's an increased risk of a lifetime of being overweight or obese, which increases the chances of diabetes, high blood pressure, cancer, and heart disease.

# 98 days to go...

**YOUR BABY TODAY**

The space between the two frontal bones of the forehead (the dark line) has now nearly closed. The bones on the left and right sides come to lie very close to each other with a small gap to allow for further growth of the head and brain.

Dreaming is a natural and healthy part of your sleep cycle, but at this stage of pregnancy unsettling dreams can be common.

**Vivid dreams are common** among women in the third trimester. You may, in fact, not be dreaming more than usual, but difficulty in finding a comfortable sleeping position and waking often to go to the bathroom may mean that you remember your dreams more than usual (you normally would not wake during the dreaming phase of your sleep cycle, so often do not recall your dreams in the morning).

It is common to dream about babies and small children in distress or danger. It is not uncommon for women to feel anxious about such dreams, but you should know that they are in no way insights into what is in store for you. Dreaming is a way of filtering any negative emotions so that you do not have to experience them first hand. Rest assured that, although disturbing, these dreams will help you cope with your natural concern for your baby's welfare.

## GOING ON A HOSPITAL TOUR

**As part of the build up** to your baby's birth, you may be offered a tour of the hospital. Not only will you be able to see first hand where you'll be delivering your baby and what the units are like, but you can also figure out the practical details, such as parking, admission procedures, what you'll need to bring, and what facilities there are, such as cafés and shops for visiting friends and family.

Ultimately, a hospital tour offers you a reassuring chance for you and your partner to prepare yourself mentally for the big day and what will follow your baby's birth.

Use the opportunity as a fact-finding mission. Ask how the hospital uses birth plans (see p.303), and when and why they might have to be adapted. Ask how many other moms there will be in the unit, and, if you want, how you can arrange a private room. There is usually a fee for this. Find out what support you'll have in the first 24 hours. Most hospitals now expect the mother to keep the baby with her during the night. Ask about visiting hours, and the number of visitors you can have at any one time. You could also ask how many babies are born at the hospital each year, and how many of these are born by cesarean (emergency or otherwise). Request information about how long the shifts are and what nurses and doctors do to provide continuity of care during labor and birth. Ask to see a delivery room and the nursery.

Are there birthing pools or baths available? Do they have TENS machines or any other form of pain relief you may be considering? What support is there for breast-feeding, and are there breast pumps available?

Finally, although you probably won't need to use it, you may want to see the neonatal intensive care unit (NICU) (see pp.452–3). If your baby needs this type of care, it can help to have seen the equipment and gained a basic understanding of what it's used for.

# Your 27th week

**YOU MAY FIND IT DIFFICULT TO SLEEP DUE TO YOUR BABY'S ACTIVITIES**

Space is now getting tight in your uterus. The baby is likely to give you a few sharp jabs with his feet and fists as he stretches and turns. However uncomfortable the kicks may be, you'll find them a welcome reassurance that the baby is thriving. Relax in bed or in the bath and watch your belly—you'll be amazed and amused at how it pops up and down and moves around.

**The eyelids** are fully open this week. Your baby responds to bright light, although he cannot focus, and he can blink.

**The baby** is taking up a lot of space in the uterus and there is less amniotic fluid surrounding him.

**The baby kicks** often and a large kick against your ribs may take your breath away.

**At 27 weeks** the average crown to heel length is 13.6 in (34.6 cm) and the average weight is 1.5 lb (660 g).

**A boy baby's testes** often descend fully into the scrotum around about now. However, in some babies, the testes remain in the pelvic cavity until after birth.

# 97 days to go...

## YOUR BABY TODAY

The coiling umbilical cord is very clearly seen in this image. The umbilical cord grows as your baby grows and will be about the same length as your baby at this stage of your pregnancy: about 13.6 in (34.6 cm).

When you settle down for a nap it can be frustrating if your baby starts exercising, but take this as a sign that all is well.

**You may have noticed** that your baby is more active at some times than at others, often when you're trying to relax or sleep! This is likely to be because when you're busy or distracted, you're less aware of your baby moving because you're not paying much attention to him as at other times. The moment you stop and sit down to put your feet up or go to bed will be the time your baby starts to do his somersaults.

Remember that, like newborns, babies still in the uterus spend a lot of time sleeping, so there will be periods when you don't feel your baby being very active—it's fine for him not to be moving all the time. Every baby has a different cycle of waking and sleeping, and there are no rules as to when your baby should be kicking and when he should be still.

If you're familiar with your baby's pattern of movements and are concerned that you haven't felt him move, try lying down on your side and relaxing or playing music to see if your baby responds. If, however, you're concerned, then call your doctor. She may want you to come in to examine you and listen for the baby's heartbeat.

Some women count their baby's kicks using a chart, noting down when they feel the baby move. Kick charts are not often used now, unless recommended by a doctor because they are thought to cause unnecessary concern. Babies have an individual pattern of movements, and it is this, rather than the number of kicks, that's important.

**I've never taken care of a baby and I don't even know how to put a diaper on one! What can I do?**
You're not alone: I had never been around babies much and was full of questions. How do diapers work? What do babies do all day? What if I drop my baby? Luckily a friend had a three-month-old who we "borrowed." As you'll soon realize, there are plenty of weary moms and dads out there, and almost certainly someone among your family and friends will be only too happy to take a break. But before you remove the baby from his comfort zone, spend time with him and his parent(s). Feed him and change diapers under his mother's watchful eye. If she's confident that you're up to the job, offer to take charge, perhaps just for a few hours at first.

If all goes well, you could build up to a day—or even overnight. It'll work wonders for your confidence and eliminate any fears you have about baby care. When it comes to taking care of your newborn, you'll have some idea of what to expect and feel more sure about what you're doing.

## AS A MATTER OF FACT

**During pregnancy your total volume of blood is 50 percent** higher than normal.

The amount of blood pumped with each heartbeat increases by about 40 percent and you make around 20 percent more red blood cells than normal.

# 96 days to go...

**YOUR BABY TODAY**

This color ultrasound shows the baby breathing the amniotic fluid (red, flowing toward the ultrasound beam) in and out. The baby is breathing a stream of fluid out through the nostrils and, at the same time, a smaller amount through the mouth.

## As the development of your baby's eyes and sense of sight continues, he reaches another milestone: the eyelids open.

**Although your baby's eyelids** formed at nine weeks of pregnancy, they have remained fused together until this week. Your baby is not in complete darkness, however, because as the uterus grows its wall thins allowing in increasing amounts of light. Now, your baby's eyes have reached a stage of development where they can open.

Even with the eyelids open, the delicate structures of the eyeballs are protected by a fine membrane that will completely disappear during the final month of pregnancy.

It's too early for your baby to respond to light in a fully coordinated way, but he may turn toward very strong lights or, if startled by a sudden loud noise, he will often respond with a blink, just as children and adults do.

The retina has just started to be lined by light-receptive rods and cones. The cones are responsible for color vision and develop later than the more numerous rods. The rods transmit an image in black and white and are used for nighttime vision and for peripheral vision. Connections form between the retina and the optic nerve, that then transmits the information it receives to be decoded in the visual cortex at the back of the brain.

Your baby will often bring his hands up to his face. However, because his limb movements are now so well coordinated, he won't touch his eyes.

### ASK A... DOCTOR

**I've got inverted nipples. Will I be able to breast-feed?** Babies breast-feed rather than "nipple feed" and if your baby latches onto your breast correctly (see p.448), inverted nipples shouldn't cause difficulties. About 10 percent of women have flat or inverted nipples. The best way to find out whether you can breast-feed is simply to try once your baby is born. There are various techniques that may help: consult your doctor if you're having problems or contact a lactation consultant. Your doctor or hospital may recommend one or the La Leche League can help (see p.480).

### FOCUS ON... TWINS

## Growth of twins in the last trimester

**In these last three months, you're likely to get very big.** As you'd expect, the more babies inside, the greater the challenge for your body to provide enough space as well as the perfect conditions for growth. You'll probably be advised to gain just under 1 lb (0.5 kg) a week for the first half of your pregnancy and slightly more each week in the second half.

From around 28–29 weeks, the growth of twins and other multiples slows down compared with that of singletons. But they still move and kick as much as possible, cushioned by amniotic fluid, which continues to increase in volume until 36 weeks.

# 95 days to go...

**YOUR BABY TODAY**

Your baby sticks his tongue out often especially before or after a particularly large gulp of amniotic fluid. Fluid doesn't enter the lungs but is swallowed into the stomach. Your baby would be completely unaware of the ultrasound scan, so is not reacting to the scanner.

It's a natural instinct that parents are fiercely protective of their children, and not unusual for this to start well before the birth.

**You may be feeling** very protective of your belly and baby. The belly almost acts as a beacon to other people, making them aware that you're pregnant. It's not unusual to feel quite vulnerable, for example in a jostling crowd or when you're out shopping. When this happens, make it clear to people that you're pregnant and, hopefully, they'll give you more space and give up their seat, if necessary.

When you're driving, you may find you're doing so even more carefully than normal, or becoming a very nervous or critical passenger. You may become more irritated than usual by people who you feel are driving without concern for your safety.

This protective instinct is a natural part of becoming a mother. It's the desire to protect and nurture your child, even before yourself. Rest assured, though, that your baby is in the safest possible environment inside your uterus. Your body is providing your baby with warmth, food, and oxygen. The baby is cushioned and protected by the amniotic fluid in which he floats, and this acts as a buffer to any shoving or bumping by crowds of people.

## ASK A... DOCTOR

**Why am I being told I need a glucose tolerance test?** In pregnancy some women develop a form of diabetes known as gestational diabetes (see p.473), which disappears when the baby is born. It may be suspected if you have signs such as fatigue and thirst and is confirmed by testing urine for glucose. If it's found, you'll be advised to have an oral glucose tolerance test (OGTT) between 24 and 28 weeks. You'll be tested earlier if you have a BMI over 35, a close relative with diabetes, or had diabetes in a previous pregnancy.

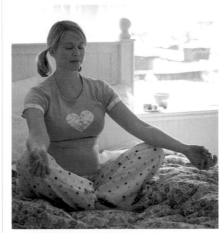

**HypnoBirthing is a great idea** but it's important that you are taught the various relaxation and visualization techniques and practice them regularly during pregnancy.

## THE LOWDOWN

## HypnoBirthing

The idea of hypnoBirthing—giving birth in such a relaxed state that you barely feel pain—sounds too good to be true. But the research extolling its benefits is impressive. Several studies have shown that self-hypnosis helps women feel less anxious about labor and birth. They also tend to require minimal pain relief and medical intervention: many women succeed in giving birth at home.

■ **You learn a series** of self-hypnosis, relaxation, visualization, and breathing techniques, which over time become second nature, enabling you to approach childbirth in a calm, positive frame of mind.

■ **By practicing hypnoBirthing,** you should feel in control of your body and able to manage the pain during labor and delivery.

■ **The key is to practice frequently,** and a supportive birth partner is invaluable for helping you perfect the techniques, and use them in labor.

■ **Ask your doctor** to recommend a course near you or visit HypnoBirthing.com.

# 94 days to go...

**YOUR BABY TODAY**

On this 3D image each finger is held outstretched in front of the face. Holding the fingers in this way for any length of time is tiring so most of the time the hands are held with the wrists slightly flexed and the fingers bent, ready to grasp any object that floats into reach.

Your baby's reproductive organs are now in place; a boy's testes have descended and a girl's ovaries have all their follicles.

**ASK A... MOM**

**Is it normal to argue all the time when we should be happily looking forward to our baby's arrival?** Expecting a baby puts pressure on even the strongest of relationships. Concerns about having a healthy baby and adjusting to parenthood were at the heart of most of our arguments. And when we started to talk about it, we found we had conflicting opinions about big child-rearing issues. I was sensitive, irritable, and moody, and often snapped when I didn't mean to.

We sat down and talked calmly and agreed not to "sweat the small stuff," avoiding areas of contention, and compromising when it didn't really matter. In the throes of a disagreement, I'd stop and think: I love this man, we're having a baby together, is this really important in the long run? We also made time to do positive things together that we had enjoyed before I was pregnant, and tried to find opportunities to laugh, to reduce stress, and to put things into perspective. By the time the baby arrived, we were both much more relaxed.

**If your baby is a boy,** it's at about this time that the testes complete their descent into the scrotum. This is often associated with a small amount of fluid around each testis called a "hydrocele." This fluid will disappear naturally either before or after birth.

The cremaster muscle, part of the spermatic cord, is able to raise the testes back into the groin. This helps to regulate the temperature within the testes after birth, relaxing when cooling is needed. If your baby is slightly cool when examined, the cremaster muscle retracts the testes giving the impression of an undescended testis in your newborn baby.

Temperature control is not required in the uterus and the testes slowly move down into the scrotum. It is by no means unusual for one testis (or both) not to have descended at birth. Your doctor will check for this as part of the routine baby development checkup and confirm that both testes can be brought down into the scrotum.

Unlike the ovary, which already contains all of the egg-producing follicles that it will ever make, the testes do not start to make sperm until puberty.

Differences in the speed of growth and weight gain become more apparent now, and boys tend to be slightly heavier than girls at birth.

**WEIGHT GAIN IN THE THIRD TRIMESTER**

**In your third trimester** gaining weight steadily is important. If you were a healthy weight before your pregnancy, you should gain 3–5 pounds in the first trimester and 1–2 pounds a week the rest of your pregnancy, for a total of 25–37 lb. Keep in mind that the largest contributing factor to your overall weight gain will be your baby, followed by extra fat, which you will need to sustain your pregnancy and when breast-feeding. Your doctor will monitor your weight gain to ensure it's healthy.

**Weight gain chart**

Your third trimester

# 93 days to go...

## YOUR BABY TODAY

This week, some babies open their eyes for the first time but this is a brief event, difficult to capture on ultrasound, so you may not see it on a scan. Some light is reaching your baby but he hasn't developed a sleep–wake cycle that corresponds in any way with day and night.

As each day passes, your baby is getting bigger and bigger and you will be more conscious of his body and movement.

**As wonderful as it is** to feel your baby move inside you, sometimes it can be uncomfortable. As your baby grows there is less and less room for him to move around, especially as he kicks or stretches against the walls of your uterus. These movements can vary from gentle paddling motions to feeling as though the baby has hiccups. Sometimes the baby will kick hard; if it's under the ribs it can take your breath away and leave you feeling quite sore. The kicking can also wake you when you're sleeping, and many women say that their babies are more active at night. If you're sitting or lying in a position that the baby doesn't like—for example, if you spend too much time on one side—your baby may well kick until you move.

Although sometimes these movements can be uncomfortable or take you by surprise, most of the time they're just a gentle reminder of your growing baby and, as such, are something to look forward to feeling.

### ASK A... DOCTOR

**If I went into labor now, would my baby survive?** Until relatively recently, babies born before 28 weeks' gestation often did not survive. Today, with medical advances in neonatal intensive care units (NICU), babies of 22 weeks' gestation have survived outside the uterus, although this is still very rare. At many hospitals, doctors won't resuscitate a baby under 24 weeks, because there is little chance of survival.

Extremely premature babies have an increased risk of disability, even with the best medical care, and often the delivery itself can put an enormous strain on the baby. Very experienced doctors and nurses are involved in the care of extremely premature babies.

If possible, the delivery should take place in a hospital with a neonatal intensive care unit (NICU) (see pp.452–3). If this isn't possible, babies are often transferred to a special center when they are stable enough to be moved. Very premature babies take a long time to "catch up" and meet developmental milestones.

Each day and week of pregnancy is a milestone, and the closer to full term (37–42 weeks) you deliver, the better it is for your baby.

### FOCUS ON... SAFETY

## Buying bedding

**Your baby doesn't need a blanket** or pillow—in fact, experts advise against them. To reduce your baby's risk of sudden infant death syndrome (SIDS), put a fitted sheet on a firm crib mattress (don't use a second-hand mattress), and keep blankets, pillows and stuffed animals out of the crib. If your baby sleeps in a Moses basket or bassinet, you should buy sheets designed specifically for these. Keep the room at a temperature that feels good to you. If you're concerned that your baby is chilly, consider a sleep sack. Many parents find them to be comfortable for their baby.

# 92 days to go...

## YOUR BABY TODAY

At this stage, thumb sucking is becoming much more coordinated as the sensitive lips and fingers meet. On scans most babies look as if they enjoy it, and there's no doubt that it provides important sensory feedback and perhaps reassurance to your developing baby.

## The thought of being off work in the last months of pregnancy is tempting, but it will give you less time off with your baby.

**As long as you're feeling in good health,** try to work into the last month of your pregnancy. It can be particularly frustrating if you finish two months before, only to find that your baby is born later than expected. Working as late as possible may also allow you to spend some time with your replacement. If you're finding work tiring, try to adapt your working day and avoid traveling during rush hour, if possible. Whenever you start your leave, colleagues may hold a party and want to buy gifts for your newborn. If you're asked what you want, suggest gift certificates since these will allow you to purchase some of the more expensive baby equipment, and prevent duplication of gifts. Many stores also offer baby registries, which are a good way to choose the items you want.

### BACK PAIN IN THE THIRD TRIMESTER

**One of the most common pregnancy complaints,** back pain is generally a reaction to your increased weight and the laxity of the joints that are an integral part of pregnancy. There are some ways to alleviate this, and anecdotal evidence suggests that women who exercise are far less likely to suffer from extreme back pain than those who don't.

It is best to try to avoid back pain by exercising your abdominal muscles which will give your back support, and keep your legs and arms strong too. See page 250 for an effective abdominal workout.

Carrying does not end when you have had your baby. You will have a car seat, baby bag, and perhaps groceries to carry, as well as your newborn. So it's best to keep your muscles strong throughout your pregnancy to prepare for this. Here are five top tips to avoid back pain in the third trimester:

■ **Stay strong:** strength training for all parts of your body (see p.196) will help you deal with the increased weight you gain during pregnancy.
■ **Support:** invest in a support belt that will give your back a break from bearing the load of your belly. It will also support your sagging stomach and may relieve discomfort in your legs. This can be particularly useful if you're carrying twins or more.
■ **Sleep:** while sleeping, place a pillow between your legs to ease the stress on your back. Buy or borrow a shaped pillow that gives your belly and back support at the same time.
■ **Stretch:** flexibility will help your back to relax and prevent your muscles from getting too tense.
■ **Sit:** keep your back supported by the back of a chair (see p.219). Use a pillow to increase the support in your lower back, if necessary. If you work at a desk, make sure your chair adequately supports your back.

**Stretching helps prevent your muscles from tightening,** so you feel less tense and more relaxed. Put on some comfortable clothes and stretch as often as you can, and always stretch before and after exercise.

# 91 days to go...

**YOUR BABY TODAY**

This baby looks quite upset. Your baby often makes strange and funny faces in the uterus. It's as if he is practicing every type of facial expression in preparation for after the birth when these will be one of the tools he uses to communicate his needs and emotions.

As you soak in a relaxing bath, it's an amazing sight to look at your baby moving and stretching your belly.

**Your belly is a marvelous thing.** It's already changed so much over the last 27 weeks and will continue to grow until you give birth.

Inside that belly your growing baby is moving around. When your baby is kicking and turning around, take the time to look down, and you may be able to see him move or even see the imprint of a foot as it kicks you.

While you're taking a bath is a good time to watch your belly—you may find that your baby is more active around this time because you're relaxed—and you can take the time to observe his movements. Keep your partner involved when your baby is active by encouraging him to touch your belly.

**Watching your baby move** is wonderful. You may even miss your ever-expanding and active belly once you're no longer pregnant.

## Are you tired too?

**Being pregnant is more tiring than most women anticipate.** In the third trimester, your partner's bladder is under pressure and this can cause her to wake during the night to use the bathroom. The size of the belly starts to become uncomfortable, and it can be difficult for her to find a relaxing sleeping position. The other changes she's going through, from shifting internal organs through to altered hormone levels, can contribute to her restlessness. And if she's having trouble sleeping, you are likely to be disturbed too. The end result is that both of you feel constantly tired.

Unfortunately there is no answer. Going to bed earlier can help, but having some time to relax together before bed is just as important. The bottom line is that disrupted sleeping patterns will now become part of the norm for both of you. There is no quick fix to this problem, but it may help to cut back on your social life in the evenings.

**ASK A... DOCTOR**

**My belly measurement has been the same for three weeks. Why isn't my baby growing?** In pregnancy your abdomen is measured to establish the height of the top of the uterus, which indicates how the baby is growing. It is important to know whether the same person is measuring you since there is an element of subjectivity depending on the technique the doctor uses. In early pregnancy, it is not necessary to measure you because this doesn't give an indication of fetal growth, but after 26 weeks, growth can be assessed this way However, even with your own growth chart and with the same person measuring you, the estimation of your baby's growth may still not be 100 percent accurate. If there are any concerns, your doctor may order an ultrasound to figure out why your measurement, called your fundal height, hasn't changed.

# Your 28th week

**EVEN BEFORE BIRTH, YOUR BABY IS ESTABLISHING A PATTERN OF BEHAVIOR**

Your baby is beginning to have regular sleep–wake cycles and her breathing, yawning, and swallowing are taking on a more definite pattern. However, your own life may seem less rhythmical. You may find things are slightly different at work and, perhaps, be seeing less of some friends because you don't always feel up to socializing. Don't become isolated, though—if nothing else, stay in touch by phone and email.

**The lungs** have established a rhythmical pattern, which helps to speed up their development.

**Eyelashes and eyebrows** are growing longer and thicker.

**The hair** on your baby's head is growing longer.

**Many babies** now move into a head-down position, though they are likely to keep turning for a few more weeks.

**At 28 weeks** the average crown to heel length is 14 in (35.6 cm) and the average weight is 1.7 lb (760 g).

**In some women**, the pelvic joint is painful at this stage of pregnancy, due to hormonal changes.

# 90 days to go...

## YOUR BABY TODAY

On a scan the space between the frontal bones of the forehead appears as a dark line on the soft spot at the top of your baby's head. This is not a line on the skin: instead where there is no underlying bone, more of the ultrasound beam passes through rather than being reflected.

**Do all you can to stay involved with medium- and long-term plans at work so that you continue to feel part of the team.**

### The difficulty of balancing

motherhood and a career can crop up even while you're still pregnant. Depending on your career, you may find yourself excluded from long-term planning discussions as colleagues assume that you won't be around, or won't come back after your maternity leave. Some colleagues may simply treat you differently just because you're pregnant, assuming you can no longer do your job in the same way. You may feel left out of future planning, or feel that your opinions are disregarded since you will not be there to implement them. This can be compounded by the fact that it can be difficult to motivate yourself if you know you won't be there to see a project through to the end.

No one can be certain of being in a job in six months' or a year's time, but you have the advantage of knowing how much longer you're going to work and you may even have a reasonable idea of when you're intending to return to work. Continue to do your job and make it clear by your actions that you want to provide input on all projects, even though you may not be there to see them through to the end. If at this point in time you're intending to return to work after the baby is born, make this clear to any colleagues who may doubt your long-term commitment.

You can also help plan for your maternity leave by, perhaps, dividing up your workload or helping to search for a replacement to cover your role. Being organized now will make the countdown to going on maternity leave much easier in the coming weeks.

---

**ASK A... MOM**

**Should we buy a baby bath or can the baby use our bath?** I thought a baby bath was an optional extra, but having bought one found it really useful. A huge advantage is that you can use it in any room (though if the room doesn't have a water supply, you'll need to transport water).

I was a bit apprehensive the first few times we bathed the baby, then experienced parents told me even they found it tricky to hold a wiggling baby safely in a bath of water. Using a smaller baby bath is less daunting and helps you develop confidence. However, a baby outgrows a baby bath by around six months and, once not in use, the bath can take up a lot of storage space (unless you can recycle

it to a pregnant friend). Many parents choose a bath seat designed for newborns in the family bath. Alternatively, enjoy a bath together, although you must keep the water tepid for the baby and you may find this too cold for you.

---

**AS A MATTER OF FACT**

**As your uterus grows, your diaphragm is compressed** with the result that you may find it difficult to breathe deeply.

In fact, you're actually taking in more air. It's important not to fight the natural tendency to hollow your back. This opens up your rib cage to let in more air, and also helps balance the excess weight of your belly.

# 89 days to go...

## YOUR BABY TODAY

Your baby may be looking happy today. Babies smile and grimace, wrinkle their foreheads, and stick their tongues out. Many of these behaviors are only becoming more apparent now as 3D ultrasound has provided a unique opportunity for their study.

## Your baby has developed a sleep–wake cycle very similar to the one she will have in the days and weeks after birth.

**Your baby's yawns** have, until this point occurred only occasionally as a single event, but they are now becoming more repetitive, with several yawns following one another. Your baby's swallowing reflexes were developed at 25 weeks but still need to become much better coordinated.

The baby's breathing movements are vital for the normal development of the lung tissue. Your baby does not breathe amniotic fluid into her lungs; The lungs are filled with fluid produced by the lung tissue itself, and as breathing movements are practiced, small amounts are expelled. With each breath, the diaphragm pushes down, and the chest wall moves in as the larynx relaxes, allowing fluid to escape. Only a tiny proportion (0.5 percent) of the fluid in the lung escapes with each breath. This compares to a fifth (20 percent) of the air in the lungs moving in and out with each breathing movement.

Your baby has been breathing for some weeks, but the pattern up until now has been somewhat random. Now, the baby's breathing patterns start to reflect her better developed sleep–wake and becomes more rhythmical.

---

### FOCUS ON... NUTRITION

## Burning calories

**During pregnancy your body will store fat**—mainly in the hips, thighs, and abdomen—to ensure there is enough energy for your baby to grow. Usually, the body relies on glucose for energy but in mid and late pregnancy, hormonal and metabolic changes facilitate the use of fat as an energy source. If you exercise regularly without adding on calories, you could be reducing the amount of stored fat. In addition, doing cardiovascular and weight-bearing exercise regularly tends to increase your metabolic rate slightly; therefore even when you're not exercising, your body will burn more calories.

It's important that you do exercise regularly during pregnancy but you need to make sure that you're taking in enough calories to meet the demands of your growing baby and your body. A simple guideline is that during your third trimester you should be taking in an extra 200 calories a day, with an extra 150 calories on the days that you exercise.

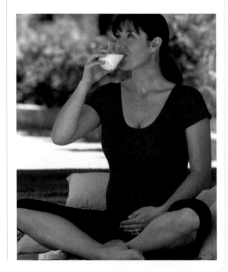

---

### TIME TO THINK ABOUT

## Prenatal care

**As your pregnancy progresses, you'll have appointments every two weeks.**

At each one, your blood pressure will be measured, and your urine tested for protein. The doctor will also check the size of your baby by measuring the height of your uterus, and she will listen to any concerns and offer you advice.

# 88 days to go...

## YOUR BABY TODAY

This baby is at the end of a yawn. Your baby is yawning in a more coordinated way now with one yawn often following another. It may look as if this image shows the fingertips in the bottom right but in fact it is a foot, nearly brought up to the mouth.

Pregnancy is a subject about which everybody has an opinion they want to share with you, whether you like it or not.

**Although you may** have become very proud and protective of your belly, it can be extremely irritating if other people become overprotective of you. You may find that everyone has an opinion on your pregnancy, and what you should and should not be doing to stay healthy. Some women find all the attention comforting, but others find it frustrating or suffocating. If you're someone who finds all the advice difficult to handle, try to remember that people mean well.

Of course, it's your body, and you'll do what is best for you and your baby. If it's all getting too much, then try talking to the main offenders, often a partner, mother, or mother-in-law. Explain that you're trying your best and that you're aware of what you should and shouldn't do while you're

pregnant and are following the advice of your doctors. Politely thank them for their input and reassure them that you're taking good care of yourself and your baby.

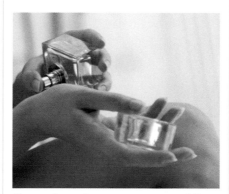

**Choose the perfume you put on carefully** since you may find that some scents, even one you're used to wearing, make you feel nauseous or light-headed during pregnancy.

## On smelling good

Are you wafting through pregnancy feeling fresh as a daisy? It's rarely discussed, but being pregnant may make you feel less fragrant than usual, not least because you will sweat more than before—although it's unlikely that anyone else will have noticed. An increase in vaginal discharge is also nothing to worry about, but if it smells offensive or is yellowish or greenish in color, you could have an infection so see your doctor. To stay smelling sweet:

- **Shower or bath regularly** and apply deodorant every time. Take handy wipes with you to stay fresh all day.
- **Use body sprays** and lotions if your usual fragrance doesn't smell "right": they tend to be lighter and are less likely to cause headaches.
- **Avoid wearing tight clothing:** wear loose clothes in natural fabrics, which absorb sweat and allow your skin to breathe.
- **Wear cotton underwear,** and change it more often, if necessary.
- **Use disposable panty liners,** if needed, to stay feeling fresh.

**FOCUS ON... YOUR HEALTH**

## Blood pressure checks

**About 8 percent of women** have problems with high blood pressure in pregnancy. High blood pressure can be caused by preeclampsia (see p.474), a serious condition that also leads to protein in the urine. Preeclampsia can affect the liver and kidneys and, if

untreated, lead to eclampsia or seizures. If you have preeclampsia, your doctor will closely monitor your blood pressure. High blood pressure can affect also your baby, so medication may be recommended. Don't stop the medication without your doctor's okay.

# Assessing fetal growth and well-being

In addition to monitoring your own health and well-being throughout your pregnancy, the doctor will also assess how your baby is growing and will refer you for further tests if she has any concerns about your baby's well-being.

**Measuring your abdomen** helps the doctor monitor your baby's growth.

## Measuring your baby

In a low-risk pregnancy, the abdomen is measured at prenatal visits to assess the baby's growth. The measurement in centimeters from the top of your pubic bone to the top of your uterus (the fundus) should be about the same as the number of weeks you are pregnant, with an allowance of up to 2 cm either way. For example, if you are 26 weeks' pregnant, you should measure between 24 and 28 cm. Your fundal height can be measured between 24 and 36–37 weeks, since once your baby "drops" into the pelvis in late pregnancy, the measurement

may not reflect his or her true size. If there is a variation of 3 cm or more, your doctor will arrange for an ultrasound to check your baby's growth (see below) and the amount of amniotic fluid. If the scan indicates a problem, the doctor will arrange for scans every two weeks since analyzing growth patterns over time gives a more accurate assessment of whether your baby's growth is normal.

In certain cases, for example if a woman is obese, in twin pregnancies, and where there are large uterine fibroids, the only accurate way to measure growth is by ultrasound.

---

**UNDERSTANDING RESULTS**

## Growth charts

**If your doctor has any concerns about your baby's growth later in pregnancy,** he or she may arrange for scans to be done over a period of time so that your baby's growth can be plotted on a chart and monitored. Individual measurements will be taken of the head, abdomen, and limbs. Measurements of the head and

abdomen are most important since an unequal growth pattern in these areas may indicate a particular problem.

The three lines on the graphs here represent different growth rates. The red line in the center, referred to as the 50th percentile, shows an average pattern of growth. The thinner lines above and below, the 90th and the 10th percentiles,

show the top and bottom ranges of normal growth. Since the head and abdominal circumferences are measured over time and plotted on a graph, a pattern of growth becomes clear. Here, the head is growing normally, but growth has slowed in the abdomen, possibly due to a placental problem that in itself may be caused by a condition in the mother. For example, conditions such as high blood pressure (see p.283) or diabetes (see p.473) can affect placental blood flow. If the blood flow to the baby is restricted, this can result in the oxygen and nutrients carried in the blood being diverted to the baby's most vital organs, the brain and heart, rather than to the abdominal organs, which results in unequal growth patterns in the head and abdomen.

**Head circumference**

cm
36
32
28
24
20
16
12
8

14  18  22  26  30  34  38  42
Weeks of gestation

**Abdominal circumference**

cm
36
32
28
24
20
16
12
8

14  18  22  26  30  34  38  42
Weeks of gestation

## Measuring growth with ultrasound in late pregnancy

By late pregnancy, the length of your baby can no longer fit on the screen and so his or her size will be calculated by combining several measurements in a mathematical formula, as is done at the 20-week scan (see p.214). Measurements include the width of the head (biparietal diameter), circumference of the head, and the abdominal circumference, which are plotted on a graph over a period of time (see box, opposite page). The length of the upper leg bone (femur length) may also be measured. If your baby is smaller than the 10th percentile or has a small abdomen, you may have more tests to assess his or her well-being (see below). A measurement above the 90th percentile can be a sign of gestational diabetes (see p.473) and will need investigating. Also, if your baby is at the larger end of the scale, your doctor may recommend you have a cesarean delivery.

## Your baby's well-being

If there are concerns over your baby's growth, you may be referred for a "non-stress" test and/or biophysical profile testing, which observe how your baby responds to stimuli and if there are signs of fetal distress. If you have a known condition that can affect your baby's growth (see box, opposite page), your doctor may arrange for you to have one or both of the above tests once or twice a week after about 32 weeks' gestation as a matter of routine, whether or not there are concerns about your baby's growth. Some hospitals also perform special scans, known as Doppler scans (see box, right) to assess placental blood flow.

**A non-stress test** This test assesses your baby's well-being. An external transducer is placed on your abdomen to listen for accelerations in your baby's heart rate that last about 15 seconds. The mother may or may not

## Doppler scans

**A Doppler scan is a special scan that analyzes blood flow through the placenta.** If the placenta is functioning well, the blood flows easily. If there is a problem in the placenta, it is resistant to the blood flow and the baby's heart has to work harder to pump blood. In extreme cases, there are periods between your baby's heartbeats of no blood flow or reversed blood flow through the umbilical cord. In this case, an early delivery may be suggested unless you're very premature.

High pressure at start of heart pumping cycle

Reduced pressure at end of heart cycle

High pressure at start of heart pumping cycle

Very low pressure at end of heart pumping cycle

**A normal Doppler reading shows the continuous blood flow** to the baby via the placenta. At the beginning of a heart cycle, the pressure is high; it then dips at the end of the cycle, but doesn't ever stop.

**An abnormal reading** indicates that there is resistance to blood flow in the placenta, resulting in very little or no flow at the end of the cycle. The baby may not receive sufficient oxygen, which can affect growth.

---

notice any fetal movement during these accelerations. The test result is thought to be "reassuring" if the heart accelerates twice over 20–30 minutes, and there are no large decelerations. About 10–20 percent of babies have a test with less than two accelerations. This doesn't necessarily mean there is a problem: your baby may just have been asleep, and the test may be repeated.

**A biophysical profile (BPP)** If, after the non-stress test, your doctor has concerns about your baby, a biophysical profile (BPP) may be done. A BPP combines the results of a CTG reading with a scan to evaluate four factors: the volume of amniotic fluid, fetal movement, fetal muscle tone and posture, and fetal breathing. Two points are given for each part of the test, so a "reassuring" BPP result would be eight points.

I've heard about "kick counts." Should I be doing these?

Fetal movement counting, or "kick counts," is one way to monitor the well-being of your baby from 28 weeks onward. However it can cause undue worry to moms and other indicators of movement are important. These include noting a change in the pattern of movement and inactivity when your baby is normally active. Your doctor may ask you to write down your baby's normal movement and call her immediately if there are any changes in the pattern.

Can my baby move too much?

Usually, the more movement the better, even if this keeps you up at night or causes discomfort. An active fetus is not a sign that you'll have a restless baby or hyperactive child.

# 87 days to go...

**YOUR BABY TODAY**

This baby's back is turned and she's facing away from the ultrasound scanner. The skin is much less transparent than before since your baby is constantly laying down fat reserves beneath it. This fat accounts, in part, for much of your baby's weight gain from now on.

## Your baby is growing eyebrows and eyelashes—and hair on her head—and making good use of all the space in your uterus.

**Your baby's eyes** are now open, and both the eyebrows and the eyelashes have grown. The hair on your baby's head continues to get longer.

It's quite likely that your baby is making use of all the space available and may well be in a breech position (bottom down), at least some of the time. This is the case in a third of pregnancies at this stage but your baby's position is unlikely to stablize until after 36 or 37 weeks.

Because the shape of your uterus naturally favors a head-down position, only 3 to 4 percent of babies remain in the breech position after 37 weeks. It may be quite difficult for you (and your doctor) to tell the position of your baby at this stage. For example, just because the feet kick you in one particular place doesn't tell you much about your baby's position. She is very flexible and an ultrasound might show that she is doubled up with her feet on her head.

### BLOOD TESTS

**Some time between 26 and 30 weeks** your blood will be tested to check that you aren't anemic. If you are found to be anemic your doctor may prescribe iron pills for you. Because of an increase in the fluid content of your blood, your hemoglobin count is likely to fall later on in your pregnancy, so it's a good idea to address this issue now. Iron pills can cause digestive problems, such as constipation or diarrhea, so if this happens to you, ask your doctor if your prescription can be changed. The liquid medications available over the counter are kinder on the digestive system than pills, so ask your doctor if one of these is appropriate for you. If a previous blood test has shown that you're Rh negative, you'll receive an injection of Rh immunoglobulin (RhIg) at around 28–34 weeks. You'll get another shot after the baby is born.

(see p.470)

### FOCUS ON... YOUR HEALTH

## Pelvic girdle pain

**You know you've got pelvic girdle pain—or PGP—**when sneezing hurts, you're waddling like an old woman, and turning over in bed is a major task (see p.470). Formerly known as SPD, or symphysis pubis dysfunction, PGP affects one in five pregnant women. It's caused by hormonal changes that change the way the pelvic joint functions and it can be extremely painful. Try the following if you have PGP:

■ Keep your legs together when getting in and out of bed or the car (place a plastic bag on the seat to help you swivel).
■ Sleep on your side with a pillow between your legs.
■ Wear comfortable shoes.
■ Avoid doing tasks that hurt, such as housework or pushing a supermarket cart.
■ Relax in warm water.
■ Ask your doctor for a support belt to help ease the pain.
■ Get some therapy: studies show that physical therapy and acupuncture may help symphysis pubis dysfunction.

# 86 days to go...

**YOUR BABY TODAY**

A finger is held close to the eye in this image. The eyes are shut for most of the time but also a simple reflex action will prevent a stray finger (or toe) from touching the eye. Furthermore, the fingernails are still well away from the fingertips at this time.

Deciding to go it alone is never an easy option, but with the right support, you can look forward happily to your baby's birth.

**It's reassuring to know** that many women have babies on their own and do not find life an endless struggle. Although it would be wrong to pretend that parenting alone is as easy as it is when you share the care, with additional support it is possible. Even if you are in a relationship, you may feel you are going it alone at times. You may have very strong reasons why you want a baby, for example your increasing age, and this determination will give you strength and focus.

It is helpful for all pregnant women to find someone to talk to and confide in. This could be your mother or a close friend or relative. As you are making far-reaching decisions about your future, it's important that you have support, accurate information, and time to think things through without fear, panic, or pressure from others. Finding somebody you really trust and whom you know can give you support when you need it—especially in labor and in the first days and weeks with your baby—may help relieve any pressure you are under. It will also enable you to think more calmly and clearly about your situation and make plans.

It's worth, even at this early stage, starting to think about who you would like to ask to be your birth partner: this is a big decision that should not be rushed.

---

**BUILDING A SUPPORT NETWORK**

**It's important for all pregnant women** to have emotional and practical support, and this is especially true if you're single.

■ **Go to all your prenatal appointments** and build a relationship with your doctor; she is an invaluable source of information.

■ **Sign up for for prenatal classes.** If you're single, you may find that daytime courses are less populated by "couples"; this gives you a chance to build up a network of female friends. Also try to go to classes, such as yoga and water aerobics.

■ **Give plenty of thought** to choosing your birth partner: a trusted friend, or perhaps your own mother, who is likely to be thrilled to be asked to share this experience with you.

■ **Don't be too proud to accept offers of help** from friends and family—most will genuinely want to be involved now and after the birth.

**You may find an added bonus** of having a baby on your own is that it reshapes your relationship with your own mother, and you may talk together more often.

# 85 days to go...

## YOUR BABY TODAY

Although ultrasound cannot show it, there is now some hair on your baby's head and her eyelashes and eyebrows have grown. The pattern and color of hair growth has a significant impact on the overall look of your baby but this is not apparent on a scan.

While women who are pregnant in the summer may find it hard to stay cool, being pregnant in the winter is also challenging.

**Most women** are understandably reluctant to buy a winter coat that will see them all the way through pregnancy and may well never be worn again. The good news is that you probably won't need one at all! You are likely to feel very warm toward the end of your pregnancy, and may find it more comfortable to wear plenty of layered knits rather than one warm coat or jacket. Layers can also be easily discarded if you become overheated while you're traveling.

You can also probably hijack some of your partner's wardrobe, and borrow a coat or jacket that will fasten over your belly if you're planning to be outside for extended periods. Alternatively, go to a local second-hand shop—you may well find a larger coat or jacket for a bargain price that will last the few weeks of your pregnancy.

Another thing to consider is wearing your own coat unfastened, with a long scarf hanging down to fill the gap.

Think about purchasing a large shawl or wrap, which will see you through the winter months, and keep you and your baby warm after the birth. Shawls and wraps are ideal for keeping you warm when your baby is in a sling, and also for unexpected breast-feeding sessions outdoors.

You'll need to be extra careful in the winter, when you're in icy conditions. Make sure you wear sensible flat shoes when you're out and about to reduce the risk of slipping and falling.

FOCUS ON... TWINS

## Practical adjustments

**If you're having two or more babies,** you'll need to consider making some adjustments to your living space. To reduce the risk of crib death, it's best for babies to sleep in the same room as their parents but you don't need two cribs. You can put both your newborn babies to sleep in one crib (see p.335), but this isn't recommended after they're three months old.

It's a legal requirement for each baby to have an individual car seat if you plan to drive them anywhere, including home from the hospital.

### ASK A... NUTRITIONIST

**My doctor has told me I'm anemic. Can I improve my iron levels through my diet?** All pregnant women should be offered screening for anemia, which is done early in pregnancy (at the first appointment), and again between 26–30 weeks (see p.286). Generally, an iron-rich diet is advised in pregnancy and this is enough to prevent or improve anemia. Eat plenty of lean red meat, beans, dried fruits, dark green vegetables, fortified cereals, and bread. Try including a vitamin C-enriched food or drink in your diet, since vitamin C helps the body absorb iron more efficiently. Vegetarians need to eat plenty of eggs, legumes, beans, and nuts to boost iron supplies.

Taking iron supplements may be recommended depending on how low your iron levels have become.

# 84 days to go...

## YOUR BABY TODAY

The amniotic fluid is approaching its maximum amount at this time and your baby will have plenty of space in which to move. Here the baby is down toward the level of the umbilical cord. Your baby is still likely to change position several times a day.

## If you're the first among your friends to have a baby, be prepared for friendships to evolve and change.

**Some friendships change** as you go through different life stages. You'll probably have had different groups of friends through school, college, and different jobs, with one or two close friends throughout. Friendships often develop with people when you're at a similar stage in your lives. This means that during your pregnancy and when you have young children you may feel most comfortable with other women in similar situations. You'll meet new friends at postpartum classes or post-partum groups, or in situations such as toddler swimming or music classes.

As you make new friends, you may find your old relationships begin to change. Friends without children may find it difficult to understand your new role as a mother, and the intense love that you have for your child, and you may start to drift apart. Of course this is not always the case; some friendships are unchanging, irrespective of whether your lives go along different paths.

### ASK A... DOCTOR

**I've seen a second-hand car seat advertised. Is there any reason why I shouldn't buy it?** Don't use a second-hand car seat unless you can be absolutely certain of its history because it may have been in an accident or damaged.

if you must use a second-hand seat, only accept one if you are absolutely certain that you know its history and that it hasn't been in a bad accident. Don't use a seat that cracked, that doesn't come with the original instructions, is missing parts, was recalled, or is too old. Don't purchase a car seat for your baby at a second-hand store or through classified ads, or on the internet.

### FOCUS ON... NUTRITION

## Choosing organic

**Eating organic food is one way to eat more healthily during pregnancy.** Organic fruit and vegetables are grown without any chemical pesticides or fertilizers. Organic meat, poultry, eggs, and dairy products come from animals that are not given growth hormones or antibiotics. For these reasons, organic foods are free from pesticide residues, additives, and preservatives. They are also usually higher in nutrients. Organic farming also promotes the use of environmentally friendly practices. Most additives are safe during pregnancy, but eating organic is a second step that can add to a healthy foundation of food choices.

The downside of eating organic food is that it tends to cost more than regular groceries. Given the price of food, many families cannot afford the extra that goes with eating organic. If you can't afford organic foods, eating whole foods in their least processed, most natural form, and plenty of fresh fruit and vegetables is the next best thing, and is still a very healthy diet.

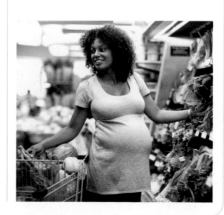

# Your 29th week

**USE THIS THIRD TRIMESTER TO GET ORGANIZED BEFORE YOUR BABY IS BORN**

You may feel a little bored and back-achey at this stage of pregnancy, but there are plenty of positive ways to take your mind off things. For example, you could start to make enquiries about breast-feeding classes, plan your maternity leave, and draw up shopping lists of baby essentials, such as diapers, a changing mat, onesies, bibs, and baby wipes, and perhaps buy a couple of items each week.

**As your belly** continues to get bigger it may put pressure on your ribs and diaphragm.

**A jellylike fluid** in the coiling umbilical cord prevents it from becoming compressed as the baby twists and turns.

**At 29 weeks** the average crown to heel length is 14.4 in (36.6 cm) and the average weight is 1.9 lb (875 g).

**Fine lanugo hairs** cover the baby's body. Most will disappear before the birth, but a few may still be seen on the baby's back when he is born.

**The brain** continues to get bigger and its surface is beginning to take on the creases and folds seen in mature brains.

# 83 days to go...

**YOUR BABY TODAY**

This week is something of a landmark in your baby's development. Although a baby born at this stage would still need help with breathing, the lungs have matured to an extent that survival chances outside the uterus are significantly better than earlier in the pregnancy.

## It's never too early to start thinking about the financial implications of maternity leave, and whether to return to work.

**When you're on maternity leave,** it may be the first occasion that you haven't worked for a long time. This change can be quite daunting, even though you know you'll soon be busy taking care of a baby. Depending on your employer, you'll be entitled to varying amounts of pay during your maternity leave. Every company has a different maternity leave policy. You may get paid or unpaid leave for a specific number of weeks or you may be able to use sick days or vacation days.

Ask a human resources representative about your options. Depending on your partner's employer, he may be eligible for the Family Medical Leave Act (FMLA), which means he could get 12 weeks of unpaid leave. Some companies are more generous than others, offering a percentage of your salary during your maternity leave. Going on maternity leave may cause a significant drop in your income. You should talk to your partner about how much money will be coming in and

going out and how you will manage a change in your finances.

Even though it's a long way in the future, you might also start thinking about plans for working after the baby is born. You may think that you have no real option financially and have to return full time, but explore the possibilities of working more flexibly, or working part time, or from home one or two days a week. You may also want to start thinking about your child-care options (see p.332).

### CHOOSING DIAPERS

**Should you opt for disposables** (use once, then throw away) or cloth (wash, dry, and use again)?

■ **Disposable diapers** are slim fitting, super absorbent, and will keep your baby dry, even overnight. However, they cost more (by some estimates, up to $1,000 per child by the time you start potty training) and there's the landfill factor to consider. Eco-friendly diapers, however, are now available—they use no polluting bleaching agents and fewer chemicals are used to produce them.

■ **Cloth** costs less—although the initial investment is greater. They also provide a softer landing for toddlers

who topple over. However, all that soaking, washing, and drying could get you down (plus this has an environmental impact). You may opt to use a diaper-laundering service each week (at a cost). Cloth diapers need changing more often than disposables. They are slightly more difficult to put on and take off, but modern cloth diapers are fastened with Velcro, not pins.

■ **Using a combination** of reusable and disposable diapers can work well: buy the occasional package of disposables for when you're out and about or for if you leave your baby with a babysitter, but opt for cloth the rest of the time.

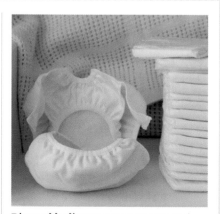

**Disposable diapers** are easy to use and ideal for when you're out and about. But they cost more than cloth diapers, which can be washed and used over and over, even for your next baby.

# 82 days to go...

**YOUR BABY TODAY**

This image shows a typical chin-on-the-chest position with an arm held up to the side of the face. A knee is just visible to the left of the image with a loop of umbilical cord above it. Your baby now is likely to be in a head down position but there's still time to change.

## The coiled umbilical cord connects your baby to the placenta, his life-support system until birth.

**Most umbilical cords** finally grow to be about the same length as the baby (although there are exceptions), reaching a final length of 20–23.5 in (50–60 cm). The umbilical cord has up to 40 turns along its length and these turns are seven times more likely to twist to the left than the right. The coiling pattern was in place nine weeks after conception, with more coils at the baby's end than the placental end; this may be a response to your baby's movements. The cord contains three blood vessels: two arteries taking

deoxygenated blood and waste from your baby to the placenta and one vein carrying oxygen-rich blood from the placenta to the baby. The cord diameter is usually less than ¾ in (2 cm) and the blood vessels are embedded in and protected by a layer of jelly. The watery composition of the jelly, together with the cord's coiling pattern, prevents compression of the cord.

After the birth, your doctor will check the number of vessels in the cord since in 1 percent of singleton pregnancies the cord contains only one umbilical artery.

---

**ASK A... DOCTOR**

**If my baby has a low birthweight, will he have health problems?**
A low birthweight is less than 5½ lb (2.5 kg) and although the majority of small babies thrive, some do have difficulties. Most low birthweight babies are small because they are premature. There are many ways you can reduce the risk of your baby being a low birthweight: eating adequate amounts of healthy food to gain the right amount of weight (see p.99), not smoking or drinking alcohol, reducing stress, and keeping all prenatal appointments so that your health—and your baby—can be monitored.

---

**FOCUS ON... YOUR BODY**

## Restless legs

**Some pregnant women experience restless legs syndrome (RLS),** whereby they have an irresistible urge to move their legs. It most commonly happens while resting, so can be very disruptive to sleep. The exact cause isn't known but it may be related to an imbalance of a brain chemical called dopamine. The level of dopamine can be affected by a lack of iron. Restless legs syndrome will pass once you're no longer pregnant. To minimize the effects of restless legs syndrome:
■ **Ensure your diet** includes an adequate intake of iron (see p.154).
■ **Taking steps to get a good night's sleep** may help you fall asleep—and stay that way. Keep your bedroom cool, quiet, comfortable, and dark. Don't watch television, use a laptop, talk on the phone, or do any work in bed, and keep a consistent sleep schedule. Also, try doing something to challenge your brain before bed (a crossword puzzle, word jumble, or Sudoku puzzle). This may help ease your restless legs.

# 81 days to go...

## YOUR BABY TODAY

This image offers the first view of the eye opening. The lids have separated and the dark pupil can be seen. There is no true reflection of color on ultrasound so the white of the eye is colored the same as the eyelids and face. The "eyebrows" are in fact shadow.

If you're starting to feel that you've been eclipsed by your belly, it's time to do something just for you.

**Like many pregnant women,** you may feel that you've disappeared behind your belly; that the essence of who you are has been lost in the guise of "pregnant woman." People may no longer ask about how you're feeling, or what's going on in your life. Instead of "How are you?", they might ask, "Is everything OK with the baby?"

It can be difficult for people, and even for you, to remember that you still exist in a role that is separate from pregnant woman or mother. If during your pregnancy you are feeling very frustrated by this, consider doing something just for you, maybe some pampering or a dinner for two, to make you feel special again.

---

**FOCUS ON... NUTRITION**

## Grazing through the day

**You need to eat plenty of good-quality protein** to encourage your baby's growth and keep you in glowing good health, so try to eat either eggs, cheese, lean meats, fish, legumes, or grains at every meal. Add to that lots of fruits and vegetables, nuts, seeds, and some unrefined carbohydrates (see p.92).

Break the food down into a plan of five to seven small meals and snacks each day. If you usually have soup and a sandwich for lunch, try a vegetable soup mid-morning, and have the sandwich later; prepare snacks such as raw vegetables, cheese, nuts, and fruit and graze on them through the afternoon. Perhaps have a bowl of oatmeal early evening, followed by fruit later.

There are no "rules" about when food needs to be eaten, so eat these "mini-meals" when you're hungry. As long as you get the nutrients you need and don't overeat, you can graze as often as you like.

---

**ASK A... DOCTOR**

**I have a sharp pain in my lower back and leg. What causes this?**

This sounds like sciatica, a sharp pain that travels down the back and leg when the sciatic nerve—the longest nerve in the body—is trapped in a joint in the lower back. This is not related to your pregnancy, although it can get worse in pregnancy. For lower back pain, warm baths and a warm compress can help, as can gentle massage by an experienced practitioner. Exercise such as yoga or water aerobics classes can help strengthen back muscles, but check with your doctor before embarking on a new exercise regimen. Watch your posture (see p.249) and wear comfortable, supportive shoes.

If you have sciatica, ask your doctor to refer you to a physical therapist. You'll be shown exercises to help relieve the pain and minimize the risk of it recurring.

Spine

Compressed nerve causes pain in the back and leg

# 80 days to go...

### YOUR BABY TODAY

The sleep–wake cycle is now more established, however just because your baby is moving you cannot assume that he is awake. He spends little time fully active with his eyes open, so many of the movements you are feeling are happening while he is asleep.

## Your baby's growth depends on many factors and its rate varies through the course of your pregnancy.

**The growth of your baby** relies on a steady stream of nutrients. Most nutrients are transferred unaltered across the placenta, but some substances are made by the placenta itself and a few are produced from scratch by your baby. These include the hormone thyroxine, the production of which depends on iodine from the mother crossing the placenta. Thyroxine has several functions and its level needs to be controlled very precisely. The placenta forms a nearly perfect barrier to thyroxine, enabling you and your baby to adjust thyroxine levels independently of each other.

In the early stages of pregnancy, genetic factors largely determined the size of your baby, but by now environmental factors are becoming more important. Overall, your baby's final birthweight is determined about 40 percent by genetic factors and 60 percent by environmental factors. Your baby grows at a steady rate from 24 weeks until the last 2–3 weeks, when growth continues but more slowly. (If you're expecting twins, your babies grow as if alone in the uterus up until 28 weeks but from this point there is a reduction in their growth rate.) Your baby's internal organs account for much of his current growth.

The liver and brain, in particular, continue to enlarge and muscle mass increases. Later, fat will be deposited under the skin, rounding out your baby's contours.

### AS A MATTER OF FACT

**The number of twin births** has been jumped 66 percent from 1980 to 2003.

The number of triplet births or more increased four-fold in the same time period. Twins are born, on average, 17 minutes apart.

---

**FOCUS ON... TWINS**

## Buying for your twins

**The clothes you buy for your twins** should be easy to put on and take off, and, of course, machine washable. You'll probably be given outfits as presents, so just buy the basics.

For each baby, you're likely to need at least:
- Six undershirts
- Six onesies
- Two jackets
- One or two hats (sun hat for summer)
- Several burp cloths and bibs.

Keep in mind when choosing diapers that twins are often smaller on arrival than a single baby, and you may therefore get through a wide range of sizes in the first few months.

It's advisable to buy a good-quality double stroller, since it will be used for quite a while. When choosing a stroller, a side-by-side model is preferable to a tandem stroller, so that your babies can see each other and communicate as they grow older.

# 79 days to go...

**YOUR BABY TODAY**

Although many babies look similar on 3D ultrasound, particularly strong features, such as those affecting the shape of the ears, lips, or nose, are easy to see. From now on these features will become more and more individualized and recognizable.

Breast-feeding may be natural but it can be tricky to get started, so try to go to a class or two now while you have the time.

**There is a lot of pressure** on women to breast-feed: breast-feeding has health benefits for both you and your baby and it helps with bonding. People may already be asking you whether you intend to breast-feed or not, and it's reasonable that you don't yet know the answer. After all, you haven't tried!

Most women want to try breast-feeding, but some feel uncomfortable with the thought of doing it, especially in public. There will likely be a lactation consultant in the hospital or you may be able to hire one. In some areas you can go to classes during pregnancy,

which will explain the benefits of breast-feeding and aspects such as positioning the baby so that you're both comfortable and the baby is latched on (see p.449).

The expectation of breast-feeding is that, because it's natural, it's easy. The reality is that until you get the hang of it, it can be a little more difficult. Ask your delivery nurse to show you how to position the baby. Most importantly, keep an open mind and try it. Once breast-feeding is established, it's beneficial to your baby's health, great for your figure, and a wonderful way to be close to your baby.

**THE LOWDOWN**

## On leakages

**Some pregnant women** experience some leakage of breast milk, perhaps when their breasts are massaged or sexually stimulated, and sometimes for no apparent reason. Some discharge in pregnancy does mean that things are working properly, but women who don't experience this symptom are perfectly able to produce and provide milk for their baby.

**FOCUS ON...** NUTRITION

## Cultured foods

**Probiotics**—such as some yogurts, miso (a Japanese paste, often used in soups), and some juices and soy products—contain enzymes and bacteria that help your body digest food, and build up friendly bacteria in the intestines. If your digestion is sluggish and you're finding constipation a problem, ask your doctor about whether eating more probiotic foods could help.

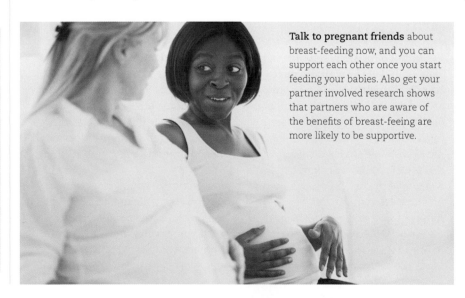

**Talk to pregnant friends** about breast-feeding now, and you can support each other once you start feeding your babies. Also get your partner involved research shows that partners who are aware of the benefits of breast-feeing are more likely to be supportive.

Your 29th week

# 78 days to go...

### YOUR BABY TODAY

Your baby's external appearance is fully formed but inside there is still a great deal of activity as many of the organs are continuing to mature. Even after pregnancy further development occurs, especially of the brain and lungs.

Back pain is not an inevitable part of being pregnant: there are lots of things you can do to help prevent and relieve it.

**Yoga and other stretching exercises** are great during pregnancy, since they strengthen key ligaments while relaxing areas that are tight and painful. Although it may seem easier to rest when you experience pain (especially back pain), and to avoid exercise, gentle stretching and movement often decreases muscle spasm and improves the function of the spine, resulting in less pain. Exercise also boosts energy levels and contributes to an easier labor, delivery, and postpartum recovery. Try stretching and relaxation techniques as a first resort for back pain.

If the pain is severe, ask your partner to massage the area. Ask your doctor if you can safely take any painkillers or if acupuncture might help ease your pain.

If the area feels inflamed and painful, try placing a cold pack on the affected area for 5–10 minutes, several times a day.

### ASK A... MOM

**I'm bored of being pregnant! How will I get through the next couple of months?** I felt the same at about six months but found the last three months went quite fast just because more was happening. Along with more prenatal visits and classes, there was planning when to start maternity leave, then finishing work, then getting the nursery ready, and buying things for the baby. And I made an effort to see all my girlfriends—it all made the time pass quickly.

### FOCUS ON... YOUR BODY

## Minimizing strain on your back

**Your growing belly shifts your center of gravity** to the front of your body. As the baby strains your abdominal muscles, and pregnancy hormones soften your ligaments, your abdominals give less support to your spine, which can result in back pain. Lifting and bending can exacerbate back pain, so try these strategies to help avoid added strain.

■ **To lift something from the floor,** stand close to the object with one foot in front of the other. Bend your knees, then straighten them, so that you use your thigh muscles to lift. Avoid locking your knees: always bend from the waist with your knees bent. If you need to pick something up, consider sitting, kneeling, or squatting to reach it to avoid putting your lower back under stress.

■ **If you have to move a heavy object** (try to avoid this if you possibly can), push it rather than pull it: that way, your legs, not your back, take the strain.

■ **To get into and out of a car,** or bed, keep your hips, pelvis, and back aligned in the same direction. To get out of bed, roll on to your side, and use your arms to push yourself up.

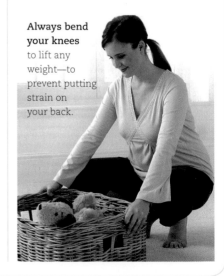

**Always bend your knees** to lift any weight—to prevent putting strain on your back.

# 77 days to go...

**YOUR BABY TODAY**

This is a close-up of how your baby's foot is looking now. Your baby will easily put his feet on top of his head one minute only to bring them down the next, so just because your baby is kicking you at one end it doesn't mean the head is at the other.

## Pregnancy can be a time of information overload, and sometimes it's difficult to know which sources are reliable.

**In today's society** women are simply overloaded with information about pregnancy, from newspapers, magazines, books, and the internet. Photographs of glamorous pregnant celebrities, who look as if they don't have a care in the world, abound in the media. Two sources on the same topic can offer conflicting opinions. Although the internet can be a wonderful source of useful information, it has drawbacks: you don't know who has written an article on a website, it may not have been written by a health professional, and some recommendations may even contradict standard medical advice.

This means that constantly scouring the internet and reading everything you find can be confusing and scary.

Articles telling you that you risk the health and well-being of your baby by doing something can make you feel inadequate. Keep telling yourself that women have been having children for centuries without the aid of the internet! If reading lots of information makes you feel empowered and better able to make informed choices, then read away, but if it makes you feel confused then don't. A sensible course might be to pick just one reliable book or information source to read instead.

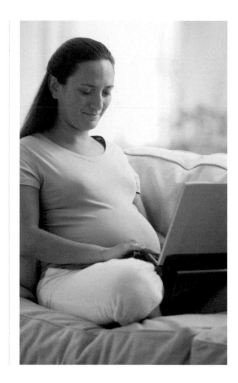

**Use the internet to gather information** about your pregnancy, using reputable health sites. However, if too much information makes you anxious or stressed, get your doctor's advice.

### ASK A... DOCTOR

**I plan to bottle-feed. What do I need to buy in advance?** You'll need plastic bottles (nipples are included), a sterilizing unit or kit (see p.449), which often has everything you need, and your preferred formula. Each comes in a range of options, so you need to decide what works best for you.

As you get to know your newborn baby, you may have to change the type of nipple and/or formula, so it's not advisable to buy too many before the birth.

### FOCUS ON... NUTRITION

## Immunity-boosting blueberries

**According to a US study,** blueberries topped a list of more than 40 fruits in terms of antioxidant activity. They are also a source of fiber, which is great during pregnancy, especially if—like many women—you suffer from constipation. Blueberries also contain nutrients that can prevent or repair damage to the body's cells. This may strengthen the body's immune system and your ability to fight infections.

# Your 30th week

**YOU'RE GETTING TIRED MORE EASILY BUT THAT PROBABLY WON'T STOP YOUR NESTING PLANS**

The nest-building instinct often kicks in as a woman approaches her due date. You may be overwhelmed with the urge to clean and decorate, but although it's natural to want a perfect home for your baby don't wear yourself out. Work, traveling, and a constant round of prenatal appointments are probably all much more of an effort these days. If you need to keep stopping to rest, listen to your body and do just that.

**You are still feeling** a lot of strong kicks, although the baby is moving around less.

**In the brain**, nerve cells are developing into distinct areas that will eventually control specific functions such as memory and coordinated movement. As yet, the neural network is very immature.

**The amniotic sac** has finished growing and is no longer forming new cells. Because the membranes of the sac are highly elastic, they keep stretching as the baby gets bigger.

**At 30 weeks** the average crown to heel length is 14.8 in (37.6 cm) and the average weight is 2.2 lb (1 kg).

**The tip** of your baby's nose is still upturned and the bridge is becoming more evident.

YOU ARE 29 WEEKS AND 1 DAY

# 76 days to go...

**YOUR BABY TODAY**

The image shows the eyes are open once more for a brief look around. It's not completely dark within the uterus and the more advanced your pregnancy, the more light can penetrate inside. Your baby will gradually be assimilating this information.

Be prepared to spend more time in waiting rooms from now on, as your care providers ask to see you more often.

**It's important to remember** that your pregnancy is a natural, healthy process, but with more regular prenatal appointments, and a lot of time spent sitting in a waiting room at the doctor's office, sometimes surrounded by people with various medical conditions, you may start to feel that you have a medical problem. Even though you're visiting the hospital so often, you are fit and well; you just also happen to be pregnant.

At every prenatal appointment you will be asked for a urine sample, which is checked for protein. If you find it's getting increasingly difficult to catch your sample in the tiny, difficult to hold bottle you're given, don't worry. Only a small amount of urine is needed, so if you can't see anything just start to urinate and then move the bottle underneath the flow to catch some.

Urine is sterile (unless you have a urinary tract infection) so don't worry about getting some on your hands — just wash them thoroughly afterward.

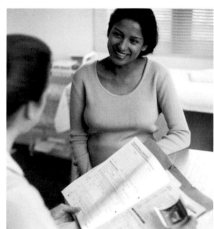

**Regular appointments with your doctor** take time out of your day, but they offer reassurance that all is well with your baby.

**ASK A... DOCTOR**

**We know our baby has Down syndrome. How can we prepare ourselves?** Knowing now will give you time to come to terms with the fact that your baby will have Down syndrome. You won't need any special equipment or toys when your baby is born, but you will need emotional support, so turn to the people now who you think will best give you this.

Contact the Down Syndrome Association (see p.480) for information and support, including getting in touch with parents of children with Down syndrome through your local support group.

**THE LOWDOWN**

## Freebirthing

Giving birth without any medical assistance from a midwife or doctor might seem a little crazy, but a small minority of women believe that so-called freebirthing is the ultimate way to welcome their baby into the world. Some moms-to-be plan an unassisted home birth after having a negative experience during a previous labor; others want their birth to be "natural," "private," and devoid of medical intervention.

■ Freebirthing is not against the law, but it is radical. The American College of Obstetricians and Gynecologists and the American Medical Association oppose home births because of the potential for complications, even in low-risk pregnancies. Complications such as the baby needing oxygen can and do happen.

■ Some women have an unplanned DIY delivery—usually because of a short labor—and in these instances the mothers and babies are usually fine. But actually choosing to go it alone is definitely not something that should be considered lightly.

# 75 days to go...

**YOUR BABY TODAY**

Now the bridge of the nose is more apparent than earlier in the pregnancy. The tip of the nose can still look slightly upturned at this stage adding to the "button nose" appearance. As the face lengthens, the tip of the nose does move downward slightly.

## Your baby's nerve cells are developing, but they are still not mature enough for her to feel pain, temperature, or touch.

**Electrical activity** can now be detected in the increasingly convoluted folds of gray matter, the part of your baby's brain that controls the higher functions, such as memory and consciousness, as well as muscle control and sensory perceptions, such as seeing and hearing.

The neurons of the cortex—the outer layer of gray matter—have started to develop into six distinct layers with separate functions, a process that will be completed in about about five weeks, although further maturing will be needed. Your baby is born with almost a full complement of neurons, but there is further growth in early childhood.

For nerves to function effectively and signals to pass along them faster, they need insulating. In a process known as myelination, the nerves are insulated with myelin sheaths of fat. Although all of the components of the nervous system are present from an early stage of development, the peripheral sensory and motor nerves, spinal cord, and brain need the entire pregnancy to develop and function as a unit.

The nerves of the brain and spinal cord carry the sensations of pain, temperature, and touch. However, the process of myelination is ongoing and will not be complete until the final few weeks of pregnancy, so your baby does not register or recognize pain, temperature, and touch at this stage.

---

**ASK A... DOCTOR**

**The reality of having to give birth is hitting me now! How can I avoid getting too anxious?** A little way into your third trimester, the reality of childbirth may sink in. You may be experiencing some pregnancy discomforts, including Braxton Hicks' contractions (see p.410), which give an indication of what is to come.

First of all, remember that the calmer and more relaxed you are, the easier your birth will be. Try to use a little positive visualization—your baby coming out easily in a "whoosh" of fluid, and focus on contractions being "positive pain" to bring your baby into the world. Remember that your baby will be fine, however long she takes to arrive, and that your pain and discomfort are all controllable. In other words, even if you decide on a natural birth now, you can get help and relief when you need it.

Try to relax and enjoy the last months of your pregnancy. Treat yourself to a massage, and keep yourself busy—perhaps undertaking a creative project for your new baby. Above all, don't worry. Think about childbirth as welcoming your baby into the world, and focus on this rather than any concerns.

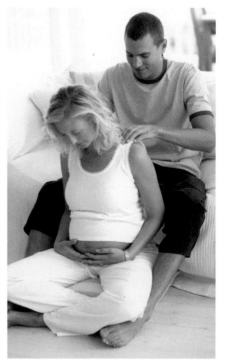

**A massage is soothing and relaxing** and can be very welcome attention as you wind down toward the birth of your baby.

# 74 days to go...

## YOUR BABY TODAY

Your baby often grasps one hand with the other or, as this image shows, grasps a foot. This helps with important sensory feedback to the brain as the nerves within the brain start to mature and become insulated along their length to carry signals more effectively.

## Start getting your baby's room ready now, while you still have the energy for shopping and helping with decorating.

**It's recommended that your baby sleeps in the same room** as you for the first six months, but many parents-to-be still like to prepare the baby's bedroom. This room can still be used for the baby's clothes and any newborn gifts you're given. You might also want to breast-feed, and set up a diaper-changing area in there.

Check out garage sales and eBay for second-hand baby equipment. This can be a good opportunity to buy some bigger items at a reduced price. If you do buy a second-hand crib, make sure it's certified by the Juvenile Product

Manufacturers Association and that the slats are no more than 2 ⅜ in apart. Hand-me down clothes, sheets, and towels also save money. If this isn't your first baby you may find that you have more or less everything you need, except for disposables, such as diapers (unless you are using cloth diapers—see p.291).

Although it's good to be prepared (and sometimes babies do arrive early), remember you won't be trapped in your house forever so you don't need to prepare as if for a siege. If you don't have something you need or you run out, you can always get it after your baby is born.

**If you don't know the sex of your baby,** opt for a neutral color scheme for your baby's room. If you do know, then you can decorate accordingly.

### ASK A... DOCTOR

**Do I need a carriage/travel system/stroller?** Most parents-to-be are unsure about the type of stroller they'll need for their baby and, since there are a number of options and types available, this can make choosing the right item difficult. You will need to buy some type of travel equipment for your baby and what you choose will vary depending on your circumstances.

If you mostly drive a car, you may want to consider a car seat that attaches to a carriage, or a car seat and separate travel crib. If you intend to walk a lot, you may find a lightweight stroller more appropriate than a carriage. Keep in mind how long your baby will be in the stroller: it must be comfortable, have a lie-flat option for the first six months, and adjustable seat options as your baby grows. The stroller must also be weatherproof.

If you do a lot of "around town" travel, you might consider a lightweight option in addition to your main system. It's a good idea to take a look around in stores and online to compare different models and get the best price.

# Planning for your birth

As your due date approaches, you may start to think in greater detail about how you would like to manage your labor and birth. Being informed will help you feel more confident about the choices you make.

## Your choices for birth

When planning the type of birth experience you would like to have, you'll need to consider a number of factors. One of the most important decisions is where you would like to give birth. You may also want to think about the details of your birth, such as which positions you would like to adopt during the birth, and what type of pain relief you might choose to use (see pp.396–407).

It's important to be flexible. You may have preferences as to the type of birth you want, but accepting that your choice may be limited or advised against because of a preexisting medical problem, or because a problem arises in labor, will help you prepare mentally and curb disappointment if events don't go as planned. It is generally accepted that the care of healthy women in labor who have had a straightforward pregnancy should be monitored and managed by their doctors at the hospital, with support given by the nursing staff throughout the process.

**The place of birth** Earlier in pregnancy, you'll probably have thought about where you would like to give birth and discussed the options with your doctor. Although you may have already stated a preference, it's important to know that you can review your choice and change your mind toward the end of pregnancy.

Where you give birth may be influenced by factors such as whether you've had complications in pregnancy, such as gestational diabetes (see p.473) or high blood pressure, that would make a hospital birth preferable. On the other hand, if your pregnancy has been

straightforward and you have become more informed about labor and birth over the course of your pregnancy, your confidence may have grown and you may decide to look into a home birth in familiar surroundings, or to investigate midwife-run birthing centers in your area.

Sometime in the third trimester you may have a hospital tour, which gives you a chance to see the labor and postpartum wards in your hospital, and to ask questions about hospital policies and what facilities are available. Ask your doctor for details of tours.

**An active labor** In prenatal classes, you'll learn a range of techniques to help you cope with pain during labor. Most methods center around breathing and relaxation techniques that help you focus during labor and birth and don't inhibit movement. Maintaining mobility and an upright position during labor is thought to help you deal with

NEW PROCEDURES

## Stem cell collection

**The collection of stem cells, which are found in the umbilical cord,** is a relatively new private service. Stem cells develop into many different types of cell in the body and can be used to treat diseases such as leukemia by replacing diseased cells (see p.310). Stem cells are collected from the umbilical cord immediately after birth and sent to a laboratory where they are frozen and stored, acting as health insurance for the baby in future life. If you want to have this done, you must make arrangements with a private company and check that the hospital has procedures to allow the collection to be done.

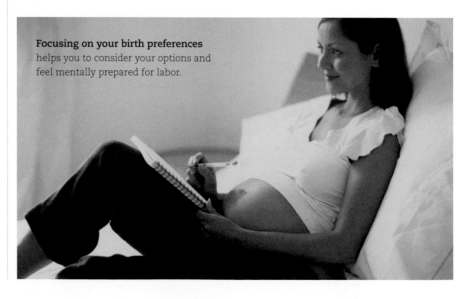

**Focusing on your birth preferences** helps you to consider your options and feel mentally prepared for labor.

contractions and to use gravity to help push your baby down the birth canal.

If you want an active birth, this may influence how you feel about the type of pain relief you want to use (see below) and about monitoring in labor. For example, continuous monitoring (see p.418) can limit your movement. If the doctor wants to monitor your labor continuously, talk to her about how you can maintain some mobility; for example, by sitting on a birthing ball, or adopting an all-fours position on the bed or on a mattress on the floor.

**Your pain relief options** Factors that may influence the type of pain relief you would like include how active you want to be (see above); what effect different drugs may have on how you experience labor; and how drugs can affect the baby.

Natural methods, such as breathing techniques, laboring in water, and TENS (see p.399), and some medical pain-relief options, such as analgesics (see pp.402–3)

allow an active birth because you won't lose all feeling or muscle movement. However systemic (IV) analgesics cross the placenta and can affect the baby's breathing at birth. Regional anesthetics, such as epidurals (see p.404), limit movement and can mean that you won't feel when you're pushing.

## Making a birth plan

Writing your preferences in a birth plan helps you to consolidate your thoughts and to pass this information on to your doctor. Or your doctor may discuss a birth plan with you. A birth plan is useful too for your birthing partner, who may need to advocate on your behalf in labor. Birth plans also allow you to state any special needs you may have, such as whether you have a disability.

Make your birth plan straightforward and accessible. Working with your caregivers as a team will help you deal well with labor and be involved in decision making, whatever the outcome.

---

# Questions to consider

When planning where and how you ideally want to give birth, you need to consider both what you would prefer and what the hospital or birthing centers can offer. The following questions may act as helpful prompts.

### Questions to ask yourself
■ Who would you like to have with you during the labor and birth?
■ Do you want an active labor?
■ What pain relief do you want?
■ If you have an assisted birth, would you prefer vacuum or forceps?
■ Do you want your partner to be present if you have a cesarean?
■ Do you want the third stage of labor to be managed naturally or assisted with drugs?
■ How do you want to feed your baby?

### Questions to ask the hospital
■ What is the policy on induction? Will the hospital monitor your baby before labor if you don't want to be induced?
■ Will the choice of pain relief and the place of birth change if you're induced?
■ Are there tubs or birthing pool facilities?
■ Will you be able to bring in aids such as massage oils or music?
■ How much privacy will you have?
■ How many people will you be allowed to invite into your labor and delivery room?
■ Will your baby remain with you throughout your stay in the hospital?
■ Does the hospital have facilities for sick babies, or are babies transferred?
■ Can you go home when you feel ready, or is there a set discharge time?

---

# Birth ideologies

In the mid-20th century, labor and childbirth in the West became highly medicalized. In reaction, several childbirth philosophies emerged that focused on empowering women and viewed childbirth as a natural rather than a medical experience. Many of these approaches are now integral to the way childbirth is managed today.

**Dr. Grantley Dick-Read,** an American obstetrician, linked labor pain to fear when he was working during the 1950s. He promoted breathing and relaxation to help cope with pain, and his methods are now commonplace.

**Dr. Ferdinand Lamaze** was inspired by the Russian scientist Dr. Pavlov, who trained dogs to have a set response to stimulus. In the 1950s, Lamaze extended this idea to childbirth, believing that women could be trained to respond positively to labor pain.

**Sheila Kitzinger,** a well-known birth practitioner who became prominent in the 1960s, believes in a woman's right to choose how to give birth.

**Frederick Leboyer,** a French obstetrician, came to prominence in the 1970s with his book *Birth without Violence.* Focusing on the baby, he believed a traumatic birth could impact negatively later in life. He promoted "gentle birthing" where the baby has skin-to-skin contact and is immersed in warm water.

**Michael Odent,** a birth practitioner, advocates active birthing, believing women act on instincts in labor. His birthing center in Pithiviers, France has the lowest national rates of intervention.

**Janet Balaskas** founded the Active Birth Movement in 1981. At her Active Birth Centre in London, she teaches relaxation, breathing, and yoga.

# 73 days to go...

## YOUR BABY TODAY

In this image a hand is held up to the forehead and, to the right, part of a foot can be seen. The groove between the nose and the upper lip is visible and the nose has the characteristic "button" shape. It looks cramped in there but there is still room to move.

Your baby is cushioned in a sac of amniotic fluid, which surrounds her until your water breaks and you go into labor.

**As your uterus** has enlarged throughout your pregnancy, the amniotic sac has expanded to accommodate both your baby and the amniotic fluid. From now on, however, the sac will grow by simply stretching rather than forming new cells.

The amniotic sac is formed from two distinct layers or membranes, an inner "amnion" and outer "chorion." The chorion originally had a blood supply of its own, but this has now been lost. The thinner amnion is able to slide over the chorion as your baby pushes against it. Neither layer contains nerve cells: this explains why it's not painful when your membranes rupture or "water breaks."

Combined, the layers are only 0.5 mm thick. Collagen fibers in each layer allow for a great deal of stretch—this is vital in these final months to avoid early rupture of the membranes. Indeed, the membranes may be so resistant to rupture that they don't break until the final stages of your labor (see p.411).

In addition to holding in the amniotic fluid and providing a barrier to possible infection through the cervix, the membranes contain substances that form prostaglandins. Prostaglandins play an important part in the initiation of labor. This is one of the reasons why labor often starts when the membranes have ruptured.

**Your baby may have** several episodes of hiccuping in a day, or only one or two—you will both be able to feel these as a series of light, rhythmic movements.

---

### AS A MATTER OF FACT

**The only reliable way** to discover the sex of your baby is to have a diagnostic test (see pp.152–3), such as amniocentesis or chorionic villus sampling.

Even ultrasound can be wrong. And despite the common belief that the size and shape of your belly indicate gender, these are in fact determined by your muscle tone, your baby 's position, and your weight gain.

---

### FOCUS ON... DADS

## Kicks and hiccups

**By now, it's possible to see and feel** your baby moving, often with kicks and punches. This may happen more often in the evenings, when your partner finally gets to sit down and relax. Watching your baby's movements can be a great way to bond with her, and with your partner.

Your baby will respond to your voice, to music, and may even jump at unexpected noises (see p.206);

it's impossible to say whether this is because these noises are enjoyed or because they're irritating.

Your baby will also hiccup sometimes (see p.204) and you have a better chance of feeling her moving while she's hiccuping than any other form of movement. This is because hiccups occur over prolonged periods of time, while kicks and punches can be fairly random.

# 72 days to go...

## YOUR BABY TODAY

The lip shape and groove between the nose and upper lip are particularly well shown here. If you or your partner has a prominent groove, or philtrum, above the upper lip, your baby may too, or she may inherit characteristics that are somewhere in between.

Regardless of your size—and that of your baby—nature won't let her grow too large for you to be able to give birth.

**Your body shape** isn't an indication of whether you'll have an easy birth. The size of your hips is not always a good indication of the size of your pelvis so having slender hips doesn't mean you'll have a difficult birth, and having larger "child-bearing" hips doesn't mean you'll have an easier birth.

What is known is that, although how big your child will be is determined genetically, women have an extra influence on the size of their babies while they are in the uterus. So, even if your child ends up growing to 6 ft (1.80 m) tall, if you're small you'll limit how big she gets in the uterus. This makes sense—if you're small, you wouldn't be able to deliver a hefty 12 lb (5.5 kg) baby, so your body limits the baby's size at delivery. Your baby will then catch up on her expected growth after the birth.

There's a condition called cephalo-pelvic disproportion in which the baby is too big or the pelvis is too small for the baby to engage. An MRI scan will be performed to get exact measurements.

### ASK A... DOCTOR

**What will happen when I go for a gestational diabetes screening?**
You'll be given a very sugary drink and asked to wait for an hour, after which your blood will be tested. If your levels are high, you'll have to take a glucose tolerance test, which is similar, but longer. If you do have gestational diabetes, you will be taught how to test your blood sugar at home. You'll likely be able to control your condition with diet and exercise.

It's reassuring to know that most women who have sugar in their urine have normal blood-sugar levels in the glucose test.

**As you marvel at the size of your belly,** you may be concerned about how you'll ever deliver your baby. But don't worry—nature is on your side.

### TIME TO THINK ABOUT

## A support network

After giving birth, your body will spring back into shape overnight; you'll be bursting with energy and raring to go. That's one scenario! The other—more realistic—possibility is that you'll find yourself struggling to get breast-feeding established and to brush your teeth before lunch time. If you don't like living in a mess, act now to prevent resentment (and the laundry) from building up in a few months' time.

■ **Talk to your partner now** about how you're going to split the chores once you're parents.
■ **Your "job" will be to nurture your newborn,** so you'll need domestic backup, if possible, particularly during the first few weeks. Recruit helpers (family and friends; or pay professionals if needed). Delegate so that you won't have to think about shopping, cooking, or cleaning.
■ **New parents need their own space,** so it's never too early to arrange for some babysitters for a few weeks after the birth. If you're breast-feeding, you'll need to express your milk.

# 71 days to go...

## YOUR BABY TODAY

Increasingly sounds enter the uterus and your baby will respond to some of the loudest. The fluid all around her can have quite an effect on the sounds that your baby can hear: the effect is similar to how you might feel when you swim with your head under water.

Your maximum blood volume won't be reached for a few weeks yet, but your circulation is working harder than ever at this stage.

**Your blood volume** is likely to be nearly a gallon and a half between weeks 25 and 35—an increase of about 25 percent. This increased blood volume means that your heart is pumping harder and faster. Your blood vessels are as relaxed as they can be by this stage of pregnancy, and will not stretch any further to accommodate this extra blood flow. You may notice that you sweat more, and that your skin feels hotter (this is the rosy glow that many women experience).

In addition to this extra blood, there is also a lot more fluid circulating around your body. This makes all your body tissues thicker. It's common and normal for your face, fingers, and ankles to be puffy or swollen (see pp.466–7). However, since puffiness is also a sign of preeclampsia (see p.474), it's important to have your doctor to check this out.

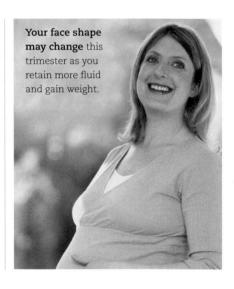

**Your face shape may change** this trimester as you retain more fluid and gain weight.

### ASK A... DOCTOR

**I've noticed that I get short of breath very easily. Should I be concerned?** No, when you're pregnant, your lungs have to work much harder to meet your body's increased oxygen needs. To help you take in more air, your ribs spread sideways and your lung capacity increases dramatically. This can make you feel breathless, particularly from mid-pregnancy.

In the last three months of pregnancy, most women find they get breathless even during mild exertion, which happens as the expanding uterus pushes up against the lungs. However, being breathless can also be a sign of anemia (see p.472), which may need to be treated. Your breathing may start to get easier when your baby engages (moves down into your pelvis ready to be born) (see p.361).

### FOCUS ON... TWINS

## Exercising safely

**If you're pregnant with twins,** it's recommended that you don't do any vigorous or aerobic exercise in the third trimester. The last three months are particularly tiring so you probably won't feel up to doing much anyway. You'll also get bigger sooner than someone who is having a single baby, and your size may preclude you from doing certain activities.

If you do want to be active, go for a gentle walk or swim, or to a pregnancy yoga or Pilates class. If you want to do anything more vigorous than this in the third trimester, check with your doctor first.

Your doctor will be monitoring your babies' progress and she may advise you on your level of activity if there is any slowdown in the babies' growth and development.

Whatever activity you're doing, always follow the guidelines for safe exercising (see p.18).

# 70 days to go...

**YOUR BABY TODAY**

Does your baby start to feel tired? Certainly on some scans it can look as if she is. In fact, your baby actually spends most of the time in a state of sleep rather than full wakefulness: it seems that during pregnancy your baby does need to spend most of the time asleep.

## You probably won't want to stop working just yet, but you may need to make some adjustments if you're feeling very tired.

**Later on in the third trimester** you may begin to feel more tired than usual. The strain on your body may begin to show itself—you may find yourself uncomfortable and easily fatigued. Things that never bothered you previously, such as standing for long periods of time or walking a lot, may get increasingly difficult. For example, your trip to and from work may tire you much more than it did previously. If that is the case, find out whether you can alter your hours to avoid traveling at the busiest times of the day and, if you find yourself traveling during rush hours, don't be shy about asking someone to

give up their seat on the train for you. If there is a room in which you can rest at work, you may be able to take a short nap in the middle of the day or early afternoon, which might help to alleviate your fatigue a little.

You may want to discuss with your employer ways to make your job less physically demanding, or ask for help, for example if you need to carry heavy files or your job involves walking long distances. With a few adjustments you should be able to keep going until the start of your maternity leave, but above all, listen to your body: if you're tired, rest; if your feet and legs hurt, sit down.

### USING A BIRTHING POOL

**Laboring and giving birth in water** can not only relieve much of the pain, discomfort, and stress of childbirth, it can also induce relaxation and reduce blood pressure. Research shows that warm water on the lower back (the area of the spinal cord that receives the nerves from the lower abdominal region) can reduce labor pain, while the level of endorphins, or natural painkillers, rises in the same environment. Whether you choose a birthing pool or a warm bath, water is a great way to deal with contractions.

If you give birth in water, your baby's umbilical cord will continue to provide her with the oxygen she needs, but she will have to be brought to the surface quickly to encourage her to breathe on her own.

Water birth should be done with your doctor's supervision, and many birthing centers and hospitals now offer the option (see p.343). Make sure you include these details on your birth plan (see p.303). Using a birthing pool will not be recommended if your birth is considered to be high risk.

### FOCUS ON... TWINS

## Cesarean birth

**You're more likely to deliver twins** by cesarean than a single baby (see pp.438–9). Many of these are elective: the decision is made in advance, and the mother doesn't go into labor. A cesarean is major surgery, but for the babies it's often the best way to arrive and a small price to pay for the mother.

Vaginal birth can be complicated for twins, especially the second twin who goes through two rounds of uterine contractions. It's considered high-risk if the babies are premature.

**A growing number of hospitals** and birthing centers offer birthing pools. If you'd like to have a water delivery, check the availability of a pool at your hospital when you tour the facility.

# Your 31st week

**EVEN IF YOU HAVE A BIRTH PLAN IN MIND, BE PREPARED TO BE FLEXIBLE**

You may have firm thoughts about what you consider to be the ideal birth experience. However, keep an open mind because many factors can influence where and how your baby is born. There's nothing unusual in a woman changing her mind, even after her labor has actually started. Your health-care team will expect you to ask a lot of questions about childbirth, so take advantage of their experience and expertise.

**The blood in the umbilical cord** contains stem cells, which have the ability to develop into specific body cells such as those forming blood, or brain, or muscle tissues.

**The baby** spends much of his time asleep. Like children and adults, babies have a sleep pattern that includes a "dreaming" stage, when rapid eye movements (REM) can be recorded.

**The legs** may be crossed or even curled up on top of the head at times but there is still space for them to be stretched out fully.

**At 31 weeks** the average crown to heel length is 15.2 in (38.6 cm) and the average weight is 2.5 lb (1.1 kg).

**Some 25 percent** of babies are lying bottom first at this stage. Most of them turn before the end of pregnancy.

YOU ARE 30 WEEKS AND 1 DAY

# 69 days to go...

## YOUR BABY TODAY

From this point in the pregnancy your baby will yawn just as often as during the first few weeks after birth. Exactly why babies yawn before birth remains unknown, but seeing your baby yawn on a scan is quite likely to make you yawn as well.

It's well worth giving some thought to where your baby is going to sleep before you actually bring him home from the hospital.

**It's recommended that your baby** sleeps in a crib in your bedroom for the first six months. See the box below, if you're considering co-sleeping. With your baby in your bedroom, you'll be close by when he cries at night and able to attend to him easily. This is especially useful if you're breast-feeding.

Remember that babies are not necessarily quiet sleepers: they may wiggle, grunt, and move around and these noises may disturb you or your partner. If your partner has to go to work the following day this extra disturbance may affect him. It will affect you, too, but you may have a chance to "catch up" on some sleep, or at least rest, when your baby naps. You should do what is best for all three of you, even if that means your partner spends some nights in the spare room. Some new parents find that they are so exhausted by life with a newborn that they sleep, regardless of whether their baby is snuffling or not.

If the baby is in his own room you may worry that you may not hear him cry, but you will if you use a baby monitor. When he does cry, yet again at 3 am, be aware that a short trip along the landing can seem like a mile.

### SHOULD YOU CO-SLEEP?

**You may want to put your baby into your bed with you,** and yet you may be concerned that you might roll over on him. For this reason, the American Academy of Pediatrics does not recommend co-sleeping. It can be especially dangerous if either of you smoke or use alcohol or drugs that make it hard to wake up, or if you sleep with the baby on a waterbed, couch, or in a chair. The safest place for your baby is in a bassinet near your bed.

### FOCUS ON... YOUR BODY

## Breast changes

**In the third trimester,** your breasts will begin to prepare themselves for feeding your baby, and you may experience some discomfort and changes that you had not anticipated. Your breasts will become fuller, and may actually feel very heavy; your areolas (the area around your nipples) will become darker, and you may feel lumps and bumps in your breasts, as the first milk, colostrum, begins to be produced. This may leak out a little (see p.295).

The small glands on the surface of your areolas (known as Montgomery's tubercles) will also become raised bumps. You may have darkened veins along your breasts, due to their increased blood supply. Your breasts may also feel more tender and sensitive than usual, especially if touched.

**Your breasts will change** in preparation for breast-feeding, whether you intend to breast-feed your baby or not. Since your breasts will feel full and heavy by this stage, it's important to wear a bra that properly supports you. Go for a fitting if necessary.

# 68 days to go...

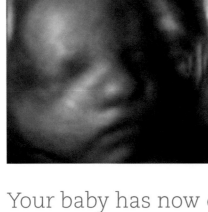

## YOUR BABY TODAY

You will be aware of times when your baby is especially active and times when he is more quiet. There is still a lot of space for your baby to move within the uterus but it is likely that there will be a favorite spot that receives more kicks than any other.

## Your baby has now developed a clear rhythm of sleeping and waking that may mimic your own or be personal to him.

**Exactly when and how** your baby develops a cycle of sleeping and waking before birth remains a bit of a mystery. It's not known whether your own rhythms influence your baby's sleep–wake cycle or whether your baby develops his own internal clock. Indeed, such a clock might be triggered in response to the small amount of light that is able to penetrate through the uterus during the last few weeks of pregnancy. It's apparent from brain scans, however, that by this stage of pregnancy, your baby does have very separate periods of activity.

There is a clear cycle, alternating between periods of quiet rest, sleep with rapid eye movements (REM), wakefulness with activity but no eye movement, and wakefulness with lots of activity and eye movements. During this sleep–wake cycle, the baby's actions becomes more coordinated as periods of activity are linked to rhythmical breathing and increased heart rate, and eye movements.

By this stage of pregnancy, electrical activity in your baby's brain shows patterns reflecting periods of sleep or wakefulness. An EEG of your baby's brain would show that the quietest period, deep sleep, takes up almost half of the time. The next most common state is REM sleep (the sleep stage

during which children and adults dream). This is a time of great electrical activity within your baby's brain. During REM sleep the baby may be quiet or making lots of movements, so it's not possible to tell whether your baby is

truly awake at this time or if he's dreaming. Paradoxically, the least electrical activity happens when your baby is most awake—in fact less than 10 percent of your baby's time is spent truly awake at this stage.

### STEM CELL COLLECTION

**The blood in your baby's umbilical cord** contains "cord blood," which is rich in stem cells. These cells are the building blocks of organ tissue, blood, and the immune system. Some parents save these cells and store them (in a private facility at a cost) in the event that their child or another family member needs their healing benefits (see p.302).

Studies have found that they are very effective in the treatment of more than 70 diseases including juvenile diabetes, cancers, heart disease, and brain injury.

Stem cells are widely used, but there is significant evidence to show that using cells from the cord blood of a sibling or other family member is more effective than using cells from an unrelated donor, or bone marrow from relatives.

Cord blood can be expensive to store. Some women choose

to donate their blood to public cord blood banks. The donated blood is stored, and this is used to treat patients who need it most. Talk to your doctor if you'd like to do this.

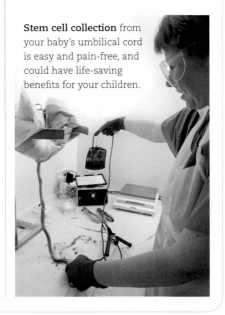

**Stem cell collection** from your baby's umbilical cord is easy and pain-free, and could have life-saving benefits for your children.

# 67 days to go...

**YOUR BABY TODAY**

It can come as quite a surprise to see that your baby will be increasingly making all sorts of expressions. Here the baby had his mouth turned down but the next minute will be yawning, grimacing, or peacefully sleeping.

Natural birth has many advocates, but the best birth is one that delivers your baby safely with minimum trauma for both of you.

**Many women want a natural delivery,** with no pain relief or other medical intervention. Giving birth naturally is for some reason perceived as the "best" way, and to do otherwise means that you somehow "failed" at childbirth. This pressure means that women can feel guilty or even depressed if they needed pain relief or a cesarean section, for example.

Bear in mind that some women have higher pain thresholds and can get through labor with simple breathing or relaxation techniques, while others need more help. Pain is subjective, no one else can feel your pain; if it is too much for you, then ask for help. Your options (see pp.402–7) will be explained to you by the doctor.

Childbirth is hard work, but the experience should not be so painful that it scars you. Being pain-free may mean that you have a more enjoyable, even empowering, labor experience. If you do decide you want pain relief, an epidural is the most common option—more than half of women having a baby in a hospital receive one.

**Having a natural birth** is high on the list of many women's priorities, but it's a good idea to prepare mentally for medical intervention, in case it becomes necessary.

---

**ASK A PANEL ABOUT...** NATURAL BIRTH

## I want a natural birth but everyone says I'll change my mind once I'm in labor. Are they right?

**Mom:** Nothing can prepare you for the discomfort of labor, and I found my carefully laid plans were unrealistic and impractical when the pain kicked in. No matter how well prepared you are, you may change your mind during labor, and it's worth being prepared for that. I did feel a bit disappointed that I couldn't manage without pain relief. It helps if you focus on what's important—delivering a healthy baby. If you achieve this aim, you've succeeded, no matter

what happens along the way. I would say to stick it out for as long as you can, but you'll be doing yourself and your baby no favors if you both become exhausted and distressed.

**Doctor:** Many women are shocked by the intensity of the birth experience, and soon forget about their idealistic birth plan. It's better for all involved that you allow for contingency plans, and keep an open mind. Pain relief (see pp.396–407) and interventions

are designed to make the experience better for you and your baby, and will not be offered unless they're necessary, or you feel that you can't do without them. Some women get through labor naturally; others need some help. A lot of women do change their mind about "going natural," and there is nothing wrong with that. A mom who has her pain under control will find that the delivery is much quicker, and she'll have much more energy for her new arrival.

# Twins

Just a few weeks to go. By now, you're probably quite large and, of course, excited at the imminent arrival of your twins, or more. However, you may also be concerned about how you will manage during and after the birth.

## Getting ready for the birth

Although multiple pregnancies and births are more likely to have complications, they are now safer than ever as advances in prenatal and postpartum care have dramatically improved the outlook for premature babies—the main concern with multiples (see below).

You can prepare for the birth by getting plenty of rest. Putting your feet up, or even having a nap during the day, helps improve the blood flow to the placenta, which in turn helps your babies grow. Practicing Kegel exercises (see p.69) is important with a multiple pregnancy since your pelvic floor muscles are under additional strain.

### THIINKING AHEAD

## Bonding with twins

**Often, expectant moms of twins or more** worry about how they will bond with more than one baby. It's true that bonding can be harder with twins, and even more so with higher multiples. After all, it's hard to fall in love with more than one person at a time, especially when you're exhausted caring for two babies or more. Being aware of this and arranging extra help for after the birth may ease your anxiety. Also, accept additional offers of help that allow you to rest or spend time with one twin. If someone offers to take the twins out, you might consider one twin going and the other spending time with you.

### TWINS

## How your babies lie in the uterus

**In the final weeks, your babies will take up their positions for the birth.** The most common position is with both babies lying vertically. With 75 percent of twins, the first is head down (cephalic); the second twin may be head down or breech, or one twin may lie across the uterus (transverse). You may suspect their position from the kicks, but only a scan confirms this.

A cesarean will be recommended if you have triplets or more, or your first twin is breech or transverse (25 percent of cases). A vaginal delivery is most likely if both twins are head down. If the first is head down and the second is transverse or breech, there are different opinions as to the best type of delivery, which you can discuss with your obstetrician.

Both babies head down (cephalic)

One baby head down, and one breech

Both babies in a breech position

One baby head down and one transverse

**A shorter pregnancy** Twins or more usually arrive earlier than singletons. Space in the uterus is one factor. In addition, with multiple pregnancies the placenta becomes less efficient toward the end of pregnancy. As a result, the average length of pregnancy is shorter: for twins 36 to 37 weeks is considered typical, for triplets the average pregnancy is 33 weeks, and for quadruplets pregnancy lasts about 30 weeks. The average birth weight for each twin is 5 lb 8 oz (2.5 kg) at full term.

You may deliver even earlier than this, since nearly 50 percent of twins are born prematurely. However, nowadays expert care for premature babies means that about 75 percent of babies weighing 3 lb 5 oz at birth, and 57 percent of babies weighing 2 lb 3 oz at birth, survive.

### Preparing for more than one

Even if your twins are identical they're individuals, and relating to them as separate people will help their development and your relationship with them. Even in pregnancy, some expectant moms notice how different their babies are from their different movement patterns in the uterus.

# 66 days to go...

**YOUR BABY TODAY**

In this 3D scan the baby's arm is held up next to the face. This type of scan shows external features but also looks inside the baby in 3D so you may see some parts of your baby "through" an arm or leg. Here, the baby's ear can be seen through the arm.

In the uterus and in the first months of his life, your baby relies on your immunity to various infections.

**If your immune system thought your baby was foreign,** it would mount an attack on him. You and your baby are designed so that this does not happen. Your baby does not have the ability to produce antibodies (which would attack you) in the uterus: he relies completely on you to protect him from infection, not only in the uterus but also after birth. Protection after birth is possible because antibodies from your immune system cross over the placenta into your baby's bloodstream, while you're pregnant. If you have immunity to a disease such as measles, mumps, polio, and many other severe infections, your baby will carry your antibodies to these conditions. This so-called passive immunity is lost with time and it is for this reason that, from two months onward, your baby will require a program of immunizations to protect against these and other illnesses.

---

**FOCUS ON...** YOUR BODY

**There have been numerous studies** over the past few years involving women exercising while they're pregnant. The bottom line is that exercise performed effectively and safely, at a moderate intensity and in healthy women, is beneficial.

In addition to being good for your health and making you feel more energized, exercising will get you into great shape for labor and childbirth, which is, in effect, a workout!

Here are the myths:

■ **Exercising will harm my baby if I move too much.** Your baby is protected by amniotic fluid and nourished by the placenta. By keeping within safe exercising guidelines (see p.18), and not doing any high-impact sports or activities where you are at risk of falling or injuries, you are not putting your baby at risk.

■ **Exercise will use up some of the nutrients my baby needs.** Your baby's growth will be monitored at doctor appointments, so you and your doctor will be able to tell whether your baby is growing at a usual rate or whether you should increase your calorie intake. If you're concerned, increase your calorie intake on the days that you exercise.

■ **Doing abdominal exercises will harm the baby.** You can do abdominal exercises but you should not do abdominal exercises lying on your back in the second and third trimesters. The risk of lying on your back is that the baby can press down on the vena cava (the large blood vessel that returns blood to your heart). This causes your blood pressure to fall and compromises the oxygen flow to the baby. The first sign of a problem will be feeling dizzy: if you roll on to your left side, any

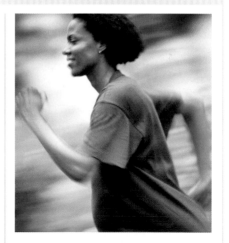

symptoms should disappear. Don't hesitate to consult your doctor if you're concerned. The abdominal exercises shown on page 250 give you some great ways of doing safe abdominal exercises that do not put you or your baby at risk.

# 65 days to go...

**YOUR BABY TODAY**

Here the hands are holding the umbilical cord as it arises from what will become the belly button, or umbilicus. The umbilical coils and its covering of firm, clear jelly protect the cord from kinking and prying fingers.

## If you want a home birth atmosphere with additional support, consider having your baby in a birthing center.

**Birthing centers** give moms-to-be a labor experience different than that of a hospital. The emphasis is on a natural birth. They can be attached to a hospital or on a separate site. Some hospitals have a birthing center facility in the maternity unit. Since the majority of women give birth without needing medical intervention, these centers provide a good alternative to a more medicalized hospital environment. The environment in a birthing center tends to be more relaxed and flexible than a hospital environment. You'll have continuous support from a combination of labor nurses and midwives. Your doctor may also be affiliated with a birthing center. Furthermore, the medical team in these centers is very experienced at handling a birth without medical intervention. All of these factors therefore increase your chances of having a straightforward birth. To be give birth in such a center, you need to have had an uncomplicated pregnancy and be unlikely to require specialized medical care or monitoring in labor and birth. If complications did occur, you would be transferred to the closest hospital, although this is rare.

**The prospect of sleeping in your own bed** and being taken care of by people who love you are reason enough to opt for a home birth. It's natural to feel less inhibited at home, and you may be more inclined to move around more and for longer, be as vocal as you like, use gravity, and try different birthing positions, all of which can make labor and delivery shorter and easier. Your midwife will explain what's involved, so seek her advice. On the big day be flexible: you may want to head for the hospital.

**ASK A... DOCTOR**

**I'm having a home birth. Can my older children, four and six, be present at the birth?** There is nothing more wonderful or miraculous than the birth of a baby, and it's natural to want your older children to be present and witness it for themselves. However, do consider this carefully before you give them the go-ahead. For one thing, even the easiest of labors are painful, and young children will be distressed to see mom in pain. What's more, they may be slightly daunted to see their new sibling emerging from your body, probably covered with various substances. Having said that, many kids handle the experience well if they know what to expect, so outline everything, and explain that any cries, shrieks, or swearing on your behalf are necessary to help get the baby out. You could also mention that you may cry or even vomit, just so they are prepared. Let them know to expect some blood, and that baby will be attached to a (rather gruesome!) cord. If they're squeamish, get them to position themselves by your head, or bring them in immediately after.

**Sit down with your partner** and discuss what you both would like to happen during the whole labor and birth experience. Then start putting your hopes, thoughts, and feelings into a birth plan that you can discuss and expand on with your doctor.

**Your baby** still has slender arms and legs and little fat under the skin. His skin is covered with fine lanugo hair and waxy vernix and he now has eyebrows and eyelashes—his first mature hairs.

**YOU ARE** 30 WEEKS AND 6 DAYS

# 64 days to go...

**YOR BABY TODAY**

Here the baby is resting on the placenta, seen at the right-hand side of the image, with the umbilical cord just below the baby's chin. The eyes are closed and this image was taken at a time when the baby was at his quietest, during deep sleep.

## Once your baby's production of red blood cells is in full swing, in theory your immune system could begin to harm your baby.

**At 30 weeks** your baby's red blood cell production switches from the liver to the bone marrow. These red blood cells are unlikely to be of the same blood group as your own. Small numbers of these red blood cells often leak across the placenta; your body recognizes them as foreign and attacks them.

Your blood group is not important because, although antibodies to blood groups A, B, AB, or O attack your baby's cells in your circulation, they are too large to cross the placenta and attack your baby. Therefore differences in ABO blood groups do not matter. However, everyone is also Rhesus positive (85 percent) or negative (15 percent). If you are Rhesus negative (see p.123) and your partner is Rhesus positive, your baby may also be Rhesus positive.

Rhesus negative women produce antibodies to rhesus positive blood cells; these are smaller than ABO antibodies and can cross the placenta. Once they do, large numbers of antibodies can attack your baby's blood cells, leading to anemia. First pregnancies are rarely affected. In pregnancy you are given an injection of the rhesus antibody "Rh immunoglobulin (RhIg)" around now—with another after the birth. The Rh immunoglobulin (RhIg) is in a form that it is too large to cross the placenta. This mops up any of your baby's blood cells in your circulation, preventing your immune system from attacking your baby.

### AMNIOTIC FLUID

**Your baby excretes and reabsorbs** about 16 fl oz (0.5 liter) of urine daily, and the amniotic fluid reaches a peak volume of 1.75 pints (1 liter) at 35 weeks. After this time the volume starts to decline and can be as little as 3.5–7 fl oz (100–200 ml) in an overdue pregnancy (see p.393).

Low levels of amniotic fluid, known as oligohydramnios (see p.473), can be a sign of a growth-restricted baby or a baby with kidney problems.

Excessive amniotic fluid, known as polyhydramnios (see p.473), may be seen in twin or triplet pregnancies, and is also associated with physical abnormalities in the baby or diabetes in the mother.

After 40 weeks, the fluid level needs to be checked regularly to ensure that there is not too steep a decline in fluid levels. If the overdue baby is thought to be at risk, an induction (see p.432) will be recommended.

**FOCUS ON... YOUR HEALTH**

## A good night's sleep

**Insomnia is a common problem** during pregnancy and can lead to fatigue, feelings of stress and anxiety, and irritability. Whether it's brought on by your increased size, back pain, heartburn, getting up to empty your bladder, or something else, insomnia is not fun. Taking a warm bath or having a small snack before bed may help, as can relaxation techniques, such as deep breathing. A calming scent in a potpourri or fragrance on your pillow may aid relaxation. Make sure to exercise during the day. If you still can't sleep, get up and do something relaxing: read a book, watch TV, or listen to calming music until you feel sleepy. And try to make up for lost sleep with daytime naps.

# 63 days to go...

**YOUR BABY TODAY**

One leg is shown here crossed over the other. Your baby can still stretch the legs out fully and even curl up in such a way that the feet can rest on top of the head: just because you're kicked on one side doesn't mean that the head will be on the other.

Epidural is a common form of pain-relief during labor and may be an option for you if you have a low pain threshold.

**Many women have decided that they want a pain-free delivery** with an epidural (see pp.404–5) even before they go into labor. It's good to know, however, that labor has to be well established before you can have an epidural, so you'll still experience some painful contractions. Epidurals generally work well, but sometimes the block isn't complete or is more effective on one side than the other. Some women decide to have an epidural because they know they're unlikely to cope well with labor pain. Many women start off saying that they don't want an epidural and change their minds halfway through—if it's your first pregnancy, you can't possibly know how you'll feel.

An elective cesarean (see pp.438–9) is one that is planned and generally performed for medical reasons—for example, because of a low-lying placenta (see p.212)—and not simply because a woman wants to have one. Having a cesarean is major abdominal surgery and in most circumstances it is safer to have a vaginal delivery. Recovery after a cesarean usually takes longer than after a vaginal birth, so one is only performed if necessary.

THE LOWDOWN

## Tocophobia

**This condition is an intense fear or dread of childbirth**. There are two types: primary tocophobia predates pregnancy and can start as early as adolescence; secondary tocophobia is associated with an earlier traumatic experience in childbirth. This fear can manifest itself as nightmares, intense anxiety, or panic attacks.

If you have tocophobia, your doctor will refer you to a consultant obstetrician who deals in mental health issues, or you may be referred directly to a psychologist to discuss your fears. Some experts believe that hypnotherapy can help to tackle any subconscious fears of childbirth. An elective cesarean (see pp.438–9) may be recommended if your fear of having a vaginal birth cannot be overcome.

**FOCUS ON... RELATIONSHIPS**

## Comfortable lovemaking

**You may need to experiment** to find lovemaking positions that are comfortable. Most women find that the missionary position becomes increasingly uncomfortable as your partner presses on your belly. You may find being on top is enjoyable and does not put pressure on your belly. Lying in the spoons position, with your partner behind you, can also be pleasurable. Other positions that don't restrict your pleasure and are comfortable include sitting together, kneeling while your partner enters from behind, and lying side by side with your legs entwined.

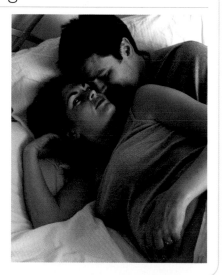

# Your 32nd week

The baby has not settled into her final birth position just yet, but an assessment of how she's lying will be made at every routine checkup. There's still room in the uterus for your baby to exercise her limbs and she's getting much stronger and more active. You'll know all about it! As your belly gets bigger, it may become more difficult to be very active and to get comfortable when you're sitting or lying down.

**The baby's movements** are mainly from side to side, and you won't know where to expect the kicks to come from.

**The baby** is likely to be near her maximum length now, since her bones have almost reached their full pre-birth growth.

**The skin** starts to look pinker and less translucent.

**Increasing layers of fat** and muscle are rounding out the baby's body, and she looks a little less skinny.

**Creases** can be seen in the skin of the wrists and the palms of the hands.

**At 32 weeks** the average crown to heel length is 15.7 in (39.9 cm) and the average weight is 2.9 lb (1.3 kg).

# 62 days to go...

## YOUR BABY TODAY

The amount of amniotic fluid within the uterus is at its maximum over the next two weeks but will subsequently start to reduce gradually. Measurements of the four deepest pockets of amniotic fluid can add up to 6–8 in, allowing space for your baby to move.

## If you listen to music while you're pregnant, your baby will be tuning in, too—and it might just benefit her.

**You might have noticed that your baby becomes more active** when you're listening to music. It's been noted that unborn babies move and even breathe in time to music, and there have been claims that by exposing your baby to certain types of music, you can enhance her brain development.

One study, relating to a "Baby Mozart" brain-enhancing product, claimed that the structure of, say, a particular Mozart arrangement, stimulated brain development to a greater extent than other genres, and even other classical composers. This theory has, however,

been debunked. Some research found that college-aged students who listened to classical music showed a brief and temporary improvement in spatial intelligence. However, the same research was not tested in children or babies. The research has not been repeated and the results are open to several different interpretations.

Whether or not it enhances your baby's intelligence, listening to classical music can relax you, which is always a good thing during pregnancy. And if you gently sway to the music, your baby may enjoy being "rocked" to sleep.

---

**FOCUS ON... YOUR BODY**

## Protruding navel

**You may be surprised to find** that by now your perfectly formed navel is protruding. This protrusion is caused by the pressure of your rapidly expanding uterus, which presses against your abdomen and literally pops your belly button out.

Some women find their protruding navel unsightly, and choose to wear skirts or pants with a high waistband to cover it; you can also cover your protruding belly button with a Band-Aid.

A protruding navel is a normal consequence of pregnancy and it will return to normal a few months after the delivery. Although you may find that, like other parts of your body, your navel sags a little more than it used to.

---

**ASK A... DOCTOR**

**What exactly is an "active birth"?**
Having an "active birth"—staying mobile during the first stage of labor and remaining upright, squatting, kneeling, or on all-fours during the second stage—can make labor and delivery easier and less painful. Working with gravity helps your pelvis to open and encourages the baby's head to press on your cervix, helping it to dilate. To get active:
■ **Practice squatting (see p.424):** it takes time to learn to do it, but it's an effective way to speed labor up. When squatting, make sure you have

sufficient support—from your partner, for example.
■ **Relax by kneeling** with a birth ball or beanbag.
■ **Use a birthing pool** if you want to relax in water for a while.
■ **If you need an IV,** because you've been induced (see p.432), ask for one with a long tube that will leave you free to move around a little.
■ **Choose a walking epidural,** which should enable you to stay active.
■ **If lying down** makes your contractions stop, get up and start moving again.

# 61 days to go...

**YOUR BABY TODAY**

Your baby's hand coordination continues to improve as her brain is better able to make sense of the feedback it receives. The eyes will often open but only for short periods at a time, reducing the chance of a stray finger coming too close.

By this stage, your baby is the length she'll be at birth, but she's still very thin and needs to gain fat and muscle.

**At this stage of pregnancy,** your baby's muscle mass and fat are continuing to increase. Her skin is now thicker and less translucent, and begins to look pink rather than red as the underlying blood vessels are overlaid with more flesh. Growth hormone is being produced by your baby's pituitary gland but before she's actually born this does not influence her growth. Instead insulin and insulin-like growth factors

are key. As your baby's skeleton is now close to its final size, her overall length is established. Your baby is still, however, very skinny.

A sonographer can make a good estimate of your baby's weight from an ultrasound scan but her final birthweight will very much depend on when she is born. She'll continue to grow throughout the pregnancy, although in the last few weeks

growth is mainly due to fat deposits rather than to muscle mass.

If you're trying to guess how heavy your baby will be at birth, the latest research indicates that the size of your baby has a lot to do with "imprinted" genes. These are genes that are marked as having come from the father, which promote the baby's growth, or the mother, which are growth limiting and attempt to preserve her resources.

---

**FOCUS ON... TWINS**

## Dressing your babies

**Twins look adorable when they're dressed alike,** so you may be buying—and certainly will be given— lots of sets of matching clothing. But it's much easier to tell identical twins apart when they're dressed differently. It also helps everyone relate to them as individuals, which is good for their development.

Also keep practicalities in mind: every time one of your twins gets dirty, are you going to change them both? You may find it pays to be flexible: if there are only two clean onesies, then that is what they'll have to wear, regardless of style or color match.

Newborns don't care what they wear, but if you get in the habit of dressing them the same, they may become conscious of it in the toddler years and get distressed if they're wearing something different.

How you dress your babies is your decision, but you could:
- **Dress your babies in matching outfits but different colors,** or the same colors but different styles.
- **Only dress them identically on certain occasions,** for instance for a family photograph or special occasion.
- **Give any identical outfits you receive to one twin.** The next batch of identical outfits goes to the other twin.

# 60 days to go...

## YOUR BABY TODAY

Here the umbilical cord is seen lying over the baby's shoulder and next to the wrist. This is very common, in fact at some time every baby will have the umbilical cord lying close, especially during these next few weeks while the baby frequently changes position.

Jolts and jostles are all part of being pregnant—and your baby probably won't even notice them.

### ASK A... MOM

**I'm finding it increasingly hard to focus at work. How can I best get through the next few weeks?**
As your baby—and you—get bigger, you may find that you have less energy and your concentration span decreases accordingly. This is normal, but it can pose problems if you have a job to do! First of all, take regular breaks, putting your feet up or closing your eyes for a few minutes to rest. Make sure you drink enough, since dehydration can affect your performance. Similarly, eating healthy snacks, little and often, can keep you from flagging. Iron-rich foods, such as dried fruit, are particularly important: low iron levels can make you tire easily.

Carry a small notebook with you, and jot down anything that you need to remember, no matter how trivial. This can help overcome lapses of memory, and keep you focused on what needs to be done. It may also help to start your day with a "to-do" list, and check your way down it in order of priority. Finally, try to get enough sleep, which will give you at least half a chance of feeling refreshed the next morning.

**Your belly is getting larger and larger.** As you walk you may notice that your belly also appears to move, swaying from side to side with each step. It can be difficult to remember that you're so much bigger than you used to be. You may find yourself trying to squeeze through tight spaces, or between tables and chairs in a restaurant that previously you would have fit through and now find yourself a bit stuck! Even if you find that your belly is getting bumped around occasionally this really is nothing at all to worry about: your baby is safe, protected by the pool of amniotic fluid that acts as a cushion against the occasional jolt. Soon enough, though, you will be back to your normal shape, or nearly your normal shape, and it can be odd to think back to having to compensate for a belly.

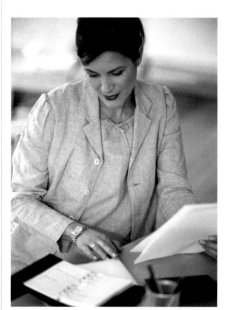

**Keep a notebook to hand** to jot down everything from what to do today, what to say when you make a call, and what you need to cover in a letter or e-mail.

### FOCUS ON... YOUR HEALTH

## Heart palpitations

**Having a run of fast heartbeats,** or missing a beat occasionally—or simply being acutely aware of your heartbeat—is defined as heart palpitations (see p.469). It's common to have these in late pregnancy. They are usually nothing to worry about and are simply the result of changes to your blood circulation, coupled with a large abdominal bulge, although unnecessary stresses and anxieties can play a part as well.

If, however, palpitations are accompanied by chest pain or breathlessness, or if you think they are occurring more frequently, mention this to your doctor.

# 59 days to go...

### YOUR BABY TODAY

Measurements around the head, abdomen, and thigh bones are used from the ultrasound image to estimate the weight of your baby. Interestingly, on average, boys are now starting to be slightly heavier than girls.

## As your baby puts on muscle and its tone improves, she begins to be capable of more complex and stronger movements.

### Your baby's muscle tone takes some time to develop fully.

By this week of your pregnancy, head control is improving and in the legs muscle tone now allows for smoother and more complex movements. For once, the arms and hands lag behind the legs and feet in development, taking another three weeks to achieve the same level of tone and movement.

In the last few weeks the familiar "fetal position" is increasingly seen on scans: this is not only due to lack of space, but also because your baby's flexor muscles (those that bend the elbows, hips, and knees) have a better tone than her extensor muscles (the muscles that extend the arms and legs) in each limb.

You will also be aware that your baby is moving more now than at any other time. You only feel the movements that hit the lining of your uterus, but there will be many more small movements of which you are completely unaware. Movements inside the uterus are important: they help your baby's coordination, strengthen her bones, and increase muscle mass. The number of muscle cells increases up until 38 weeks. From this point on, individual muscle cells lengthen and expand in response to exercise, further increasing muscle mass and strength.

**There is no need** to feel left out when all around you are partying: enjoy fresh fruit juices over ice, topped with soda, tonic water, or ginger ale to add a little fizz.

### NON-ALCOHOLIC DRINKS

**Here are some ideas** for delicious non-alcoholic drinks:
- Cranberry juice/orange juice/lemon juice/ginger ale
- Grapefruit juice/cranberry juice/soda or tonic water
- Sparkling apple juice/lime juice/sugar to taste
- Orange juice/bitter lemon
- Lemon juice/pineapple juice/orange juice/grenadine/soda
- Diced lemon/diced lime/diced orange/ginger ale/sugar to taste
- Apple juice/pear juice/ginger ale.

### ASK A... DOCTOR

**Will having an orgasm cause me to go into labor?** In a pregnancy without problems, an orgasm will not cause premature labor (see p.431), and at full term orgasm will only cause the onset of labor if it's going to happen anyway. If you have had any signs of premature labor, or your water has broken (see p.411), you'll be advised to avoid sexual intercourse. This is because the hormone oxytocin increases during sexual arousal and oxytocin causes the muscles of the uterus to contact. Orgasm may increase practice, or Braxton Hicks', contractions (see p.410).

If you've gone past your due date and are at a point when your body is ready to go into labor, then sexual intercourse may help things to start for two reasons: the prostaglandins in semen will help the cervix to soften at this stage of pregnancy, and the contractions stimulated by orgasm have more chance of developing into early labor contractions.

# 58 days to go...

## YOUR BABY TODAY

This image shows a furrowed brow and an open-eyed expression. Just as the muscle tone in the limbs is strengthening, so the muscles of the face are being used and tested. This can produce some unusual expressions that do not necessarily reflect your baby's emotions.

## How your baby is positioned can affect your delivery, but there is plenty of time at this stage for things to change.

**Each time you are examined** your doctor will assess your baby's lie and presentation (see p.336). Many babies are in the breech position earlier in the pregnancy, but most turn into the head down position by the end of the pregnancy. Still, breech births occur in about one in 25 full-term births. Between 32 and 37 weeks is the best time for your doctor to try to turn a breech baby. This is because there is plenty of room for the baby to turn around. After the 35th or 36th week, the baby is unlikely to change position since there is less room for large maneuvers. If your baby is breech, your doctor may try to turn the baby, a process called version and she may recommend an extra ultrasound scan at 37–38 weeks of pregnancy to check the baby's position. It may be difficult to be completely sure, on examination alone, whether the doctor is feeling the baby's bottom or head. If your baby is breech, your doctor may suggest a cesarean delivery.

---

**FOCUS ON... DADS**

# Getting the balance right

**Much of later pregnancy** involves your partner doing less than normal. This may range from doing less exercise to not doing household chores. It may be challenging for your partner to realize that she's not able to do things as easily as before and, to a certain extent, is less independent.

You can be a great help to her in the final weeks of pregnancy, but be aware that there's a fine line between being supportive and being overly protective. Deep down you may want to turn into "superman" and do everything, but it might frustrate your partner if you become overly protective. Try to take the lead from her and give her help as and when she needs it, as well as space to do her own thing.

# 57 days to go...

**YOUR BABY TODAY**

You can see from this image just how much amniotic fluid is around your baby at this time. Ultrasound displays the fluid as black on the screen. Sometimes there will be speckles within the fluid: these represent skin and hair cells that are shed as your baby grows.

## If your third trimester coincides with the summer months, staying cool and comfortable can be a real challenge.

**When the weather is hot**, your baby makes it sweltering! Keep yourself hydrated by drinking lots of cool water. Consider carrying a spray bottle of water (keep it in the fridge overnight so that it's nice and cold next day) to spritz you when you're too hot.

Opt for sleeveless clothing that is made of natural fabrics, such as linen and cotton, which will help keep the air circulating. If you want to keep some or all of your arms covered, wear short-sleeved jackets or cotton cardigans. Wear a sun hat and sunglasses, especially if you're in direct sunlight for any length of time.

Opt for flip-flops or low-heeled sandals to let your feet breathe—these can also be a good option if your feet are swollen (see pp.466–7).

(see pp.466–7)

### FOCUS ON... YOUR BABY

## Listening to your baby's heartbeat

**From the very earliest stages of pregnancy,** your baby's heart will be beating, and there can be nothing more uplifting and reassuring than hearing this for yourself. Your doctor can use a variety of instruments to hear your baby's heartbeat, including a stethoscope and a Doppler monitor (which uses ultrasound technology). A baby's heart beats between 120 and 160 times per minute (with slight variations)—quite a few more than your own heartbeat, which is normally under 100. The sole purpose of listening to the heartbeat is to ensure that it falls within a normal range, and to reassure moms-to-be that all is well. If there's an unusual rhythm or the heartbeat speeds or slows unexpectedly, your doctor can arrange for tests to confirm that all is well. Some women feel that hearing their baby's heartbeat helps the bonding process in advance of the birth.

### THE LOWDOWN

## First hours and days

To help you prepare for what will follow the birth of your baby, here's a few interesting facts you might like to know:

■ **You may shake all over** just after giving birth and don't be concerned if you vomit, this is quite normal and nothing to worry about.

■ **Newborn babies don't always master breast-feeding** (see pp.448–9) immediately. Just like you, they need to practice.

■ **After pains** (the clamping sensation in your uterus when your baby nurses) can hurt almost as much as contractions.

■ **The first time you urinate** and defecate after giving birth can be uncomfortable.

■ **You may feel very vulnerable,** and in need of your own mom, in the first few days of parenthood.

■ **Lochia** (after-birth bleeding) can be a challenge at first, even if you're using larger-sized sanitary pads.

■ **Bonding with a newborn doesn't always happen** immediately for all mothers, but it's worth the wait.

# 56 days to go...

**YOUR BABY TODAY**

The blood flow in the umbilical cord is highlighted in this image. The colors show the direction of flow. The smaller umbilical arteries that carry blood toward the placenta are seen in blue as they wrap around the more central umbilical vein (in red).

## The best way to make sure you get enough sleep is to find ways to slow down mentally and relax.

**You may find that you're having difficulty sleeping,** partly because your belly makes it uncomfortable to lie down in certain positions, but also because you have lots to think about at the moment. Try to take some time out with your partner each evening relaxing and bonding together with your belly. Even spending 10 minutes doing nothing except focusing on yourself, your body, your partner, and your baby can be invigorating and rejuvenating.

Get yourself in a comfortable position, and try to focus inward on your body, turning your mind away from all your external worries. First focus on slowing down your breathing. Then turn your thoughts to a place and a time when you felt relaxed and happy—for example, when you were on vacation, walking on the beach. Next focus on clenching and then relaxing each set of muscles in turn, or imagine a ball of heat passing slowly through your limbs and body making them feel warm, heavy, and relaxed.

You might want to involve your partner, perhaps he could sit with you with his hands or head on your belly and try to adjust his breathing so it's in sync with yours. Just lying next to your partner, even without talking, can relax you and bring you close together.

### DRESSING FOR EXERCISE

**In this last trimester,** dressing appropriately for exercise can make all the difference to your activities and the way that you feel.

During pregnancy it is possible to look good in your workout clothes, while still supporting your belly and your breasts. Ensure you wear the correct size clothes—trying to squeeze into a size you outgrew three months ago will be uncomfortable and restricting.

There are some great pregnancy exercise clothes on the market, which are cut well and have ample room for your belly. If, however, you'd rather

cover up while you're exercising, just wear a large T-shirt and baggy athletic pants or loose-fitting shorts. Wear whatever makes you feel confident and comfortable.

There are some good support belts available, which may make your cardiovascular exercise that much more comfortable. If you're carrying twins or more this will be even more of a welcome addition to your workout wardrobe. Most of the support belts are made from elasticized fabric with Velcro fastenings that can be adjusted to suit your belly size. These belts, available at many maternity stores, are inexpensive and can help ease back pain, too.

Your breasts will need additional support by this stage of pregnancy, but especially when you're exercising. A well-fitting sports bra is vital for any activity as the delicate breast tissue can weaken due to the increased pressure of your larger and heavier breasts. If your breasts are very large, and you feel they're unsupported by just wearing a sports bra, try wearing it on top of your usual bra.

# Your 33rd week

**IT'S HARD TO IMAGINE HOW LIFE WILL BE WITH A NEW BABY**

All prospective moms, and not just first-timers, find it difficult to envisage the future after the arrival of the baby. The imaginings, dreams, and hopes of the last few months are about to become realities—which may be very different from what you expect. You may find that it helps to concentrate on practical matters, such as the birth celebrations and future child care. You could make plans for recovering your pre-pregnancy figure. The belly won't be with you forever, even if it feels like it!

**Calcium from your diet** is crossing the placenta and being used to help the hardening of your baby's bones.

**With bottom up**, head down, and chin tucked into his chest, a baby is in an ideal position for the beginning of labor. Of course, not all babies are so obliging.

**Fingernails** have grown long enough to reach the tips of the fingers.

**At 33 weeks** the average crown to heel length is 16.2 in (41.1 cm) and the average weight is 3.3 lb (1.5 kg).

**The amniotic fluid** swallowed by the baby passes through the stomach and intestines in the same way as food travels through a mature digestive system. Waste is stored in the baby's colon to be excreted after birth.

# 55 days to go...

## YOUR BABY TODAY

In this image the hands are folded over beneath the chin and there's a foot up by the mouth and nose. It can look as if your baby is quite a contortionist but because he is still quite skinny, the joints allow for a great deal of flexibility.

If you feel you have little control over your own body, it's natural to think your figure will never be normal again—but it will!

**At this stage of the third trimester,** you'll still be gaining 1–2 lb (0.5–1 kg) per week but weight gain tends to slow down in the last few weeks of pregnancy. By now, your belly will have stretched and your belly button may have popped out—this can be quite protruding and may be seen through your clothes (see p.319). You may have developed a linea nigra in your second trimester, a dark line of pigmentation down the center of your abdomen (see p.170).

Like most women you are probably happy and excited about having a baby but a little concerned about getting your figure back after the birth. Some women get quite upset at the thought that their abdomens may not return to their previous shape, and this is completely normal. Rest assured that with a bit of hard work and exercise and the continuation of your healthy pregnancy diet after the birth, your figure can return to its pre-pregnancy state and your belly button should pop back to its normal shape of its own accord. The key is to remember it will take a bit of time: it did, after all, take nine months to gain the weight.

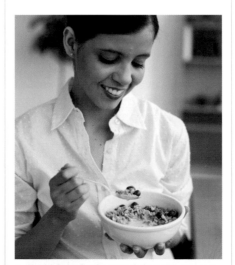

**A diet rich in foods containing** fiber is good for health at any time of life but especially during these three months to relieve common symptoms such as constipation. Snack on whole-grain breads and cereals.

### ASK A... DOCTOR

**I want to work right up to the birth—is that allowed?** Yes. Many women do, so they don't waste any maternity leave before baby. Check with your doctor to make sure it's okay for you. Think carefully before making this decision. Late pregnancy can be extremely tiring and, if your job is mentally and/or physically taxing, it may be better to begin your leave before your due date. You will also need time to prepare for the arrival of your baby.

### FOCUS ON... NUTRITION

## Fabulous fiber

**Fiber is very important** in the third trimester, since it will help your digestive system work more efficiently. Dietary fiber—the indigestible part of plant foods—is the best natural way to keep the bowels regular. Most pregnant women who eat a diet based upon whole grains, fruits, and vegetables, are likely to be getting enough fiber.

Pregnant women should aim for 1 oz (25 g) of fiber daily. To give a sense of what it takes to achieve this, there are around 3 g in a medium avocado or banana, or a serving of broccoli, blueberries, brown rice, or beans. Eating three or four servings of fruit a day, vegetables with your meals, and eating whole-grain breads and brown rice will provide plenty.

Fiber makes you feel fuller sooner and longer, and can help to prevent overeating and excess weight gain. It also contributes to the management of diabetes, lowers cholesterol, and decreases the risk of heart disease.

Your 33rd week

# 54 days to go...

## YOUR BABY TODAY

During this week your baby's fingernails have become fully developed and now approach the tips of the fingers. Bathed in amniotic fluid, the nails are kept very soft: it's only after birth that your baby might tend to scratch and need to wear mittens.

Every 40 minutes, your baby swallows enough amniotic fluid to fill his stomach, before emptying it back into the amniotic sac.

**Your baby is swallowing** and recycling almost half a liter of amniotic fluid each day. In addition to providing him with nutrients, especially proteins, this fluid is important for the healthy development of the gut. Your baby's sense of taste is thought to have developed to such an extent now that if you have eaten spiced food he can distinguish this in the fluid he drinks.

Amniotic fluid does not enter the lungs but travels down the esophagus into the stomach where it is stored for a short time. At this stage, the stomach fills every 40 minutes, but, from 35 weeks, as the stomach enlarges, this rate slows down to every 80 minutes. Muscle contractions move the fluid in waves into the small and then large bowel. As it travels along the bowel, water is reabsorbed so that only waste material or "meconium," enters the colon, the final section of the large bowel. This meconium accumulates in the large bowel, which is completely full by the time your baby is born. Babies don't usually pass meconium before the birth but do so soon after. Meconium consists mainly of skin cells, lanugo hairs, and vernix. It has a greenish color due to the presence of bilirubin, a breakdown product from red blood cells.

---

### FOCUS ON... THE BIRTH

## False alarms

**In the next few weeks,** as you and your partner await your baby's arrival, you may experience one or two false alarms, especially if it's your first baby. A false alarm can come at any time of the day or night and it won't respect important meetings or deadlines.

It can help if you—as well as your partner—familiarize yourself with all the signs that indicate labor may be starting (see pp. 409–11). If, however, you're ever in doubt, do contact your doctor to ascertain that labor has not started, rather than assuming that this is the case. She will be very experienced in dealing with false alarms and won't mind you contacting her.

---

### ITCHY SKIN

**Having itchy skin on your belly** is common: as the skin there stretches and thins, it can become dry. You could try using a moisturizing lotion to soothe this.

If, however, you have severe itching on your abdomen, or on the palms of your hands or soles of your feet, see your doctor. This itching can be a sign of obstetric cholestasis (see p.473), a rare pregnancy condition involving the liver, which causes bile salts to enter the bloodstream, making the skin (especially on the hands and feet) itchy, although there is no rash. The condition may also cause a vitamin K deficiency. Vitamin K helps the blood to clot, so a deficiency increases the risk of bleeding for both mother and baby. Medication to bind the bile salts and vitamin K supplements are effective treatments. Some studies suggest early induction of labor (at around 37 weeks) helps avoid complications. The condition resolves after delivery, usually without any long-term liver damage.

Your third trimester

# 53 days to go...

**YOUR BABY TODAY**

Your baby's position in the uterus is influenced by your own posture. Gravity has some effect on your baby, so whether you are standing or sitting, and which side you lie down on affects the way your baby's back is turned and which side he rolls onto.

## As your belly grows, it's normal to feel you want to support it when you're walking around.

**You've probably had to change** the way that you exercise by now due to your growing abdomen. You may well have had to replace jogging on the treadmill, for example, with going for long, brisk (or not so brisk!) walks. If you find that even walking makes your belly and pelvis sore or uncomfortable, you may find you naturally hold up your belly with your hands to try to give it some extra support and to give your pelvis and back a break. Some women say it feels as if the baby "might fall out."

You might want to invest in a pregnancy support band; made of stretchy fabric, this useful item supports the belly and can help prevent lower back pain.

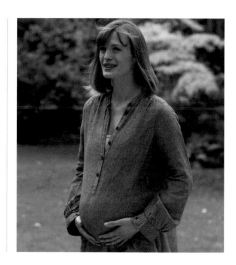

**Walking at a comfortable pace** when you are heavily pregnant will cause your belly to shift around and your instinct may be to support your baby with your hands.

### BUYING A BABY MONITOR

**There are hundreds** of monitors on the market, so choosing one can be daunting. Although monitors vary, they have the same basic components—a minimum of two units: one to transmit your baby's sounds, and one that stays with you so that you can hear if your baby is crying or fussing.

Additional features include: video screens, a moving lights-sound display, low power and out-of-range warnings, the option to use electricity or batteries, a talk-back function, and a temperature sensor. Some have a night-light function. With all these features available, your choice largely depends on your personal preferences and your budget. If your house is small, you don't necessarily need one.

### FOCUS ON... YOUR BABY

## Repositioning your baby

**Your movements during late pregnancy** can affect the position of your baby. Ideally, he'll lie head down, facing your back, with his chin tucked into his chest. You can encourage this optimum fetal position by:
- **Spending time on all fours,** wiggling your hips from side to side; or arch your back, then drop your spine down.
- **Sitting with your knees lower than your pelvis,** and your body tilted slightly forward.

- **Kneeling on the floor,** leaning over a beanbag, cushions, or birth ball.
- **Sitting on a birth ball,** with your legs positioned slightly apart and knees lower than your hips, then rocking your pelvis.
- **Assuming the tailor pose:** sit on the floor with your back straight and the soles of your feet together. Let your knees fall to the side and rest your elbows on your inner thighs.
- **Swimming:** breaststroke helps to open the pelvis.

# 52 days to go...

**YOUR BABY TODAY**

This image shows that the bridge of your baby's nose is now more fully formed. The face is taking on a more rounded shape and some babies may look quite chubby from now on. Shadows around the top and sides of the head will increasingly give the illusion of hair.

By this stage of pregnancy, your baby's fingernails have grown and reach the tips of his fingers.

**By now, your baby's fingernails** have reached the tips of the fingers. The fingernails first appeared at 12 weeks, and since the development of the arms is consistently ahead of the legs, the toenails started to develop four weeks later. The future nail begins at the tip of each finger or toe, where a nail fold is formed. At the base of this nail fold, the cells start to harden into nail,

in a process known as keratinization. The nails grow from new cells formed in the soft nail bed. It takes nine weeks for the nails to reach the fingertips and it will be another four weeks before the toenails reach the tips of the toes.

The nail is actually all the same color, but the white part of the nail appears white because it does not have the nail bed, with its rich blood supply, beneath

it to give the illusion of color. Since the nails already reach the fingertips, it probably won't be long after the birth before your baby's nails need trimming—they are very fine and soft and you may find it easier to trim them by nibbling them away rather than trying to cut them. Or cut them with baby nail scissors while your baby is asleep and not wiggling around.

---

**FOCUS ON... YOUR BODY**

**Yoga is excellent exercise** for the mind and body while you're pregnant, and may be a cornerstone of your birth preparations if you choose to take active birth classes (see p.333). An instructor will tailor a routine for your body and the stage of your pregnancy. The individual stretches shown

below are ideal for opening up the pelvis and strengthening the legs. By practicing them while you're pregnant, you'll be able to use them more effectively and confidently during labor. When you're practicing squatting, it may help if your partner supports you from behind.

**Get into a squatting position.** Squat only if you find it easy to hold this position with your heels on the floor and your back straight.

**Sit with your left leg stretched out in front of you** and right leg bent. Gently twist your body, placing your hands on the floor for additional support.

**Sit with one leg stretched out behind you,** and the other tucked beneath your belly. Stretch upward, breathing deeply throughout.

YOU ARE 32 WEEKS AND 5 DAYS

# 51 days to go...

## YOUR BABY TODAY

In this image of the baby lying on his side, the arm is positioned beneath the head and is partly outside of the 3D view. This allows the ultrasound scan to look within the arm. Part of the bones in the elbow and forearm are seen here as bright reflections.

To get used to the fact that your newborn will arrive very soon, start focusing on life after the birth.

**Friends and family** might now begin talking about what will happen after the birth and what it will be like for you to have a baby.

If this is your first baby, you probably can't really envisage what it will be like to be a mom, and even if you have had a baby before you've never had a second or third and so don't know what it will be like to have another one. Of course you know that life will continue, but it can be difficult to see past the labor to the realities of life with a newborn. As ever, keep talking to those close to you about how you feel, be it excited or scared and unprepared (usually all three in rapid succession). Talk about what you think or hope it will be like after the baby is born, for example when are grandparents and other key people going to visit, and whether you would like a christening or naming party—or perhaps neither of these. This may help you get used to the idea that not only are you pregnant but there is a baby coming.

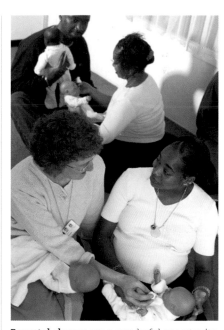

**Prenatal classes** are a wonderful opportunity to swap ideas and information with a group of people in the same position as you. Long-term friendships can be made here.

## ASK A... DOCTOR

**How will I benefit from going to prenatal classes?** You'll get the opportunity to share information, ideas, fears, and concerns about childbirth in a comfortable environment, and to discuss and decide upon issues that will affect the way you choose to give birth. You'll also meet other parents-to-be. Often friendships formed at classes continue after the birth as you support each other in your new parenting role. In most classes, you'll be given advice about:
■ **Tried-and-tested labor techniques,** such as breathing through the pain, massage, suitable sustenance, and some positive visualization exercises
■ **Pain-relief options** and a range of natural alternatives (see pp.396–407)
■ **How to present** (and preserve) your birth plan (see p.303)
■ **The practical and emotional support** a birth partner can offer
■ **The items required** for a hospital or home birth (see pp. 341 and 358).

You'll be advised on how to prepare yourself for the birth, what to expect in the first few days, and how to encourage healing afterward, as well as being given tips on caring for a newborn, including diaper changing, bathing, and establishing breast-feeding.

## AS A MATTER OF FACT

**In a first birth,** the cervix dilates by about 0.5 cm every hour, compared to 1.5 cm an hour for subsequent babies.

First-time moms push for around an hour, compared with about half an hour for a second baby.

# 50 days to go...

**YOUR BABY TODAY**

This image may show the start of a smile. Your baby will often be smiling inside, sticking his tongue out, and making all sorts of faces. He may also still be experiencing hiccups that may be something that you are now becoming aware of.

## The days and nights fly by with a newborn, so it's a good idea to start thinking about child care well before you need it.

**It may seem impossible** to believe that you should be considering child care before your baby is even born, but it can be useful to think through the options while you have the time. There are two main types of child care: in and out of your home. In the first case, you can have a live-in or live-out nanny or mother's help, an au pair (which may be acceptable if you work from home, for example, and can supervise), or perhaps a family member or friend who is prepared to come to your house to take care of your baby. If you choose outside child care, there are a number of options including day-care centers, relatives or babysitters in their homes,

or on-the-job day care. Before you set your heart on one particular type of care, it's a good idea to investigate the costs and the availability in your area. You may want to pay a visit to some of the nurseries or other facilities close to you, just to get a feel for what's available, and establish now what you do and don't want. Secondly, remember that good-quality child-care facilities and babysitters are usually in demand, and, even if you aren't entirely sure when you will be going back to work, it's probably a good idea to put your baby's name (or last name, at least!) down for a few, to give you options when the time comes.

**CALCIUM INTAKE**

**Your baby's skeleton began** forming at the end of the first trimester, but the majority of your calcium is transferred to the baby from your body in the third trimester. This happens regardless of your calcium intake. If a mother-to-be's diet is low in calcium, it will be taken from the reservoir in her bones, which can affect her bone density.

The recommended amount of calcium in pregnancy is 1000 mg daily. Calcium needs to be accompanied by vitamin D in order to be absorbed by the body.

Dairy products are a rich source of calcium, and some, such as margarine and low-fat spreads, are often fortified with vitamin D. Vegetarian sources of calcium include tofu, leafy green vegetables, dried fruit, seeds, and nuts.

**FOCUS ON... DADS**

## Being at the birth

**Many dads-to-be are anxious** about being with their partners during labor and birth. This is often because they will be witnessing their partner experience one of the most intense things a woman can ever do and they may be unsure of how to help.

There are plenty of ways in which you can support your partner during labor: being aware of her wishes, speaking for her if she is unable to,

and repeating what doctors have said if she didn't hear clearly; passing her a drink; rubbing her back; holding a warm cloth to her face; switching music on or off; being encouraging and reassuring her.

Going to prenatal classes can be useful (see p.331). You will learn more about labor and birth, and how to support your partner physically and emotionally.

# 49 days to go...

**YOUR BABY TODAY**

Soon your baby will be approaching a time when the lungs can fully support him after birth. At 33 weeks though, most babies would still need some help with breathing if born this early. Your baby will be regularly practicing these breathing movements inside.

Choosing who will be present at the birth with you is a big decision, so start thinking about it in good time.

**You can choose whoever** you like to be your birth partner, though the doctors and nurses might object if you have a team of people! If you do want more than one partner, get approval ahead of the birth and put this in your birth plan (see pp.181 and 303). You may want to ask your mom, sister, or close friend in addition to your partner. You might also find that your partner is unable to be there, for example if he is unavoidably going to be out of the country. If you're comfortable with it and feel that you will benefit from someone else being there, then ask away. You can put who you want to be

your birth partner or partners on your birth plan. Of course, if you're going to ask someone else other than, or in addition to, your partner to be present, discuss it with him first. He might not be so thrilled at the idea of your mom being present, but explain why you would like her there. Remember that this is a special occasion for him as well and he may have his own preferences for who is or is not present at the birth.

Now might also be a good time to discuss things like whether you want a video made of the birth, but you may prefer that your partner supports you, rather than handling the camera!

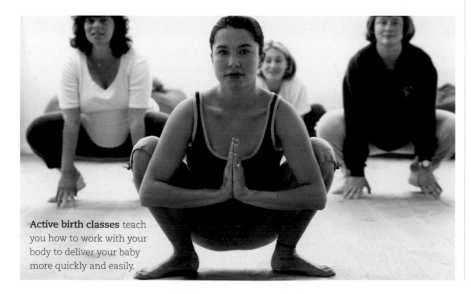

**Active birth classes** teach you how to work with your body to deliver your baby more quickly and easily.

TIME TO THINK ABOUT

## Active birth classes

The goal of active birth classes is **to make women feel good about their bodies and give them the confidence that they have the mental and physical reserves to have a successful birth experience.** Classes are generally appropriate regardless of fitness level, flexibility, and your stage of pregnancy.

■ **Active birth classes** promote the benefits of yoga and exercise as both physical and mental preparation for childbirth.
■ **Yoga strengthens the body,** improves posture and circulation, and teaches how to use relaxation and breathing techniques to relieve stress.
■ **Like prenatal classes,** active birth classes allow you to meet other parents-to-be and share their pregnancy experiences.
■ **The downside** is that these classes aren't widely available, so they get booked quickly and can be expensive. Ask your doctor about local classes. If you can't find a class in your area, read an active birth book or consider taking a prenatal yoga class.

# Your 34th week

**YOUR BABY IS ALMOST FULLY EQUIPPED FOR THE OUTSIDE WORLD**

If your baby was born this week, she'd still need some help with breathing and feeding. But it's reassuring to know that basically she's in pretty good shape for survival. However, you are unlikely to go into labor this early. Now is your chance to start practicing the relaxation and pain-relieving exercises that you've been learning at your prenatal classes. The more familiar you are with the techniques, the more they will help you during labor.

**The amount** of amniotic fluid surrounding the baby varies in individual pregnancies. At this stage, the fluid has reached its maximum level.

**The position of the baby** is unlikely to change between now and the birth if this is your first pregnancy.

**At 34 weeks** the average crown to heel length is 16.7 in (42.4 cm) and the average weight is 3.7 lb (1.7 kg).

**The fundus,** or top of the uterus, is high in your abdomen and the pressure under your ribs may make it impossible for you to enjoy a full meal without discomfort.

**Your baby's gut** would be able to process food if she were to be born this week. All the digestive enzymes are now active.

# 48 days to go...

## YOUR BABY TODAY

Your baby may well be head down by this stage. The head is the heaviest part and gravity plus the shape of your uterus favors a head-down position. Ask your doctor at the next visit if she can determine the position for you.

Premature labor is highly likely in a twin pregnancy, so your doctor will be on alert and monitoring you closely.

**There's still six weeks to go until the due date** for a single pregnancy, but if you're expecting twins they may arrive any time from now. Most singleton pregnancies are 38 to 42 weeks, but if you're carrying twins, 37 to 39 weeks is optimal. But more than half of twins are born before 37 weeks. Women expecting twins are at higher risk of high blood pressure, preeclampsia, placental insufficiency, gestational diabetes, and premature labor. That said, many women do go on to deliver twins naturally and many doctors will allow you to continue to 40 weeks, after which time an induction or cesarean might be suggested.

If the babies are in any position other than "head down," or the placenta is in an awkward position, such as near the neck of the uterus, a cesarean may be recommended. Some doctors prefer to deliver twins by cesarean because the second twin may run into difficulties during the delivery, particularly if she is not head down. Premature babies are more at risk of complications than those who go to full-term. A cesarean delivery ensures the babies are delivered quickly without having to go through hours of potentially stressful labor.

Sometimes, one twin is born vaginally and the other by cesarean. This often happens if the lower twin is in the "head down" position and the higher twin isn't.

### AS A MATTER OF FACT

**The average birth weight** of twins is 5 lb 5 oz (2.6 kg).

This is compared to 7 lb 8 oz (3.5 kg) for singleton babies. It's not unusual for there to be a difference in birth weight between the babies. In fact, one twin may weight 2 to 3 lb more than the other.

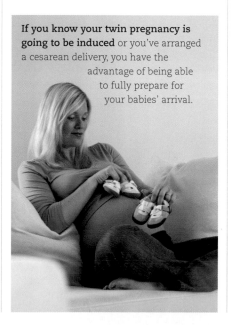

If you know your twin pregnancy is going to be induced or you've arranged a cesarean delivery, you have the advantage of being able to fully prepare for your babies' arrival.

### ASK A... DOCTOR

**I'm having my twins in a couple of weeks. Can they sleep in the same crib?** Having shared the same tight space in the uterus for many months, it seems natural to allow twin newborns to sleep together and, in fact, research indicates that it may have some benefits. Not only has it been found to be safe for twins of roughly the same size to sleep together until three months of age, but one study found that putting newborn twins in the same crib helped regulate their body temperature and their sleep cycles.

They can be placed side by side, or head to head. To be safe, don't overdress them or use blankets, bumpers, or pillows. Make sure the mattress is firm with a fitted sheet over it. Like singletons, twins should be put to sleep in the safe sleeping position, on their backs (see p.444).

A double crib, which will last until your twins are old enough to move to a bed, but many experts believe twins should be given their own sleeping space from three months, so they can be given individual attention and the opportunity to develop their own sleep patterns.

# 47 days to go...

## YOUR BABY TODAY

Shadows give the impression of hair on the eyebrows and eyelashes on this 3D image. Because this baby was lying head down, the view of the top part of the head is lost in the shadows caused by the mother's pelvis.

## With well-developed hearing, your baby may not be getting as much peace and quiet as she would like in the uterus.

**Although some quieter high-pitched sounds** don't penetrate the uterus, it is not quite as peaceful for your baby as you might think. There will be a constant background noise produced by your heart beating, your breathing, and your stomach rumbling. While the uterus and amniotic fluid will prevent many quieter sounds from reaching your baby, voices do penetrate quite easily. Your baby has already learned to adapt to repetitive sounds but is now acquiring a memory for familiar noises. The most familiar sound is, of course, your voice. Your baby will startle and turn toward loud or unfamiliar sounds and these will also cause her heart rate to increase.

---

**FOCUS ON... YOUR BABY**

## Lie and presentation

**Your baby's lie and presentation will be assessed by your doctor** at every prenatal appointment.

Your baby's "lie" means which way round she is lying, vertically or horizontally—a horizontal lie is known as transverse. The "presentation" refers to which part of the baby is closest to the pelvis, and would come out first.

The most common presentation is head down, bottom up, called the cephalic presentation. Breech presentation (see far right) is when the baby is bottom or feet down with the head upward. A footling breech means that the baby is head up, with one leg and foot extended downward while the other is tucked in.

In an anterior presentation (see below), your baby's head is down and faces your back. In a posterior presentation, your baby's head faces your belly, which can prolong labor and may increase the chances of an assisted delivery.

**Cephalic presentation**     **Breech presentation**

---

**ASK A... DOCTOR**

**What is perineal massage and how do I do it?** Spending just five minutes a day massaging your perineum (the area between the vagina and anus) with oil could reduce your risk of tearing or having an episiotomy (see p.427) during the birth. It also means you're less likely to experience pain in that sensitive spot after the birth—even after having an episiotomy.

**Here's how to do it:**

■ Wash your hands. Apply a mild lubricant, like K-Y jelly, to your thumbs, then slide them an inch inside the vagina. Gently stretch the vagina until you feel a slight stinging sensation.

■ When you feel that sensation, hold the pressure steady until you no longer feel the stinging. Then gently massage the lower half of the vagina with your thumbs. With your thumbs hooked in the vagina, pull forward to stretch the skin.

■ Not sure you're doing the first part properly? Insert your fingers into the corners of your mouth and pull your mouth open to the sides for a similar "burning" sensation.

# 46 days to go...

## YOUR BABY TODAY

At this stage it is simply no longer possible to see the whole baby on a scan. The ultrasound scan cannot not step far enough back to include the whole baby in a single view. Instead it is necessary to move the probe around, to examine one area at a time.

## Most women want to wait as long as possible to start maternity leave, but you must make the decision that is right for you.

**Your blood pressure will be monitored regularly** at this stage because a high reading can be a sign of preeclampsia.

### FOCUS ON... YOUR HEALTH

## Essential checks

**Some of the regular tests** you will have in the third trimester are designed to check for preeclampsia (see p.474). A combination of high (or rising) blood pressure and protein in your urine can be an indication of preeclampsia; another sign of this condition is extreme swelling, particularly of the face and/or ankles.

**There is generally no risk in working up to the final month** of your pregnancy. You may decide to work right up until you deliver, but by this week you are highly likely to find it increasingly tiring. If you are feeling exhausted and you think you might want to start your leave sooner, speak to your boss without delay. Hopefully, he or she will be understanding, but realize that if you start your maternity leave early, you may have to come back to work sooner (see pp.348–9). But if you are struggling to cope with the discomforts of late pregnancy, the decision to take sick leave during the last four weeks may be the right move for you. Talk to your doctor and your employer as soon as you make this decision.

Another desirable option is to work flex-time, so that you can travel to work at a less busy time and, if it's possible with your type of employment, work from home sometimes to cut out some of the commuting.

### ASK A... DOCTOR

**Will I have to give back my maternity pay if I decide not to return to work after the birth of my baby?** This is a little bit complicated, and it's a good idea to get some legal advice.

In a nutshell, if you do not want to return to work after your maternity leave, you must resign.

Bear in mind that every situation is different, and every company has a different set of rules and guidelines. You should let your company know of your decision as soon as possible. Make an appointment with your human resources representative to discuss your company's policies with you so you have plenty of time to think about your options. Also keep in mind that if your company let you take vacation or sick days that you haven't yet accrued as part of your leave, they may ask you to reimburse them for those days if you're not returning to work.

This happens quite often, and your boss may not be surprised to hear that you're not returning to work. And if you're not 100 percent certain about not returning to work, it may be a good idea to ask your employer about coming back to work on part-time basis or working from home one or two days a week, if that's feasible.

# 45 days to go...

### YOUR BABY TODAY

A foot is shown here with the toes spread out. Not all of the movements that you feel will be due to kicks, some movements will be shrugs or punches and some from the bottom or head as it touches the sides of the uterus.

## The size of your belly will increasingly be due to the baby alone as the amniotic fluid now reduces slightly each week.

**The amount of amniotic fluid** that surrounds and protects your baby is now at its maximum and the placenta has almost completed its growth.

Amniotic fluid is essential for your baby's lung development, gut maturation, protein requirements, and temperature control. Adequate fluid also allows your baby to move easily since she is in an almost weightless state. There is about 800 ml of amniotic fluid around your baby. The range, however, is quite wide and "normal" can be anywhere between 300 ml and 2 liters. Sometimes there is too little, a condition known as oligohydramnios

(see p.473), or too much fluid, a condition known as polyhydramnios (see p.473), surrounding the baby. In this situation you would be closely monitored and premature delivery may be necessary.

It's not surprising that the size of your uterus may not reflect the size of your baby since there can be so much variation in the quantity of fluid.

As the amount of amniotic fluid reduces in late pregnancy, your baby is not as well cushioned and her movements may become more obvious, although you should bear in mind that increasingly, as she grows, she has less space in which to move around.

### AS A MATTER OF FACT

**One of the most common concerns for women** in late pregnancy is that their water will break in public.

The reality is that the amniotic fluid is unlikely to gush out. It is much more likely to trickle out because in a head-down position, the baby will press down on the cervix and prevent the liquid from escaping. If it does happen in public, don't worry—you won't be short of people offering help.

---

### FOCUS ON... DADS

## What's in your hospital bag?

**Once your partner's labor begins,** your attention will need to be focused on helping her both practically and emotionally. So in addition to helping your partner prepare her maternity bag (see p.358) in advance, it's a good idea to prepare a bag of your own.

Understandably, dads are not always well supported in delivery units, and certainly don't get fed. You'll also find that you're at the hospital for several hours.

**Consider packing the following:**
- Snacks
- Drinks
- A pillow
- Something to read or play
- A reasonable amount of change to pay for parking and to buy snacks, juice, and soft drinks if they're in vending machines
- A list of phone numbers, or enter them into your cell phone now
- A camera.

**Text messaging is an effective way** to inform some family and friends about the birth. Make sure you've entered all the numbers into your phone before the big day.

YOU ARE 33 WEEKS AND 5 DAYS

# 44 days to go...

## YOUR BABY TODAY

At this stage your baby may lie transversely (see p.336) across your uterus as here, but such a position becomes increasingly less likely as the pregnancy advances. The more babies you have had the more likely it is that the shape of your uterus allows this lie.

You may be learning breathing and relaxation techniques at prenatal classes, but practice them at home, too.

**When you are tense and frightened,** pain can feel much worse, so teaching yourself to relax and stay calm can help. With around six weeks to go, you still have plenty of time to try out some of the breathing and relaxation techniques that will help you during labor. It's true that practice makes perfect and it can take some time to train your mind to relax at will, especially if you are in pain.

Spend a short period of time as often as you can, every day if possible, practicing your breathing—close your eyes and slow your breathing down, breathing in through your nose and out through your mouth. As you breathe in, imagine your breath entering your body and relaxing you and as you exhale you

breathe out any pain or tension. You might want to involve your partner by asking him to breathe with you or count your breathing, a slow count to three or five for every inhale and exhale.

Some women like to practice using the techniques while pinching their arm temporarily to simulate a contraction—although of course it won't mimic the pain exactly! Practicing these techniques in a calm, relaxed manner in late pregnancy will help you to use them effectively on the big day.

**A banana is a fabulous fruit** to eat before exercising because it gives you a slow and steady release of energy.

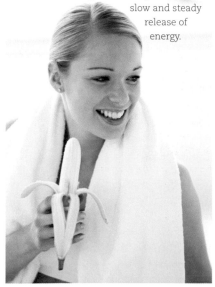

## FOCUS ON... NUTRITION

## Fuel for fitness

**Demand for nutrients is higher** when you're exercising and even higher when you're pregnant. This is not the time to reach for low-nutrient, high-calorie snacks; ensure you make careful choices when it comes to the nutrients you put into your body.

You should be eating a snack before you exercise, consisting of a complex carbohydrate and a protein. You should also eat frequent small meals and snacks if you are feeling hungry. It's fine to snack throughout the day.

Some healthy snack ideas are as follows:
- Half a bagel spread with two teaspoons of peanut butter
- An apple or banana and a handful of raw almonds
- A pear with two slices of Cheddar cheese
- Carrot, celery, and cucumber sticks and/or breadsticks dipped into two tablespoons of humus
- Cottage cheese or cream cheese spread on two large crackers or whole-wheat toast.

# 43 days to go...

**YOUR BABY TODAY**

Your baby is now capable of producing all of the enzymes that will process food within the digestive tract. If born early, your baby could now feed normally although some will still require help since they need to fine tune the coordination of their suckling reflexes.

## Your baby is naturally nourished inside the uterus and her own digestive tract is now functioning well.

**Eighty percent of your baby's energy needs** are met by carbohydrates, mainly in the form of glucose, and almost 20 percent from protein. Fat is not used as an energy source but it is used for growth. All mineral, vitamin, and calcium needs are met from your own reserves and your diet. Two possible exceptions are iron and folate, a water-soluble vitamin

that occurs naturally in foods; folic acid is the synthetic version. Folate does not easily cross the placenta to reach and nourish your baby. Your own iron reserves may already be low if you eat little or no red meat or if this pregnancy has followed on quickly from your last one. Your baby needs iron (and folate) to make red blood cells and because only a small percentage of iron in your diet

is absorbed, iron supplementation is often recommended at this stage.

While all of your baby's gut structures were present by 20 weeks, it is not until this stage that all the enzymes needed for digestion are activated and the absorptive surface of the gut is established to a degree that would enable your baby to feed if she were born now.

### GETTING UP FROM LYING DOWN

**After you've exercised on the floor, or have been resting in bed,** you may find it a struggle to get up from lying down. This simple maneuver can put a strain on your abdominal muscles, which are stretched, and it isn't helped by your altered center of gravity. The technique shown below was

originally devised by yoga teachers to help you get up safely from a lying down position.

As with any strenuous maneuvers at this stage of pregnancy, always take your time and remember to breathe slowly and deeply throughout.

**Step one:** With your knees bent, roll on to your right side bringing the knee beneath you up to waist level. Keep your right hand aligned with your bent knee.

Align arm with knee

Bring your knee to waist level

**Step two:** Shift your weight onto your left hand and knee. Position your right knee under your right hip and your right hand under your shoulder and come up slowly on all fours.

Raise your head slowly as you get up

Place the weight on your left-hand side

# 42 days to go...

**YOUR BABY TODAY**

A close-up of the baby's face clearly showing the lip shape and slightly separated eyelids. The slight shadowing seen to the left of the image is from the wall of the uterus, which at this stage of the pregnancy will always be very close to your baby.

If you've made the decision to have a home birth, you'll need to ensure you're fully prepared in good time.

ASK A... DOCTOR

**What additional things do I need to think about if I'm having a home birth?** Have all the items you need for labor and birth gathered in the place you intend to deliver, and organize your items separately from the baby's items.

As well as practical items, such as clothing, toiletries, and sanitary pads, you may also want to have on hand music, phone numbers, and a camera. It's a good idea to have a well-stocked fridge so make a list of nutritious foods to stock up on before your due date. This will help you during labor and in the first week of parenthood. Your baby will need diapers, cotton cloths, onesies, clothing, sheets, and blankets.

If you have other children, you may need to make arrangements for them to be taken care of.

Even though you're planning to have your baby at home, there are circumstances in which you may need to be transferred to a hospital. This can happen before, during, or after labor and so, even though you may not want to contemplate this outcome, have an emergency bag packed (see p.358) just in case.

**Women had their babies at home for generations;** it was only in the 20th century that women began to have hospital births. If you're considering a home birth, remember that the majority of pregnancies and deliveries are normal and do not need any medical intervention.

Be reassured that if you have decided to have a home birth and then change your mind, for example if you decide you want an epidural, or your midwife advises you that the baby needs help, you will be transferred to a hospital.

**Your relationship with your midwife** is even more important if you're giving birth at home as she will be your sole medical support.

**TIME TO THINK ABOUT**

## Group B strep test

Ten to 30 percent of pregnant women carry the strep B bacteria in the vagina or rectal area. Known as GBS (group B streptococcus), it is usually harmless in adults, but can cause a rare and serious infection in newborn babies if untreated.

■ **Many women are now routinely screened for GBS,** at 35–37 weeks of pregnancy. If the result is positive, antibiotic treatment can be given during labor that will reduce the risk of the baby becoming infected. Some hospitals don't screen but if the bacteria is detected in a urine test or a swab is taken for another reason and is positive, antibiotic treatment may given in labor.
■ **The test is very straightforward** and involves taking a swab of the area around your vagina and rectum with results usually within 24–48 hours.
■ **If GBS is detected,** and treatment given as soon as labor starts, there is little risk to the baby.
■ **It is possible to be infected with GBS** in a second pregnancy, even if you didn't have it first time around.

# Your 35th week

**TRY TO STAY ACTIVE, EVEN THOUGH YOU MAY BE WADDLING BY NOW**

Getting exercise is probably the last thing you want to do, but it's worth the effort. The more you move, the more energy you will gain. Gentle exercise will also help relieve some of the aches and twinges of late pregnancy. The baby's movements may change as he has less room to move around. Instead of kicks, he may be shuffling around. He's busy, though, practicing for the outside world, teaching himself to suckle and focus his vision.

**The baby has less room** to maneuver and will have periods when he is very quiet, but you will feel some movements every day, and he can still manage some strong kicks.

**The lungs** are filled with fluid which will disappear when the baby takes his first breath.

**The pupils** of the eyes now dilate in response to light filtering into the uterus.

**By practicing suckling** movements, the baby is teaching himself how to feed when he is born.

**At 35 weeks** the average crown to heel length is 17.2 in (43.7 cm) and the average weight is 4.2 lb (1.9 kg).

# 41 days to go...

**YOUR BABY TODAY**

This profile of the baby shows the tip of the nose touching the placenta. Your placenta will not be growing any more and now thins slightly. Within, the placenta continues to mature and it remains a highly efficient means of supplying your baby's energy needs.

## As your size begins to have an impact on your daily activities, you'll find that a few practical adjustments are necessary.

**Your posture will change** as your belly continues to grow. To compensate for the heavy weight you're carrying, you might find that you lean back slightly, especially when you're walking downhill. You might also waddle when you walk as you shift your weight from side to side. In a few weeks' time, when the baby begins to engage into the pelvis (see p.361), you may find that you waddle even more.

It's normal at this late stage of pregnancy to move more slowly than normal. You may find yourself struggling to get out of bed or out of a chair, and picking something up off the floor can be more difficult than usual. Tasks such as tying your shoelaces or painting your toenails can seem impossible. You can overcome tasks such as these; for example by putting your feet on a stool to tie your shoelaces so you don't have to bend down so far. If you need help, there's no shame in asking. It can be difficult to be reliant on others but remember it's only temporary.

### ASK A... DOCTOR

**Can I have a water birth in the hospital?** This depends on the maternity unit: some have birthing pools; others have facilities for you to rent a pool. More hospitals and birthing centers are offering this birthing option, so ask about renting a pool and bringing it in, but realize that just might not be an option. Some hospitals only allow you to labor in a pool, but not to deliver.

If your maternity unit does have a birthing pool, bear in mind that it may already be in use when you go into labor.

### FOCUS ON... YOUR HEALTH

## A diabetic pregnancy

**Whether you develop diabetes in pregnancy (known as gestational diabetes—see p.473),** or have preexisting diabetes, you'll require special care from your doctor. She will work out a plan for you, since diabetes poses risk in pregnancy.

In the mother, risks include high blood pressure, blood clots, preeclampsia (see p.474), diabetic kidney disease, and diabetic retinopathy, a condition that affects the retina in the eye. For the baby, there is an increased risk of congenital abnormalities and growth may be too fast or too slow.

The key to a healthy pregnancy and baby when you have diabetes is good blood-sugar control since your insulin requirements will change throughout pregnancy. Controlling blood-sugar levels reduces the risk of birth defects and stillbirth, or of you having a larger than expected baby, which can lead to problems during the birth.

If you have gestational diabetes, you will need to adapt your diet to include carbohydrates and fiber and reduce your intake of fats and sugar. You may also need insulin injections (see below) to help control your blood-sugar levels.

# 40 days to go...

**YOUR BABY TODAY**

At the back of your baby's eye, nerve cells that identify either black and white or color are maturing. The cells that respond to color signals are the last to develop but will eventually process more than half of the information that the eyes receive.

## Your baby is blinking and learning to focus, and his pupils will dilate in response to light filtering through the uterus.

**Your baby's eyes first began to develop** two weeks after conception and then all of the major eye structures are formed over the following four weeks. The eye, however, keeps growing during the pregnancy and the optic nerve continues to develop after birth.

The eyes have been opening since 26 weeks of pregnancy but, until now, eye movements have been poorly coordinated. Eye movements are first seen at 18 weeks but they are random and infrequent. Movements become more frequent from 26 weeks and now, in the final few weeks, movements settle into a cycle of rest alternating with rapid eye movements (REM).

Some light does get through into the uterus and your baby is now much more responsive to strong lights.

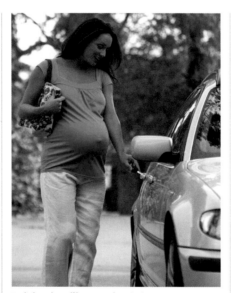

**Driving is still an option** in late pregnancy, but you may find it uncomfortable to be in the car for long periods.

ASK A... MOM

**I'm concerned my maternity leave substitute will do a better job than me. Are these fears normal?** Yes, completely normal. I remember being worried that the man filling in for me would outshine me. The amazing thing was that once my baby was born, anything work related was eclipsed by my new role. Far from losing skills, I think I became an efficient multitasker and when I returned to work, found the job easier than taking care of a baby.

Try not to worry. Not only do you have legal rights regarding the safety of your job (see pp.348–9), but you will have your chance to shine once again when your baby has settled into child care. In the meantime, enjoy your leave. It goes quickly, but also presents you with an opportunity to hone some important life skills.

**GETTING OUT AND ABOUT**

In most cases, it's perfectly safe to drive in the months leading up to the end of your pregnancy. However, if you feel that you're not able to concentrate at the wheel, or driving makes you uncomfortable, then give it a pass. When driving, it's very important that you position your lap belt directly under your belly (see p.253), to ensure that there is no danger to your baby if you are involved in an accident.

Traveling by public transportation is fine, too, but make sure you take full advantage of your condition to pointedly request a seat. Being jolted around on a train or bus is not ideal—not because it will damage your baby, but because your center of gravity has changed and you are more likely to fall or experience embarrassment and discomfort. Long periods of standing can also cause your ankles and feet to swell.

If you're feeling uncomfortable or dizzy, get off the train or bus and sit down in a cooler environment, preferably with your feet up, for about 20 minutes. Always carry water with you when you're out.

# 39 days to go...

**YOUR BABY TODAY**

Your baby will often stick his tongue out, as part of the development of the reflexes needed to feed. The rooting reflex enables your baby to find the nipple, then the strong suckling reflexes take over to coordinate breathing, feeding, and swallowing.

As maternity leave approaches, you might be looking for ways to save money, so here are ways to find baby clothes on a

**Dressing your newborn baby doesn't have to be expensive.** Don't be shy about asking friends and family members for hand-me-downs. Those who aren't planning any more children will probably be glad to get rid of them. Get together with your women in your prenatal class, and arrange a swap session—many moms may have older children of a different sex than the new baby, and have no need for pink T-shirts, or polo shirts! While the idea of your baby wearing "used" clothing may take some getting used to, rest assured that most babywear is hardly worn.

Look on the internet for end-of-season sales, and even on some of the auction sites, where you can often pick up designer goodies for a fraction of the original price. Visit your yard sales or garage sales. Shop around; you don't have to pay a lot for items such as sleep sacks and will find inexpensive prices in the supermarket. Make a purchase with your weekly grocery shopping and you won't notice the cost as much.

Remember, too, that you will probably receive numerous gifts of clothing when your baby is born. If you know exactly what you'd like, you may like to create a gift registry from a favorite store or ask people for gift certificates for that store. When looking for more expensive

**Knitting your own baby clothes** is a great way to save money, and it can be rewarding to see your newborn in your own creations.

items of clothing, head for the three- to six-month-old rack, so that your baby will get plenty of use out of them. It can be disappointing if your newborn only gets a couple of weeks' wear out of an outfit you like.

**FOCUS ON... DADS**

## A little squeamish?

**It's quite normal to feel concerned about getting through labor** on the day, and focusing on your partner and attending to her needs may help keep you distracted and reduce your anxiety. If possible, try to develop a good relationship in the coming weeks with your partner's caregivers. This way you'll feel more able to express any worries you're having, and hopefully get the reassurance and information you need.

If you find yourself feeling woozy on the day, try to leave the room since the nurses and doctor will be focused on caring for your partner. If you don't have time to leave the room to seek help when you feel faint, sit down immediately, with your head lower than your hips, or lie down with your feet raised. Try to stop yourself from panicking by taking slow, deep breaths. You'll find that the feeling passes quickly.

A good tip is to ensure that you are not too hot and to eat and drink regularly to prevent your feeling faint due to low blood sugar.

# 38 days to go...

### YOUR BABY TODAY

This 2D ultrasound has captured the moment that the baby is sucking his thumb. Your baby is gradually learning to coordinate this complex activity with breathing movements even though surrounded not by air but by the amniotic fluid.

Inside the uterus your baby is already practicing the suckling reflex, which will enable him to feed when he's born.

---

### ASK A... DOCTOR

**My mom has offered to stay with us after the birth. Is this a good idea?** Some couples prefer to get to know their baby on their own, taking the first few days to settle in and get used to the idea of being new parents. It's also good to try to do things your own way when it comes to caring for your newborn. Having said that, you'll find an extra pair of hands invaluable.

It really depends on your relationship with your mom: if it's good and you feel she'll be supportive, then it's more likely to help than hinder. However, gently establish some guidelines—namely that while you welcome her help, you'd like to do things your way and have space to bond with your baby. Encourage your mom toward helping around the house, rather than just with the baby, not least so that your partner doesn't feel excluded at this important time.

**By this stage of pregnancy** you may not feel up to spending hours shopping for equipment and clothes for the baby. You can save a lot of time by getting catalogues from the major stores and making some preliminary decisions from the comfort of your armchair.

**The suckling reflex is present earlier in pregnancy** but it is known from assessing premature babies that it's usually not until around this time that the baby is strong and coordinated enough to suckle with ease. Your baby regularly practices suckling and this, in combination with the rooting reflex, will enable your baby to feed.

After birth you will see the rooting reflex as your baby turns toward anything that strokes his cheek. The head will turn, and your baby will move his mouth in a series of gradually diminishing circles until the object is found. Once feeding is well established,

at about four months, the rooting reflex disappears. From this point on, your baby has much more control over the process, able to turn and directly latch on (see pp.448–9) to the nipple.

While in the uterus, there is no chance of your baby accidentally swallowing amniotic fluid into the lungs. The lungs are already filled with fluid and the high pressure of this, together with your baby's larynx, keeps out amniotic fluid. After birth, babies have a series of reflexes designed to keep breathing and drinking separate. To help with feeding, babies always breathe through their nose.

---

### ARE YOU READY FOR THE BABY?

**You may find that you soon become too tired to shop.** Try to buy items gradually, but there are certain things that it's worthwhile purchasing by around 37 weeks, just in case you go into labor. First, buy those small baby-care items you'll need right after the birth (see p.269) plus a car seat and a Moses basket or crib. You won't need a carriage immediately after the birth.

If going out shopping becomes difficult in late pregnancy, consider buying some items online.

# 37 days to go...

**YOUR BABY TODAY**

This is an MRI image showing a cross section of the entire pregnancy. The mother's spine is on the left of the image, and the baby is lying head down within the pelvis. An MRI is rarely needed during pregnancy, but if recommended, it is entirely safe.

You'll probably find yourself analyzing every ache and pain in these final weeks of your pregnancy.

**By this stage of pregnancy** every time you get a twinge you may worry that it's the onset of labor. This is a normal concern, but try to remember that, even though you're heavily pregnant, most aches and pains are still likely to be due to constipation, or stretching ligaments, rather than labor.

You may begin to have Braxton Hicks' contractions; these practice contractions occur as the uterus tightens as a warm up for labor. They also help direct more blood to the placenta in the final weeks of pregnancy. Some women are unaware of them, while for others they can be quite uncomfortable. Relaxing the uterine muscles by changing your position, walking around, or taking a warm bath can help.

If you're unsure whether the pains you're having are Braxton Hicks', always consult your doctor.

---

**ASK A... MOM**

**What will I need if I'm planning to breast-feed?** I found all the following items really useful when I was breast-feeding my baby:
- **Nursing bras** that can be unclipped at the front (see right) or have zip-open cups. Get properly fitted (bearing in mind that your breasts will be bigger once your milk comes in). You'll need at least two nursing bras and, thankfully, it's possible to get some attractive styles.
- **Nipple cream**: this is soothing if you have cracked nipples.
- **Breast pads** (disposable or washable). Slip them inside your bra to absorb any leaks between feedings. Alternatively, breast shells slot inside your bra to catch any excess milk.
- **Breast-feeding pillow:** a V-shaped pillow isn't essential, but it will help you and your baby to get comfortable.
- **Burp cloths** to catch dribbles.
- **Breast pump** and bottles or bags for storing expressed milk.

---

**TIME TO THINK ABOUT**

## Breast-feeding

If you've decided to breast-feed, it's the best choice for you and your baby (see pp.448–9). However, it doesn't always come naturally so make it easier by being prepared:

- **Read all about it.** If you're expecting some of the discomforts, they won't come as such a shock and you may be able to take measures to prevent them. It can help, for example, to know how to latch on your baby correctly (see p.448).
- **Address any concerns** before your baby is born: ask your doctor, or friends who've breast-fed.
- **See how it's done** by visiting a breast-feeding group (ask your doctor to recommend one). You may have been concerned about breast-feeding in public, so it can help to see how discreetly it can be done. You could also ask a friend to let you watch her position and breast-feed her baby.
- **Look for a lactation consultant**—available from your doctor, or maybe a friend can recommend one, or contact the La Leche League (see p.480) for a list of counselors.

# Your rights and benefits

Having a baby is a huge life change and many new parents find time and money are in short supply. Maternity and paternity leave and pay can help ease the transition, so it's worth finding out what you're entitled to.

**Finding out about your maternity benefits** can give you peace of mind that you will have some security during your maternity leave.

## MATERNITY LEAVE EXTRAS

### Paid leave: the facts

**Some states have passed laws that offer new parents paid maternity leave and, in many cases, paternity leave.** California was the first state to pass such legislation. Through its Paid Family Leave Program, employees who participate in the State Disability Insurance Program can receive up to six weeks of partial pay for time off within the first year of their baby's birth. Two other states, Washington and New Jersey, have passed similar legislation, and other states may follow suit. Find out about the laws in your state.

## Your rights

When you have a baby, you can take up to 12 weeks off work during a 12-month period and retain your right to return to the same, or an equivalent, position, including equivalent pay and benefits, if you are eligible to be covered by the Family and Medical Leave Act (FMLA). Employees eligible for FMLA have worked for their employers for at least 12 months, including at least 1,250 hours during the previous 12 months. Additionally, the employee must work within 75 miles of where 50 or more employees work. FMLA leave is guaranteed unpaid, but employers or employees can opt to use paid vacation or sick time, when this is allowed by an employer. Both men and women are eligible for FMLA leave, which applies to private employees, all state and local government employees, and some federal employees. Your employer is required to continue your health insurance coverage during your FMLA leave. If you've been paying a portion of your health insurance premiums, you'll have to continue doing so during your FMLA leave. If you don't want to take all 12 weeks of FMLA leave in a row, you may be able to break it down into shorter blocks of time, or even a shorter work week or work day. When possible, employees who are planning to use FMLA leave are required to tell their employers 30 days before the leave would begin. But if you have pregnancy complications that require you to stop working before the baby is born, the 12 weeks of FMLA leave would begin then.

## PAID LEAVE: THE FACTS

### Better breaks for parents abroad

**A recent report from researchers at Harvard University and McGill University** found the US lags behind most other countries when it comes to paid maternity and paternity leave. Out of 173 countries studied, 168 offered working women guaranteed paid maternity leave. The US was one of only five countries that did not, along with Lesotho, Liberia, Papua New Guinea, and Swaziland. Sixty-six countries offered men paid paternity leave; the US did not.

## Maternity pay

According to 2008 data from the US Department of Labor's Bureau of Labor Statistics, just 9 percent of all workers were eligible for paid family leave. According to the Institute for Women's Policy Research, which analyzed 2006 rankings for America's 100 most family-friendly employers, 93 percent of those best-ranked companies provide at least one week of paid maternity leave, but 52 percent of the companies pay for six weeks or less. Every company has its own policies for maternity leave. If an employer does provide compensation, the amount you'll receive may depend on what you earn and how long you've been working for the company. The best way to find out what you may be eligible for is to meet with a human resources representative or read the

If I have to take a pregnancy-related absence, will my employer hold my job for me or will I be left without my job when I'm ready to return to work?

According to the Pregnancy Discrimination Act, employers must hold open a job for a pregnancy-related absence for the same length of time that jobs are held open for employees on sick leave or on disability leave.

What happens to my eligibility for a bonus if I go on FMLA leave?

You'll still be eligible. The Family and Medical Leave Act requires an employee to be given her same, or an equivalent, position, and that would include eligibility for bonuses, including perfect attendance bonuses. If you don't miss days before or after your FMLA leave, you will still be eligible for that bonus.

I've just been offered my dream job, but I'm eight weeks' pregnant. Should I keep mum or should I say something to my new employer?

The Pregnancy Discrimination Act states that employers cannot refuse to hire a woman because of her pregnancy or a because of a pregnancy-related condition.

employee handbook. You may be allowed to use paid sick time, vacation days, or the company's short-term disability coverage, in addition to paid leave.

## Dads at home

Far fewer employers offer paid paternity leave to new dads than paid maternity leave to new moms. According to the Institute for Women's Policy Research, only 50 percent of 2006's 100 most family-friendly companies offered paid paternity leave. Of them 35 percent paid for one to two weeks leave, and no companies paid for more than six weeks of paternity leave. Dads who want to be home for a newborn's earliest days may be able to use paid vacation or sick leave, or they can take FMLA leave.

## Going back to work

Before returning to work, consider the following:
■ Will life as a working mom be easier if you switch to a flexible working arrangement, such as a job share or part-time work? Give your employer ample time to consider any request.

■ If you're breast-feeding, will your employer provide a private, clean, and safe room for you to express milk? If not, would it be possible for you to pump inside a bathroom stall?
■ You're entitled to time off (which may be unpaid) for family emergencies.
■ You may be eligible for working and child tax credits, which can help with child-care costs.

## Breast-feeding

Most states (47 of them) have laws that protect a mother's basic right to breast-feed her child. But women still experience negative reactions when they nurse in public. Nearly half of the states (21 of them) have laws that protect women's rights related to lactation and employment. Being able to pump at work prolongs the amount of time that you can breast-feed your baby, so these protections are important to breast-feeding moms. According to La Leche league, during an 8-hour workday, many moms find time to pump three times a day: during morning, lunch, and afternoon breaks. Since time is a premium at work, many moms get by by double-pumping with

electric pumps, which should supply enough milk for the following day. La Leche League recommends that working moms should breast-feed their babies when they are at home mornings, evenings, and weekends.

## Child care

If you will be returning to work, you will likely need child care for your baby. It is wise to look into your child care options while you are still pregnant, because it may take time to make a decision and some programs may have long waiting lists. Contact a local child-care resource and referral center for recommendations.

Some employers offer flexible spending accounts to employees that reduce salary by a set amount to pay for tax-preferred expenditures like day care. You won't pay taxes on the set-aside funds. Check with your human resources department to see if a flexble spending account is available to you.

# Baby and child benefits

**Your baby will need health insurance coverage just like you do.** When your baby is born, you'll need to add him to your health insurance plan so he can get the coverage he will need. Most health insurance companies make the process easy. Typically you'll just need to call your health plan and tell them your baby's name and the date of your baby's birth, and your baby be automatically added to your plan. For most insurance plans, you will have 30 days to give notice of the birth. From then on, your baby will be covered for doctor appointments in the same way that you are.

# 36 days to go...

**YOUR BABY TODAY**

The placenta, shown in red above the baby's green profile, is now receiving half a liter of blood each minute from your circulation. In order to accommodate this increase your blood volume expanded dramatically in the first few months of the pregnancy.

It's never too late to improve your fitness and whatever you do now will stand you in good stead for labor.

### ASK A... DOCTOR

**Why are some babies born prematurely?** There are certain factors that may increase a woman's likelihood of having a premature baby. These include a previous obstetric history of prematurity of either themselves or a mother or sister; illness during pregnancy; the state of a woman's health prior to pregnancy; having a multiple pregnancy; fetal problems, such as reduced growth, which may be due to lifestyle factors such as smoking, and other fetal disorders.

**You might be in the final few weeks** but you still need to stay active. Exercising regularly and consistently will enable you to reap the rewards of your efforts: increased fitness, higher self esteem, and much more energy.

Find activities that you enjoy: swimming and walking are often favored by pregnant women in this late stage. As well as helping improve fitness, both of these activities will help you relax and unwind.

It is difficult to put an exact figure on how long you should be exercising for, but bear in mind that this will be determined by how hard you exercise—the two are linked. Consider the difference between a sprint and a marathon—each will have their own energy needs, one is short and has a very intense need for energy, while the other needs slow and sustained energy.

Always listen to your body and stop if you're in danger of overexerting yourself. It's important to eat plenty if you're exercising: choose snacks that will fuel your body (see p.339), especially given that the third trimester is the most demanding in terms of your baby's nutritional needs.

### KANGAROO CARE

**If your premature baby goes into a Neonatal Intensive Care Unit (NICU)** (see pp.452–3) you may be able to take care of him using a method called kangaroo care. You will be asked to hold your baby on your chest between your breasts with his head turned so that his ear is next to your heart.

Developed in Bogota, Columbia, in response to a lack of incubators, kangaroo care is shown to have many benefits for NICU babies—mainly that their heart and breathing rates regularize quite quickly, allowing them to sleep for much longer periods. The baby's temperature is regulated by the temperature fluctuations in your breasts, meaning he doesn't have to expend energy keeping himself warm.

This, in addition to the extra sleep, preserves his energy for other vital functions, such as brain development and weight gain. Breast-feeding is also more sucessful and some kangarooed babies lose none of their birth weight.

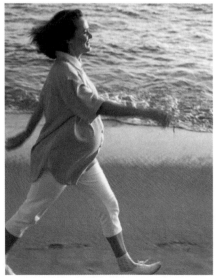

**If you go for a daily walk** you will feel energized and it will be good preparation for all those strolls you'll be doing with your baby.

# 35 days to go...

## YOUR BABY TODAY

Your baby's brain continues to mature. This ultrasound image shows that the folding pattern overlying the cerebral hemispheres has now developed giving rise to the familiar folds and grooves on the brain's surface. The bright reflections are from the bony skull.

**The reality of being a mother will begin to hit you in these final weeks, and you have everything to look forward to.**

**Before the birth,** it can be difficult to imagine having a relationship with your baby, even though you may feel a close bond during pregnancy.

Fortunately, bonding is a chemical process in your brain when you give birth. Other people's babies may leave you feeling cold, but it's highly likely that your own baby will spark all kinds of feelings that you never even knew you could experience. It's normal to worry about being a mother—coping with the responsibility, taking care of a helpless baby, being "good enough," and making lifestyle changes. However, when your baby is born, your priorities will become abundantly clear, as will your affections—although bonding may not always be instant.

In some cases, postpartum depression (see p.475), or even the short-term baby blues (see p.450), can interrupt the natural progression of feelings a mother has for her newborn baby.

### ASK A... DOCTOR

**Will I be able to breast-feed my twins?** Yes, but if possible, arrange for a lactation consultant with experience in feeding twins to be available after birth. If you get the positions correct and know how to latch on your babies (see p.448) at the outset, you'll feel much more confident continuing on your own.

Many moms of twins find that feeding them simultaneously, using a specially designed breast-feeding pillow, is the easiest way to manage. This is something you may want to buy now. There is a variety of effective breast-feeding positions for twins that the consultant or a midwife can show you.

### FOCUS ON... YOUR BODY

## Pamper yourself

**You may not feel particularly lovely,** but that's all the more reason to pamper yourself. There's unlikely to be time for beauty rituals once the baby is born.

■ **Treat yourself to a manicure,** but don't have nail extensions for when your baby is born—sharp implements and babies don't mix.

■ **Indulge in a facial:** it will make you feel good and help you relax.

■ **Have your hair cut** since it may be some time before you get to the hairdresser again. It's a good idea to opt for a style that will be easy to manage once your baby arrives.

■ **If you have aches and pains,** book a massage with someone who specializes in pregnancy.

■ **Have a pedicure** a week or two before the birth. You'll be thrilled once your belly has gone and you're able to see your feet again.

**If you're keeping a photographic record of your belly,** you'll want it to look as good as possible. Gently exfoliating and moisturizing will ensure the skin is as smooth as possible. It won't, unfortunately, prevent stretch marks but it will improve the appearance of the skin.

# Your 36th week

**GET TOGETHER WITH YOUR PARTNER AND TALK THROUGH YOUR BIRTH PLANS**

Don't leave crucial arrangements until the last minute. Have an action plan ready for when you go into labor—it might be sooner than you think. Babies can arrive ahead of schedule, so make sure you and your partner feel confident about managing. Figure out practicalities, such as arranging care for other children, or even the cat. Rope in your parents or friends to help if need be, pack your hospital bag, and relax.

**The uterus** has very little remaining space, so most babies lie curled up, with their limbs folded closely against their bodies.

**The lungs** are structurally complete and the air sacs, or alveoli, are producing a lubricant called surfactant, which will help keep the sacs open when the baby takes her first lungful of air.

**The head** may be starting to engage, dropping down lower in the pelvis toward the birth canal in readiness for the start of labor. Your doctor will be keeping a close check on the baby's position.

**At 36 weeks** the average crown to heel length is 17.7 in (45 cm) and the average weight is 4.7 lb (2.1 kg).

# 34 days to go...

### YOUR BABY TODAY

Your baby's hair and eye color are all determined genetically and set before birth. Unfortunately, however detailed an ultrasound image is, it can only show the shape of structures and will never be able to show true color information.

## You may be surprised to find that your social life is already changing, and the baby hasn't even arrived yet!

**If you've become a homebody recently,** be reassured it's quite normal. Wanting to stay at home is common in the final stages of pregnancy. You may be reluctant to plan social engagements for the next few weeks, just in case. For example, you don't want to spend money on a theater ticket that might not get used. Do, however, pencil in dates with friends because they will understand if you cancel last minute. You'll also find that once you're on leave, you're glad to get out of the house in the evenings.

Take the opportunity to go out with your partner in these last few weeks since dinner dates may not be on the agenda once the baby arrives.

---

### ASK A... DOCTOR

**My feet are swollen and tight; can I do anything about it?** Swollen feet and ankles, known as edema, is due to excessive fluid seeping into the tissues because of the increased volume of blood (see pp.466–7). By late pregnancy, as blood volume continues to rise, this is a common problem. The swelling is usually worse later in the day and when the weather is warmer.

There are steps you can to take to help reduce the swelling, such as elevating your legs when sitting, rotating your feet, and lying on the floor with your feet up the wall. Wearing support hose (see p.225) also improves circulation. Make sure you drink plenty, particularly water, since this improves the kidney function and reduces water retention. Don't take diuretics—studies have found that these can adversely affect an unborn baby.

---

### FOCUS ON... YOUR BODY

## A soothing swim

**Although you may feel too big to be exercising,** swimming is a great activity for late pregnancy. The water supports the weight of your belly, so you may feel much lighter than you do normally. Try to do some gentle swimming as well as just relaxing in the water. Also consider going to prenatal water aerobics classes, which have exercises tailored for pregnant women.

**When the weather is hot,** relaxing in a swimming pool can be the best place to be. Use a float to support yourself and enjoy the wonderful feeling of weightlessness.

# 33 days to go...

**YOUR BABY TODAY**

This MRI scan shows detail of the baby's brain. MRI is particularly good at showing structures within the central nervous system. Taking and interpreting these images remains difficult and time consuming, however, so they are not part of routine testing.

Although the color is developing in your baby's eyes, the final color will not be known for some time.

**What color will your baby's eyes be?** The iris controls the amount of light that enters the eye and gives the eyes their color. Eye color is determined by the amount of melanin within the iris; this is the substance in the skin that gives different skin tones.

It certainly doesn't follow that your baby will have an identical eye color to that of you or your partner. Most fair-skinned babies will be born with only a small amount of melanin in the eye and the iris will appear gray or blue. If dark-skinned then there is a great deal of melanin and the color is usually dark gray or brown. The color continues to change after birth as melanin is produced in response to light. Your baby will be a year old before the final color of her eyes is fully developed.

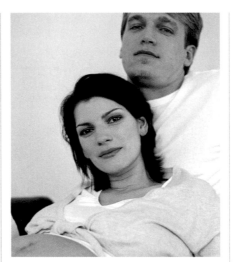

**You may have started to wonder** whether your baby will have the same eye color as you or your partner. Her eye color may resemble either of yours, or it may be different than both of you.

**PRACTICING VISUALIZATION**

**Visualization is an effective and positive way** to help prepare for labor. Try practicing it in these final weeks, beginning with a basic relaxation exercise. So start at the top of your head and gently flex and relax every muscle down to your toes, concentrating on each muscle, and your breathing, as you do so. Now imagine the birth, with every step given a positive connotation. For example, your baby is floating in water, and is gently rocked as the contractions begin; the tightening you feel is the strong walls of your uterus, guiding your baby into the world; the contractions are waves on which you and your baby are riding, as your baby is washed out—you are both swimming together with the tide.

**FOCUS ON... YOUR BODY**

## Cesarean birth

**If you know you're going to have your baby by cesarean,** it's good to being aware of what to expect following the birth. Although you should remain mobile after cesarean surgery, it's also important to get plenty of rest. Keep in mind that a cesarean section is major surgery so you will need to avoid lifting and carrying heavy loads for the first few weeks. Since this may be difficult if you have other small children or you are at home alone, you should try to recruit as much help as possible after the surgery. You should avoid doing any shopping since this usually involves carrying heavy bags. Order online if you can.

The advice is not to drive for six weeks. If you feel up to it before this time, check with your doctor that it is okay and make sure you're comfortable wearing a seatbelt and doing maneuvers, including emergency stops.

It is generally thought to take up to six weeks to fully recover from a cesarean delivery.

# 32 days to go...

**YOUR BABY TODAY**

In this week, the lungs become almost fully functional and able to support the baby if delivered early. This baby at this time is still considered preterm and it is not until 37 weeks that the baby's maturity is such that full term is reached.

Don't forget this is a life-changing time for your partner, too, so find positive ways to involve him in the time preceding the birth.

**There is, understandably, a lot of focus on women** in the lead-up to childbirth, but it's important not to neglect the dads-to-be. Your partner may be getting anxious about the birth itself, fearing that he might not manage well with being in the delivery room or just concerned about how it will affect him to see you in pain. Some men feel guilty that they cannot take their share of the pain and help more during labor.

Aside from thinking about the birth, your partner may be anxious about the fact he'll be responsible for a newborn baby in just a few weeks!

Talk to your partner if he appears anxious and involve him as much as possible—from helping you cope with pregnancy discomforts to preparing for the birth. If you've written a birth plan (see pp.181 and 303), go back over it now and discuss what might happen and how your partner could help on the day.

You could practice positions and breathing techniques for labor so that he feels more confident about helping you manage. If possible, he could go to your final prenatal appointments with you, where he can discuss any concerns he has with the doctor.

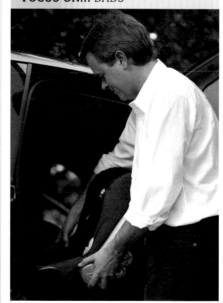

FOCUS ON... DADS

## Getting ready

**Have you done all your dad-to-be jobs?** These include:

■ **Buy a car seat** and make sure you know how to install it safely in the car. You can't leave the hospital with your newborn without one.

■ **Assemble the crib** if you're going to use one in the early weeks.

■ **Ensure there is storage space** for the baby's clothes, bedding, diapers, and other bits and pieces.

**ASK A... DOCTOR**

**I'm having my twins next week, but will I be able to love them both equally?** Although this can be a concern, it is more likely to be the case that rather than favor one child over the other, a parent gives more love and attention to the baby who needs it most at that time.

It is also possible that the strain of having two babies in the house may increase the likelihood of delayed bonding, although this can also happen if the birth has been traumatic; if the mother or indeed the father is exhausted; or if one baby has taken time to establish feeding, or is more fractious than the other. This does not mean that bonding will not take place over time.

In every family, there are bound to be ebbs and flows of love between parents and children. When a parent has two children born at different times, that parent may love one child differently than the other, but this does not mean that the love a parent has for one child is to the detriment of the other. If once your babies are born you still have concerns, speak to your doctor.

# 31 days to go...

## YOUR BABY TODAY

Your baby's heart will beat quite fast, at between 110 and 160 beats every minute. Even after birth, your baby's heart will continue to beat at this speed. It will be several years before the heart rate is 70 or so beats per minute, the same as an adult.

## The lungs don't become fully functional until these final weeks, but important development is taking place now.

**If you imagine the lung as a tree,** then the windpipe or "trachea" is the trunk of the tree. This then forms several branches or "bronchi," which divide several times, like twigs, to then produce the most delicate structures: the alveoli or leaves of the tree. It is within the alveoli that gas exchange will take place.

The alveoli began to develop at 24 weeks but they continue to increase in number throughout the pregnancy. The alveoli contain surfactant-producing cells to keep them open and these now become fully functional.

### PRESCRIBED BEDREST

**Toward the end of pregnancy,** there are some circumstances when you may need to be admitted into the hospital for bedrest.

- **If you have contractions,** but your water hasn't broken.
- **If you develop preeclampsia** (see p.474). Measures will be taken to reduce your blood pressure.
- **If you have placental abruption,** where the placenta separates from the uterus (see p.473).

**You may be closely monitored in hospital** toward the end of your pregnancy if there is any concern about your health or that of your baby. A fetal monitoring machine will be used to check your baby's heartbeat.

### FOCUS ON... YOUR BODY

## Getting strong

**Maintaining muscular strength,** stretching, and doing gentle exercise right up until you give birth will help your posture—minimizing backaches, reducing stress on your skeleton, and making you feel more energized and relaxed.

As long as you feel good and adhere to the guidelines set out on page 18, you can continue with your activities.

Most importantly, at this time you should use common sense and listen to your body. If you're in pain, feel fatigued, or have dizzy spells, see your doctor immediately and stop exercising. You'll be feeling tired carrying around all that extra weight so adjust your activities accordingly. This could mean that you lower the intensity of your exercise and exercise for a shorter time, but if you feel good don't stop exercising entirely.

Look at the routines on pages 90 and 250, but don't do any exercises at this stage that require you to lie on your back.

YOU ARE 35 WEEKS AND 5 DAYS

# 30 days to go...

## YOUR BABY TODAY

Many babies will still have a good volume of amniotic fluid around them, but shadows from the placenta or side of the uterus, coupled with the curled up fetal position, will make imaging the baby harder and harder.

It's a good idea to make practical arrangements now for what might happen if you go into labor.

**With only around four weeks to go,** now is the time to make sure you have all your partner's contact details and know exactly how to get hold of him in case you go into labor when he's at work. He might want to be extra careful to ensure he has his cell phone switched on and at hand in these final few weeks, and that he's not traveling too far away.

If you have other children or other dependants (pets, for example, a dog) then you should arrange what will happen to them when you go into the hospital. You may want to explain to any older children what is going to happen so that they are prepared for when they go to stay with Grandma, or whoever will be taking care of them.

If you're having a cesarean, you might also want your older children taken care of once you're home from hospital.

Reassure your children that you will be coming back and that you're not sick, but that you have to go to the hospital when the baby comes. Depending on the age of your children, you could go with them to buy a present for the baby or you could give them a special job such as opening all the new gifts. Presents from the newborn to her elder siblings is also a good gesture.

**In the lead-up to the birth, ensure your toddler spends time** with any family members who will be taking care of him while you're in the hospital. This will help him manage without you without getting upset.

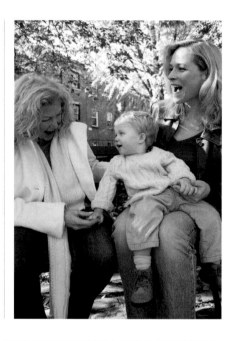

## AS A MATTER OF FACT

**In one study of women** who anticipated that they would not need pain relief, 52 percent actually used it.

According to recent research from NICE (National Institute for Clinical Excellence), women underestimate how much giving birth will hurt, and don't find out enough about the pain-relief options available (see pp.402–7).

## ASK A... DOCTOR

**My baby was premature and is in the neonatal intensive care unit. I'm trying to express milk—am I helping?** Yes, very much so. Breast milk helps ensure that the mother's natural immunity is passed on to her baby via her milk. Since premature babies are more prone to infection, expressing your breast milk is a great way to help your baby while she is in the NICU. Breast milk is much easier for a baby to digest: this is important for premature babies since their digestive tract may be less developed than a full-term baby's.

This is also a great way for you to bond and develop a relationship with your baby. It's likely to be a time of considerable stress for you and you may feel helpless, so knowing that you're doing such a great thing to help your baby will help enormously.

# 29 days to go...

**YOUR BABY TODAY**

Most babies will now be positioned longitudinally (lying straight up and down, with their head well in the pelvis). Even now, when space is limited in these final weeks, there is still time for the position to change to head down if your baby is bottom first (breech).

Complex developments are taking place in your baby's lungs that will enable her to breathe unaided once she is born.

**The blood flow to your baby's lungs** mirrors the development of the airways. Blood leaves the right side of the heart through a one-way valve into the main pulmonary vein. This then divides to give a pulmonary branch to each lung, and also a duct that allows blood to bypass the lungs and travel to the body directly. This will close soon after birth as the lungs expand and their resistance to blood flow falls.

Because your baby doesn't use his lungs for gas exchange in the uterus, the blood supply to them is quite small—only 10 percent of the post-birth supply. At this stage of pregnancy, the lungs' blood supply has completed its development, branching into finer and finer vessels as they come to lie closer to the alveoli.

When your baby is born, her chest is compressed in the birth canal and this helps to push the fluid out of the lungs in preparation for that incredible first breath. If your baby is born by cesarean, she will need first to bring the fluid up by herself. This is not a problem but for this reason the first breaths of a baby born by cesarean can be full of mucus.

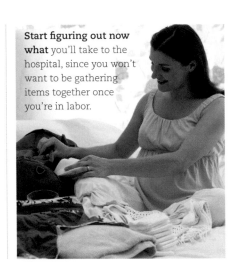

**Start figuring out now what** you'll take to the hospital, since you won't want to be gathering items together once you're in labor.

---

**ITEMS FOR YOUR HOSPITAL BAG**

**Make sure you have all the items you need for your hospital bag.** Remember to include items for yourself as well as the baby and, if you know you're having a cesarean, pack enough items for a few days.

**For yourself:**
- Pajamas
- Underwear
- Nursing bras
- Slippers
- Dressing gown
- Hairbrush
- Toothbrush
- Toiletries

- Maternity sanitary pads
- Breast pads and nipple cream
- Comfortable loungewear in case you stay in and want to get dressed.

**For your baby:**
- Undershirts
- Footed onesies
- blanket
- Diapers
- Diaper bags
- Cotton pads
- Diaper cream, such as Desitin
- Baby wipes if you intend to use them
- Hat and cardigan for going home—you can also use the cardigan if your baby

needs layers to keep warm while she's in the hospital.

**Other useful items:**
- Camera—still camera and/or video camera
- Music for the delivery room
- Books and magazines
- Massage oil
- TENS machine (see p.399)
- Washcloths.

Your partner should also get a bag ready for himself (see p.338) and ensure the car seat is installed. Pack snacks and drinks closer to the time, but think about what you might need.

# 28 days to go...

## YOUR BABY TODAY

You may notice a change in the character of your baby's movements, reflecting the reduced amount of amniotic fluid and, consequently, space to move around in. Each movement is more likely to be felt, however, as he touches the side of your uterus.

All pregnant women need support in the final weeks, but if you're single this can be even more important.

### THE LOWDOWN

## Baby showers

Throwing a baby shower to celebrate the imminent arrival is a great opportunity to get together with the girls. Arrange it yourself, or ask your best friend to do the honors. Note to best friend: surprise parties are great, but consider whether the mom-to-be will want to be the center of attention.

Think about:

■ **A pampering theme:** the guests could give each other manicures and pedicures, or you could even hire a beautician for the afternoon.

■ **Chipping in together to buy the mom-to-be something useful,** such as a car seat, or indulgent, such as a relaxing day out at a spa.

■ **Games you could play,** such as inviting guests to guess the baby's sex, weight, and date she'll be born.

■ **Refreshments:** Champagne, non-alcoholic drinks, nibbles, and a "birth" day cake.

**Whether you're single by choice,** or have unexpectedly found yourself in this position, you may be experiencing mixed feelings about the weeks to come. There is no doubt that going solo involves extra responsibilities and worries, but with a little help from your close friends and family, you can make these final few weeks of your pregnancy positive.

If you're concerned about going into labor alone, line up a close friend or family member who is on call at all times. He or she might want to get permission from their place of work to take leave to be with you should you go into labor. Keep yourself busy before your baby arrives, planning plenty of activities during your maternity leave.

Don't be afraid to ask people for help with shopping for last-minute baby buys or getting your home ready for your new arrival. Most people will be delighted with the honor of being asked to keep you company, and helping you get things ready.

Most importantly, take care of yourself: get organized by preparing meals you can freeze so you have plenty of healthy food in store for the weeks after the birth.

**At your baby shower** you'll probably receive lots of gifts. It's common for there to be presents for both mom and the newborn.

# Your 37th week

**YOUR BELLY MAY LOOK AS THOUGH IT'S STARTED TO SLIDE DOWNHILL**

You're now about as big as you're going to get. Soon—maybe this week—the baby will drop down lower into your pelvis, ready for birth. Your belly may shift downward, too, giving you a different shape. This doesn't necessarily mean that labor is imminent, so don't worry about the baby "falling out." You're likely to still have some time to enjoy maternity leave and get organized.

**Some of the pressure** under your rib cage may be easing off as the baby continues to descend into the pelvis.

**Short, very fine hairs,** called vellus hairs, are growing in place of lanugo hair on most parts of the baby's body.

**Your baby turns** toward a familiar sound and practices looking for its source: your voice is the most familiar sound to him.

**The baby is still gaining weight** as more fat covers his limbs and abdomen. As a newborn, he will look much the same as he does now.

**At 37 weeks** the average crown to heel length is 18.2 in (46.2 cm) and the average weight is 5.2 lb (2.4 kg).

# 27 days to go...

## YOUR BABY TODAY

When scanned, this baby was lying with his back to his mother's. This "back to back" position is common at this stage but becomes less so as the pregnancy continues. Your doctor will be able to feel for the position of your baby's back from this point on.

You're in the home stretch now, and may start maternity leave soon. This can be a relief, but also a time of mixed emotions.

**Going on maternity leave is a significant pregnancy milestone.** As you leave your working role, the reality of beginning your role as a mother may hit you—but you hopefully have a few more weeks to get used to the idea!

It can be a welcome respite to take it easy and not have to rush around in the mornings, and you'll feel less tired by not having to travel to work. Although you need to take it easy, it's a good idea to plan some outings, since not having a routine can take some getting used to.

Although it's good to stay in touch with colleagues, try not to fall into the trap of logging on to work emails or staying up-to-date with what's happening at work. You might be worrying about losing some of your identity while you're on maternity leave; this is a common feeling but you'll find that before you know it your leave is over and you're settled back into work again.

Try to enjoy this lead-up to the birth and make the most of the time (see p.366) to get organized and prepare for your new arrival.

### ASK A... DOCTOR

**Will I feel different when my baby drops?** You will feel lighter, in that your breathing will be easier, with more room for your lungs to expand. Your abdomen may seem smaller, with your belly shifting down and forward, as your baby's head enters the birth canal. With pressure on your bladder, you may need to urinate more. You may also experience some pelvic pain.

### WHEN YOUR BABY DROPS

**Engagement is when your baby's head starts to move down into the pelvic brim** in preparation for birth, and this can occur any time in these final few weeks of pregnancy, until the start of your labor. In the last weeks of pregnancy, your doctor will check to see if the head has started to engage, or drop, sometimes called "lightening."

Your doctor will do an examination to check to see where the baby's head is. This is called the station, and it's measured from -5 (the baby's head is floating above the pelvis) to +5, the head is at the opening of the vagina. This last stage is called crowning.

When your baby drops, you may find it easier to breathe, since your lungs will have more room to expand, or the need to urinate more because of more pressure on your bladder.

Your belly is high and facing forward

Mostly above the pubic bone, a -5 station

**Not engaged:** The baby's head has started to move into the pelvis, but more than three- or four-fifths can be felt above the pubic bone.

Your belly is lower, relieving pressure on your ribs

Once halfway through the pelvis, he's at 0 station

**Engaged:** The baby has dropped into the pelvis in preparation for birth. This causes your belly to change position and shape.

# 26 days to go...

### YOUR BABY TODAY

Although almost invisible in the image, a very thin layer of vernix covers your baby. At first this helped to reduce the amount of water leaving your baby's skin, but now it helps to prevent direct contact with the skin and amniotic fluid.

## Have you started nesting? The need to provide a safe, comfortable space for your new baby is a primitive desire.

### THE LOWDOWN

## Plaster casts!

Preserve your belly for posterity by making a plaster belly cast. You can either buy a kit or (far cheaper) purchase the plaster separately; it's all available online.

You will need:
- Plaster of Paris bandages, cut into several strips
- Large tub of petroleum jelly
- Bucket of warm water
- An assistant or two (not essential, but can be useful for speeding up the process and bringing refreshments).

Here's how to do it:
1. Strip down except for some old underwear (the smaller, the better)
2. Apply petroleum jelly liberally to your belly and breasts
3. Assume a comfortable pose
4. One by one, dip the plaster of Paris strips into the water, then apply, overlapping the layers until you have a thick coating
5. Sit and wait for it to dry—it's a good excuse to take a rest
6. Slip it off, when it's rock hard and paint it if you'd like.

**The nesting instinct usually begins** in the final weeks of pregnancy, accompanied by a surge of energy and an uncontrollable urge to get your home in ship shape.

Give in to your inner domestic goddess: cook, clean, organize, and de-clutter, but take it easy. If you spend hours on your hands and knees scrubbing, you may find yourself in labor sooner than you'd expected.

Some men develop a nesting instinct, but unfortunately this tends to be associated with cars and garden sheds. If this happens to your partner, at least you can look forward to a sparkling-clean car, spruced-up patio, and manicured lawn.

Nesting not happening for you? Pay the professionals to do a spring cleaning. Or forget it: your baby won't care whether the cupboards are clean.

**Every nook and cranny of your home** will get your attention once the cleaning bug hits you!

# 25 days to go...

**YOUR BABY TODAY**

A short portion of the umbilical cord is lying close to the mouth, which makes this baby appear to have a rather grumpy looking expression. The placenta is seen to the right of the image partially obscuring the view of the face.

You'll find that your beautiful belly is intruding on your life more and more, affecting your movements and eating patterns.

**You might be getting a little frustrated** by your size around now, which can make everyday activities more difficult. Simple maneuvers, such as fitting through doors or getting off the sofa, can be more difficult and you may find that everything takes a bit longer to achieve. All you can do is be patient and focus on getting through the next few weeks. You'll soon have your body back to normal.

## THE LOWDOWN

### VBAC

**Doctors used to think that if you had one baby by cesarean,** all future babies must also be born that way. But doctors now know that 90 percent of women who delivered by cesarean are candidates for VBAC, or vaginal birth after caesarean. Depending on the reason for your prior cesarean, you may be able to deliver vaginally, especially if you have no major medical problems, the baby is healthy and in head-down position, of normal size, and any condition that necessitated your last cesarean isn't present. If you have diabetes, high blood pressure, or are pregnant with multiples, you are not a candidate for VBAC.

During pregnancy, it's common to eat more often than previously but to eat less at each meal. This is because your uterus has grown so much that all your other organs have moved around and are squashed into much less space. Your stomach simply has less room in it to fit the food so you can't eat as much before feeling full. When your stomach empties you may find yourself hungry again. It's fine to snack, but make sure you're reaching for healthy foods and not the cookie jar!

**Getting comfortable behind the steering wheel** will become increasingly challenging in the late stages of pregnancy. Keep trips as short as possible or take regular breaks if you need to travel for any length of time. Always wear your seat belt (see p.252).

## FOCUS ON... YOUR BABY

### Working out with Mom

**Your baby will usually move several times in the 20 to 30 minutes** after you exercise. By keeping the intensity of your exercise at a moderate level you will not compromise the oxygen supply to your baby. When you exercise too hard and for too long, you may compromise this exchange and the result is the baby's movements will fall below their usual levels.

If you're concerned and unsure, keep a log of how much your baby is moving and compare this to the activity levels after exercise. If the level falls below what you consider to be "normal," speak to your doctor.

# 24 days to go...

## YOUR BABY TODAY

Your baby is now more suitably equipped for the time after the birth: his ears are fully formed on the outside and inside and he is used to hearing the sound of your blood circulating and your heart beating, and he recognizes your voice.

Your baby is losing the downy hair that he's had for several weeks, but if he's born now there may still be some visible.

**Lanugo is extremely fine hair** that covers your baby's body and, unlike adult hairs on the body, it is not associated with sweat glands. Lanugo hairs begin to be shed now since they are lost into the amniotic fluid in the last few weeks before birth. Your baby then swallows these lanugo hairs in the amniotic fluid but this is not a cause for concern: these hairs provide your baby with an important source of protein, essential to his development. It's been estimated that two-thirds of the protein in the fluid is swallowed and absorbed by the baby's gut each day, providing 15 percent of his protein needs.

The fine lanugo hairs are gradually replaced by vellus hairs, which are short, soft, nonpigmented hairs (often seen more on women and children). Terminal hair is the thicker, coarser, and longer hair that first grows on your baby's eyebrows, then his eyelashes, then his scalp. In adults, facial hair (beards), armpit, and pubic hair, is terminal hair.

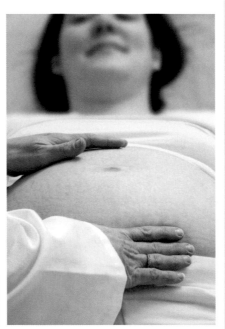

**The doctor will examine your abdomen in late pregnancy to check the position** of the baby. If the baby is breech, an ECV (see right) may be recommended to turn him into a head-down position. If he doesn't turn, a cesarean delivery may be necessary.

### FOCUS ON... YOUR BODY

## Desperate for a toilet

**In the third trimester you'll be frequenting the bathroom regularly,** as you did in the first trimester. At this stage it's due to the increasingly heavy baby pushing down on your bladder from above. If you find that it hurts when you expel urine, you may have a urinary infection and should contact your doctor for a test.

### ASK A... DOCTOR

**I've heard about doctors "turning" breech babies. How does this work?** Some obstetricians may try to turn a baby in late pregnancy using external cephalic version (ECV), which has a success rate of around 65 percent. The obstetrician tries gently to guide the baby into a head-down position by pressing his hands on the mother's abdomen, using an ultrasound as a guide. You may be given medication to relax the uterine muscles. You will be scanned first and if the baby is in an awkward position the procedure may not continue. If your baby is large this can affect the procedure, as can the amount of amniotic fluid: a low amount of fluid offers less protection to the baby.

If you're Rh negative, you may get an injection of Rh immunoglobulin (RhIg) after the version because of the small risk of a bleed around the placenta. An ECV is not recommended if you have a multiple pregnancy, have had bleeding, your placenta is low-lying (see p.212), your membranes have ruptured, or there is a known problem with the baby.

# 23 days to go...

**YOUR BABY TODAY**

3D views at this stage of the pregnancy will be extremely clear. Every part of the face is fully developed and your baby will be very expressive. Your baby is only a few days away now from being full term.

## Don't be concerned about embarrassing yourself in labor—your caregivers will have seen it all before.

**Many women worry about losing control** during labor—for example that they will urinate or defecate when they are pushing. You might well pass a bit of stool when you're pushing but you probably won't notice; your doctor will put on a pair of gloves and use gauze to remove it.

The reality is that when you're in the throes of labor, you really won't care— you'll just want that baby out!

**Keep an open mind about pain relief** since you won't know how you'll handle the pain or what your pain threshold is until you're actually in labor.

### ASK A... PANEL

## What if I can't deal with the pain of labor?

**Doctor:** If you're concerned, take time to investigate the pain-relief options in advance of labor, so that you're aware of what's available, even if you don't plan to use it.

There's no shame in deviating from what you requested in your birth plan; the ultimate goal is to deliver a healthy baby, and to keep your energy levels and your spirits high. It's also important to ask for pain relief as soon as you feel that things are getting away from you.

**Mom:** When I was in labor, the pain literally took my breath away, and I really did feel that I would be unable to continue. Changing position, walking around, and using a birthing ball proved to be a good distraction, even if they passed the time rather than provided relief, and I chanted to myself, over and over, "You can do it!"

I dimly remembered that when the pain is at its worst you've hit "transition," which signals the beginning of the delivery itself, and it did help to know I was near the end, even if it did seem a long time in coming. Focus on how much you want your baby in your arms, and view every contraction as one step closer to that moment.

**Midwife:** Moms who are prepared for the pain seem to find that it isn't as bad as they thought it might be, and are able to cope using breathing exercises and massage. The best advice is to know your limits. If you find the pain unbearable, then ask for some pain relief. Ask the doctor or nurse what pain options are available to take the edge off of the discomfort, and make the process more bearable.

No woman can anticipate how her labor and delivery will proceed, and sometimes babies make things difficult by presenting themselves in awkward positions, or simply enjoying life inside a little too much to arrive promptly. Take things one step at a time, and when you know you've had enough, conserve your energy by getting the help you need. Any woman who delivers a healthy baby has had a successful delivery, and that's what's most important.

# 22 days to go...

## YOUR BABY TODAY

Your baby will be able to recall and recognize the frequency and pattern of the most familiar sounds he hears within the uterus—your voice. Also, you might have noticed that loud noises may startle your baby during these final weeks.

If you're lacking in energy, try carb loading. This is also an effective measure in the days leading up to labor.

**The idea behind carb loading** comes from endurance athletes, who get 70 percent of their calorie intake from carbohydrates for three days prior to a big event. This enhances muscle uptake of fuel so that muscles are fully loaded with glycogen, the form in which carbs are stored in the body. If you're feeling tired, and especially prior to being active, ensure you take on plenty of carbohydrates.

In the days before your due date, base meals on carbohydrates, so that this food group provides up to 70 percent of your total calories. Include cereal or bread for breakfast, sandwiches for lunch, and include pasta, rice, or potatoes at dinner.

**A baked potato** is a great mini-meal, providing you with carbohydrates. Try different carbohydrate foods in the lead-up to labor to see which you like best.

### MAKING THE MOST OF MATERNITY LEAVE

**Maternity leave offers a great opportunity** to prepare yourself for the birth of your baby.

■ **Take time to rest.** While it may seem like the optimum time to rush through a long "to-do" list, it's important to conserve your energy for the birth, and the weeks afterward.

■ **Prepare your hospital bag** (see p.358), or anything you may need for a home birth (see p.341).

■ **Make a list** of everyone you'd like contacted after the birth.

■ **Put together some natural remedies** to help you through labor and its aftermath. Lavender oil can be sniffed during labor to relax and calm. You may need ice packs if you end up having an episiotomy (placing ice pads or chilled witch hazel pads on the area may soothe your pain). Ask your doctor about safe pain medications for after delivery, or, if you want to avoid medications, ask him or her for drug-free suggestions.

■ **Prepare a few freezer meals.** There can be nothing better than having an already prepared, healthy meal on hand that can be taken right from the freezer when your arms are full with your new baby, and you lack the time and energy to get dinner on the table.

■ **Sort your baby's new clothes** into sizes, so you don't find yourself searching through piles to find something that fits.

■ **Get ahead** by preparing your birth announcements—address and stamp envelopes, or design something that can be sent via email, so that you only need to slot in your new baby's photo and details at the last moment.

■ **Get a manicure, pedicure, or massage.** Not only will time be tight after your baby arrives, but money may be, too! Take the opportunity to lift your spirits and feel your best.

■ **Produce something creative**— paint your baby's nursery, cross-stitch a little pillow or picture, make a crib bumper, start a scrapbook, or simply write a letter to your baby to put in a keepsake box. These personal touches are satisfying, and will be treasured for years to come.

■ **Catch up with friends and family for lunch.** It may be some time before you feel like going out again once you're getting used to being a parent and enjoying your new baby in the comfort of your home.

# 21 days to go...

**YOUR BABY TODAY**

This baby is lying in the breech position, with the umbilical cord seen as is travels toward the placenta in the top left-hand side of the image. Approximately 3 in every 100 babies will be in a breech position after 37 weeks.

## Your baby is now able to hear many sounds that will all be familiar to him once he's born.

**In this late stage of pregnancy, sounds penetrate the uterus** easily and there is no doubt that the baby can hear and respond to these before birth. Your baby will startle at loud sounds but now also turn toward familiar sounds, and practice looking for the source of the sound. Your baby is not only recognizing a wider range of sound frequencies, but also discriminating between different sounds as well as learning and remembering familiar sounds, such as your voice and that of your partner.

Your baby breathes more quickly when he's concentrating on sounds and his heart rate increases. Although the baby can hear at birth, the ear drum continues to thin out, at the same time becoming more mobile and responsive to sounds. Your voice will be the most familiar sound to your baby at birth.

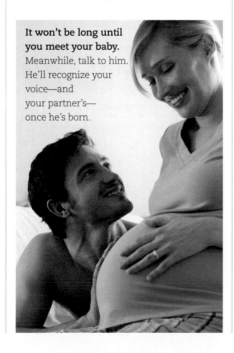

**It won't be long until you meet your baby.** Meanwhile, talk to him. He'll recognize your voice—and your partner's— once he's born.

---

### ASK A... DOCTOR

**What if I can't breast-feed?** It's normal to have doubts but be reassured that most women have enough milk, and with some help with positioning the baby can breast-feed without any problems. By this stage, you may even be leaking colostrum (see p.295).

Try to keep an open mind and remember that the breast milk does not come in straight after the birth (see p.448). Even if you have problems, try to persevere and don't feel pressured to give up just because it's convenient for the hospital staff or your partner, or because a friend or family member tells you it's not necessary.

Even if you don't end up breast-feeding, you can still get close to your baby by bottle-feeding.

---

### FOCUS ON... DADS

## The final weeks

**You aren't alone if you're a dad-to-be who's feeling a bit bewildered** and shell-shocked by the imminent arrival of your baby. To begin with, you can expect a lot of changes at home. Once your partner starts maternity leave, she may start a whirlwind of activity in preparation for the new arrival, and will need your help to get everything ready.

While supporting your partner both practically and emotionally will be important in the coming weeks, take care of yourself, too. Take every opportunity to get some rest. Even if you've agreed that your partner will do the majority of the nighttime baby care, your sleep will still be disrupted in the weeks after the birth. Catch up with friends now, but not to the point where you tire yourself out, and keep up your exercise routine, if you have one.

It's normal to feel anxious about what's ahead—both being a birth partner and a dad—but be reassured that somehow everything will fall into place. Focus on the thought of holding your newborn baby.

# Your 38th week

**EVEN IF YOU HAVE ENJOYED YOUR PREGNANCY, YOU MAY BE LONGING FOR IT TO BE OVER**

The baby is nearly ready, you are more than ready, so when is the birth going to happen? Probably not yet—especially if this is your first pregnancy. For another week or so, the uterus is still the best place for your baby while the finishing touches to her development take place. If you have other children, you can tell them that their new brother or sister won't keep everyone waiting much longer.

**Parts of the skeleton**, particularly the long bones of the arms and legs, have hardened, a process known as ossification.

**The placenta** has reached its full size and is spread out like a plate. It will continue to function for the full duration of the pregnancy.

**The hands** may be curled into fists, grasping the umbilcal cord, or free-floating with fingers outstretched. The grasp reflex is very strong.

**At 38 weeks** the average crown to heel length is 18.6 in (46.2 cm) and the average weight is 5.8 lb (2.6 kg).

**The head** may now be fully engaged. At this stage there are several normal variations in position and the direction in which the baby is facing.

# 20 days to go...

## YOUR BABY TODAY

Full term has been reached and your baby's features are now very clearly formed. To a certain extent from now on your baby is simply growing and putting on weight—factors necessary to provide energy after birth and help with temperature control.

Start preparing for the birth now: by being practical and positive, you can make it memorable for all the right reasons.

---

### AS A MATTER OF FACT

**Being hypnotized during pregnancy** can make you more confident in the lead-in to labor.

A study found that first-time pregnant women also experienced a shorter labor. The average amount of time they pushed in the second stage was one hour, compared with the usual two hours for a first baby.

---

**Probably the most effective way** to remember as much as you can about your labor and the birth of your baby is to try to remain as healthy and rested as possible prior to the start of your labor; this will give you the best chance of staying strong and clear-headed throughout.

Feeling strong and having plenty of energy may also help you remain upright and active during the course of your labor, reducing the need for pain relief such as Demerol (see p.403), which can sometimes cause memory loss that makes it more difficult to remember the finer details of the birth. It's also helpful to have your birth partner with you throughout your labor so that he or she can help to fill in any blanks later. Photographs and videos are also good prompts.

After the birth, if you find that there are parts you can't remember, you can ask your doctor to let you see your birth notes. You might want to write up your experience in a journal.

---

### FOCUS ON... DADS

## Health professionals and you

**When you get closer to the birth, and especially during labor,** you will find that there is inevitably more contact with health professionals. These individuals are a source of reassurance and a font of knowledge, but as a male you may sometimes feel that you're being sidelined or that your opinion doesn't count. This can be very frustrating if you want to be highly involved in the pregnancy and birth.

Bear in mind that the health professionals are trying to provide care for the person who needs it the most—namely your partner. If you want to be heard, it's a good idea to write down any questions that you may have before you meet with health professionals. Labor nurses will make every effort to help you to feel involved, and support you in supporting your partner.

Try to keep in mind that the most important relationship your partner has is with you, and that a positive attitude on your part can make a substantial difference to your partner's pregnancy and birth. So be patient and persistent but not pushy.

**Ensure you get plenty of rest** in the next few weeks to get you in the best frame of mind for labor and birth.

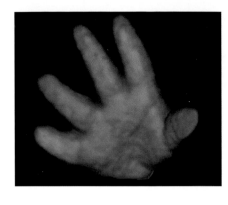

# 19 days to go...

### YOUR BABY TODAY

A 3D close-up of the hand shows the skin folds. Just as fingerprints are unique, so are the deeper skin folds seen on the hands and feet. The grasp reflex is strong and your baby will start to grasp anything that touches the palm of her hand.

Your baby will benefit from extra time in the uterus, but her development is almost complete and she's now "full term."

### THE LOWDOWN

## Hair down there

**One dilemma that's rarely discussed**—but much pondered— among moms-to-be is whether they should shave or trim their pubic hair before giving birth.

It's really a personal choice and depends how much it bothers you: just because your best friend had her pubic hair waxed, you shouldn't feel pressure to do the same—aside from anything else, itchy regrowth will not be welcome in the days following the birth of your baby.

You might want to trim your pubic hair or use tweezers or shave any stragglers, though, in the interests of postpartum hygiene. Postpartum blood loss will cling to the hair.

If you've arranged to have a cesarean, the top inch (at least) of your pubic hair will be shaved in hospital, so you may prefer to do this at home yourself.

**There is now less space for your baby to move** and she will soon, if she hasn't already, settle down into a comfortable head-down position. The shape of the uterus encourages this head-down position and, once in it, turning would be a major effort for your baby. Plenty of amniotic fluid remains to cushion and protect your baby, who will still be attempting to be very active in this more confined space.

Your baby's behavior is now exactly the same as a newborn: she'll turn toward light and yawn just as much as a newborn, and she'll continue to practice breathing the amniotic fluid in and out with regular rhythmical movements.

**Your baby will be very cramped** in the uterus. It won't be long, however, until she's positioned head down and begins to engage in the pelvis as she prepares to make her entry into the world.

# 18 days to go...

**YOUR BABY TODAY**

With each day that goes by delivery is becoming ever more likely. You may experience Braxton-Hicks' contractions, which help to soften the cervix and prepare for labor. The amniotic fluid that surrounds your baby ensures she'll hardly notice these mild tightenings.

## It's a good idea to give some thought to life after the birth, and ensure you have adequate help and support lined up.

**Even at this late stage of pregnancy,** it may still be hard to imagine your baby being born and living in your home. You and your partner may settle into life with your newborn with ease, and manage without any help, but it's still a good idea to have backup support just in case.

What you may not be prepared for is the fact that you're likely to be exhausted after weeks of poor sleep during pregnancy, and the rigors of labor itself. Add to this interrupted nights' sleep and the whole adjustment to being a new parent, and you may well find you'll need to call on people to help practically and emotionally.

It can help enormously to have a good support network set up in advance. Ideally, this will be close family and friends who you know you can rely on to drop in to help, but who will also know when you need to be left alone. Even an hour's help to prepare you a nutritious meal, or hold your baby while you get a much-needed rest or a shower, can give you some welcome respite.

Have the number on hand for your lactation consultant, so that you can ask for advice. Also get on the phone to moms-to-be whom you've met at prenatal classes; they more than anyone will be able to relate to how you're feeling.

Don't be too proud to accept help with housework and shopping. Knowing these tasks are taken care of will help you relax and focus on your baby.

Try to limit the number of guests you have in the early days, and make sure that they are warned that visits will be short. Although you will be desperate to show off your new baby, visits can be draining so it's better to wait until some routines are more established.

---

**FOCUS ON... NUTRITION**

## Healthy snacking

**Large meals are likely to leave you feeling uncomfortably full,** especially late in the third trimester. If you go long periods of time between meals, you may become light-headed and feel weak from hypoglycemia—low blood sugar. This is because the baby is constantly drawing glucose from your bloodstream.

Healthy snacking is the key to eating well and comfortably:

■ **Keep lots of fresh fruit** on display in a bowl so you'll remember to eat it.
■ **Stock your cupboards** with a variety of dried fruits and nuts.
■ **Hard boil eggs** and keep them in the fridge. Try eating them with a sprinkle of salt to quell that salt craving.
■ **Buy or make some frozen juice pops** and keep them in the freezer. Some women also find it refreshing to suck on these during labor.

**Yogurt is a nutritious and healthy snack** for any time of day. For variety and additional nutrients, sprinkle granola or dried fruit on top.

# 17 days to go...

## YOUR BABY TODAY

What exactly triggers the start of labor is still a mystery. Does the signal come from your own body or does the baby play a part in the decision? Every labor is different, and the timing of your first labor can be quite different from your second.

Gradually, each of your baby's bones is becoming strengthened thanks to adequate amounts of calcium.

**Your baby's bones are strengthened** by the process of ossification in which hard bone is formed from calcium. To meet this increase in demand, you absorb calcium much more readily from your diet.

By this stage of pregnancy, the baby's humerus in the upper arm, femur in the upper leg, and tibia in the lower leg have undergone this process. As ossification occurs at specific weeks in your pregnancy, ultrasound can use these as markers to estimate the date of the pregnancy, if necessary.

The time at which this ossification occurs may be seen a few days earlier in girls than boys and, interestingly, the patella (knee bone), does not ossify until after birth.

### AS A MATTER OF FACT

**Just because your partner weighed above average at birth,** it doesn't mean your baby will too.

The birth weight depends on the mix of genes your baby inherits. So, if your partner is tall and big boned and you're petite and were a tiny baby, keep your fingers crossed that you have the more dominant genes!

### ASK A... DOCTOR

**I've had a small amount of bleeding. Should I be concerned?**
Bleeding in late pregnancy may be serious since it can be due to the placenta partially, or totally, detaching from the wall of the uterus, known as placental abruption (see p.473), or to a low-lying placenta, known as placenta previa (see p.212). If you have a mucus discharge tinged with blood in late pregnancy, this may be a "bloody show" (see pp.391 and 411).

Always seek medical advice for bleeding at any stage of pregnancy to rule out any problems.

### BACH FLOWER REMEDIES

**Flower essence blends are designed to calm and center your energy,** which some think can help you relax and encourage you to focus. Rescue Remedy and Emergency Essence, types of Bach Flower Remedy, are thought by some to be effective when used in labor, and in the weeks prior to and after the birth. The remedies are taken for a variety of symptoms including anxiety, shock, worry, stress, or simply for a boost during a long or painful labor.

A few drops may be taken on your tongue as required or mixed in water, as shown above. Both of these blends also come in cream form, to apply topically, or as a spray, to spritz yourself, and your environment.

Ask your doctor before you try these or other natural remedies, since they haven't been thoroughly studied.

**One way to take Bach Flower Remedies** (see below) is to put four drops into a glass of water and sip it at intervals. Alternatively, you can put the drops directly on to your tongue using the pipette. Always talk to your doctor before using any remedy.

# 16 days to go...

**YOUR BABY TODAY**

The size of your uterus may have reduced slightly as your baby's head becomes more deeply engaged within your pelvis, allowing her body to move down. This can take some of the pressure away from your ribs, which is a welcome relief at this stage.

When there's going to be a new arrival on the scene, it's important to prepare the little members of your household.

**How you handle introducing the new baby** to your children will depend on their age. A toddler might be totally indifferent and unfazed, being more interested in your new baby's toys than the fact that she has a new brother or sister. An older child might be shocked and jealous by the arrival of a new baby, who appears to steal her limelight, and usurp his mommy and daddy's attention.

It's a good idea to prepare your little one several weeks in advance, explaining that the new baby will need a lot of time and attention, will need to be fed and changed regularly, and probably not be much fun for a few months. Focus on how your child can be a great helper, and show her what the new baby will need when she is born. Take some books out of the library that explain how families change when a new baby is born, and ask your child to talk about how she's feeling, and how she thinks things will be different when the baby arrives.

Encourage your child to choose a gift to give to the baby, and find something your child really wants as a gift from her new sibling. Ask grandparents or close friends to arrange a few treats or outings for your child both now and after the birth, so that she's occupied, and getting extra attention.

---

**ASK A... DOCTOR**

**My mom had a difficult delivery with me. Am I likely to have the same experience as her?** Like many women, you're obviously aware of the details of your own birth.

Some say you'll have the same sort of delivery your mom had with you—for example, your baby will be early or late or you'll have a very quick labor or a slow, assisted one. This isn't necessarily true.

Remember, depending on how old your mom is, there have probably been significant developments in obstetrics since your mom's days and, even if you face the same hurdles during your labor, they might be managed differently.

Also, you might be healthier and stronger than your mom was, so don't assume you're in for a difficult labor just because she had one.

---

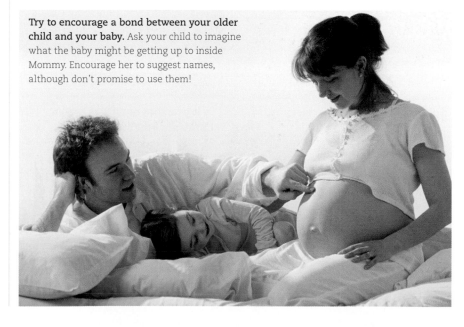

**Try to encourage a bond between your older child and your baby.** Ask your child to imagine what the baby might be getting up to inside Mommy. Encourage her to suggest names, although don't promise to use them!

# 15 days to go...

## YOUR BABY TODAY

Estimating your baby's size by measuring from the top of the uterus to the front of your pelvic bone can give you an idea of size, but this is less accurate now. Your baby may not yet have moved down into the pelvis and the amount of fluid around your baby is variable.

Newborn babies can tightly hold someone's finger because of the grasp reflex, and this is already functioning in the uterus.

**Inside the uterus your baby has developed a strong grasp reflex.** The grip is so strong after birth that it could support your baby's weight. This grasp reflex persists until your baby is about six months old; she will then have more choice over whether to grasp an object or not.

Interestingly, your baby also has a similar reflex in the foot. This is the "plantar reflex" and it causes the toes to attempt to curl around your finger if the sole of the foot is stroked. The plantar reflex takes slightly longer to disappear after birth, typically persisting until 12 months of age. Another reflex action causes the toes to spread out if the side of the foot is stroked. These reflexes and others seem to be quite primitive in nature and although they are thought to protect the baby, the precise function of each reflex is not fully understood.

### AS A MATTER OF FACT

**Second labors are usually** shorter in duration than first labors.

This usually means an easier labor, but a second baby could be bigger than a first, or positioned differently. There are many factors to consider.

**In addition to being an effective way to relax,** using a birthing pool can speed up labor. It is thought that water sets off a surge of the hormone oxytocin, which triggers contractions.

### ASK A... DOCTOR

**Is it true that natural or water births are best for the baby?** Most childbirth experts would agree that a straightforward vaginal birth is the safest form of birth for both mother and baby. It is also generally considered safe to use water as a method of relieving the pain in uncomplicated labors.

However, it is sometimes not possible to achieve a straightforward vaginal delivery due to certain situations that can arise during, labor and birth. If a problem with either the mother or baby occurs, the medical team will advise you on the safest way of delivering the baby.

It's important to think about the type of birth you would prefer and are comfortable with, but be prepared to be flexible and to see how labor unfolds. Speak to your doctor to find out if there's a birthing pool you can use at your hospital.

### THE LOWDOWN

## Owls!

Could owls give us an insight into pregnancy and birth? It's doubtful, but these myths are entertaining!

- **If a pregnant woman** hears the shriek of an owl, her child will definitely be a girl.
- **An owl living in the attic** of a house will cause a problem with the baby.
- **When the time comes to give birth** there should be no owls in the delivery room—if they hoot at the moment of birth the child will have a miserable life.

# 14 days to go...

**YOUR BABY TODAY**

The back of the hand is held up against the mouth in this image. Your baby will be practicing suckling at every opportunity, but this will be with parts of the hands, thumbs or fingers, since it's no longer easy to reach the toes.

## If you haven't found out the sex of your baby, the excitement will be building; if you have, you can get very organized!

**Knowing the sex of your baby** enables you to decide on the name, buy specific outfits, and even decorate the nursery, if you have one, in a certain way. Remember, however, there's a chance that the scan (see pp.214–15) gave you misleading information. The only way to be absolutely certain of the baby's gender is if you found out following a diagnostic test, such as amniocentesis or chorionic villus sampling (see pp.152–3).

### THE LOWDOWN

## Boys and girls

Still wondering what you're having? Well, to help you guess, you might want to bear in mind a few more old wives' tales...

■ **If you have soft hands** you're having a girl, rough hands you're having a boy.
■ **If the father-to-be is nervous,** it's a girl, if he's relaxed it's a boy.
■ **If the mother picks up her coffee cup** with two hands it's a girl, if she picks it up by the handle it's a boy.
■ **If you have a sensitive belly button** it's a girl, if you have cold feet it's almost certainly a boy!

If you know the sex, you won't have the same incentive of a surprise at the end of your labor, but you may feel you can bond more closely with your baby during pregnancy and picture what he or she will be like as a newborn.

If you don't know the sex yet, then you will have a well-earned surprise after your hard work in labor. Some women who don't know the sex of their babies say that they have a strong instinct that the baby is a particular sex, but may be quite surprised when they have a baby of the opposite sex.

Try to keep an open mind and not raise your hopes about having a baby of a certain gender—the odds are slightly in favor of you having a boy.

**While knowing the sex of your baby helps you make decisions,** such as should you buy pink or blue, not knowing gives you a greater sense of anticipation.

### ASK A... DOCTOR

**My baby is in a posterior position. How will this affect my labor?** In the posterior position the baby faces your belly instead of your spine (see p.336). This position may prolong your labor, which can be tiring, and cause more of a backache. If this is the case, you can try the same methods as for turning a breech baby (see p.329) to encourage your baby to move into an anterior position.

Sometimes the baby turns with the help of contractions when you are in fully established labor. If she doesn't turn, intervention such as the use of forceps or vacuum (see pp.436–7) may be needed.

### AS A MATTER OF FACT

**Your body** is designed to handle the pain of labor!

Nobody likes pain, but your body's endorphin levels will increase during labor to help you cope with it. So it's reassuring to know that as the intensity of the contractions build, so does your ability to handle them.

# Your 39th week

**TIME MAY FEEL AS THOUGH IT'S STANDING STILL AND EVERY SMALL TWINGE HAS YOU ON THE ALERT**

Know the signs that mean labor is really about to start. You may have some false alarms, so don't hesitate to call your doctor for advice and reassurance. Excitement will be competing with nerves—and that goes for your partner as well. No one can predict how labor is going to turn out, but before the big day it's helpful to agree on what your partner's role should ideally be.

**The eye** is large and well formed, although its neural networks are not yet sophisticated enough for the baby to focus. Vision in newborns remains poor for a few weeks after birth while the eye continues to develop.

**The head** may be covered with hair, a few wispy strands—or no hair at all.

**At 39 weeks** the average crown to heel length is 19.1 in (48.6 cm) and the average weight is 6.3 lb (3 kg).

**Breathing** is now rhythmical, with your baby making around 40 breathing movements every minute.

**The baby** is so low down in your pelvis that you have probably exchanged discomfort in your upper abdominal area for pressure on your bladder.

# 13 days to go...

**YOUR BABY TODAY**

This baby's hand is in the same position as in the image opposite, with the fist held tightly in front of the face. All of your baby's movements help build muscle strength and aid coordination, whether it's a kick or simply curling and uncurling the fingers.

With labor imminent, you'll be playing the waiting game. Staying active will help the time pass much more quickly.

**You'll be resting a lot in the next two weeks.** As your figure expands and you become more tired, it's natural to want to sit out the remainder of your pregnancy at home with your feet up, and put the answering machine on to field all the "Has it arrived?" inquiries!

It's fine to do this but it's good to remember that the very best way to stimulate labor is to keep active. What's more, the hormones produced by even gentle walking will lift your mood and help you feel more positive when your labor begins.

Try giving yourself one or two small tasks each day—perhaps meeting a friend for lunch, going for a very gentle swim, or purchasing some last-minute items for baby—being careful to stop and put your feet up when you feel tired. Be sensible about the type of activities you undertake, and avoid anything that could be exhausting or potentially dangerous; for example, bear in mind that your center of gravity is way off balance at the moment, and that wallpapering the nursery or carrying heavy groceries should definitely not be on your to-do list.

It may feel as though your life is on hold at the moment so that's why it's good to fill your time as best you can. Don't forget, however, that in just a couple of weeks you'll have your newborn occupying all your time.

THE LOWDOWN

## The power of music

**Research has shown that women who listen to music during labor** tend to feel less stressed and are less likely to need pain relief. There's also some evidence to suggest that babies born to the accompaniment of music are calmer.

One study compared different beats and found that classical, instrumental sounds were the most relaxing. Familiar tunes and rhythms could distract you from the pain and—if you choose the right track—help you focus on your breathing. Line up a selection of tunes on your iPod well in advance of labor.

**Try out a selection of music** to discover what you find most soothing, or invigorating. Labor is a bit like a mini-marathon and listening to the right tunes might just help you get to the finish line.

# 12 days to go...

### YOUR BABY TODAY

Although your baby's head is deep within your pelvis, it will remain rounded in shape. It is not until labor starts that the bones of the skull move closer to each other, elongating the shape of the head, and allowing your baby to pass more easily along the birth canal.

## Although your baby will be born with beautifully big eyes, it will be some time before he will see clearly at a distance.

**Your baby's eyes are almost their adult size at birth.** Although the eyes continue to grow very slightly until adolescence, and the lens within the eye grows throughout life, the eye is three-quarters of its adult size at birth. Both color (cones) and black and white visual cells (rods) are present in the retina but vision is still rather poor—

equivalent to being able to just see the top letter of the optician's chart. This is referred to as 20/400 vision. This means than if the baby could read, then he could read a letter at 20 ft (6 m) that a person with perfect vision could read when 400 ft (122 m) away. Because of this, your newborn may not seem to pay much attention at first; he'll have some difficulty focusing and his eye muscles will be quite weak. He will, however, be able to see objects 12 in (30 cm) away; since this is roughly the distance between your breast and face, it means your baby can see your face as he nurses.

He'll be six to eight weeks old before fixing onto and following an object, four months before he can judge distances, and two years of age before his vision has perfected to 20/20.

**Your baby will have gained weight steadily** during these final weeks, with fat being laid down under the skin. If born now, he would have a plump, rounded appearance.

### AS A MATTER OF FACT

**95 percent of babies don't arrive on their due date**—of these 25 percent come early and 70 percent late.

There's a four-week window between 38 and 42 weeks of pregnancy that's regarded as normal and safe in medical circles.

A month is a long time to wait, so put a message on your voicemail along the lines of "We'll be in touch as soon as the baby's arrived." Keep yourself busy: have your hair done (much easier without a newborn in tow), catch up with friends, and, most importantly, get some sleep!

### ASK A... DOCTOR

**I don't often swear but is it true that I'm likely to subject my partner to verbal abuse during labor?**
Possibly, but no one will blame you if you do! Giving birth can be incredibly painful, and you may feel emotional, irritable, shaky, and even nauseous. Don't worry too much about what you say and do: try to stay focused on the birth and ask for pain relief if you

need it. Most birth partners will be forgiving and are unlikely to take the abuse personally. They will realize that you might not quite be yourself during childbirth—and if they've been by your side throughout labor will be fully understanding of what you're going through. You may also be irritable with your caregivers, but they will be used to this!

# 11 days to go...

**YOUR BABY TODAY**

This image demonstrates how your baby has laid down fat reserves, nicely rounding out the cheeks. The exact weight of your baby will depend now on which day you deliver since your baby will continue to grow in the uterus, although at a slower rate than previously.

## If you're having a home birth, you can make the midwife's task as easy as possible by being well organized.

**If you're having your baby at home,** spend this week ensuring that everything is in order and that the room in which you plan to give birth is clean, comfortable, and adequately heated.

Your midwife may bring around a pack about now, which contains all the items she will need. To make her task easier, make sure the bed on which you're going to deliver (if you plan to use a bed) is easily accessible from all sides. You might also want to ensure you have plenty of extra pillows on hand as well as several changes of bed sheets.

Even if you plan to labor in dim lighting, there needs to be a good source of light for the midwife, especially after the birth when you may need stitches.

**Learn to catnap** for 10–20 minutes. This will help you rest and revive you, and it's a good technique to use once the baby is born.

### THE LOWDOWN

## On pushing

**Is pushing the baby out natural and instinctive?** All women will feel an urge to push during labor, but because it's painful they might resist doing so. Medications, such as an epidural (see pp.404–5), will interfere with the sensation of needing to push. Your midwife will help you throughout and guide you as to when it's safe and most effective to push.

### ASK A... DOCTOR

**I'm so tired already. How will I ever get through labor?** First of all, take every opportunity you can to rest—even if this means napping several times during the day. Every bit of sleep you get will make a difference to your energy levels, especially if you're having broken sleep at night.

When you are feeling active, try to do some gentle exercise since this can encourage healthy, restful sleep. Swimming can be a great way to expend energy, and take your mind off things and it puts little or no pressure on your belly or your aching muscles and joints.

Try eating food containing tryptophan (see p.177) before you go to bed, which can encourage sleep, and make sure that you get plenty of high-energy carbohydrates (see p.92) during the day, to keep your blood-sugar levels stable and prevent energy slumps.

# 10 days to go...

### YOUR BABY TODAY

Your baby's neck muscles have strengthened, so the head can be held well away from the chest wall. Once delivered though, the buoyancy provided by the amniotic fluid will be lost and you will need to support your baby's head at all times while holding him.

## Could your baby be dreaming already? A lot of his movements are occurring when he's fast asleep.

**Your baby has been practicing breathing** since the 10th week of pregnancy but now the pattern has changed from short practice bursts lasting 10 seconds or so, to a regular rhythmic breathing pattern of approximately 40 breaths per minute, just as the baby will breathe after birth.

Eye movements have also matured with periods of rapid eye movement (REM) lasting for just over 25 minutes at a time and rest periods lasting just under 25 minutes. REM sleep is closely coupled with periods of increased activity and a faster heart rate. So, just because your baby is moving it doesn't always mean that he's awake.

Although your baby cannot stretch out as freely as before, movements of at least 10 times a day should continue in the same familiar pattern and are a reassuring sign of a healthy baby.

### FOCUS ON... NUTRITION

## Fuel for labor

**Most hospitals don't allow women in labor to eat or drink,** because if you need general anesthesia, there's a risk of aspiration. But in 2008, the American College of Nurse-Midwives issued a clinical bulletin stating that allowing a woman in labor to eat or drink provides her with hydration, nutrition, comfort, and can even reduce stress. Ask your doctor if you can eat, and if so, what. A few suggestions: Choose something light, such as soup or broth, popsicles, applesauce, or ice chips—which you can chomp on even if you're not allowed food. And your partner should snack to keep his strength.

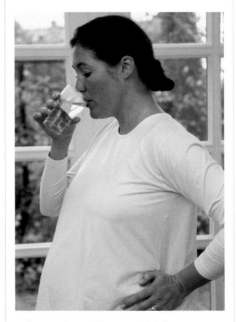

**Ask your doctor if you can drink** or eat during labor. Drinking will keep you hydrated while your body is working hard.

### ASK A... DOCTOR

**What is "stripping the membranes" and could I have this instead of being induced if I end up being overdue?** Depending on your health and the baby's condition, and many other factors (for example, you're more than 42 weeks along, you have high blood pressure, you have an infection), your doctor may induce labor. There are many ways to do this, including stripping the membranes. With a gloved finger, your doctor checks your cervix and sweeps her finger over the membranes that connect the amniotic sac and the uterine wall. The goal of this is to stimulate the release of hormones that may start labor contractions. Although this is likely to be an uncomfortable procedure, it should not cause you actual pain; you will also experience a mucus/bloodstained "bloody show" (see p.411)—following stripping of the membranes, which is quite normal.

The procedure can be done at your doctor's office or in the hospital (see p.432). Your doctor will advise you closer to the time.

YOU ARE 38 WEEKS AND 5 DAYS

# 9 days to go...

## YOUR BABY TODAY

In many ways you will be the best judge of the likely size of your baby, especially if you can compare it with a previous pregnancy. An ultrasound scan can estimate the weight, but as with all other measurements at this time it has a fairly wide margin of error.

Don't just wait for contractions—it's worth familiarizing yourself now with the signs that may mean labor is imminent.

### FETAL MONITORING

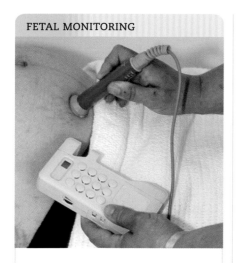

**If there are no complications or reasons for concern,** your baby's heartbeat will usually be monitored using a handheld device much like the one used during your prenatal appointments. You may be hooked up throughout the entire labor and birth, or your doctor may listen to your baby's heartbeat every 15 to 30 minutes, which means that you can move around as much as you like in between these checks.

If you've had complications in pregnancy, or problems develop during labor, the doctor may monitor the heartbeat using a CTG (see p.418).

### When does labor actually start?

If it's your first pregnancy, it can be difficult to recognize the signs that the baby is on his way. Some women get lower back pain that is minor before becoming painful. You might notice a bloody show (see p.411), which can happen well before true labor actually starts. Your water may break as the sac containing the amniotic fluid bursts open. Even if your water breaking is not accompanied by contractions you should still inform your doctor of what is happening.

Finally, the most obvious sign is contractions: these painful tightenings of your uterus will increase in intensity and become more regular as labor progresses. Contractions are associated with the dilation and shortening of your cervix, so your doctor will examine you to see how far you've progressed (see pp.414–15).

If you think that you have gone into labor, stay calm and telephone your doctor and listen to her advice. Inform her of your symptoms and, especially, describe your contractions. If you are having contractions every 5 minutes that last for one minute (time them), and they're so uncomfortable that you're forced to stop what you're doing, you should think about going to hospital.

### ASK A... DOCTOR

**How long am I likely to stay in hospital after the birth?** In most maternity units, there's a degree of flexibility as to how long you remain in hospital. If you want to stay for as brief a period as possible, talk to your doctor. It depends on many variables, but federal law says insurance companies can't force you to check out before 48 hours for a vaginal delivery, or 96 hours for a cesarean. It is recommended that a healthy newborn stay in the hospital for at least 48 hours.

How long you stay in hospital will largely depend on your type of delivery. If you have a vaginal birth, you should be able to go home after six hours, but a cesarean may mean you need to stay in for about three days. If your baby is born early, is unwell, or is struggling to feed or maintain his temperature, you'll be advised to stay in the hospital. If your baby has to remain in the hospital for a long period, you would have to go home and visit him in the neonatal intensive care unit (see pp.452–3).

# 8 days to go...

## YOUR BABY TODAY

The movements that you feel will usually be concentrated in a few areas since your baby cannot readily change position. Although the character of these movements will have changed, you should still experience many movements each day.

Because you're heading into the final week, you're bound to feel a little anxious, but hopefully excited, too.

**It's normal to feel a little jittery** about your impending labor, especially if it's your first baby. Try not to keep your feelings bottled up: share anxieties with your partner, since you might find he's in need of reassurance, too. If you have specific concerns, call your doctor. She'll be used to handling these worries and will be able to put your mind at rest. Find ways to occupy your mind, even if it's just doing crosswords, since this will stop you from worrying.

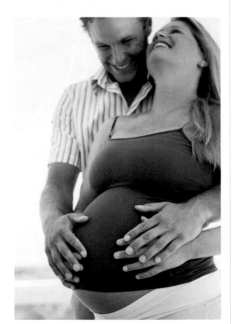

**You're in it together** and will need each other more than ever in these final two weeks.

---

**FOCUS ON... DADS**

## The stages of labor and you

**There is so much variation in the time taken** to complete the first stage of labor (see pp.408–21) that for one pregnancy a woman might be in labor for days, whereas a subsequent labor might be a matter of hours.

As your partner's primary support, you have the difficult job of trying to take charge, exude calm, and give emotional and practical support. Don't hesitate to call the doctor for advice—a short discussion with her may help you to gauge how far through the first stage your partner has progressed. You must allow plenty of time to get to the hospital and you should be familiar with the route well beforehand (see box, below).

There may be periods when your partner is not lucid, but you will know what she wants better than anyone else. It's therefore your role to advocate for her and to engage with medical staff when she can't do so herself. You'll also know how to reassure and encourage your partner in the right way.

You'll need to support her in whatever position she chooses to use during the second stage (see pp.422–7)—when she's delivering the baby—and provide lots of encouragement. In the third stage (see pp.428–9), once the baby is born, you may cut the cord and might be holding your new baby while the placenta is delivered.

---

**ASK A... DOCTOR**

**What are the signs that it's too late to go to the hospital?** Generally speaking, if you're having an uncontrollable urge to push, then that's the point where it may be too late to reach the hospital before your delivery. If you did find yourself in this situation, call your doctor who will advise you. He or she may arrange to send paramedics to you for the delivery of the baby. Or you can contact the emergency ambulance services yourself and follow their advice while you wait for their arrival.

# 7 days to go...

### YOUR BABY TODAY

This baby can easily be seen at this late stage in the pregnancy because there is ample amniotic fluid present. The amount of amniotic fluid at this point is still extremely variable, but it is usually in the region of 0.75 pint (0.5 liter).

## Use this time in the lead-in to labor to get your partner fully up to speed on how he can help you on the big day.

**It's a good idea to prepare your partner in advance,** and figure out what may help the proceedings once labor does begin. If you're planning on listening to music during labor, laboring in a tub, or walking around, inform your partner ahead of time what you think you'll expect from him.

Practice some massage strokes, and teach him how to do them (see p.163). Some women can't bear to be touched during labor, but others find it helpful to have their back, or even just their hands and feet, massaged. You won't really know what works for you until you're in labor but practicing massage now won't harm.

If your partner has been going to prenatal classes with you, he'll be familiar with the breathing and

relaxation techniques so practice these together and, if necessary, get advice from your doctor about techniques.

It may be helpful for your partner to speak to male friends or relatives who have recently become fathers. Hearing the experiences of others and learning some do's and don'ts of being a birth partner might be useful.

**You may find it relaxing to have your feet massaged** in the early stages of labor, even if you don't want your back or shoulders touched. A massage helps to relieve tension.

### AS A MATTER OF FACT

**Whatever their weight,** most babies at 40 weeks are approximately the same length.

Ninety-five percent are between 17.7 in (45 cm) and 21.6 in (55 cm) long. The length of newborn babies is remarkably consistent and relates to skeletal growth, whereas birth weight may vary considerably.

### FINAL PREPARATIONS

**It's amazing that even after 40 weeks of pregnancy,** when labor begins there is still a scramble to get everything organized as you head off to the hospital. So to avoid any last-minute panic:

■ **Make sure your bag is packed** (see p.358). You may also want to pin up a list of any extras you need to include at the last minute.

■ **It's advisable to keep a small bag of change** in your hospital bag to pay for parking, and drinks from vending machines.

■ **Decide who will do what:** so, for example, perhaps your partner could prepare snacks.

■ **Do a trial run** of the trip to the hospital—anticipating areas where there is likely to be traffic, seeking out shortcuts, and figuring out where you are most likely to find a parking space. It can also help to time the run at various points in the day, so that you can avoid school-run hotspots or commuter traffic. Also find out how to get into the maternity unit at night.

■ **Above all, don't panic.** The majority of parents-to-be do get to the hospital in plenty of time.

# Your 40th week

**ALL THE MILESTONES ARE SAFELY PASSED AND YOU WILL MEET YOUR BABY ANY DAY NOW**

Like many moms-to-be, you may have to linger in suspense beyond the "last" day of pregnancy. Without a doubt, the big event is about to happen very soon and it will be worth the waiting, wondering, and worrying. Once you see and hold your baby, you won't spend much time looking back over the past 40 weeks, but you'll certainly marvel at the miracle of it all.

**The membranes** of the amniotic sac will rupture once labor starts, and the fluid that has cushioned the baby for months will drain away.

**Shortly after** the baby is born, further contractions will separate the placenta from the wall of the uterus. The doctor may gently deliver it by pulling on the umbilical cord.

**The umbilical cord** is about the same length as your baby.

**At full term** the baby has the rounded chubby cheeks typical of new babies.

**At 40 weeks** the average crown to heel length is 19.6 in (49.8 cm) and the average weight is 6.8 lb (3.1 kg).

**The skull bones** are separated by membranes that allow for movement between bones and an easier passage of the head through the birth canal.

# 6 days to go...

**YOUR BABY TODAY**

If you are having a planned cesarean delivery, this is usually offered now—in order to balance the chance of labor starting unexpectedly with that of delivering your baby too soon. It is best for babies to be delivered as close to the due date as possible.

## It's good to revisit your birth plan at this late stage since you may feel differently now about some of the requests you made.

**A birth plan is usually filled in earlier in pregnancy,** and you may not have given it much more thought since (see pp.181 and 303). Now that the birth is imminent, look over it with your partner to figure out whether you've changed your mind about anything. For example you may be veering toward a more natural birth or, conversely, you may now be certain you want an epidural. Adapt it as you wish and discuss it with your doctor, if necessary.

Since your partner will be your advocate in labor, putting your requests forward to your labor nurses and doctor if you're unable to express them, it's important that he understands your wishes and that they're fresh in his mind.

Remember, though, that you won't really know how you'll feel or what you want until you're in labor, so keep an open mind and be prepared to adapt your plans on the day if it's in the best interests of your baby's well-being.

Get your partner's view. Remember that this is a big event for him, too: the moment when he'll meet his baby for the first time. He may have anxieties and concerns and want reassurance about what his role will be on the day: tell him how you think he can best help you, whether it be a massage or just holding your hand throughout. Discuss how you both are feeling in the preparation for the birth—your concerns, hopes, and expectations.

---

### ASK A... MOM

**How many visitors can come see the new baby in the hospital?**
Check the hospital's policy, but this is generally up to you. If you want your friends and family to come, by all means you can invite them— just be sure to check the visiting hours. Right now, you might think you want a roomful of visitors, but you may change your mind after you've been through labor and delivery, so wait to make your decision. You might just want to sleep or spend time alone with your partner and the baby. Remember, too, that young children (other than immediate family) may not be allowed to visit.

### STAYING CLOSE

**It can be difficult to think of anything** but the birth and meeting your baby when you are this close to the end of pregnancy. Try to focus on other things, too:

■ **Spend time with your partner:** Enjoy quality time together while it is still just the two of you, before the baby makes demands on your time, and exhaustion sets in. Share your hopes and fears about how your lives are going to change.
■ **Make love:** you might feel you are too big, or too tired, but it is good to remind yourselves of your sexual relationship. And, you never know, making love could just get your labor started (see p.393).

# 5 days to go...

### YOUR BABY TODAY

This close-up 3D ultrasound view shows that this baby's earlobe is particularly prominent. The dark flecks around the ear look like hair, but are in fact shadows (although many babies have hair at this stage).

## Your baby's bones have hardened to a certain degree, but this process will continue right up to the teenage years!

**Your baby's skeleton has gradually transformed,** from soft cartilage to bone, a process called ossification (see p.372). This process starts in the center of each bone spreading outward. By the end of pregnancy, ossification is complete along the length of each bone but the ends of the long bones and the tips of the bones in the finger and toes remain as cartilage. This is necessary to allow later bone growth as the child develops.

The bones in the upper part of the skull are slightly different, developing from membranous structures rather than cartilage. These do not fully fuse until several years after birth and remain separated from each other by connective tissue. This connective tissue forms areas called sutures and where more than two bones meet, wider spaces called fontanelles. Their function is to allow space for movement or "molding" between the skull bones making it easier for the head to descend into the pelvis during labor. It is also these suture lines and fontanelles that help your doctor determine the position of the baby's head during labor.

After delivery you will notice that your baby's head shape is often elongated, but this soon changes as the bones realign back into their usual positions.

**This MRI (magnetic resonance imaging) scan** shows a fetus approaching full-term. The baby's brain, spinal column, heart, liver, and lungs are visible, and the umbilical cord can be seen to the right of the image.

### THE LOWDOWN

## Placenta on toast?

**The thought of eating the placenta** may turn your stomach, but some women choose to do exactly that. The organ is revered for its spiritual properties, and devotees of placentophagia believe the nutrients it contains, including vitamin B6, will help prevent them from developing postpartum depression. However, the evidence in favor of the health benefits of consuming a placenta is purely anecdotal.

An alternative and less controversial custom involves dressing the placenta with herbs, then burying it at a party to celebrate the baby's birth: this is thought to be an important bonding ritual for the extended family.

Art is another option: press the placenta against a piece of paper and you'll get a tree-shaped print.

Some cultures use the dried organ to make medicinal herbs.

Not sure how to cook placenta? Well just look online and you'll find plenty of placenta recipes, from pâté to lasagne, but, understandably, these might not be to everyone's taste.

# 4 days to go...

**YOUR BABY TODAY**

Once labor starts your baby will no longer have room to place her hands on top of her head or by her face although, interestingly, she is still moving around—you probably won't notice these movements since you will have other things on your mind.

The inquiries may begin flooding in this week and it will feel as though the whole world is awaiting news of your baby's arrival.

**In this final week of your pregnancy,** the weight of expectation can be immense. It can feel as though everyone is waiting for you to pop, especially if it's your first baby.

You'll no doubt cope with it this week—and you may even enjoy getting all the attention—but if you happen to go overdue you might get frustrated by the constant calls and by having to repeat yourself. Try to be patient and remember people are simply excited for you and are just as frustrated with waiting as you are.

Matters aren't helped by the due date. Everyone will have this estimated date in mind, but unfortunately not many babies stick to a schedule and they enter the world exactly when they are ready (see p.378). Up to 42 weeks isn't really considered that late in medical circles. If it all becomes too much, rely on others close to you to field all the calls and make it clear that you promise to be in touch with an announcement just as soon as there is any news.

**Text messaging** can be a useful way of staying in touch with people in the final days. Sending out a circular "baby hasn't arrived yet" message is a good idea.

FOCUS ON... YOUR BODY

## False labor

**You may experience deep and painful twinges,** and practice contractions, known as Braxton-Hicks', particularly toward the end of pregnancy. It's easy to mistake these for the real thing, and you may find yourself rushing to the hospital when your body is really still practicing. You may also experience regular contractions for a period, which then stop. All of this is normal.

One sure sign that labor is imminent is that you lose your mucus plug (see p.411), another is your water breaking. In some cases, however, neither of these events takes place until labor is established, so don't panic if they don't happen to you.

You'll definitely know you're in labor when your contractions are occurring regularly, approximately every 15 minutes—time the gap between them. True contractions will get longer, stronger, and closer together as time goes on, and won't go away when you walk around or change position.

**ASK A... DOCTOR**

**Is it worth paying extra for a private room when I'm in the hospital?**
This is entirely up to you. It is expensive; it can cost a few hundred dollars a night, but some women find it money well spent. In addition to giving you more privacy and private time to bond with your new baby and your partner, a private room will be quieter, and you won't have as many interruptions, since you won't have medical staff coming in to treat a roommate. A private room can also make a difference in getting good rest at night, especially if you are a light sleeper.

Your 40th week

# 3 days to go...

## YOUR BABY TODAY

This image shows that even at this time your baby will be able to reach down and touch her toes (see the foot on the right and the hand on the left). Because there is less space your baby will no longer be able to place her feet on top of her head.

## Don't be too concerned if your baby hasn't engaged yet since this won't have any bearing on the final delivery date.

**There are many reasons why** your baby may not have engaged yet: the shape of your pelvis may mean that you need the pressure of the contractions to get the baby's head to engage. Very athletic women tend to have babies who engage late because their taut muscles hold the baby in a different position. Second and subsequent babies tend to engage later because the abdominal muscles are very loose, so the baby may move freely without feeling any need to get her head down. A big baby may not descend into the pelvis until the contractions start.

### HOW YOUR BABY IS POSITIONED

**Once the baby is head down and moves into the pelvis** there are several positions she may adopt: six of the most common are shown below. The position is determined by where her back and occiput (the back of her head) are lying. The most usual position is LOT. If the baby is breech (see p.433), the position is determined by how the bottom is lying.

LOT: left occiput-transverse

LOA: left occiput-anterior

LOP: left occiput-posterior

ROT: right occiput-transverse

ROA: right occiput-anterior

ROP: right occiput-posterior

**LOT (left occiput-transverse):** the back and occiput are positioned on the left-hand side of the uterus at right angles to the spine.

**LOA (left occiput-anterior):** the back and occiput are positioned closer to the front of the uterus on the left-hand side.

**LOP (left occiput-posterior):** the back and occiput are toward the spine on the left-hand side of the uterus.

**ROT (right occiput-transverse):** the back and occiput are at right angles to the spine on the right-hand side of the uterus.

**ROA (right occiput-anterior):** the back and occiput are toward the front of the uterus on the right-hand side.

**ROP (right occiput-posterior):** the back and occiput are toward the spine on the right-hand side of the uterus.

# 2 days to go...

**YOUR BABY TODAY**

This great image of the hands even shows the fine folds that have formed in the palms. Every baby has a unique pattern of folds on the palms and on the soles of the feet that you'll see when your baby finally arrives.

You'll be in labor very soon and it's normal to be anxious about what you need to go through to meet your baby.

**You're bound to have mixed emotions about going into labor.** While you'll want your baby to be born, you may be apprehensive about going through childbirth. Most women are understandably concerned about the pain, and may worry about their health and that of the baby. Remember that the majority of deliveries are normal and without complications and the majority of babies are fit and healthy.

Even though you've spent the past nine months preparing for the birth, you may still feel that you're not ready for the baby and that you won't be able to manage. Some of this will be the fear of the unknown—you have not yet met your baby and it's impossible to predict what the labor—and the weeks that follow it—will be like.

Although you may not feel fully prepared, be confident that you'll know how to take care of your newborn. In fact, you'll have probably already started the process of becoming a mother, wanting to nurture and protect your baby even before she's born, and this natural instinct will continue.

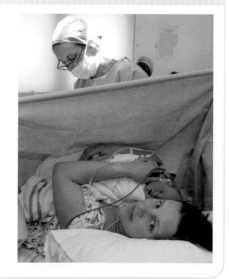

**ASK A... DOCTOR**

**What's the difference between an emergency and elective cesarean?**

An elective cesarean is when a planned decision is made during pregnancy to deliver the baby by cesarean section before the onset of labor. This is usually decided upon for medical reasons, although some women may decide to have an elective cesarean for practical reasons or to avoid having to go through labor.

An emergency cesarean is when a situation arises, usually in labor, that means the safest route for delivery is by cesarean section.

**MRSA: IS IT A RISK?**

**There's a great deal of media coverage of "superbugs,"** such as MRSA. This is a bacterium that can live harmlessly on the skin of healthy people, but can lead to infection in vulnerable individuals. Good hygiene, particularly in the form of precautions such as hand-washing, is an effective method in the prevention of MRSA and your chances of acquiring the infection in hospital are low.

If cutlery and plates are washed using detergent and hot water this removes MRSA, and the risk of acquiring MRSA through contact with curtains, sheets, and pillows is very low. Health-care workers use antiseptic solutions, such as alcohol hand rubs, and more recently many hospitals are taking steps to prevent transmission of MRSA.

In addition to general hygiene measures, hospitals prevent the spread of MRSA by treating those infected with antibiotics, and by detecting cases early so that they can isolate affected patients. Infected patients are moved to a private room or to a room with others who have MRSA.

The final details of your baby's appearance—including eyebrows, eyelashes, and nails—are now in place and all her internal organs are sufficiently developed for life outside the uterus.

# 1 day to go...

## YOUR BABY TODAY

It's been wonderful to see your baby's progress and facial features as each day of the pregnancy has passed by. 2D and 3D ultrasound images, as well as MRI, have all played a part in giving us a glimpse into the fascinating and complex world of life before birth.

Your newborn's stomach will be fully developed, but low acid levels mean she can only be fed milk for the first few months.

### RASPBERRY LEAF TEA

**Raspberry leaf tea is a traditional remedy in Europe.** European studies have found that drinking this tea in the months prior to delivery (not before week 30) helps shorten the second stage of labor by helping the uterine muscles to contract more efficiently, so that contractions are more effective.

The tea is also said to reduce the risk of having an assisted delivery, such as emergency cesarean or vacuum (see p.437).

In addition to this, raspberry leaf tea is believed to help the uterus to contract back to its normal size after the birth, and encourage the flow of breast milk.

As always you should talk to your doctor, before drinking any herbal teas or or taking any kind of herbal remedies.

**Unlike an adult, your baby produces** little gastric acid and keeps amniotic fluid in the stomach longer; it is this fluid that helps keep the acid content of her stomach low. While your baby is in the uterus hiccupping, turning upside down, and trying to coordinate breathing with swallowing, not having much hydrochloric acid in the stomach is a good idea.

After birth the acid content of your baby's stomach will increase quickly in the first 24 hours but not reach adult levels until three months. This is why solids aren't introduced until a baby is at least four months old, although six months is the current advice on when to start weaning. Babies have a reflex to spit out solid food if it's introduced too early and will only be able to take about 20–25 ml of food before the stomach is full. So it's easy to see how the stomach can quickly be overloaded, resulting in spitting up, which is when the baby brings the food and some milk back up.

### THE LOWDOWN

## Take a break

**Getting to know your newborn** can be difficult if there's a constant stream of visitors bearing gifts and good wishes. Why not shut out the world and spend a few days home alone? Your newborn baby will sleep a lot, so take the opportunity to do the same. There will be plenty of time for people to meet the new member of your family.

Your hormones will be all over the place, so expect to experience lows as well as highs, especially when your milk comes in (see pp.448–9).

Your partner also needs time to bond with his baby, nurture you both, and come to grips with diaper changing.

So stick a message on the front door, switch on the answering machine, and snuggle up with your new family.

### ASK A... DOCTOR

**What exactly is a "bloody show"?** During pregnancy, a plug of jellylike mucus seals the lower end of your cervix and this prevents infection from getting into your uterus (see p.411). This "plug" comes away toward the end of pregnancy—known as a "bloody show"—and although this can mean that labor is going to start soon, it can also dislodge up to six weeks before your labor actually starts.

YOU ARE 40 WEEKS EXACTLY

# 0 days to go...

**YOUR BABY TODAY**

Your baby is now ready for the outside world. Sudden changes will take place with that first breath after delivery, as she immediately adapts from her time within the fluid-filled environment of the uterus to life in the air outside.

You've reached 40 weeks exactly! It may have seemed like a long wait, but it will be worth it once you're holding your baby.

**Congratulations! If you don't yet have your newborn baby in your arms,** you soon will, and your life will be changed forever. Even the longest pregnancy seems unaccountably short when your labor begins, and the reality begins to hit that you'll soon be holding your newborn.

You'll get through the labor; and you'll forget about the discomfort after a few good sessions detailing it to family and close friends. In fact, everything that precedes that moment when you hold your newborn baby for the first time becomes inconsequential when you realize that you have created the most wondrous thing of all: a new life. So good luck and well done! This is only just the beginning of the most amazing years of your life.

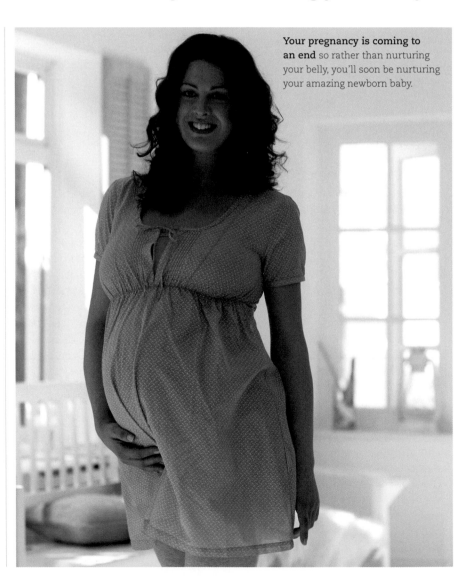

**Your pregnancy is coming to an end** so rather than nurturing your belly, you'll soon be nurturing your amazing newborn baby.

**AS A MATTER OF FACT**

**58 percent of parents questioned in a recent survey** believed that the name they gave their baby would contribute to his or her success in life.

More found it easier to name a boy than a girl, and just 3 percent said they would change the name they'd given their baby if they could.

# Overdue baby

Your baby is described as being overdue if you have not gone into labor by the time you are 40 weeks' pregnant. This is not unusual since most women do not go into labor at exactly 40 weeks, and anything between 37 and 42 weeks is considered to be normal.

**Why labor is late** As the exact trigger that sets off labor is unknown, it's not clear why some women are overdue. You are more likely to be overdue if this is your first baby, if you've had an overdue baby before, or if the condition runs in your family. Some think it's more common in well nourished women, and there is even evidence that pregnancies are longer in the summer than in the winter. If your due date was figured out from an early ultrasound, this gives a more accurate dating of pregnancy than the date of your last menstrual period, and you'll be less likely to be classified as overdue.

## What will be done

After 41 weeks, there is a slightly increased risk to your baby's health that may be due to the reduced efficiency of the placenta. After 42 weeks the risk increases, but is still small. Depending on hospital policy, you will be offered an induction around 41 weeks (see p.432). The following may also be done.

**Stripping the membranes** After 40 weeks, your doctor may do an internal examination to "strip the membranes." She'll insert a gloved finger into the cervix and pull the membranes in a circular pattern. This can soften the cervix and increase the chance of you going into labor by 30 percent in the next 48 hours. It's safe for you and your baby, but can cause cramps and slight bleeding.

**Assessments after 42 weeks** Many doctors induce labor by 41 or 42 weeks. If your pregnancy goes beyond 42 weeks and you don't want to be induced, your

**Going over your due date** can be stressful, but it may help to remind yourself that it's also extremely common and quite normal.

doctor may offer monitoring with scans to measure the baby's pulse and volume of fluid around the baby; or you may have a NST (see p.418) once or twice a week until labor to pick up any signs that the placenta is failing. If a problem is found, you'll be advised to have a cesarean or an induction of labor.

## How you're feeling

You might find the physical and mental stress of being pregnant beyond your due date considerable but it can help to know that unless you have a medical condition, being overdue does not significantly increase your health risks. You may worry that your baby will grow too large, causing difficulty in labor, but your baby isn't likely to put on enough weight in the last week or so to make a big difference and most overdue babies have a normal birthweight.

---

**AT-HOME STRATEGIES**

## Bringing on labor

Although no "home" or alternative remedy has been proven to bring on labor, there are several harmless techniques that are thought to assist the body's natural processes.

■ **Probably the most enjoyable way to try to bring on labor is to make love** with your partner. Sperm contains prostaglandins that may act as a natural uterine stimulant, although the evidence that this works is inconclusive. Making love is not dangerous to your baby, unless your doctor has specifically told you to refrain from intercourse for a medical reason, such as fetal growth restriction or placental bleeding.

■ **Nipple stimulation during sex** or by itself can cause the release of oxytocin from your pituitary gland, which is linked to contractions and cervical ripening.

■ **Walking and exercise** may cause a mild increase in uterine contractions by helping the baby move down the pelvis, putting pressure on the cervix.

■ **Raspberry leaf** has been associated with increased uterine activity. Very little research has been done studying the use of raspberry leaf in pregnant women, so it's best to avoid this herbal remedy unless your doctor gives you the go-ahead and your pregnancy is already full-term.

As the moment you've so eagerly anticipated approaches, you may have increasing concerns about what lies in store for you during the labor and delivery, and doubts as to whether you'll be able to cope with the physical and mental demands during this crucial time. Being as informed as possible about the progress of labor and your options for pain relief are both important first steps in enabling you to face labor and birth with a positive mindset.

# Labor
# and birth

# Pain relief options

**A PRIOR KNOWLEDGE OF PAIN RELIEF WILL HELP YOU MAKE INFORMED CHOICES IN LABOR**

Once in labor, in addition to needing emotional and physical support, which your doctor, nurse, or midwife and birth partner will provide, you may also need some form of pain relief to help you cope. They will help you work with your labor pain by employing natural methods such as breathing techniques. If you need stronger pain relief, they'll advise you on medical methods, such as analgesics or an epidural (see pp.402–407).

# Coping with pain

To help you cope with labor and birth, it's important to have an understanding of the progress of pain during labor.

Labor pain is unique and quite different from everyday chronic and acute pain. Generally, pain is a warning sign that something is wrong, but labor pain acts as an "alert" that the birth process is underway and that you need a safe environment in which to give birth. Some women prefer a homelike environment, which has been shown to have many benefits, including reducing the need for medical forms of pain relief. For this reason, many labor rooms in maternity units and especially birth centers have homey decoration and furnishings to make them feel less medicalized. Other women need the reassurance provided by hospitals that stronger forms of pain relief and medical backup are available.

**Being informed about the pain of labor** can reduce your anxiety and help you manage.

## How women react to pain

No one really knows what starts labor and every woman's labor is unique. Likewise, the pain associated with labor can vary enormously between women. Some women have relatively painless labors, while some describe the pain as moderate, and others experience severe pain. One thing that does seem clear is that anxiety and fear increase the levels of adrenaline, which in turn can increase the intensity of the pain experienced. The strength of labor pain can also be affected by factors such as your emotional state and anticipation of labor; your previous experiences, if any; cultural beliefs; and, in particular for first-time mothers, the fear of the unknown. Thorough preparation prior to labor and sensitive and caring support throughout labor and birth can help reduce anxiety and fear considerably.

## Thinking ahead

The sensation of pain is different during the different stages of labor, and as labor progresses the intensity and duration of the pain increases. The most effective methods of dealing with pain will also change as your labor progresses (see box, left).

The more familiar you are with the methods of dealing with pain and with the several natural and drug-induced methods of pain relief available (see following pages), the easier it will be for you to manage during labor and birth. To make decisions about pain relief, you will also need to understand the changes that take place in your body during the three different stages of labor (see pp.408–29).

---

### PAIN RELIEF THROUGHOUT LABOR

**Your pain-relief requirements may change during labor,** so it helps to be aware of when different types of pain relief can help.

**Early first stage** In this phase, the cervix begins to dilate. Contractions are mild, and you may find that natural methods, such as massage and breathing, are helpful. If you need stronger pain relief, you may be given analgesics, which dull pain but allow you to remain active since you won't lose all feeling or muscle movement.

**Active first stage** The cervix now starts to dilate more quickly and contractions are stronger and closer together. Some women are happy to continue with natural or analgesic pain relief; others may need stronger relief and an epidural may be given at this point (see pp.404–5).

**Transition** Contractions are intense and frequent as the cervix dilates fully. Systemic (IV) analgesics aren't usually given this close to the birth since they could affect the baby. If you have an epidural already in place, this can be topped off.

**Second and third stages** Stage two lasts from full dilation of the cervix until birth; contractions are strong and longer lasting, but easier to manage since you start pushing. Analgesics may be used. In the 3rd stage, delivery of the placenta, contractions are mild and you shouldn't need pain relief.

# Natural pain relief

Many women opt for natural pain relief in labor, or choose to complement medical pain relief with natural methods.

During your labor, encephalins and endorphins (feel-good hormones) are released to provide you with some naturally induced pain relief. Many women now are also more aware of natural techniques, such as staying active, and of the availability of complementary therapies that they can use in addition to, or instead of, medical pain relief during pregnancy, childbirth, and following the birth. Some of these therapies are self administered and some are practitioner administered. A knowledge of the benefits of different therapies and how to use them is important if you are considering using them to deal with pain in labor.

## Staying active

Being active in labor has been shown to help women to deal with pain and reduce the length of labor. Historically, women have been active in labor for centuries, but a medicalization of childbirth in the West led to an acceptance that women lie in bed, and a common image of a laboring woman is one lying in bed. Although during labor you may want to rest on a bed between contractions, many women find that when they feel supported, they will instinctively move around and do not cope well lying down, which can increase pain and hamper the progress of labor as your baby pushes against gravity. You may find it helpful to take a walk, roll on a birthing ball, rock in a rocking chair or change positions when you get too uncomfortable. There are certain interventions, such as the use of electronic fetal monitoring (see p.418), IVs, and some types of analgesia, that will limit your mobility.

---

**RELAXATION TECHNIQUES**

**There are various techniques you can use to help you relax during labor;** if you're relaxed, it will be easier to stay calm and in tune with your body. These techniques include focusing on your breathing (see below); listening to music (perhaps humming to the beat of a favorite tune during a contraction); and listening to a meditation CD.

Learning how to breathe slowly and steadily in labor helps you focus and stay calm. Usually, your breathing responds to how you're feeling and may increase slightly during a contraction, or you may hold your breath, which can make you feel light-headed. If this happens, you need to focus and steady your breathing. Your nurse will remind you to breathe slowly and steadily. Breathing in for five and out for seven slows your breathing down, helps you relax, and stops you from panicking.

**Concentrating on your breathing** in labor is calming and helps you focus (top). **Leaning forward while breathing** steadily can be comforting during contractions (bottom).

**Listening to some of your favorite music** in the first stage of labor is a great way to relax between contractions, enabling you to let go and reserve energy for later in labor.

**Once the electrodes for TENS** are positioned on your back, you will be free to move around and find comfortable positions.

## TENS

TENS stands for Transcutaneous Electrical Nerve Stimulation, and is a small electrical device that reduces pain signals sent to the brain. In addition to being used in labor, the device can also be used at the end of pregnancy (after 36 weeks) if you have a backache or uncomfortable Braxton Hicks' contractions (see p.410).

The battery-operated TENS machine has thin wires that are connected to four electrodes, or sticky pads, which are taped to the lower back. The machine is thought to work by sending electrical impulses from the machine along nerve roots to the pain pathways in the brain, thereby blocking pain impulses. It's also thought to stimulate the brain to produce "feel good" encephalins and endorphins, which can modulate the pain.

TENS is most effective in early labor, particularly for lower back pain, and it is therefore important to have the device available at the beginning of labor. It's therefore worth finding out if your hospital has TENS machines or whether you need to rent one in advance. You can hold the device or have it near you in labor and can increase the strength of the electrical impulse with a button as your contractions get stronger.

There are several advantages to TENS. It has few side effects; it allows you to remain active; and it can be used in combination with other types of pain relief. The disadvantages are that there hasn't been much research done about its safety for the baby, so a theoretical risk exists, and it is generally effective with just mild to moderate pain; the sticky pads mean that a back massage is not possible; and it isn't possible to labor in water or have an epidural inserted while using the device.

## Water

Many women find being in warm water during labor very soothing and an excellent way to cope with labor pain. The warmth of the water soothes muscles, promoting relaxation, and being in water aids buoyancy, which can help relieve the pressure on your pelvis. Over the last decade or so, this natural method has become more available for women and many hospitals and birth centers provide bathtubs. Whether or not you can actually deliver your baby in the water will depend on the hospital's policy and whether there are any doctors or midwives trained in water births (see p.427). You can also purchase or rent a birthing pool.

## Hypnosis

Self-hypnosis, using visualization and breathing techniques to induce a state of deep relaxation and banish fear, is an increasingly popular means of dealing with labor, and is referred to as "HypnoBirthing." This is based on the "fear-tension-pain" syndrome of

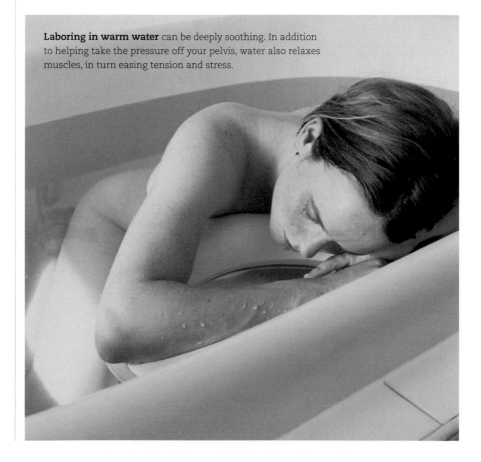

**Laboring in warm water** can be deeply soothing. In addition to helping take the pressure off your pelvis, water also relaxes muscles, in turn easing tension and stress.

## QUESTIONS AND ANSWERS

**Will I be able to stay active in labor?**
Yes, most women are able to remain active through labor and are encouraged to do so, perhaps using props such as a chair, beanbag, or birthing ball. Staying active can help since this can speed up labor, and changing your position can help you deal with labor pain. When you arrive at the hospital or birth center, discuss your birth plan with the doctor and inform her that you want to be as active as possible.

**Will I lose control if I use hypnosis during my labor?** No, you will simply feel deeply relaxed, but will still be in control and know what you are doing. Don't worry—self-hypnosis will help you be less anxious and frightened during your labor, which will help you to deal with labor pain. With preparation, your partner can help you stay focused and use some hypnotic techniques too.

**I've had a previous cesarean. Does this mean that I won't be able to labor in water this time?** It depends on the procedures that your health-care provider follows for women who have already had a cesarean. After a cesarean, the doctors will want to monitor you and the baby either continuously or frequently during labor, because there is a very small chance that your uterus may rupture, which is often only detected through a change in the baby's heartbeat. But waterproof monitoring systems are widely available and many practices perform WBAC— water birth after cesarean.

**At what point can I get into the birthing pool?** This is up to you. Relaxing in warm water is often suggested in the early stages of labor, as long as your contractions are progressing. You can sit in the warm water for 1½ to 2 hours for pain management, but then get out. Changing your environment helps keep your labor active.

childbirth first described by the English obstetrician Grantly Dick-Read (see p.303), who believed that fear prevents the release of the "feel good hormones," endorphins and encephalins. He maintained that when fear is eliminated, most women can give birth naturally. With HypnoBirthing, you are fully aware of what is happening around you, but may feel as though you're daydreaming or drifting off to sleep. You and your birth partner can attend HypnoBirthing classes anytime during pregnancy to learn the techniques before labor. To find a class in your area, visit hypnobirthing.com/findapract.htm.

## Acupuncture

This uses fine needles placed at specific points on the body to reduce pain by stimulating the production of endorphins. Acupuncture is a traditional form of Chinese medicine that believes there are channels within the body through which energy, or "chi" runs. Blockages can occur in these channels, and so by inserting needles at certain points, energy is unblocked, relieving pain and restoring balance to the body. Many women find acupuncture helpful to treat mild pregnancy symptoms, and some women use this therapy during labor. Acupuncture has no harmful side effects for the mother or baby and in labor, needles will usually be inserted in points that do not restrict your movement, for example in the ear. If you want to have acupuncture during labor, you will need to look for an acupuncturist who specializes in this area and arrange to have him or her with you during labor.

## MASSAGE AND TOUCH

**Many women find massage helpful in labor** to induce relaxation, bring about a sense of well-being, and alleviate pain. Your birth partner may find it relaxing and therapeutic too. Ideally, he or she will have had a chance to see massage techniques demonstrated in prenatal classes and to practice before labor. Massaging the lower back helps relieve pain in this area; head, neck, and shoulder massage is beneficial for relieving tension and fatigue.

The touch therapies shiatsu and acupressure can also help relieve pain and tension. They involve application of pressure to specific points to increase endorphin levels. You or your partner will need to learn the techniques from a trained practitioner. Ask your doctor if she can put you in touch with a practitioner.

**Your partner can use** the heel of his hand to apply firm pressure to your sacrum. The hands can be alternated to stroke around the lower back.

**Using the thumbs** to massage the lower back in a circular motion, working from the base of the spine down to the buttocks, can release tense muscles.

**Applying deep pressure** to the buttocks and lower back with the thumbs can help you focus and release held-in tension during contractions.

## Homeopathy

This is based on the principle of treating like with like. Talk to your doctor before using any homeopathic products during pregnancy or labor, since homeopathy is an area of complementary and alternative medicine that's associated with much debate and scientific controversy. If your doctor gives you the okay, a certified homeopath can prescribe remedies based on your individual needs. There is a lack of scientific evidence on the effectiveness of homeopathy, although many women find the remedies helpful.

## Aromatherapy

Aromatherapy (essential) oils are derived from plants and used for their therapeutic properties. The use of these oils in childbirth can stimulate, refresh, and soothe you and to some extent your partner. There is some evidence that oils, such as lavender, reduce anxiety in labor, which in turn helps you cope with pain. Hot and cold compresses with essential oils added to the water used to wet the cloth can be soothing and massaging diluted essential oils (in a carrier oil) into the skin is therapeutic. Many experts recommend against aromatherapy during pregnancy and labor because some scents may be hazardous to pregnant women. The effects of most plant oils on pregnant women is unknown.

## Reflexology

Reflexology involves massaging reflex zones on your feet that correspond with different parts of your body to improve your blood circulation and relax any tension you may be feeling. Reflexology is gaining some popularity as a coping technique in the early stages of labor. However, because many women naturally want to be active and move around during their labor, this may be more helpful in between early contractions.

---

### BIRTH STORY: A NATURAL HOME BIRTH

Jenna is a 31-year-old mom and this is her second labor. She had a straightforward birth with her daughter, now three. This pregnancy was uneventful, so she decided to have a home birth this time.

**Jenna's story:** When I was eight days overdue, my midwife did a "stretch and strip" (see p.393) of my cervix to encourage labor. I then had a couple of bloody shows (see p.411) and irregular contractions. In the night I woke with contractions 20 minutes apart. I couldn't get back to sleep, so I had a warm bath, took a couple of acetaminophens, and went back to bed. My daughter woke at 6:45 am and we had breakfast. My contractions were every 10 minutes and getting stronger, so my husband stayed home.

By 8:00 am, my contractions were every 5 minutes, stronger, and lasting 50–60 seconds. My husband called the midwife. She said she was on her way and advised me to stay active. I started to use the TENS machine (see p.399) on a low setting, which helped me focus. I found standing and rocking my pelvis back and forth and from side to side helpful and I used a birthing ball. My husband was supportive, massaging my shoulders and under my abdomen where it hurt most; I found the heat from his hands soothing. My daughter held my hand.

At 8:40 am, the midwife arrived. She checked my blood pressure, pulse, and temperature, felt my belly, listened to the baby's heart, and took a urine sample, which relieved some pressure in my pubic area. She confirmed that I was in established labor since my cervix was 5 cm dilated. My cervix was thinning, the head was pressing down, and my membranes were intact. I remained active, using TENS, and leaning forward. My husband put on a relaxing CD.

At 9:50 am my contractions were every two minutes, very strong, and lasting 60 seconds. I tried walking and marching on the spot. My mom arrived and took my daughter to the park. I felt hot and so I had a cool drink and my midwife dabbed my face with a cool, wet cloth. I found kneeling on all fours, rocking and arching my back, helpful.

By 10:30 am my contractions were very painful. My midwife listened to the heartbeat intermittently.

By 11:00 am I felt an urge to push. My water broke and my contractions were very strong and each minute. I felt panicky, but my midwife encouraged me, saying she thought the baby would be born soon; my husband helped me focus by breathing slowly. My midwife confirmed that I was fully dilated and ready to push. I somehow found the energy to bear down and felt the head emerge. I took a breath, concentrated, and pushed my baby out. My baby boy was born at 11:14 am, 8 lb 2 oz, and my husband cut the cord once it had stopped pulsating. I delivered my placenta without drugs (see p.429). My midwife advised me to put my baby to my breast to stimulate the hormone oxytocin, which causes contractions and helps the placenta to come away. My placenta was delivered at 11:40 am.

---

**The midwife's comments:** Jenna and her husband prepared well and worked as a team. Jenna was active for most of labor, and stayed focused. Her feelings of panic in the transition period were normal, but her husband and I gave her extra support. By working with her instincts she found inner strength and had a normal birth. Her labor was nine hours, about average for a second-time mom.

# Drugs for pain relief

Various types of medication are available for pain relief during labor; many can be used alongside natural forms of pain relief.

**Up until 150 years ago,** there were few options for pain relief during childbirth.

The history of modern obstetric pain relief began in the mid-19th century with the discovery of chloroform. Nitrous oxide and opioids followed and at the start of the 20th century, enthusiasm for pain-relieving drugs was so great that they were overused, with women in labor in a state of near-unconsciousness. The natural childbirth movement in the 1960s and 1970s was a reaction to such overuse of drugs. In the 1970s another revolution was at hand as epidurals became available.

**Discussing different pain relief options** with your doctor prior to labor can help you assess the merits of each type and to think about what type of pain relief you would prefer.

For some, natural pain relief may not be sufficient to enable them to deal with the increasing intensity of contractions, and they may choose to use medication in combination with natural techniques. In some situations, for example if labor is induced (see p.432) or augmented (see p.415), contractions may start strongly rather than build up gradually and a stronger type of pain relief may be needed.

There are several types of medical pain relief available, which fall into two groups. Analgesic drugs dull the perception of pain, while anesthesia, which may be regional or general, numbs pain totally. In regional anesthesia, also known as a nerve block, local anesthetic drugs are injected around nerves that supply a particular area. There are several types of regional nerve block: epidurals and spinal blocks numb sensation in the abdomen and are used to reduce the pain of contractions; a pudendal block numbs sensation in the vagina and perineum and may be used in a forceps delivery. Occasionally, a general anesthetic is given during a cesarean.

Since all labors are different, it's not possible to have a "one size fits all" approach to pain relief. Being flexible and informed will help you feel in control. Read any literature from your doctor, go to prenatal classes, and ask questions. Try to eliminate any worries by increasing your knowledge, for example by asking if it's possible to attend a childbirth education class at the hospital that discusses the pros and cons of each type of pain relief. Keep in mind that some childbirth classes, like Lamaze and the Bradley method, can teach you breathing and relaxation techniques that may help reduce your need for pain medication during labor.

## Natural pain relief

Whether you're still at home and it's too early in labor to get pain medication, or you're trying to wait it out at the hospital to see if you really need drugs, you can try any or all of the following techniques that may help to relieve pain without medication:

- Taking a warm bath or shower
- Changing your position
- Meditation
- Hypnosis
- Getting a back massage from your partner
- Walking around
- Meditation

## Pain relief plan

Having a birth plan ahead of time that outlines the circumstances during which you would resort to using medication for pain relief may be helpful for some women. For example, you may want to try to remain medication-free unless the pain is so intense, it interferes with your ability to hold a normal conversation, or it doubles you over in pain. Perhaps you'll seek relief if your labor drags on hours longer than you expected and you need some respite to sleep for a while to regain your strength for the upcoming pushing that you'll be doing. Whatever the case, you may feel more in control if you know ahead of time what your limits are and when you want to say yes to pain medication, rather than being overwhelmed by the situation, if you don't give it much thought beforehand.

## Opioids

These belong to a group of drugs called narcotics (which literally means sleep-inducing), which includes morphine.

They attach themselves to receptors in the brain or nerves and block the transmission of pain.

**Tranquilizers** These drugs don't relieve pain, but they can help to relieve anxiety and help a women relax for several hours during early labor. Some women who are very anxious about the impending pain or of labor and childbirth may seek this sort of medication. Tranquilizers may be given orally, intravenously, or injected into a large muscle. Oral dosage takes the longest to take effect. Some women dislike what tranquilizers do to them, since they may feel drowsy and out of control. If the dose is very high, women may nod off between contractions. It may be hard for a woman to fully remember her labor experience if she's taken tranquilizers. The drugs also effect the baby, decreasing his activity and muscle tone during and after birth. For these reasons, tranquilizers are not for everyone, but in certain circumstances, they can help a woman feel less anxious about labor.

---

### ASPIRIN: NOT FOR LABOR PAIN

**When you start to experience the pain of labor contractions** at home, no matter how tempting it may be, do not reach for an aspirin to relieve your pain. Aspirin can be extremely dangerous during pregnancy, particularly in the third trimester and leading up to labor and delivery. The drug interferes with your blood-clotting ability, which means that your risk of a hemorrhage during delivery increases if you take aspirin in the weeks leading up to your baby's birth. Taking too much aspirin in the last trimester may actually prolong labor. Bleeding problems may even develop in your newborn. Taking aspirin regularly toward the end of your pregnancy can also

affect your baby's heart or blood flow, so it's best to avoid aspirin, unless your doctor recommends you take it. Your best bet for dealing with labor pain at home is to keep active until it's time to head to the hospital. While you wait, do something to distract yourself from the pain, whether it's counting the length of time between contractions, packing your bag for the hospital or anything else that feels right. Ask your partner for a massage or try a warm shower. No matter what you do, refrain from drug use. This way, if you need pain relief when you get to the hospital—many women do—you won't have any medication in your system.

---

# Opioids

### Advantages

■ Opioids help you to relax during labor, which can help you to conserve your energy between contractions.

■ Opioids can produce a feeling of well-being, which many women find beneficial during labor.

### Disadvantages

■ Many women report feeling nauseous with opioids, which can be an unexpected and unpleasant side effect on top of your pain and contractions.

■ Opioids can cause dizziness, and this can be can be disorientating during labor.

■ Some women have reported feeling out of control with some opioid medications and therefore out of touch with how their labor is progressing.

■ Opioids cross the placenta easily and pass into the baby's bloodstream. This can have the affect of sedating the baby and can affect the baby's breathing after the delivery. The administration of opioid medications therefore needs to be carefully timed during labor so that they are not given too close to the time of the delivery of the baby.

■ Opioids can depress the mother's breathing during labor. However, this side effect is more common when the mother has a preexisting respiratory illness, such as asthma or emphysema.

■ Opioids cause a delay in emptying the bowels and therefore increase the overall risk to the mother should general anesthesia be needed later on (see p.406).

## PROS AND CONS

# Considering an epidural

### Pros

■ An epidural provides absolute pain relief in 90 percent of cases; 10 percent of women have some degree of residual pain, but still have a marked improvement in their overall discomfort.

■ Epidurals do not pose any risk to your baby.

■ The presence of an effective epidural means that if intervention is needed at any time, the epidural can be topped off with anesthetic for either an assisted delivery with forceps or vacuum, or a cesarean delivery. This also reduces the likelihood that a general anesthetic will be needed.

### Cons

■ Around 1 in 10 women do not experience absolute pain relief with an epidural.

■ Some women develop a headache that persists after an epidural (see p.406).

■ A rare complication is patches of heaviness in the legs or feet.

### There are a few very rare risks with an epidural

■ In common with all invasive procedures, inserting an epidural can result in infection. Meningitis occurs in around 1 in 100,000 women and an epidural abscess occurs in about 1 in 50,000 women.

■ There is a 1 in 170,000 risk of developing a blood clot in the epidural space (epidural hematoma).

■ There is a 1 in 100,000 risk of the epidural tube moving into the fluid around the spine and resulting in unconsciousness, and there is a 1 in 250,000 chance of the epidural causing some form of paralysis.

## Epidurals

An epidural is a regional anesthetic that can be given at any stage of labor to numb the abdomen and therefore block the pain of contractions, but it's typically given when the woman is at least 4 cm dilated. In some cases, if a woman's labor progresses very quickly and she doesn't request one right away, she may not be able to get one before delivery. Epidurals are the most popular form of pain relief during labor in the US, with more than half of pregnant women delivering in hospitals choosing this treatment.

**How epidurals work** A hollow needle is inserted between two vertebrae in the lower back. A tiny plastic tube is then passed through the needle and into the epidural space surrounding the spinal cord. A local anesthetic is injected into the needle and flows through the tube into the epidural space so that the nerve roots carrying the pain stimulus to the brain are coated with anesthetic and pain is reduced or completely blocked. This will affect sensation in your legs so that you need to remain in bed and your baby will be closely monitored. A stronger epidural also affects sensation in your bladder, so you will need to have a catheter. Used late in labor, a stonger epidural may mean that you need help to push the baby out, since the pelvic floor muscles will be heavy and ineffective. In this case, your doctor will put a hand on your abdomen to feel when a contraction starts and will tell you when to push. In some cases, an assisted delivery (see pp.436–7) becomes necessary.

**When are epidurals used?** Epidurals can be used throughout labor, but they're typically given during active labor when a woman is 4–5 cm dilated. Since everyone has varying pain thresholds, the time when one is requested varies. There are factors to bear in mind should you opt for an epidural late in labor. To minimize the risks, you must remain completely still during the placement of the epidural tube. If your labor has progressed too far to enable you to do this, the anesthesiologist may refuse to proceed with an epidural for your own interest. Also, if you choose to have an epidural late in labor, it may be necessary to give a high dose so that it takes effect in time, which has disadvantages (see left).

If you're considering using an epidural, inform your doctor early in labor so that she can consult the anesthesiologist. The anesthesiologist may then discuss this with you and take a brief medical history to ensure that it's safe for you to have an epidural. She will discuss any risks, and answer any questions that you or your partner has, all of which can save time later on if you decide to go ahead.

There are occasions when an epidural is not advised. These include cases where a woman has had spinal surgery or is taking blood-thinning medication. Rarely, a woman may have an infection that could be exacerbated by an epidural.

**Side effects** There are a number of minor side effects. The medication can cause blood pressure to fall, so this will be monitored (see p.405). If it does fall, you'll be given fluids and medication, and subsequent doses may be reduced.

It's common to expericene itching with epidurals, caused by the release of histamine from the opioid component of a mobile epidural. Histamine is a substance released by the body during an allergic reaction that can cause itching. The itch can be treated, but in most cases it gets better on its own. If you develop an itch, a greater concentration of local anesthetic alone will be used.

It's not unusual to shiver with an epidural, although this is a more common side effect if a concentrated local anesthetic is used, as is the case for a cesarean delivery.

Epidural pain relief can cause a rise in temperature. If this occurs, you'll have a

**If you opt for an epidural**, the doctor should explain the procedure to you, and you should have the opportunity to ask the anesthesiologist any questions.

**Getting ready for an epidural** Before starting the epidural, a plastic tube will be placed in a vein in the back of your hand or in your arm, to which an IV containing fluid will be connected. You are given fluids during an epidural to stop your blood pressure from dropping. The doctor will then help you into the correct position to receive the epidural, which will either be sitting up with your legs over the side of the bed leaning forward, or curled up on your side on the edge of the bed. The position may depend on the preference of the anesthesiologist.

Your lower back will be cleaned with antiseptic and a drape placed over the rest of your back to reduce the risk of infection. Before the epidural needle is inserted, a local anesthetic will be given into the skin and surrounding tissues. This creates a numb patch to ensure that the insertion of the large epidural needle is not painful. When the local anesthetic is injected, you may feel a scratching sensation and experience a very short-lived sting in the area between the vertebrae bones

**The procedure** Since it's important for you to remain still during the procedure, the anesthesiologist will insert the epidural between your contractions. If this is difficult, you should try to concentrate on your breathing and remain as still as possible until the procedure is completed. You will feel a pushing sensation in your back while the anesthesiologist is trying to find the very small epidural space with the hollow needle. When the space is located, a tiny plastic tube will be fed into it through the needle. The epidural needle is then removed and the tube, which is secured onto your back with sticky tape, remains in the epidural space. The tube remains in place until your baby is delivered and, because it is very thin, soft, and pliable, it is perfectly safe to lie on the tube and to move around.

**Managing the epidural** Once the epidural tube is successfully in place, the anesthesiologist will give the first dose of medication through it by means of a syringe. Once she is satisfied that the epidural is in the correct position and is working effectively, all subsequent doses, or "top ups," can be given without another injection. Your blood pressure will be taken once the epidural is in place and will be monitored for the next half an hour or so, and then regularly thereafter, including after each top up. Each dose of medication takes around 10–20 minutes to take its full effect and can last between one and two hours. The epidural will be topped up as required, usually around every three to four hours, to keep you comfortable throughout your labor. An anesthesiologist should be available 24 hours a day to manage any concerns or problems that may arise with the epidural.

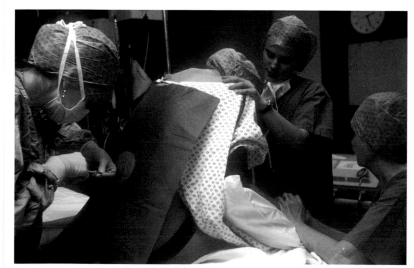

**Before the epidural is given**, your back will be covered with a sterile sheet and then a local anesthetic will be given to numb the area so that you don't experience pain when the larger epidural needle is inserted.

**The anesethetic** is given through a tube that is inserted into the epidural space, avoiding the spinal cord and its covering.

Vertebra

Epidural space

Syringe attachment

Plastic tube

Spinal cord

Drugs for pain relief

blood test to eliminate an infection since this can also cause your temperature to rise. You will be given preventative antibiotics while waiting for the blood test results, and acetaminophen to bring your temperature back to normal.

**Problems with epidurals** In addition to side effects, there can occasionally be problems with the effectiveness of an epidural. The anesthetic may not spread evenly in the epidural space, which may be caused by the epidural tube sitting on one side of the epidural space. This can mean that pain relief only occurs on one side of the body. If this occurs, the anesthesiologist will try to reposition the tube and give another dose of anesthetic. If this doesn't work, the only other solution is to redo the entire epidural.

Sometimes, one spot can remain painful, usually in the groin area or low down in the front of the abdomen, which is referred to as a "missed segment." This results from a single nerve root not being coated with the local anesthetic. Again, the anesthesiologist may reposition the tube. Sometimes, a stronger local anesthetic or an opioid is used to numb the area. If a persistent missed segment is too uncomfortable, the anesthesiologist may do a combined spinal epidural block, known as a CSE (see opposite).

It's thought that epidural pain relief may prolong the second stage of labor. It also increases your chances of having an assisted delivery, especially if a high dose of anesthetic is given toward the end of labor, which affects your ability to push. However, an epidural doesn't increase the chance of a cesarean and doesn't, despite common misconceptions, cause long-term backache after the birth.

## Spinal block

This is similar to an epidural in that a needle is put in your back and pain relief is achieved by blocking nerve fibers that supply the pelvic organs. However, in a spinal block, the needle is passed through the epidural space to pierce the membrane covering the spinal cord (the dura) so that anesthetic can be injected into the fluid around the spinal cord; no tubes are left in place. The needle used for a spinal block is smaller than that used for an epidural, which means it's less painful to insert. There is still a risk of a headache as with an epidural (see left) and the side effects should be treated the same way.

A smaller dose of anesthetic is needed and it works very quickly: pain relief is almost immediate, whereas an epidural takes 10–20 minutes. However, the use of a spinal block is limited because only a single dose of medication can be administered. As a result, spinal blocks are usually reserved for use during a cesarean, or for an assisted delivery when an epidural isn't in place.

## Combined spinal epidural (CSE) or "walking epidural"

This involves both a spinal injection and putting an epidural in place. It's sometimes done when problems are encountered with an epidural (see left) and is also used for a cesarean. A CSE gives pain relief throughout labor. However, it's a specialized technique and isn't offered in all units.

## Pudendal blocks

This type of regional anesthesia involves injecting a local anesthetic into the vagina where the pudendal nerves are located to reduce pain in the vagina and perineum. The pudendal needle is quite long and thick, so before the injection is given, a cold anesthetic spray is applied to the area. The anesthetic has no effect on the baby and can be used with other medications. It takes effect very quickly and is sometimes used just before birth to aid an assisted forceps delivery.

## General anesthesia

Most cesareans are conducted using regional anesthesia. However, in some cases general anesthesia, where the mother is put to sleep, is necessary. This may be because of a failure of regional anesthesia, blood-clotting problems in the mother, an infection in the mother's bloodstream, or persistent fetal distress.

---

### AN EPIDURAL "HEADACHE"

**Some women report a headache after an epidural, which can develop more than 24 hours** after the delivery and tends to be at the front of the head. It is made worse by sitting up and moving around and is much improved by lying down. This occurs in around 1 in 100 women and is caused by the epidural needle moving too far forward and cutting the dura sheath, the membrane maintaining the fluid around the spinal cord and brain. This small hole results in a loss of fluid from the sheath, which causes a headache. The risk is hugely reduced by remaining still during the placement of the epidural. In around 70 percent of women, the hole heals on its own.

You will be advised to drink plenty of fluids and to take simple painkillers, such as acetaminophen and ibuprofen and you will be reviewed at regular intervals by an anesthesiologist.

If the headache persists, a procedure called a "blood patch" will be done. This is done in the sterile environment of an operating room by two anesthesiologists. One places an epidural needle in your back, while the other takes around 20 ml of blood from a vein in your arm. The blood is then passed down the needle into the epidural space. This forms a clot that seals the hole and prevents further leakage of fluid from around your spine, therefore relieving the headache.

Alice was having her first baby. Her pregnancy had been uncomplicated and she had written a birth plan with her husband outlining her desire for a natural childbirth by keeping active and using TENS and then warm water to deal with contractions. Alice also stated that she wanted to avoid an epidural if possible.

**Alice's birth story:** My husband and I arrived at the delivery suite in early labor. I started to use a TENS machine for pain relief. However, as my labor progressed, I became very distressed since I hadn't anticipated that the contractions would be so painful. When I was around 3 cm dilated, I decided to remove the TENS machine and get into the bath. My husband gave me a back massage and provided emotional support. However, I think he struggled to understand my discomfort and he needed support from the nurse. After 15 minutes, I decided to get out of the bath since it was providing little pain relief. I used a birth ball to stay active and my husband gave me more massage and acupressure. I coped well for the next hour, but then became increasingly exhausted and upset. When I was

examined, I was only 5 cm dilated. We both felt despondent because we had hoped I was further along.

My nurse then suggested that I talked to the anesthesiologist about my options for further pain relief, and as a result of my conversation with the anesthesiologist, I decided to have an epidural. I told the anesthesiologist that I'd had an epidural a few years ago for knee surgery and how it had provided excellent pain relief, but that I had itched for hours afterward. The anesthesiologist surmised that the itch was caused by one of the painkilling medications (fentanyl) in the epidural top up and agreed that this medicine wouldn't be used.

The anesthesiologist agreed to do a low dose combined spinal epidural that gave absolute pain relief within five minutes. My legs were a little heavy at first, but they felt fine within an hour. I felt that we were both able to take time out after the epidural and that I was able to refocus on my labor. I felt pleased that I'd managed a large part of my labor without pain relief, and was happy with the decision to have an epidural when I did. I had an unassisted delivery later that evening and gave birth to a beautiful baby girl.

**The anesthesiologist comments:** Alice kept an open mind regarding pain relief and understood that different methods of pain relief could be used at different times during labor. After the epidural, she no longer felt that her labor was an endurance test and was able to focus again on her labor and on delivering a healthy baby.

**A low dose "mobile" epidural** means that you maintain some feeling in your legs and can remain active during labor.

**The procedure** Precautions are taken to minimize the risks to you and your baby. You'll be given an antacid to reduce stomach acid. Often a catheter is inserted into the bladder and antiseptic is applied to the abdomen before you're put to sleep to minimize the baby's exposure to the anesthetic.

As the mother is put to sleep, a face mask is held tightly over her nose and mouth. Because a major risk during general anesthesia is undigested food or liquids in the stomach re-entering the mouth and going into the lungs (which can cause damage) you'll likely be told

not to eat or drink anything once labor begins (because labor usually slows digestion), in case you need general anesthesia. You may be able to have ice chips, though. Once asleep, an anesthesiologist inserts a tube through your mouth and down your throat so that oxygen can easily reach your lungs. You may therefore have a sore throat when you wake up.

During the surgery the anesthesiologist cares for the mother, giving painkillers and anti-nausea medicine when needed. The baby is cared for by the doctor. Depending on hospital procedure, your

partner may or may not be present for the birth. However, no hospitals allow the partner to be present while the mother is being put to sleep.

**After the surgery** The procedure takes about an hour. The mother is woken 5–10 minutes after the surgery. The baby is kept with the mother at all times unless he needs extra care.

Since general anesthesia doesn't give localized pain relief, it's normal to need pain relief afterward. Oral medicine will be given regularly and morphine-based medication may be given for a day or two.

# 1st stage of labor

**WAITING FOR YOUR LABOR TO START CAN BE BOTH FRUSTRATING AND TERRIBLY EXCITING.**

You may be anxious to get your delivery over with, or feel that you aren't ready for labor. This can be an emotional time, so try to stay calm. This section helps you identify the symptoms and signs of labor and takes you through the changes that occur as your body gets ready to give birth.

# Approaching labor

As your pregnancy comes to an end, your cervix starts to soften as your body prepares for the forthcoming labor and birth.

As labor approaches, your body starts to prepare itself for the task ahead and you may notice various physical symptoms and signs that labor is about to start. Not every woman experiences labor in the same way, and certain signs can occur either before labor starts or during labor.

## Common physical symptoms

Toward the end of your pregnancy, you may experience a sensation of building pressure or cramping in your pelvic or rectal area. This pelvic cramping can feel very similar to monthly menstrual cramps. A dull pain in your lower back that comes and goes is common too. You may also notice an increase in heartburn (acid reflux) and gassiness. Unless you have a high-risk pregnancy, there is no need to go to the hospital or call your doctor if you experience any of these symptoms in the later stages of your pregnancy.

## Your emotional state

This is a time of waiting and many women busy themselves with household tasks. These bursts of activity are often thought to be instinctual, as the mother prepares the home for the new arrival, referred to as "nesting." The anticipation of what will happen during labor can give rise to a mixture of emotions, from fear and anxiety to excitement and impatience. Women may feel fearful about how much pain they will feel or how uncomfortable they will be with bodily functions. Nothing can prepare you fully for how you will feel in labor, but the more you understand about pain relief options (see pp.397–401) beforehand, the more confident you will feel about your ability to manage. It's also thought that by being informed and prepared, you are likely to reduce your anxiety during labor, which in itself can enable you cope better with the pain of contractions.

### Preparing for labor

The period before labor starts can last for hours or even days, particularly with a first labor. So that you can manage when you go into labor, you need to take care of yourself during this pre-labor stage.

■ **Stay well rested** so that you aren't completely exhausted when you go into labor.

■ **If you're having trouble resting,** possibly because of anxiety or discomfort, try practicing relaxation techniques, such as breathing or visualization techniques, whereby you focus on a tranquil setting to induce a state of calm.

■ **Continue eating to keep your energy levels up** and provide fuel for the days ahead. You may not feel like eating a large meal; instead eat little and often. Opt for wholesome snacks such as dried fruit, nuts, or a whole-wheat sandwich, and drink lots of fluids.

■ **If you're suffering with back pain, try showering in warm water or taking a warm bath.** However, be careful when showering, since pregnancy increases your chances of feeling dizzy, and avoid a prolonged bath in very hot water since this may not be good for your baby.

■ **A lower back massage is comforting** and a good way to relax and ease discomfort—ask your partner to give you a soothing massage.

**To prepare your body for the task ahead,** ensure that you get plenty of rest and relaxation. In addition to getting a good night's sleep, take a light nap during the day if you feel fatigued.

**No one is sure** exactly what triggers labor, but it seems the process varies with each species.

In sheep, a drop in progesterone signals the start of labor. In mice, babies release proteins to signal their maturity, which in turn triggers labor. In humans, little is known about the signals that start labor although there are many theories. Studies suggest that the production of hormones such as corticotrophin-releasing hormone (CRH) by the uterus and placenta may play a role. It's also thought that an increase in pro-inflammatory substances known as cytokines may be involved. Whatever the trigger, it's likely that the onset of labor involves a biological communication between your baby and your body to indicate that your baby is ready to be born.

## Braxton Hicks' contractions

One of the most common symptoms of approaching labor is an increase in the strength and frequency of Braxton Hicks', or practice, contractions (see p.387), which may be occurring up to four times an hour. The purpose of these practice contractions is to prepare your uterus to deal with real labor contractions so that labor progresses smoothly. Some women find Braxton Hicks' relatively painless, while others find these practice contractions fairly uncomfortable, especially if the baby is quite low and contractions cause increased pelvic pressure.

Apart from the level of pain, one of the main ways to distinguish Braxton Hicks' from real contractions is that Bracton Hicks' are irregular and they fade away, whereas labor pains occur at regular intervals and gradually become stronger, more intense, and closer together. The other main difference between Braxton Hicks' contractions and real ones is that, unlike Braxton Hicks', real contractions cause your cervix to dilate, which indicates that labor is beginning.

## Engagement of the head

With a first baby, dropping down of the baby's head into your pelvis, known as engagement, usually means that labor is likely to start soon. In second and subsequent pregnancies, engagement may not occur until the start of labor.

You can usually tell that your baby's position has changed in two ways. First, you may notice that you have less discomfort in your upper abdomen or around your ribs because the downward movement releases some pressure. Second, you may notice increased pressure or pain in your pelvic or vaginal area as the baby's head moves into position. Your walking may become more of a waddle and you may have to use the bathroom more frequently than before. In some cases, your baby's head may pinch some of the nerves that run through your pelvis and you may

---

SIGNS OF APPROACHING LABOR

**Although each woman's experience of labor differs** and there are no hard and fast rules as to what will happen when, there are signs that indicate that labor is likely to start either imminently or within a matter of days. One of the classic signs that labor isn't far away is a "bloody show" (see opposite), when you lose the plug of mucus that has protected your baby during pregnancy. The other indisputable sign that labor will be shortly underway is that your cervix begins to dilate, although of course this will only be visible during an internal examination.

One other sign that labor may be about to start is if your water breaks (see opposite). However, for the majority of women this happens later on during established labor.

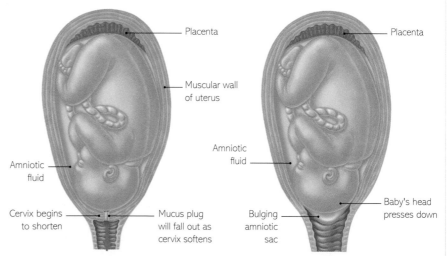

**As the cervix starts to soften and shorten,** the thick plug of mucus that protected your baby from infection during pregnancy comes away and falls out of the vagina, an event referred to as a "bloody show." When this happens, you may notice a yellowish discharge.

**The amniotic membrane bulges through the cervix** as the baby's head presses down. When the membranes break (water breaking), labor is imminent, or may have already started. The amniotic fluid may pass out as a gush of fluid or a trickle.

CHECKLIST

# When to seek help

Make your way to the hospital or seek advice if any of the following occur:

■ **You have vaginal bleeding** that is like a period or heavier.

■ **You're leaking amniotic fluid** or leaking greenish fluid that could indicate the baby is distressed.

■ **The baby isn't moving as expected** (ask your doctor for advice).

experience sciatica, a sharp electric pain that runs down the outside of your leg to your outside toes (see p.470).

## The "bloody show"

In pregnancy, a plug of mucus forms at the end of the cervix to prevent infection from entering the uterus. At the end of pregnancy, as the cervix softens and widens, this plug is dislodged and comes out through the vagina. When this occurs, you may see a discharge known as the "bloody show"; although some women don't notice anything. The discharge may appear as a thick, clear or yellow clump that looks like mucus from your nose. It's common for small amounts of blood to be present due to small tears in the cervix as the plug comes away.

Losing the plug of mucus usually means that labor will begin soon and you should make plans to leave for the hospital in the near future (within 12 hours). However, if loss of the plug is accompanied by other symptoms, such as painful, frequent contractions, heavy bleeding or leaking fluid (indicating your water has broken), you should call your doctor or hospital immediately.

## Water breaking

Rupture of the amniotic membranes, called the water breaking, usually occurs once labor has started, but it can happen earlier. If this happens, it often means that labor is imminent. For some, a big gush of fluid is a clear sign that their water has broken, while for others there may be a trickle and it can be hard to determine if the amniotic fluid is leaking. Also, since many women have trouble controlling their bladder in pregnancy, telling the difference between urine and amniotic fluid can be hard. One way to tell is to wear a sanitary pad. If the pad quickly becomes soaked, your water has probably broken. Amniotic fluid also has an odor that is different than urine, even to nonprofessional noses.

### Monitoring after the water breaks

If you think your water has broken but contractions haven't started, contact your doctor or the hospital for advice. If you're due, there are no complications, and your baby's head is engaged, you may be advised either to stay at home for a while to see if labor starts, or will be asked to be seen at the hospital. This is because, once your water has broken, your baby has lost the protective membrane surrounding him or her, which means there is an increased risk of an infection reaching your baby. The doctor should check your file to see if you're Group B Strep (GBS)-positive, and if you are, you'll be admitted and started on IV antibiotics. She may also monitor your baby's heartbeat (see p.418) to check that your baby isn't distressed. If you're GBS-negative and all is well, you may be able to return home, or stay at home, for a set amount of time and an appointment will be made to see how you're progressing. If labor doesn't start within 24 hours (the timeframe may be shorter in some hospitals), the hospital may suggest an induction (see p.432).

### Early contractions

As your body prepares to go into labor, you will start to experience mild and irregular contractions. These differ from Braxton Hicks' since they build gradually and will soften and dilate the cervix.

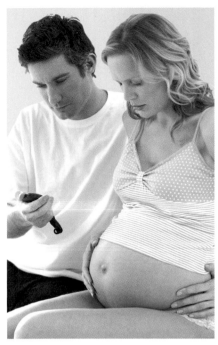

**As you approach labor**, you will experience irregular contractions; these will increase in strength and regularity as labor progresses.

CHECKLIST

# When am I in labor?

A common concern of many women is how they will know when they are in labor. The following are indications that labor is truly underway.

■ **You are having contractions that are becoming stronger** and more intense, lasting longer, and the interval between the contractions is getting shorter.

■ **Changing your position or** walking around doesn't ease the intensity of the contraction.

■ **The contractions start high in your abdomen and** move down through the uterus and lower back, rather than occurring only in the lower abdomen.

■ **Your water breaks** (see left) while you're having contractions.

# How labor progresses

Stronger and more regular contractions continue to stretch your cervix until, at around 10 cm, it is fully dilated.

## SUDDEN BIRTH

**Although uncommon, labor and birth can occur unexpectedly fast**, resulting in an unplanned home birth or a birth on the way to the hospital. Sudden birth is more likely to happen in second and subsequent labors or if you've had a previous sudden birth.

**If you're alone at home**. Try to stay calm and phone the emergency services for an ambulance. Also ask them to contact your doctor, whose number should be in your address book. Try to contact a friend, relative, or a neighbor who can help. If someone is with you, ask him or her to contact the ambulance and doctor.

Wash your hands and gather newspapers, clean towels, or clean clothing, or if you have an assistant ask him or her to prepare in this way. If there is time, the floor or bed should be covered with a plastic sheet, open trash bags, or newspapers and have a plastic bowl for the amniotic fluid and blood.

If you have an urge to push, breathe slowly; panting and blowing can help. Sit or kneel on the floor or your bed on top of a clean towel so that your baby doesn't fall onto a hard surface. Your water may break and an assistant can watch for a sudden bulging of the perineum and for your baby's head to appear, at which point you can push.

Once the head is delivered, you will feel another contraction and can push the body out. You may be able do this alone, or an assistant can put his or her hands either side of the head and apply gentle pressure. If your baby is born in the amniotic bag, this can be punctured with fingers; the baby's face will need wiping so that the airway is clear. Try to record the time of birth. Give your baby immediate skin-to-skin contact to keep him warm; then dry him and wrap him in a towel or blanket. Putting him to your breast stimulates contractions to deliver the placenta. An assistant can watch for a gush of blood or lengthening of the cord, a sign that the placenta has come away. Put the placenta in a towel in a bowl to be checked. Clamp the cord with string or a shoe lace; the doctor or paramedic will cut it when he or she arrives.

**If you're in a car.** If you feel an urge to push, your partner should pull over and put the hazard lights on. If your baby is born in the car, your partner can put him on your belly for warmth. If you have towels, dry your baby, wrap him in a clean towel, and call an ambulance.

**If you have an uncontrollable urge** to push on your way to the hospital, you may need to pull over and call emergency services.

Since every woman's experience of labor is different, it's hard to say exactly what your experience will be like. However, the stages of labor are common for all women. The first stage, when labor becomes established, starts when contractions start to open, or dilate, the cervix (see box, p.415). For some women, especially those who don't want strong pain relief, this is the hardest part of labor. Waiting for the cervix to dilate can be a long process with your first baby, and there isn't much you can do to hurry the process. The first stage of labor can be broken down into different phases, referred to as the early, or latent, phase, and the active phase (see below). After these phases comes transition, when your cervix becomes fully dilated and before you start to push your baby out (see p.416).

**The early (latent) phase** During the early phase, which can last for over a day or so in a first labor, your contractions gradually become more uncomfortable, but still relatively mild, and occur more frequently, although they may be irregular. During this phase, your cervix gradually shortens, a process known as effacement (see box, p.414) and begins to dilate. When the cervix is approximately 3–4 cm dilated and you're having regular, strong contractions, the active phase has begun (see below). The changes to your cervix during the early phase can be slow or fast and are hard to predict.

**The active phase** The active phase of the first stage is the individual point for each woman where cervical change happens more quickly and predictably.

**Many couples feel unsure about when to go to the hospital.** If your pregnancy is low risk, you will almost certainly be more comfortable at home at the start of labor and should wait until you're in active labor, when your contractions are regular, occurring every 5–10 minutes, and painful, before going to the hospital. At this stage, the hospital will want to assess how your baby is responding to strong contractions, and you may want some medication for pain. This needs to be administered in a setting where you can be monitored and, in the case of an epidural (see p.404), can only be given in the hospital.

If your pregnancy is high risk, you have had a prior cesarean, have a breech baby, or carry the streptococcus B bacterium, call the maternity ward to discuss when to go to the hospital.

Once you're in active labor, a final reason to go to the hospital is to make sure your baby is born there. An unplanned home (or car) birth is not best for you or your baby. This is unusual in a first pregnancy, but with subsequent births women are more likely to arrive at the hospital quite dilated or to have an unintended home birth.

**Getting to the hospital** Arrange for someone to drive you to the hospital, either your partner, or a friend or relative; don't consider driving yourself. Map the route ahead of time, consider a dry run before the big day, and have a bag packed with everything you will need for you and your baby (see p.358).

**Admission procedure** When you get to the hospital, you'll be checked in and will be put into a labor room if you look like you're in active labor, or into an assessment bed if this isn't clear. Usually you will be asked for a urine specimen, and a nurse will check your temperature, pulse, and blood pressure, check your cervix, and review your pregnancy history. If you're in early labor, you may be sent home. This doesn't mean you were unwise to come in; it's good to ensure all is well.

Once you've been admitted, you and your baby will be assessed by a doctor or nurse. Sometimes an intravenous (IV) line will be placed and blood tests may be done. You can make your room comfortable with items from home.

**On your arrival at the hospital** you will be assessed to see if you are in established labor and should remain at the hospital.

However, exactly when you enter active labor can be hard to establish, even for a doctor. For most women, active labor occurs at around 4 cm dilation. Your contractions are regular and may be every 5 minutes or so and getting closer together until they're 2 to 4 minutes apart and lasting from 45 seconds to one minute or more. From the start of active labor to the birth can last for around 10 to 12 hours, although this may be considerably shorter in a second labor.

In active labor, the nature of your contractions change, with pain becoming less concentrated in the lower abdomen, instead starting higher in the abdomen and moving down toward the pelvis and lower back as your baby is pushed down. Contractions are caused by a painful tightening of the muscles that may start off feeling like a severe period pain and

## As labor begins

**If you're having a home birth, your midwife will have talked to you in advance about how to contact her once you're in labor.** Since she will be traveling to you, bear in mind local traffic conditions. If the streets might be busy, it's worth phoning her in early labor. She may ask you to phone again when your contractions are closer together.

While waiting for the midwife, you may want to move around, or relax in a warm bath. If you've purchased or rented a birthing pool, ensure that this is ready to use. Ask your partner to lay down old sheets or plastic sheeting over the floor. Eating small, nourishing snacks and drinking water will provide energy for the hours ahead.

Home births are not for everyone. They're only an option for you if you're having a healthy, low-risk pregnancy, and you may need to be transferred to a hospital before delivery if complications arise. The American College of Obstetricians and Gynecologists opposes home births because of the potential for complications, even in low-risk pregnancies, as does the American Medical Association. Only 6 out of every 1,000 U.S. births are home births.

## CHANGES TO THE CERVIX

**The cervix is comprised of firm muscle that forms a strong base at the bottom of the uterus.** For your baby to be born, the cervix needs to stretch and soften so that it can open, or dilate, and your baby can pass out of the uterus and into the vagina.

Toward the end of pregnancy, substances in your blood called prostaglandins start to soften the cervix so that it becomes more malleable. While you are pregnant, your cervix is usually around 2 to 3 cm long. In late pregnancy or

early labor, Braxton Hicks' practice contractions start to shorten the cervix, a process known as effacement. Most women have a cervix that has shortened to 1 cm during the very early stages of labor. This is also referred to as 50 percent effaced. As the cervix continues to shorten, the cervix is gradually drawn up by the uterus, and by the time it is 100 percent effaced, the cervix will have started to open. Eventually the cervix becomes fully dilated (see box, opposite), and the baby can be pushed out.

**As labor approaches,** the cervix starts to lose its firmness and starts to soften in response to the presence of prostaglandins in the blood.

Lower segment of uterus

Cervix

**Once the cervix has softened,** it starts to shorten. This process is referred to as effacement and needs to occur before the cervix can begin to dilate.

Cervix drawn up by uterus

Cervix shortened

## THE "STATION"

**The "station" refers to the position of your baby's head** in relation to your pelvis. This is recorded as a number between -5 and +5. Zero station means the head is "engaged" and has entered the vaginal canal within the pelvic bones. A negative number (-5 to 0) means that the head isn't engaged in the pelvis. A positive number (0 to +4) means that your baby's head is moving down the pelvis and +5 means your baby is crowning (being born). Ideally, you should not push until the head is engaged in the pelvis, even if you're fully dilated.

-5

0

+5

**The position** of the head in relation to the pelvis is marked on a scale of -5 to +5.

---

increase in intensity as they reach their peak. Your doctor will assess if you're in active labor by observing your pain levels, the frequency and strength of contractions, and by using a tool called a labor curve, which plots cervical change and the position of your baby's head in relation to your pelvis over time (see partograms, p.419).

It's important for your doctor to determine when you enter active labor so she can assess how labor is progressing. For first labors, 90 percent of women have a cervical dilation of about 1 cm per hour, whereas labor moves faster in subsequent births. If you've had an epidural (see p.404),

labor may be slower. Once it's established that you're in active labor, the doctor can predict when you may deliver. However, since women vary widely in how long it takes them to have a baby, bear in mind that this is only an estimate.

During active labor, you may want to have medical pain relief if you haven't so far, such as analgesics or an epidural (see pp. 402–6).

## Abdominal and vaginal examinations

You will have several internal vaginal examinations and your abdomen will be palpated to assess the baby's position. If your doctor is assessing if amniotic fluid

is leaking, a speculum examination may be done, but in most cases this isn't necessary. Usually, the doctor uses her fingers to assess the baby and the progress of labor. She will try to check you often enough to make sure that your labor is progressing, but not so often that it causes you extra discomfort or increases your risk of infection. The following are assessed during a vaginal examination.

**The station** The doctor will check how far the head has descended into the pelvis (see box, above).

**Cervical effacement** The doctor will assess how your cervix is shortening, known as effacement (see box, top left). Once the cervix is sufficiently shortened, it begins to dilate, or open.

**Cervical dilation** The doctor assesses how dilated, or open, your cervix is (see box, below). Active labor is established at 3 to 4 cm dilation and full dilation occurs at around 10 cm. You can't push your baby out until you're fully dilated.

**Fetal position** Fetal presentation refers to the part of your baby that is coming out first. Babies can be born head first or bottom first (breech) (see p.433). Your doctor will also assess which way your baby is facing in the birth canal. The easiest way for a baby to be born is head down with the back of the baby's head (occiput) and spine toward the front (anterior) of your uterus, known as an occiput anterior position. Your baby can also be born vaginally from an occiput posterior position (back of baby's head and spine toward the back of your uterus), but

this can take longer and be more painful. Vaginal tears are more common when babies are born in the occiput posterior position. A final position is when your baby faces your side, known as occiput transverse. Full-term babies can't be born in the transverse position since the head is too big to fit this way. However it's not uncommon for babies to rotate around during labor, although this would need to happen before you start to push. If this doesn't happen, labor may need to be assisted with forceps or a vacuum and suction cup (see pp.436–7).

**Descent with contractions** Although most of the time your doctor will try to examine you inbetween contractions, sometimes it helps to see how much the baby's head comes down in the pelvis during a contraction, referred to as the descent. If there is a good descent during contractions this means that the baby is fitting well into your pelvis and that your contractions are efficient.

## DILATION

**Once your cervix is stretched and softened** (see box, opposite), it begins to open, or dilate, so that your baby can pass through into the vagina to be born. Regular contractions cause the cervix to dilate, and in first labors the cervix dilates at an average of 1 cm per hour; this rate is often faster for subsequent labors. You cannot push your baby out until you are fully dilated, which occurs at 10 cm.

**At 2 cm dilation,** the cervix has shortened and is beginning to open. Contractions may still be irregular.

**At 6 cm dilation,** you are in active labor. Your contractions will be more frequent, regular, and stronger.

**At 10 cm dilation,** you are fully dilated. Contractions may be almost continuous and you are nearly ready to start pushing your baby out.

### QUESTIONS AND ANSWERS

**Am I likely to have medical interventions in labor in the hospital?**
The reality of a hospital birth is that medical interventions may be suggested, some of which may be more helpful than others. Procedures that can be done include artificially breaking the water; inserting a catheter or an IV line; and speeding up labor with drugs.

**Is artificial rupture of the membranes routine in the hospital?**
Artificially breaking the bag of water, known as amniotomy or ARM (see p.432) is offered routinely in some hospitals in labor. This is a painless, low-risk procedure that is thought to shorten the time of labor by one to two hours, reduce the chance of a low early APGAR score in your baby (see p.428), and significantly decrease the chance that you'll need drugs to speed up labor (see below). ARM is usually optional. The one time it is necessary is if a fetal scalp electrode needs to be put on the baby's head (see p.419) since this cannot be done without breaking the water. It may also be done as part of the induction process (see p.432).

**How is labor speeded up with medication?**
A slow labor may be speeded up with the medication oxytocin, a procedure known as augmentation. Oxytocin is naturally released from your pituitary gland in labor. Synthetic oxytocin can be given via an intravenous (IV) line to strengthen contractions. When this is done, it's usual to have continuous fetal monitoring (see p.418) since, if the contractions become too strong, your baby may show signs of distress. Since oxytocin is quickly cleared from your system once the IV is turned off, contractions that are too strong can be weakened quickly. Oxytocin is also given during an induction of labor (see p.432).

## Transition

Transition is the end of active labor as your cervix becomes fully dilated and you ready yourself to begin pushing. This is one of the shortest stages of labor, lasting from 15 minutes to two hours, although on average it's about 30 minutes. This can be one of the most challenging parts of labor because your contractions intensify and can begin to feel continuous since they now occur every 30–90 seconds. If you haven't had an epidural, transition can be especially difficult since you may feel a lot of pressure on your lower back and rectum and have an overwhelming desire to push, but will be unable to push until your cervix is fully dilated. Even if you've had an epidural, you may notice increasing pelvic pressure. If you do push before your cervix is ready, you may tear your cervix or cause your cervix to swell and thicken, which will prolong the process of labor.

It's not uncommon to vomit now, a side effect of the stretching of your cervix and the pelvic pressure. You may also tremble or shake and have hot flashes.

**How you can cope** You may feel very uncomfortable during this period as your contractions become stronger and you try to hold back from pushing. Significant pelvic pressure during the transition phase can make it difficult to relax between contractions, and you will therefore need plenty of support from your birth partner and nurse at this time, since you may be feeling exhausted, out of control, possibly frightened, and may even think that you can't continue.

Work with your nurse to find the best position for you. This is the one stage of labor where it can be helpful not to adopt an upright position, since you can take some of the pressure off the pelvis. Sitting or being on all fours with your bottom raised may help. Keep breathing during your contractions; your nurse may show you how to pant and breathe shallowly to help resist the urge to push. If possible, moving around during contractions can sometimes help since you will focus on doing something else until you can actively push. You could try rocking on a birthing ball or in a rocking chair. If there is time between your contractions, ask your partner to massage your lower back if this helps relieve pressure.

It can be easy to lose sight of the purpose of labor at this point, so try to focus on the fact that your baby will soon be born.

**Pain relief** Your doctor may not give you intravenous pain relief now, since these can cause your baby to be too sleepy if they are given close to the birth. Depending on hospital procedure, you may or may not be able to have an epidural now (see p.404).

---

## Support in the first stage

**During the first stage,** your partner has a varied and important role. In adddition to helping you feel comfortable and assisting you with positions, your partner can also support you mentally. This is especially important at the end of the first stage, when you reach transition (see above), a point when women often feel panicky and out of control. Your partner can offer reassurance that you're doing well and that the delivery of your baby is not far off. He can also improve your comfort, for example by applying a damp, cool washcloth to your face and neck, and he can help you focus on your breathing, reminding you to pant or blow to help you resist the urge to push before the cervix is fully dilated.

**During transition, you may be overwhelemed** by the strength and frequency of your contractions. Your partner's support is crucial during this stage and his encouragement can help keep you focused on your labor.

**If your cervix is not dilating, or your baby is not descending, as quickly as expected during the first stage,** your doctor will try to assess why this is and if something can be done. Usually, your doctor will assess the three P's: the passenger (the size of the baby and his position in the uterus); the powers (the efficiency of your contractions); and the passage (the size and shape of your pelvis). These three elements work together and each one is important for your labor to progress smoothly.

There are several reasons why a labor may not progress. These include if the baby's head is too large for the mother's pelvis, known as cephalopelvic disproportion (CPD); if contractions are inefficient; and if the baby is in a posterior position with his back facing the mother's back.

## Cephalopelvic disproportion

Sometimes CPD may be suspected before labor, in late pregnancy. This may be the case if the doctor thinks that you have a narrow pelvis or a prominent sacral bone, both of which may make birth slower or more difficult. However, an assessment of the pelvis alone is not an accurate way to predict if you'll be able to have a successful vaginal birth and, even if the pelvis is not an optimal shape, the doctor may be happy for you to continue trying for a vaginal birth. This is because it's not the shape of your pelvis alone that is important, but the interaction between your baby (the passenger) and your pelvis.

If CPD is suspected, but the baby's head has engaged, a vaginal birth can still be attempted. The labor will be monitored with a labor graph (see p.419) and if there are signs that the baby is in distress, an emergency cesarean may be performed. If the head hasn't engaged toward the end of labor, a planned cesarean may be offered.

If your doctor suspects CPD in labor, she will reassess the baby's size to check if she originally underestimated his or her weight. Even though the combination of a large estimated weight and a slow labor can suggest that there may be delivery problems, often labor proceeds normally.

**Inefficient contractions** If your labor isn't progressing because your cervix is dilating slowly or has stopped dilating, your doctor will assess the frequency of your contractions, which should be every 2 to 3 minutes. She'll also assess how strong the contractions are by palpating your abdomen: the firmer it feels during contractions, the more likely they are to be effective. If contractions are more widely spaced than they should be and their strength indicates they're unlikely to be effective, she may use one or two techniques to speed up labor, known as augmenting labor. First, she may artificially rupture the membranes if they haven't already ruptured, a process known as ARM (see p.432). This can shorten the duration of labor by around one to two hours.

If ARM has no effect, you may be given the drug oxytocin to increase the strength and frequency of contractions (see p.432). Initially, a small dose is given and then increased over time until you're having three or four moderately strong contractions every 10 minutes. If this is done, you'll have continuous electronic fetal monitoring (see p.418) to check that the baby is not distressed by the sudden onset of stronger contractions.

If your labor is still not progessing several hours after the drugs have been started, then a cesarean may be recommended.

**Posterior presentation** The best position for your baby in labor is an occipito-anterior position with the back of the head (occiput) facing your front. If the back of the head faces your back (occipito-posterior) this can make it hard for the baby to turn and move down the birth canal and can prolong labor. The doctor may suggest that you change positions to encourage the baby to turn. If the baby fails to rotate, forceps or vacuum may be needed to aid the delivery (see pp.436–7).

Pelvic inlet 5⅛ in (13 cm)

Pelvic inlet 4¾ in (12 cm)

**A gynecoid pelvis** is the name given to a pelvis that has a circular shape. The generous proportions of this more typical "female-shaped" pelvis provides room for the head to pass through during the birth.

**An android pelvis** is the term used to describe a pelvis that has a more triangular shape. This reduces the room available for the baby's head to pass through and is more likely to cause problems during a vaginal delivery.

# Monitoring during labor

Throughout labor, your baby's heartbeat and your contractions will be monitored to make sure that your labor is progressing as it should be and that the well-being of you and your baby is not threatened.

**A handheld device** can monitor your baby's heartbeat at intervals, leaving you free to move around during labor.

Your baby's heart rate is an indication of how well your baby is dealing with labor and it is monitored at regular intervals, called intermittent monitoring. If a problem is found or you have a high-risk pregnancy, then you may be advised to have fetal electronic monitoring, in which your baby's heart rate and your contractions are monitored continuously by a electronic fetal heart monitor (see box, below). All the information about your labor is recorded on a chart, called a labor graph (see opposite).

## Intermittent monitoring

This is done using a handheld battery-operated device known as a Doppler sonicaid, which is held against your abdomen to listen to your baby's heartbeat. When you are pushing in the second stage of labor, the fetal heart needs to be monitored more frequently.

## Electronic fetal monitoring

In this type of fetal monitoring, two devices monitor your baby's heart rate and the strength and frequency of your contractions. Your baby's heart rate is monitored with a circular ultrasound-like device. If you want, you can hear the heartbeat, or ask that the volume be turned down if this is distracting. Your contractions are monitored with a small plastic circular device. One or two elastic belts are placed around your abdomen to secure the monitors. You should be able to stand, sit, or squat with the monitors in place, and some hospitals

---

**HOW MONITORING IS DONE**

## External fetal monitoring

**The baby's heartbeat and the strength and frequency of your contractions** are measured by devices strapped to your abdomen with wires that connect to a machine that produces a printout of the readings and an ongoing digital log on the computer.

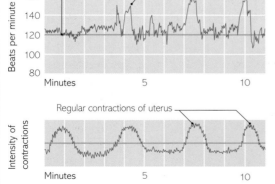

Baseline rate 120 bpm
Increase in rate with each contraction

Beats per minute: 160, 140, 120, 100, 80
Minutes 5 10

**Your baby's heartbeat** is recorded against a baseline measurement of 120 beats per minute. The heart rate rises and falls naturally with contractions; unusual variations can indicate fetal distress.

Regular contractions of uterus

Intensity of contractions
Minutes 5 10

**A separate reading** records the strength and duration of each contraction. This can detect weakening contractions and can be useful with an epidural when you're unable to feel contractions.

**Continuous monitoring of your baby's heart rate and your contractions** is done by means of monitors strapped to your abdomen.

## Scalp electrode

**If there are concerns** about the baby's heartbeat, a small electrode attached to the scalp can give a more precise reading than external electronic fetal monitoring The electrode is passed through the cervix and attached to the head.

Electrode is attached to baby's head

have monitors that allow you to walk around and be monitored by radio signal.

**Internal monitoring** If your baby's heart-rate reading indicates the baby is distressed or the signal from an electronic monitor is poor, the doctor may suggest internal fetal monitoring. In this technique, a small electrode is attached to the baby's scalp and detects the electrical impulses of his heart. A wire from the electrode comes out via the cervix and attaches to the EFM machine (see box, left). You still wear a strap around your abdomen, which holds the device for detecting the rate and strength of your contractions.

The electrode is placed during a vaginal examination and is no more uncomfortable than this. Placing a scalp electrode may be mildly uncomfortable for your baby and there is a small risk that your baby could get a scalp infection, which can be treated with antibiotics. Even though these risks are small, a

scalp electrode should not be placed routinely. Your doctor should discuss how it works before it is placed, and you should understand why it's being done. Electrodes should also be avoided if you have a viral disease that can be transmitted to your baby during labor, such as hepatitis B or C, or HIV. Once a scalp electrode has been placed, you can't move far from the monitor, although you may be able to change position.

If a EFM reading from the scalp electrode indicates that your baby is distressed, a blood sample may be taken from the scalp to check acidity levels. If these are high, a cesarean or assisted delivery may be suggested.

### Labor graphs

A labor graph is a large chart that contains several graphs which provide information on your labor, allowing the doctor to monitor the progress of your labor. One of the most useful tools in this chart is a graph showing your labor curve. This plots cervical change and the position of your baby's head in relation to your pelvis over time. The graph enables the doctor to establish when your labor became active. Also recorded with your baby's heart-rate monitoring are your blood pressure, pulse, temperature, and the rate of your contractions, as well as your pain levels.

## Should you have electronic fetal monitoring?

**Although monitoring during labor is an important part of the care of you and your baby,** there is some debate as to the benefits of continuous monitoring and some believe there may be associated maternal risks. As a result, most hospitals suggest intermittent fetal monitoring. Although you can refuse monitoring entirely, the staff may be unhappy about this and ask you to sign a form or statement releasing them from liability if anything goes wrong during the labor and birth.

**Risks** Studies suggest that women who are monitored continuously are more likely to have a cesarean section or an assisted delivery with forceps or vacuum (see pp.436–7). This is because your doctor may see changes in the fetal heart rate that concern her. Some changes, such as a faster heart rate (more than 160 beats a minute), known as tachycardia, or decreases in the heart rate that occur after your contractions, can be caused by decreased oxygen to your baby. If

your doctor sees these changes, she may be unable to determine if they were caused by low oxygen or if your baby is actually fine.

If it's thought that your baby may be at risk, an emergency cesarean section may be recommended. If there are fetal heart rate changes while you are pushing, a forceps or vacuum delivery may be offered.

**Benefits** The benefits of continuous electronic fetal monitoring are not entirely clear. You are able to hear your baby's heartbeat and some women may find this comforting. Also, experts agree that continuous monitoring reduces the chance that your baby will have a seizure after the birth, a symptom of brain injury from low oxygen. Seizures are rare, occurring in around 2.5 per 1000 births with monitoring and 5 per 1000 births without monitoring. It is harder to prove that electronic fetal monitoring can prevent rarer complications such as cerebral palsy or fetal death.

# Positions for first stage of labor

Being active during the first stage of labor is thought to help labor progress. If you're well prepared and practice different postures and positions for labor during pregnancy, you will instinctively be able to use these during childbirth.

**Leaning forward onto a pile of cushions** with your knees apart is a soothing and relaxing position, and can also encourage your cervix to dilate.

Many different postures and positions can help you in the first stage, and there is evidence that changing your position in this stage increases the effectiveness of your contractions and reduces the pain. Assuming upright positions in particular uses gravity to assist the descent of the baby.

## Active positions

Positions that allow you to remain active are thought to help labor progress. Some women find rocking the pelvis backward and forward, and then rotating the pelvis in a clockwise and then counterclockwise direction while standing or sitting on a birthing ball, helps ease the pain. Adopting an all-fours position on your hands and knees can help you stay focused and also allows you to rotate your pelvis. Moving backward and forward in a rocking chair can also be comforting. Many women find walking in place and walking around helpful.

## Supported positions

Supported positions can be especially helpful if your baby is in an occiput-posterior position (baby's back to your back). Leaning forward with your hands on a table or chair during a contraction and breathing slowly and steadily helps you focus. If you find it comforting, your partner can massage your shoulders and back at the same time. A lot of women find either sitting astride on a chair facing the back of the chair or sitting on a toilet and facing the tank with a pillow for their head and arms, a comfortable position. This also allows you to "catnap" between contractions.

**Using a birthing ball during labor** enables you to adopt upright positions while feeling supported. While sitting on a birthing ball, or adopting a supported kneeling position with one, you will be able to rotate your hips to encourage the progress of labor.

**Kneeling in an all-fours position** helps take the weight off your back. This position also allows you to move your hips back and forth or rotate them, which can be comforting during early contractions.

**Kneeling and leaning forward** onto cushions with your bottom raised also helps ease a backache and can be a helpful position to adopt during transition (see p.416) when you may need to resist the urge to bear down.

**Sitting astride a chair** can be a relaxing position because this enables you to lean forward with your legs astride while remaining supported.

**Lying on your side** with your knee bent and supported with pillows can be a relaxing position between contractions, enabling you to rest and re-energize. You may also want to adopt a supported lying position during some contractions.

# 2nd and 3rd stages

**THE MOMENT OF DELIVERY IS WITHIN SIGHT AND YOU WILL SOON MEET YOUR LONG-AWAITED BABY**

The second stage begins when your cervix is fully dilated and your baby has moved deep into the pelvis. These signs may be accompanied by an overwhelming urge to bear down and, once your doctor is satisfied that you are ready to do it, you will be able to push your baby out. The third stage, the delivery of the placenta, marks the end of labor.

# Delivering your baby

In the second stage, your labor starts to accelerate as you actively push your baby out into the world.

As you enter the second stage of labor, you will probably experience an overwhelming desire to bear down. Once your doctor has established that you are fully dilated and are ready to start pushing, you may start to feel more in control of your labor since your pushing helps move your baby farther down into the pelvis.

## The second stage

The second stage of labor starts when your cervix is completely open, at about 10 cm, and ends with the birth of your baby. This stage usually lasts for around 45 minutes to two hours during a first labor and from 15 to 45 minutes in subsequent deliveries. The second stage is intense and during this time your contractions will become stronger, but may occur less frequently, occurring around every two to five minutes. At this point you may feel a sensation of fullness in your vagina or bowel and have a strong urge to push. Many women find labor pains more bearable

### THE MECHANISMS OF LABOR

**The birth passage,** far from being straight, involves a series of rotational maneuvers known as the "mechanisms of labor."

This curve, known as the "curve of Carus," is thought to result from the evolution of humans from being on all fours to being upright. This caused the spine to curve, the pelvis to tilt, and gave a curve to the birth canal. Your pelvic floor muscles help the head rotate through the birth canal.

FOCUS ON...YOUR BIRTH PARTNER

## Support in the second stage

**In the second stage, your partner's support is invaluable.** His or her role is to make you feel supported and safe and to offer lots of encouragement.

Your birth partner can provide verbal support to help you deal with the strenuous task of pushing your baby out with each contraction. There may be times when you're not lucid and your partner will need to speak for you and liaise with medical staff.

In addition to emotional support, your birth partner can act as your physical support in whatever position you adopt in the second stage, whether this is a squatting position or another position that you find comfortable. Your partner will be able to massage your back if this is helpful, and can hold you and comfort you and help you focus on your breathing during and between each contraction.

Your partner can also watch as your baby's head crowns and describe what he or she can see, or hold a mirror for you to see the baby's head, which can be deeply reassuring as you realize that the end is in sight.

**The emotional and physical support provided by your birth partner** can be crucial during the second stage of labor, the time when you are having to exert yourself physically to push your baby down in your pelvis and out through the birth canal.

**In a kneeling position,** both your partner and the nurse can support you as you bear down (top left). **Being on all fours** with the hospital bed for support can be a comfortable position (bottom left).

**An upright squatting position** is good for pushing and can be adopted if you have firm support from your partner. He can support you under the arms while you put your hands around the back of his neck.

in the second stage since they can now actively work with the contractions and push their baby out. Other women find this a particularly hard part of labor because they start to feel exhausted from the effort of prolonged pushing.

## Second stage positions

Although you may be tired and want to lie down, it's recommended that you resist this urge in the second stage. Your partner and nurse can give you plenty of support to help you adopt the most comfortable position.

**Staying upright** Adopting an upright position during the second stage of labor has several advantages. The main one is that you are using gravity to assist your baby's descent, which will also help you bear down and push. Being upright can also improve the alignment of your baby in the birth canal; can increase the efficiency of your contractions; and widens the passageway through the pelvis.

There is also evidence that adopting upright positions in the second stage of labor can reduce the length of time you

take to bear down and give birth, and make it less likely that you will have an instrument delivery or episiotomy (see pp.436–7 and p.427).

**Which positions to adopt** Upright positions during the second stage of labor include upright sitting and squatting positions.

If you prefer a sitting position, try to sit in an upright or semi-recumbent position. If you adopt a sitting position on a bed, sitting at a 45-degree angle can help your breathing and reduce the risk of a condition known as aortocaval compression, which can affect how well your blood is circulated around your body and to your baby. This is caused by the weight of your uterus and the baby pressing on major blood vessels (the aorta and vena cava), reducing the amount of oxygen that circulates around your body, which makes you feel light headed and dizzy. If this happens, you will be advised to lie on your left side to relieve pressure and increase the amount of oxygen circulating.

Because kneeling or squatting increases the pelvic outlet, many women will naturally adopt a squatting or all-fours position to give birth since they find that this is the most comfortable and easy position in which to deliver their baby. Upright squatting and kneeling positions help increase your pelvic outlet by around 28 percent compared to when you're in a lying-down position. This means that there is more room for your baby to descend through your pelvis and into the birth canal. Some women find it hard to squat down comfortably because they are not used to being in this position and tire easily. If this is the case, ask your partner to support you as you squat.

Alternatively, you may find that lying on your side is your preferred position; your partner can help you by supporting one of your legs to keep your pelvis as open as possible. There is also some evidence that lying on your side can protect your perineum from tearing.

**Using props** Some women find using props such as a beanbag, birthing ball, pillows, or a large cushion while kneeling and leaning forward helpful.

## When to push

Your baby will start to rotate his or her head and shoulders to enable these to descend through your pelvis to be born, and you will feel the urge to bear down and push as this is happening. Your doctor will help you focus and

# Coping in the second stage

**The second stage of labor can be a time when instinct takes over** and you may find that you are oblivious to everything around you as you follow the overwhelming urge to push. You may have been concerned before labor about how you would behave during the delivery. Some women are worried that they will defecate while they are pushing. This is actually very common and it's natural to pass a stool during the delivery; you should rest assured that the nurses and doctors will be completely used to this. You may not even notice yourself that this has happened.

Rather than be concerned about how you will act, try to take encouragement from the fact that you now have more control over your labor and are actively pushing your baby out. You may find that you want to grunt or moan while pushing, or you may push quietly and intensely. Focusing on the imminent arrival of your baby will help you to persevere.

encourage you to push when you feel the urge, which will come naturally with a contraction. With each contraction, you will need to concentrate on pushing down deep into the pelvic area and bottom. It can help to put your chin on your chest and to bear down for as long as possible during a contraction, during which time you may need to take several steady breaths. You may feel like grunting and making noises when bearing down, or you may prefer to breathe deeply and quietly; you should do whatever you find helpful and works best. You will need to work with your body's instincts and adopt the position you find most comfortable and easy to give birth in (see above). Pushing your baby out into the world takes a huge amount of effort and energy, but you have the ability and are very capable of doing this.

Your doctor and birth partner will encourage and support you throughout this stage and help you to believe in your ability to give birth.

## Your baby's descent

The time it takes to push your baby out once he or she is deep within the pelvis can take around 30 minutes to one hour for a first labor, although this time may be considerably reduced in subsequent labors, sometimes taking just a few minutes. The combined force of the contractions (which are now around every two to five minutes) and your pushing moves your baby farther down into the pelvic outlet. As this occurs, the pressure on your back and rectum will intensify and you may experience a stinging sensation as your vagina becomes fully stretched. Your doctor may tell you to stop pushing at this point so that your perineum can thin further and so that the baby's head isn't delivered too suddenly, which could

### PUSHING WITH AN EPIDURAL

**If you have had an epidural, this can affect your awareness** of when to bear down and push. If this is the case, your doctor will first check that your baby isn't showing signs of distress, and may then decide to wait a while for the epidural effect to wear off slightly so you can feel when to bear down and push. Alternatively, the doctor will feel the top of your uterus so that she is aware of when a contraction is starting and will then guide you to bear down and push.

**The crowning of the head** means that the delivery of your baby is imminent and within one or two contractions the head will emerge.

**Your baby's neck** will extend backward as the head is delivered and your baby will turn to one side to aid the delivery of the first shoulder.

**Once both shoulders** are safely delivered, the rest of your baby's body will slip out fairly quickly.

**This is an emergency situation during a delivery** that occurs when the baby's head has been successfully delivered, but the shoulders appear to be stuck. Since the head may be delivered fairly easily, the problem is often not discovered until this point in labor, and immediate action is then needed to deliver the rest of the body safely. The danger is that, if the baby is not delivered rapidly, he may be starved of oxygen. The doctor will need to apply firm traction on the baby's head and neck to encourage first one and then the next shoulder to be delivered. An episiotomy (see opposite) may need to be performed to assist the rapid delivery of the baby.

Shoulder dystocia is more likely to occur where the baby is particularly large, where the mother has a small pelvis, or in women with diabetes or who are obese. If this condition has occurred in a previous pregnancy, then an obstetrician may be necessary at the birth.

**As the head crowns**, the doctor will check that the cord isn't around the baby's neck, and may then apply gentle traction to the sides of the head to help deliver the shoulders

**Your baby will emerge** covered in blood and the thick, greasy substance known as vernix that provided a protective covering for your baby's skin in the uterus.

cause serious tears. She may tell you to pant or blow instead to help you resist the urge to bear down.

**Crowning** Initially, the head will descend with each contraction and then move slightly back up the birth canal. Eventually, it will descend far enough to be visible through the vagina at the height of a contraction, known as "crowning," before it once again moves back up and disappears. As contractions continue, the head finally stays in the vaginal opening, and from this point it won't be long before your baby is born.

As your baby descends, the chin will be tucked down toward the chest and the head will rotate slightly so that your

baby is facing your back; this enables the largest part of your baby's head to pass through the widest part of the pelvis. As the head passes out of the vagina, it extends backward so that it almost touches his or her back. The doctor will check whether the cord is around the baby's neck. If this is the case, it will be lifted up and away from the neck. The doctor will remove any mucus from your baby's nose and mouth. Once the head has been delivered, it will return to its normal position.

**Rest of the body** After the delivery of the head, your baby will turn slightly so that the first shoulder can be delivered in the next contraction. Your doctor

may help by applying gentle traction to your baby's head at the side to help the first shoulder emerge. Once the first shoulder has been delivered, your baby will turn again slightly so that the second shoulder can be delivered. After this, the rest of the body will slip out and the delivery of your baby will be complete.

## Monitoring you and your baby

In the second stage, the the baby's heartbeat and your contractions are monitored. If the second stage is becoming prolonged, with the possibility of you becoming tired from pushing, an assisted delivery may be suggested with forceps or vacuum (see pp.436–7).

## Episiotomies

An episiotomy is a cut made between your vagina and anus to aid the delivery. Around 30 years ago, episiotomies were routine since it was assumed that a cut prevented worse tears. This has been shown since not to be the case, and today, an episiotomy is only done by a doctor to aid a forceps delivery or in an emergency, for example if the baby is in distress; if the baby is large; or if the perineum is tight. Before doing the procedure, the doctor should explain why they think it is necessary and should obtain your verbal consent.

Before you're cut, you'll have a local anesthetic to numb the area. The cut is usually done at an angle between the vagina and the rectum and will be stitched after the birth. The doctor will insert a long absorbable stitch in the posterior wall of the vagina, in your perineal muscle layer, and under the skin layer. If you feel discomfort, the stitches can be snipped or taken out.

You may be given oral analgesics for pain relief after you've been stitched, and anti-inflammatory medication may be recommended. Ice packs or a maternity cooling gel pad can ease pain and swelling, and bathing can be soothing.

## Perineal tears

Some women tear naturally during the delivery of their baby and this tends to be more common in a first labor. Spontaneous tears are classified by their severity and the tissue layers involved. A first degree tear involves the skin layer only; a second degree tear involves the skin and muscle-tissue layers; a third degree tear involves skin, muscle, and the anal sphincter. Fourth degree tears are uncommon and involve a tear through to the rectum. A first degree tear usually doesn't need stitches, but second, third, and fourth degree tears do. Second degree tears are the most common. Only, a small number of women sustain third or fourth degree tears, which are usually associated with assisted deliveries.

Becky is a 22-year old woman in her first pregnancy. She'd had no problems and at her 36 week appointment, she discussed her birth plan and told her doctor that she wanted a water birth at the local birth center.

**Becky's birth story:** By the time I was two days overdue I was having irregular contractions. I'd had a bloody show and had a backache. The next day I woke at 6:30 am with regular contractions. I coped using breathing techniques, stayed active, and used a birthing ball. When my contractions were every 5 minutes and lasting a minute, I called the birth center since I felt I needed to use the pool. They said they would get it ready.

At 11:35 am, my partner and I reached the center and met the doctor. She felt my contractions, listened to the baby's heartbeat and did a vaginal examination. She said I was in established labor since I was 5 cm dilated, my cervix was 50 percent effaced, and the head was descending. In the pool, I was able to move around and change position. The warm water eased my backache and contractions. I felt calmer and started to relax. I found kneeling in the water and rocking my pelvis back and forth and from side to side helpful. My partner supported me and periodically the doctor listened to my baby's heart rate.

At 3:20 pm, my contractions were every 1 to 2 minutes and very strong. The doctor and my partner reassured me and I managed to focus. I began to feel the urge to bear down. At 3:50 pm, my baby's head was born and a couple of minutes later I pushed my baby out into the water. The doctor gently lifted my baby up to me and we stayed in the water a few moments. I got out to deliver the placenta, which I did without drugs. At 4:20 pm my placenta was delivered and I didn't need stitches.

**The doctor's comments:** Becky found the warm water helped her deal with contractions, and she stayed calm. She tried different positions and the water kept her buoyant. She and her partner were focused. Her labor progressed well and was just under 10 hours. It was wonderful to observe.

**Kneeling in warm water** helped ease the pain of Becky's contractions.

**After the birth** the doctor lifted the baby to Becky's breast so she could breast-feed.

# After your baby is born

Shortly after your baby's birth, the cord will be cut and your uterus will start to contract again to deliver the placenta.

### The third stage
This is from the birth of your baby until the delivery of the membranes (the amniotic bag that surrounded your baby) and placenta. The placenta can be actively managed with the help of drugs or delivered without drugs, known as passive management or a physiological third stage. Your doctor will discuss these options with you before labor.

### Cutting the cord
Once your baby has been delivered, it may be left for two to three minutes before it is cut. Allowing the cord to pulsate for a few minutes means your baby receives more blood from the placenta, which boosts his or her oxygen supply and blood volume. The cord will be clamped in two places, about 1 cm and 4 cm from the baby's belly, and is cut with scissors between the clamps.

### Delivery of the placenta
How your placenta is delivered depends on your doctor. Many wait for it to happen naturally, but others offer an intramuscular (IM) injection of an oxytoxic drug in your thigh to make the uterus contract so that you can deliver the placenta and membranes quickly. Helping the uterus contract in this way reduces the risk of heavy bleeding occurring during the third stage, known as a postpartum hemorrhage (see box, right) and speeds up the delivery of the placenta, which can happen within 5 to 15 minutes after the birth of the baby. The risk of a postpartum hemorrhage occurring is the reason many units advise an active delivery. If you have a fibroid, active delivery will be advised because there is a heavy risk of bleeding.

Your doctor will place one of her hands just above your pubic bone to prevent the uterus from being pulled

**The umbilical cord will be clamped and cut**, a few minutes after the birth, severing the link between your baby and the placenta.

**The disc-shaped placenta, weighing** around 1 lb 2 oz (500 g), has a network of blood vessels surrounding the umbilical cord in its center.

## FIRST CHECKUPS

### Apgar score

**At 1, 5, and 10 minutes,** your baby's breathing, pulse, movements, skin color, and responses are assessed. In South Asian and black babies, the color of the mouth, palms of the hands, and soles of the feet are checked. Each is given a score between 0 and 2, called the Apgar score. A total of 7 or more at 1 minute is normal; under 7 means help is needed.

| Apgar score | 2 | 1 | 0 |
| --- | --- | --- | --- |
| Skin color | Pink all over | Body pink; extremities blue | Pale/blue all over |
| Breathing | Regular strong cry | Irregular, weak cry | Absent |
| Pulse/heart rate | Greater than 100 bpm | Less than 100 bpm | Absent |
| Movements/muscle tone | Active | Moderate activity | Limp |
| Reflexes after given certain stimuli | Crying or grimacing strongly | Moderate reaction or grimace | No response |

downward when she pulls on the cord. With her other hand, she will then apply gentle traction to the cord to help deliver the membranes and placenta. This is known as "controlled cord traction" (CCT).

**Delivering the placenta naturally** If you decide to deliver the placenta without drugs, known as a physiological third stage, this can take up to an hour. Your doctor will encourage you to bear down and you may find squatting helps. The doctor will check the placenta to ensure it's complete and that none of it remains in the uterus, which can cause a postpartum hemorrhage (see box, below).

## How you feel after the birth

After the huge effort of giving birth, it's common to have a physical reaction. Many women experience uncontrollable shaking or shivering, and some feel nauseous and may even vomit. In addition to your physical reaction, you are also likely to be feeling overwhelmed and emotional. Once you and your baby have been given the all clear, you should be given some quiet time alone to get to know each other.

### POSTPARTUM HEMORRHAGE

**A postpartum hemorrhage** describes the loss of up to 1 pint (500 ml) of blood after the delivery. This is often associated with a retained placenta, when the placenta remains in the uterus for a prolonged period of time, which is most likely to occur during a natural delivery of the placenta. It can also occur after an assisted forceps delivery; after a prolonged labor; or following a cesarean. Improvements in the treatment of this condition with antibiotics and blood transfusions has meant that the incidence of complications following a hemorrhage has fallen considerably over the years.

### YOUR BABY'S APPEARANCE

**Newborn babies are usually surprisingly unattractive.** Fortunately, as parents, we usually think they are beautiful. Newborns are covered in a waxy substance called vernix, together with amniotic fluid and blood from the birth canal. Babies who have passed meconium before the delivery may also have brown stained skin and nails.

In addition, newborn babies often have a molded, elongated head, with a swollen area on top known as a "caput," which is due to the pressure on the baby's head as it passes through the birth canal. Also, the nose may be squished to one side and the eyes may be swollen. Sometimes the genitals are swollen too. Rest assured that all of these features are temporary and within 24 hours or so the molding will work itself out and your baby will

**Your newborn baby may have a squashed appearance,** but this will smooth out within a day or two.

begin to look more like the baby you were expecting to meet.

Many babies are born with birthmarks that are referred to as "stork marks." These are red birthmarks on the eyelids and at the nape of the neck, which fade in time.

**Skin-to-skin contact** with your newborn baby will help keep her warm—newborns don't have very good temperature control—and will also help the two of you start bonding.

# Special cases

**EACH LABOR IS DIFFERENT AND THERE ARE TIMES WHEN SOME TYPE OF INTERVENTION IS NEEDED**

You may know in advance that a condition or factor in your pregnancy means that intervention, such as an induction or a cesarean section, will be needed. At other times, events can occur in labor that mean assistance is needed, or a premature labor can mean that your baby needs special care. In all cases, rest assured that procedures are in place to ensure your own and your baby's safety.

# Premature birth

The term "premature" describes both the time of birth, before 37 weeks, and how well prepared your baby is for life outside of the uterus. Premature births account for 12.7 percent of U.S. births.

Your baby may be born prematurely either because an early delivery is advised on medical grounds (see below), or you go into spontaneous preterm labor. The earlier the birth, the higher the chance of complications in the baby, such as breathing problems or infections. Nowadays, however, huge advances in the care of premature babies means that babies born as early as 23 or 24 weeks may survive. If your baby is premature, he may need to spend time in a neonatal intensive care unit (NICU, see p.452).

## Advising an early delivery

A decision may be made to deliver a baby early if the mother's or baby's health is in danger. For example, an early delivery may be recommended if the mother has a medical problem, such as a heart condition that could increase her physical stress, or preeclampsia (see p.474), which could endanger her own and her baby's health. An early delivery may also be advised if a scan shows that the placenta is not functioning well and the baby is not receiving enough oxygen. Forty-seven percent of babies in the US delivered before 32 weeks are born by cesarean, as are about a third of babies born between 34 and 36 weeks.

## Spontaneous preterm labor

The cause of spontaneous labor before 37 weeks is often unknown. However, it is more likely if a woman has a major abnormality of the uterine wall, such as large fibroids (see p.218), a weakness in the cervix, which may have been present from birth, or have occurred after surgery to the cervix or is pregnant

**Seeing your tiny baby hooked up to monitors and tubes** can be alarming, but take comfort from the fact that these are helping your baby to breathe and feed and in turn to develop.

with more than one baby. Infections like bacterial vaginosis can also set off contractions at an early stage.

**What might be done?** Preterm labor can't be stopped, but medication can slow the process and reduce some risks.

Steroids can promote the production of a natural chemical in the baby's lungs that reduces the effort of breathing. They must be given 24 to 48 hours before the birth to have maximum benefit.

You may also be given oral medicine or an injection to reduce the frequency of contractions. This can prolong pregnancy for a few days, during which time the steroids can take effect. Also, if necessary, you can be transferred to a hospital with NICU facilities.

Finally, you may be advised to have injected antibiotics since preterm babies are susceptible to bacterial infections caught via the cervix during birth.

---

### PREDICTING PREMATURE LABOR

**It's hard to predict** who will go into labor prematurely. However, if you've had a previous preterm birth, tests may be done to find out if it is likely in your current pregnancy. A cervical scan may be done around 23 weeks since a shorter cervix increases the risk of early labor. Pelvic swabs detect bacteria that are linked to preterm labor, and "fetal Fibronectin" test between 24 and 34 weeks shows whether a protein is present that, during the second half of pregnancy, generally can't be detected until 1–3 weeks before labor and delivery. Sometimes, a short cervix is strengthened with a stitch. Antibiotics can be given if abnormal bacteria are found. Progesterone may be given to stop contractions.

# Induction of labor

For 22.3 percent of women in the US, labor is started by artificial means, or induced, to reduce the risks to mother and baby.

An induction may be offered if it's felt that continuing the pregnancy poses a risk to your health or to the health of your baby. The most common reason for an induction is the continuation of a pregnancy beyond 41 or 42 weeks, in which case the placenta may begin to fail. Induction may be offered earlier if you have twins, or a medical condition such as diabetes. Before setting a date for induction, your doctor may offer to strip your membranes (see p.393) to help you go into spontaneous labor.

Induction is not the same as an augmentation of labor, which is when drugs are used to increase the efficiency of your contractions when you've already gone into labor spontaneously (see p.415).

## Assessing the cervix
Before an induction, you'll have an internal examination to assess the cervix. Induction is easier if your cervix is short and soft, described as "favorable" or "ripe," rather than long and firm. The findings may be logged in a table called the Bishop's Score, which also assesses how far the cervix is dilated (see p.415), the position of the cervix, and the station of the fetal head in the pelvis (see p.414). A total score over six indicates good conditions for an induction of labor.

## Softening the cervix
If your cervix isn't ripe, it can be softened with prostaglandins. These are naturally occurring chemicals that help stimulate contractions. Artificial prostaglandins can be given in the form of vaginal tablets of gel, which are placed at the top of the vagina near the cervix, or a vaginal suppository or an oral pill. This is usually effective, but sometimes prostaglandins fail to soften the cervix and may be tried again after a few days. On the other hand, some women experience dramatic effects after a small dose.

## Breaking the water
Amniotomy, or artificial rupture of the membranes (ARM), is one of the most important steps in the induction process, often referred to as "breaking the water" and it's done once the cervix is soft and slightly dilated, and the head has started to enter the pelvis. A thin plastic probe is passed through your cervix and used to make a small hole in the amniotic membranes, which allows some of the fluid around your baby to leak out. This softens the cervix even more and can provoke contractions in the muscular wall of the uterus. If contractions don't become established after ARM, then you'll require treatment with Syntocinon or Pitocin (see below).

## Oxytocin, Syntocinon, Pitocin
Oxytocin is a natural hormone that stimulates the uterus, increasing the frequency and strength of contractions. A synthetic form, Syntocinon or Pitocin, is used with the same effect. It's diluted in fluid then dripped into a vein in your arm or injected into a large muscle. This is safe and effective when used correctly; however, it must be used with care since excessive contractions can reduce your baby's oxygen supply in labor. Your contractions and your baby's heartbeat will be continuously monitored (see p.418).

### QUESTIONS AND ANSWERS

**Are medical interventions more likely with an induction?**
If your labor is induced, the chance that you will need an assisted delivery with forceps or vacuum (see pp.436–7) or a cesarean is increased. This is even more likely if you are having your first baby, if the cervix is unfavorable, or if you're being induced relatively early in your pregnancy. The reason for these medical interventions is usually that the labor is proceeding too slowly, or that it cannot be started at all, despite all of the steps taken. Also, concerns about the baby's well-being during the induction process can sometimes lead to intervention.

**Is induction of labor more painful than a spontaneous labor?**
Some women find that they experience strong contractions very quickly after an induction. Since they haven't been able to build up gradually to more painful contractions, they may be less able to tolerate the pain, which can result in an increased need for stronger types of pain relief such as an epidural.

**The synthetic hormone syntocinon** is given via an intravenous line to stimulate the strength and frequency of your contractions.

# Breech baby

At 32 weeks, 15 percent of babies are breech (bottom first). With time, most turn, with just 3 percent remaining breech at term.

Breech labors and births are usually more difficult, so if your baby is still in a breech position in late pregnancy, you may be offered a procedure to turn your baby (see below).

## Turning your baby

The procedure to turn your baby, external cephalic version (ECV), is usually offered at around 37 weeks if a baby is still in a breech position. The doctor presses on the lower part of your belly to elevate your baby's bottom out of the pelvis. Pressure is used to rotate your baby until he is head down. The procedure may feel uncomfortable, and you may be given medication to relax the uterus. A scan is often done before and after the procedure.

The success rate for ECVs is often over 50 percent. Complications, such as bleeding behind the placenta and premature rupture of the membranes, are rare. If an ECV is unsuccessful and you want to try for a vaginal birth, you will be advised to deliver in a hospital so help can be provided quickly if needed. In some cases, the position of a breech baby is likely to make vaginal delivery difficult and a cesarean will be advised.

## Breech diagnosed in labor

Occasionally it isn't discovered that your baby is in breech until you're in labor. This happens because it can be hard to distinguish between a baby's head and bottom by feeling your belly alone.

If a breech is diagnosed in labor, you can still have an ECV but at this stage it has a lower success rate. An ECV may not be possible in labor if the water has broken, if you're in advanced labor, or if there's no one to do the procedure.

## Delivery of your baby

If you try for a vaginal birth, you should be in a hospital with an ob/gyn present, since you may need an assisted delivery or an emergency cesarean. Fetal monitoring should be done throughout labor, since babies in distress will need to be delivered by cesarean. Sometimes a breech baby has problems getting oxygen and blood through the umbilical cord, if it's squeezed into the wrong position.

You'll be advised to have your baby's heartbeat monitored throughout labor, and you may have an IV in case you need a cesarean. You may be asked to lie on your back with your feet in stirrups so that the doctor can access the baby. An alternative position is to stand or be on all fours. Your bladder may be emptied with a catheter and an episiotomy cut may be done to prevent a more serious tear (see p.427). The doctor may apply gentle pressure to the baby's arms or legs during birth, but you're unlikely to notice this. Except for these differences, the birth is likely to feel the same as the birth of a head-first baby. During the birth, the head will be eased out of the birth canal either by hand or with forceps. to control the speed of the birth, which should be neither too fast nor too slow.

A cesarean is likely if complications arise, for example the baby shows signs of distress; the cord slips below the baby's bottom; the cervix dilates too slowly; or the baby isn't descending.

---

### POSITIONS OF A BREECH BABY

**A breech baby can lie in one of three positions,** known as extended (frank); flexed (complete); or footling. With an extended breech, the hips are flexed, knees extended, and the feet are by the head. A vaginal delivery is most likely with this type of breech. With a flexed breech, the hips and knees are flexed, with the feet above the buttocks, and a vaginal birth may be possible. In a footling breech, the hips are extended with the feet below the buttocks, so a vaginal delivery is unlikely.

Extended (frank) breech     Flexed (complete) breech     Footling breech

# Multiple births

Carrying twins or more increases the risk of complications during birth and you and your babies will be closely monitored.

Twin pregnancies occur naturally in around 1 in 53 women, but some factors increase the chance of you conceiving twins or more, including the use of some fertility treatments, becoming pregnant when you're older, already having children, and having a family history of twins.

## Monitoring during pregnancy

Because multiple pregnancies are high risk, you'll receive extra monitoring; the type of delivery depends on the position of your twins and other complications. A concern is whether twins will be born prematurely with a small birth weight, which can mean spending time in a neonatal intensive care unit (see p.452).

Toward the end of pregnancy, you may have extra scans to monitor the babies' growth, since the ability of the placenta to provide oxygen can be reduced in a twin pregnancy. The volume of the fluid around each baby and their heart rates may be measured to check their well-being.

## Possible complications

Certain complications with the babies or the mother can influence the delivery and mean that a cesarean is planned.

**Fetal complications** Twin-to-twin transfusion syndrome (TTTS) is a condition unique to identical twins who share a placenta (see p.51). It occurs if there is a direct link in the blood supply between the babies and can put the lives of both at risk. Babies with TTTS need specialized treatment that may involve reducing the fluid around one baby or using a laser to separate the circulations.

Rarely, twins can develop in the same sac, known as monoamniotic twins. The main risk of this condition is that the cords become tangled, affecting the oxygen supply. The twins may have heart traces at the end of pregnancy and are delivered early by cesarean.

**Maternal complications** When you're carrying twins, you're at a higher risk of

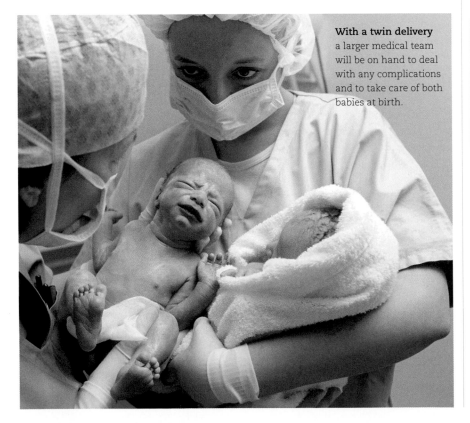

**With a twin delivery** a larger medical team will be on hand to deal with any complications and to take care of both babies at birth.

---

### QUESTIONS AND ANSWERS

**Will I have a say in how I deliver my twins?**

If you are having twins, you will get the chance to discuss your plans for giving birth with your obstetrician during the pregnancy. Your decision to have a vaginal birth or a cesarean section will probably be based upon several factors, such as the position of the babies. Once you have been given enough time to consider all of the relevant information, safety is the most important factor.

**Can I have a home birth with twins?**

Home births in the US are very rare, and organizations like the American College of Obstetricians and Gynecologists and the American Medical Association recommend against them because of the potential for complications, even in low-risk singleton pregnancies. For the safety of your babies, a hospital birth is recommended.

Gillian found out she was having twins at an early scan. At first she was worried that the pregnancy and birth would be hard, but her confidence grew as she saw her babies growing well. She went into labor at 35 weeks.

**Gillian's story:** I was shocked when they told me I was carrying twins, since none of my family has had twins. The pregnancy was tough because I was so tired and I had such a big belly. I enjoyed the scans though because they were really reassuring.

I went into labor at just over 35 weeks. After initial contractions, my water broke at 2 am. My husband got me to the hospital in 15 minutes; I think he was in a bit of a panic. Jonathan, our first twin, was born just after 4 pm, so the first part of my labor was quite long. I managed without much pain relief medication. Celia came 20 minutes later. They broke my second bag of water since her heartbeat was low, but she was fine at birth. I remember the birthing room being crowded, and even though people introduced themselves to me, I couldn't have told you who they were. However, they all disappeared soon after the birth and left us to spend some time alone with our babies. That was the best time. All the worries disappeared and we could just get on with being a mom and a dad.

**The doctor's comments:** Like many women with a twin pregnancy, Gillian was worried about what might happen to her and her babies during labor. She had talked at length to me and the doctor during her pregnancy, but still felt anxious. When she arrived on the labor ward however, she could see that the people caring for her were highly professional and experienced. This gave her the confidence to deal with events as they unfolded. Both babies were doing very well when they left the hospital and Gillian was making an excellent recovery too.

**Despite being higher risk,** a twin birth is most likely to result in the safe delivery of both babies.

complications, such as preeclampsia (see p.474), possibly because of the additional strain on the kidneys; the liver condition cholestasis (see p.473), for reasons that are unclear; and thrombosis, because there is an additional strain on your circulation. These conditions may also mean that an early cesarean is recommended.

## Going into labor

You're more likely to go into labor early and your babies may be lighter than average. With twins, you're likely to go into labor around 37 weeks; with triplets around 33 weeks; and with quadruplets around 30 weeks. The average birthweight for twins is 5.5 lb (2.5 kg); triplets and quadruplets are almost always low-birthweight.

## Labor and birth with twins

Current recommendations are that an obstetrician should attend a twin birth.

If you're planning to have a vaginal birth, the labor should be almost as quick as it is with one baby.

Continuous monitoring of both heartbeats is recommended during a multiple labor. This is usually done by putting one strap around your belly for each baby, but sometimes the second baby is monitored in this way and the first baby may have a scalp electrode put on his head (see p.419), which gives a clearer picture of the first baby's heartbeat if it has been difficult to find.

**Delivering the first twin** For your first baby, the chance of using forceps or vacuum is the same as for a singleton birth, although the birth of the first twin may need to be assisted so that the doctor can gain quick access to the second twin. After the first twin's delivery, his cord is clamped and cut, but the placenta usually remains in the uterus until the second baby has been born.

**Delivering the second twin** The medical team will confirm whether your second baby is head- or bottom-first, either by feeling your abdomen, doing an internal examination, or by scanning you. As the second baby's head or bottom enters the pelvis, the second bag of water may be broken to encourage strong contractions. A normal birth should follow in about 30 minutes, and forceps or vacuum are only used if problems arise. If the second twin is bottom-first, a doctor should be on hand to help. It's unusual for the first twin to be born vaginally and the second to be born by a cesarean, but this may happen if the second baby needs an urgent delivery and a vaginal birth seems unsafe.

**Delivering the placenta** There is a greater risk of postpartum hemorrhage with twins, which means that an active management of the third stage may be advised (see p.428).

# Assisted birth

In the US, 4.8 percent of babies has an assisted birth. These are considered safe and can prevent further complications.

## UNDERSTANDING WHY

### Reasons for an assisted birth

There are several factors that can make an assisted birth more likely.

■ **Your baby has an abnormal heart rate,** which suggests that he might be in distress.

■ **You have been pushing a long time,** but your labor is progressing slowly.

■ **You're exhausted** and can't manage any more pushing.

■ **You have a medical condition** and have been told not to push for long.

---

An assisted birth is a birth in which either forceps or a vacuum suction cup (also called a vacuum or ventouse extractor) are used to aid a vaginal delivery. There may be some mild side effects such as bruising after an assisted birth, but major complications are rare.

As with all medical interventions, the use of forceps or a vacuum extractor will only be offered when it is thought to be necessary for the health of the baby and/or mother.

### The procedure

First, your doctor will discuss with you the need for the procedure and may also explain to you the potential complications. You may be asked to sign a consent form, although not all hospitals insist on this. Before the birth takes place, you will probably be given an episiotomy and local anesthetics or epidural anesthesia. Fresh covers may be placed over your legs and abdomen and a catheter will be inserted to empty your bladder. The doctor will then place the forceps around the baby's head or attach the vacuum cup and will encourage you to start pushing again when you have a contraction. Your baby should be born within around another 20 minutes from this time. There is less of a risk for a vaginal injury with a vacuum extraction than there is with forceps.

### Forceps

Modern surgical forceps were invented by the British doctor Chamberlen in the seventeenth century and so have been in use for hundreds of years, although they have been modified over time. Forceps are an effective and reliable way to assist a delivery, but they have to be used with care by a properly trained doctor.

The forceps are placed so that they hold the sides of the baby's head near the ears and cheeks. The operator of the forceps then gently pulls the baby's head downward while you push during a contraction, and then will guide the baby out of the birth canal.

Forceps can also be used to adjust the the baby's head before the birth if the baby is lying in an occiput posterior position, which is with his back facing the mother's back (see p.417), toward the end of labor. After turning the baby's head and body, delivery is then completed as in the same way as described above.

## METHODS OF ASSISTING BIRTH

**Assisting your baby's birth with vacuum or forceps** is a safe, well practiced procedure, which can prevent the need for an emergency cesarean. Whether you have forceps or vacuum may depend on the particular expertise and experience of the doctor doing the procedure.

**With forceps,** your baby's head is cradled on either side with metal tongs that guide him down in time with your contractions.

**With vacuum,** a soft suction cup is attached to your baby's head and then your baby is gently guided out.

**Pros and cons of forceps** There are several advantages of forceps over vacuum. First, they do not rely on any kind of machinery that could cause a problem during the birth. They also work well even if your contractions are weak or if you are finding it hard to push due to exhaustion. Lastly, forceps have a low failure rate: if the doctor can get the forceps around your baby's head easily, he will usually be able to complete the vaginal birth of your baby without having to resort to a cesarean. The disadvantage of forceps is that you may be more likely to have vaginal or perineal damage than with vacuum.

## Vacuum extractor

The vacuum, or vacuum extractor, was invented in the 1950s. It consists of a cup attached to a tube that connects to a suction pump. The cup, which can be hard or soft plastic or metal, is placed on top of the baby's head and held in place while the suction creates a vacuum that makes the cup adhere to the baby's scalp. The doctor pulls downward while you push during a contraction.

Vacuum births are known to be very safe as long as you are at least 34 weeks pregnant. Before this time your baby's head may be too fragile to deal with the suction and few doctors use a vacuum before 32 weeks.

**Pros and cons of vacuum** The vacuum has some advantages over forceps; it is often a little easier to apply and may be less uncomfortable for you. It is also less likely to cause vaginal and perineal damage and you will be less likely to need an episiotomy. However, vacuum fails in up to 20 percent of cases, and it is especially likely to fail if your baby is not in the ideal position for the birth. Some doctors think it is also more likely to fail if your contractions are weak, if there is already a lot of natural swelling on your baby's head, or if you are too tired to push. If a vacuum does come off during the

**In the majority of cases, both the mother and baby** are perfectly well after an assisted birth, but occasionally complications are encountered.

**Problems during the delivery** A condition known as shoulder dystocia, in which the baby's shoulders become stuck during the birth, is more common with a forceps or vacuum delivery. If the shoulders get stuck, simple maneuvers usually release them without great difficulty, but very rarely, a shoulder dystocia can turn into an emergency, and your doctor may have to perform special maneuvers or even an emergency cesarean to complete the baby's birth.

**How your baby may be affected** Forceps can leave a temporary bruise on the side of your baby's face and can even put pressure on a nerve near the eyes, stopping the baby from being able to blink properly for a day or two. In contrast, the vacuum tends to leave a bruise on the top of the head rather than on the face (and the head may appear elongated at first where the suction pressure was applied). This can look a little alarming, but it will disappear after

a couple of weeks. More severe complications for your baby, which can include a fractured skull bone after a forceps delivery, or bleeding inside the skull after a vacuum, are very rare.

**How you may be affected** You're more likely to be given an episiotomy cut, particularly during a forceps delivery, to protect your back passage from more severe damage during the birth. This is usually successful, but in some cases an extra tear may occur in the back passage and careful stitching, after delivery is required to repair the area. Stitches may also be used if you get other tears in or around the vagina.

**A medio-lateral cut** is usually done into the muscle, angled away from the vagina and the perineum.

birth, it can be reapplied, or the doctor can reach for a pair of forceps instead. Sometimes, however, a cesarean section has to be performed if the vacuum fails.

## Pain relief

It can be painful having an assisted vaginal birth, so it is important that you have sufficient pain relief to help you cope with the delivery. In some situations, an injection of a local anesthetic in and around the vagina is sufficient to help you deal with the pain, particularly if the doctor is anticipating the birth to be fairly

quick, and if your baby has already traveled most of the way through your pelvis. For more difficult assisted births, for example where the baby is not in an occiput anterior position (see p.417), an epidural may be given (see p.404). This is especially useful if you're going to give birth in the operating room instead of the delivery room because forceps or vacuum have a high chance of failing, leading to the need for a cesarean. Finally, if you already have an epidural in place, this can be topped up with additional medication if necessary.

# Cesarean section

A cesarean delivery may be suggested if there is a potential benefit to your own or your baby's health, or sometimes both.

A cesarean section is the delivery of your baby by means of a cut in the abdomen. A cesarean rate of around 10–15 percent is thought to be reasonable, although in most Western countries the rate has risen beyond 20 percent and around 30 percent of all babies in the US are now delivered by cesarean, an all-time high.

The increase is due to a higher incidence of cesareans in first-time mothers and a lower incidence of vaginal birth after cesarean (VBAC) in subsequent pregnancies. Some women may think that cesareans are safer for the baby than a vaginal birth. In fact, if you've had an uncomplicated pregnancy, a cesarean is hard to justify on medical grounds.

## Types of cesarean

Cesareans are either emergency or planned procedures. The doctor will assess its urgency with a grading scale. A Grade 1 cesarean is one that is done if there is an immediate threat to the baby's or mother's life. A Grade 2 cesarean is one where there is concern for the baby's or mother's well-being, but no immediate threat to life. A Grade 3 cesarean is done when there is no immediate concern for the mother or the baby, but an early delivery is advised, perhaps because of a condition in the mother or baby. A Grade 4 cesarean is an elective delivery planned to suit the woman and the hospital.

**Emergency cesareans** A Grade 1 cesarean is most commonly carried out when the baby is thought to be at risk, for example if the baby's oxygen supply has been reduced and there are signs of fetal distress. In this case, the staff will try to do the cesarean rapidly—within 30 minutes when possible, although it's important that shortcuts aren't taken that could put your own health at unnecessary risk.

Grade 2 and Grade 3 cesareans take place when there's no immediate threat to life, and these are more common than Grade 1 procedures. A Grade 2 cesarean may be done if your baby's heart rate is causing concern very early in labor and the prospect of a vaginal delivery taking place within a reasonably short time is low. An example of a Grade 3 cesarean is one that is done because of a failed induction of labor.

**Elective cesareans** Around one third of cesareans are elective, or Grade 4 procedures, and the number of these has increased greatly in recent years. Reasons for an elective cesarean

**Your baby is gently lifted** out of the uterus and the cord is clamped and cut.

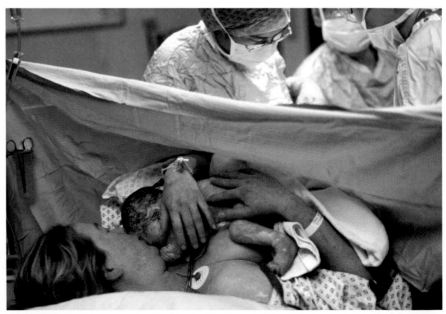

**You or your partner can enjoy the first hold of your baby** while the surgical team completes the operation by delivering the placenta and stitching the incision.

include a breech baby; a tear involving the back passage, or another traumatic event, during a previous vaginal delivery; a previous cesarean; a larger than average baby; and maternal choice. In these situations, although a cesarean is reasonable, an attempt at a vaginal birth is also reasonable with the right precautions. It's uncommon for maternal choice to be the sole reason for a cesarean, and there's likely to be another factor, such as one of those cited above.

In some situations, it would be hazardous for either you or your baby if you were to try for a vaginal birth; for example you've had multiple previous cesareans or other major surgery to the uterus; the baby can't be moved from lying horizontally; the placenta is lying very low (see p.212); or there are severe pelvic abnormalities in the birth canal. Some maternal medical conditions also mean that vaginal birth is not advisable.

## Giving your consent

The doctor will need your consent prior to doing a cesarean. He should tell you why the procedure is being proposed, and what its benefits and risks are. Ideally, you should have plenty of time to decide whether you want the surgery or not, although with an emergency cesarean, the time to think things over may be limited. Even so, you are always within your rights to say no to a cesarean, even if this means that your life or that of your baby is at risk.

## Your anesthesia

Before the surgery, you will meet an anesthesiologist, who will make sure that you have no pain during your surgery and will help you with pain control afterward. Most women are awake during a cesarean. An injection of medication into the spinal fluid in your back, called a spinal block, numbs any sensation of pain (see p.406). Or, if you've been using an epidural for pain relief in labor (see p.404), this can be used for the surgery. After your anesthetic has

been given, the anesthesiologist will check that it is working properly.

Being awake usually means that your birthing partner can stay with you and it's also a little safer for you and for your baby than a general anesthetic. Very occasionally a general anesthetic is needed (see pp.406–7).

## The surgery

Before the surgery, an IV line will be put in your hand or your arm so that fluids or medications can be given intraveneously if necessary. Also, the pubic hair on your belly may be shaved downward by about 1 in (3 cm) to clear the way for the cut. Both of these may be done before you go to the operation room or after you arrive there.

Once the anesthesiologist is assured you're pain free, a catheter will be inserted into your bladder and will stay in until the next day while your sensation recovers. Your abdomen will be cleaned with an antiseptic solution and sterile drapes will be placed over you, which prevent you and your partner from seeing the surgery.

During the surgery, a 4 in (10 cm) long cut will be made, usually horizontally, on the abdomen wall, across the bikini line, although occasionally an up-and-down cut below the belly button is done. Your bladder will be pushed down and the front of the uterus opened so that the doctor can access the baby. If your water hasn't already broken, this will be done now before the baby and placenta are delivered. The surgeon will release the baby's head from the pelvic brim and lift the baby out. Sometimes, another member of the team needs to put pressure on the uterus to assist this. You'll be able to see your baby when the cord has been cut, and once initial checkups have been done on your baby, either you or your partner should be able to hold him while the surgery is completed. After the umbilical cord is cut, your doctor will remove the placenta.

To finish the cesarean, the uterus will be closed up with one or two layers of

stitches, then the abdomen wall will be stitched in separate layers. This takes about half an hour, although it can take longer, especially if you've had previous surgeries. You may have dissolvable stitches, or stitches that have to be taken out after four or five days; less commonly, small staples may be used. The choice is usually made by the doctor, but if you have a preference, make this known to the team caring for you before the surgery starts.

## Your recovery

Your nurses will encourage you to get out of bed the following day, and by the day after this you may be well enough to do most things for yourself, with help. Women usually go home on the fourth day after the cesarean.

You've spent the last nine months anticipating this moment, but nothing can quite prepare you both for how you'll feel when you meet your baby. In the coming weeks, you'll recover from the birth, but your world will change dramatically as you grapple with your baby's everyday care. You may feel an array of emotions, from pure joy to frustration at your level of exhaustion. Most importantly, you'll be getting to know your tiny baby and marveling at this new addition to your family.

# Life with your new baby

# The first 12 hours

A few minutes ago you were a couple—and now you are parents! The moment you have been dreaming of for nine months has finally arrived… so what happens next?

Of course your experiences will depend on your labor and birth and local procedures, but here is what usually occurs in your first 12 hours after birth.

🕐 **1–2 hours** As long as he is well, your baby can be placed in your arms, and you can cuddle him and make the most of these first magical moments. The doctor or your partner will cut the umbilical cord after a few minutes, or once it stops pulsating. You may feel elated, relieved, or just exhausted. Don't be alarmed if you start to vomit, shake vigorously, or feel too exhausted to even hold your baby at first. These are all very normal post-birth sensations.

If your baby is fine and you want to breast-feed, put him to the breast, but he may just nuzzle at first. Snuggle him close, skin to skin: the warmth of your body is all he needs right now.

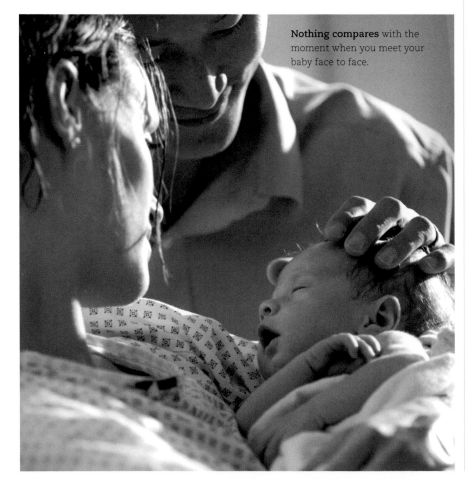

**Nothing compares** with the moment when you meet your baby face to face.

At 1, 5, and 10 minutes, your baby will be observed and given an Apgar score (see p.428). He will be wiped with a soft towel and his fingers and toes checked. He will then be weighed and his head circumference measured. He will also have a hearing test in the first hours.

But you also have work to do. As soon as your baby is born, you have to push once more to expel the placenta. You'll have milder contractions that detach the placenta from your uterus. After about 10 or 20 minutes (sometimes longer), you'll be done (see p.428).

If your perineum tore, or you had an episiotomy (a cut to ease your baby out), you may need stitches. You'll be given a local anesthetic, unless you already have an epidural, so you don't feel a thing. Your partner can hold your baby and sit close by while you are stitched.

🕐 **2–3 hours** Time to refuel: many women say their first drink of water and snack after giving birth are the best they've ever tasted… enjoy.

If you're feeling fine and there are no concerns about your condition, you'll likely be moved to the room on the maternity ward where you'll spend the remainder of your time in the hospital. You'll be taken there in a wheelchair with your baby in your arms. (In some hospitals, you'll never leave the room where you deliver; some labor and delivery rooms are designated as postpartum rooms, as well.)

🕐 **3–4 hours** After the exertion of giving birth, you'll be sweaty, sticky, and in need of a shower, which you can have now if you didn't have an epidural. Ask a nurse or your partner to walk with you if you're wobbly. Afterward you'll feel like a new woman and can put on a breast-feeding bra for comfort.

**5–6 hours** Off to the bathroom? The first time you urinate it can sting, especially if you had stitches, so pour a cup of warm water over your perineum as you urinate. The hospital needs to know everything is in good working order before you leave its care. You'll need to use sanitary pads to soak up the vaginal blood loss (lochia).

**7 hours** This might be the first chance you've had to look at your baby's tiny toes, scrunched-up legs, or fine head of hair. There may be traces of greasy vernix on his skin. Perhaps he has long, flaky fingernails that need trimming or a downy fuzz of hair called lanugo on his back. He's unique and gorgeous.

**8 hours** If your baby is awake, he may be hungry. At this stage, you're producing nutrient-rich colostrum, a fluid containing antibodies. Position him at the breast: he should open his mouth wide and take the entire areola, known as "latching on." Breast-feeding stimulates the release of the hormone oxytocin, which contracts the uterus. This can cause afterpains, more noticeable in second and subsequent births, which can feel like contractions. The only consolation is that with each contraction, your uterus—and hence your abdomen—shrinks back down.

**9 hours** If you're up to it, you might be ready for visitors, either at home or on the unit, to admire your baby. Don't let them tire you out, though.

**10 hours** Your baby's newborn checkups will take place when he is between 4 and 48 hours old. A staff pediatrician at the hospital will examine him from top to toe; listen to his heart,

## THE FIRST MEDICAL CHECKUP

**In the first 12 hours** a pediatrician will give your baby a checkup. In addition to a head-to-toe examination, there will be checks made on skin color, temperature, and muscle tone, and on reflexes, such as sucking and grasping.

**Heart and lungs** are checked to ensure they sound normal.

**Head shape** and fontanelles (soft areas between the skull bones) are examined.

**Hands and feet** are checked for reflexes, and fingers and toes are counted.

**Mouth and palate**—the separate sections should have fused together.

**Hips** are rotated and the legs are bent upward to check for signs of dislocation.

**Spine** is checked to ensure it is straight and free from abnormalities.

check his hips (and testes in a boy); and ask about the contents of his diapers.

**11 hours** In many hospitals, you can spend your first night as a new family together, since rooming-in with the baby is a common practice and new dads often sleep over. This lets the nurses see how mother and baby interact. If you need to get a few hours of uninterrupted sleep after a long or difficult labor, a nurse can collect the baby from you.

**12 hours** After a whirlwind of agony, ecstasy, and sheer hard labor, you need to rest when you can. If your baby is sleeping, fend off visitors, draw the curtains around your bed, or take the phone off the hook, and sleep.

## AFTER A CESAREAN

# Your recovery

Although you've had major surgery, you'll be encouraged to get up to get your circulation going. After an epidural, this will be as soon as you've regained the feeling in your legs. After a general anesthetic, you'll be encouraged to get up when you no longer feel sleepy, usually within an hour. You won't be able to shower yet, but your nurse or midwife can give you a bed bath to help you freshen up.

You'll probably feel very tired and sore, so ask for help with positioning your baby at the breast, and take pain medication when you need it.

# Getting acquainted

## YOUR BABY TODAY

In the first 24 hours, your baby should pass urine and meconium, the first black, sticky feces, that are made up of waste products and bile. You'll be changing plenty of diapers, and in no time, you'll be a diapering pro.

Finally, your baby is in your arms! As you recuperate in the hospital, you'll get to know the baby you've waited to meet.

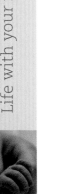
### CHECKLIST

## Safe sleeping

Crib death is a concern for all new parents. Follow the guidelines from the National Institutes of Health's "Back to Sleep" campaign to minimize the risks.

■ **Put your baby on his back** to sleep.

■ **Don't let your baby get too hot.** He really doesn't need a blanket. If it's chilly, add layers and make sure his feet are covered, but don't go overboard. In the summer, he may be most comfortable sleeping in just a onesie—but make sure the fan or air conditioning vent isn't directly overhead.

■ **Don't let anyone smoke** around your baby.

■ **Never sleep with** your baby on a sofa or armchair.

■ **The safest place for your baby to sleep is in a crib or co-sleeper** near where you sleep. If you bring the baby into your bed to breast-feed, put him back in his crib or co-sleeper when done.

■ **Keep all soft objects, like pillows, toys, and loose bedding out of the baby's crib.** A firm mattress covered by a fitted sheet is best.

**At last, you're a mom!** You may feel love at first sight, when you first hold your baby after the birth, but for many women bonding takes place over the next few days or weeks. For both parents, skin-to-skin contact with your baby helps the bonding process and is particularly beneficial for premature babies (see p.452). Try not to be anxious when you pick up your baby. In the first few weeks, your baby has little head control, so support him with a hand under his head and shoulders, or both hands under his arms and with your fingers supporting his head.

**The nurses** in the maternity ward are there for help and support. You'll be asked if you've urinated and will be given help with breast-feeding if needed. A lactation consultant will likely also be on hand to guide you through the initial difficulties you may encounter when nursing is unfamiliar. If your hospital offers "rooming in," you'll get to spend most of the day with your baby present, except when he is taken by the nurses for routine testing or examinations by the staff pediatricians. You'll also be visited by your doctor every day that you're in the hospital so he or she can check on your progress.

### YOUR BABY'S REFLEXES

**Newborn babies have reflexes** that form part of their survival skills. In addition to the rooting and grasping reflexes shown here, babies also have a startle reflex, whereby they will fling out their arms if unsupported, and a stepping reflex, which means they will step their feet up and down if held upright on a surface.

**Rooting reflex:** If you touch or stroke your baby's cheek, he will turn toward that side with his mouth open in search for food.

**Grasping reflex:** If you place your finger in the palm of your baby's hand, he will instinctively tightly grip your finger.

# Settling in

## YOUR BABY TODAY

Newborn babies sleep around 16 hours a day, although some sleep for most of the first few days while others seem awake and fretful. If your baby is very sleepy, you may need to wake her for feedings, which should be at least every four hours.

## You may be feeling anxious about your new responsibilities, but be reassured by the support network around you.

**Your ob/gyn** will visit in the hospital today. She will ask how you are managing and check that you have emergency contact numbers. You may be asked to watch short films or read brochures about the risks of Shaken Baby Syndrome and/or Sudden Infant Death Syndrome. A pediatrician will also examine your baby in the hospital today.

**It's important that you** eat a healthy diet and rest during the day whenever possible. Kegel exercises (see p.69) are vital to strengthen your muscles. If you were given painkillers or anti-inflammatory medicine, take these as necessary. If you get visitors, make sure they wash their hands before touching the baby.

### Do I need to clean the cord stump before it drops off?

Your baby's cord stump, which is the end of the umbilical cord, will shrivel up and fall off naturally around 7–10 days after the birth. Many parents feel uneasy about touching the stump and are unsure whether or not to clean it. Some pediticians recommend swabbing it regularly with rubbing alcohol but others say to leave it alone. However, if it does become dirty, clean with soap and water and dry well. If the cord stump or the surrounding area are sticky, inflammed, or smelly, contact your doctor for advice. It's important to keep the cord stump dry. Exposing it to air at times helps avoid the risk of infection.

While you're in the hospital, you may get lots of visitors. And while it's fun to show off your beautiful baby to friends and family, make sure that you take time to sleep, because once you bring your baby home, you won't have much opportunity to sleep. Many hospitals let you decide whether the baby will sleep in the room with you at night or in the nursery. There's no wrong decision; do what feels best for you and your baby.

---

### BURPING YOUR BABY

**Burping simply means helping your baby burp after a feeding.** After a feeding, air bubbles in your baby's stomach need to rise to the top and you can help this happen by sitting her on your lap or holding her upright against your shoulder. You don't need to rub or pat her, but this often feels right and babies seem to like it! It's a good idea to burp half way through a feeding and again at the end, especially for bottle-fed babies, since air fills up the stomach, slows down the feeding, and makes a baby more likely to vomit.

**Holding your baby upight** over your shoulder after a feeding can help your baby burp and therefore ease discomfort.

---

### EASING DISCOMFORT

## Stitches and hemorrhoids

The following can increase comfort.

- When you urinate, pour warm water over the area to ease stinging.

- Sit on an inflatable ring.

- Apply a cooling gel or ice pack.

- Take a warm bath or spray water on your stitches in the shower.

# Going home

## YOUR BABY TODAY

A new baby's skin is often quite dry in the first few weeks. This is normal and the skin will eventually correct itself. Although you don't need to put moisturizer on a baby's skin, if you want you could gently massage in some baby or olive oil.

Once your breast milk arrives, your baby may start to appear more relaxed and contented and go longer between feedings.

**Your first day at home** with your tiny new baby can be daunting. You are also probably feeling tired after feeding and changing your baby at night.

Keeping your baby's crib close to your bed can make life easier at night when you feed or change her. A crib with sides that can be lowered put next to your bed lets you feed her and place her back in her crib without actually getting out of bed. Try to deal with night wakings with a minimum of fuss. Keep lights low and don't talk much or stimulate your baby. Only change your baby's diaper if it is really necessary and, once the feeding is done, put her right back down in her crib.

You'll discover that babies don't like being dressed—especially having clothes pulled over their head. Keep life simple by buying machine-washable, front-fastening onesies and only change outfits if a diaper leaks. In the first weeks, there is no need to change her into a daytime outfit. If she is cold, simply add layers.

**Today, you may notice** that swelling in your hands and feet subsides as you pass more urine. However, you still need to drink plenty of fluids—two to three quarts a day—to prevent bladder infections, avoid constipation, and help breast milk production. Today or tomorrow may be the first time you move your bowels since giving birth. Eat lots of fruit and vegetables and adequate amounts of fiber to help bowel movements return to normal.

Until now, your breasts have produced colostrum, the watery premilk rich in nutrients and antibodies. By the end of the third day your milk will come in and your baby will start to feel more satisfied. Once your milk is in, your breasts will likely feel engorged and uncomfortable. As feeding establishes over the next few days this discomfort should start to recede.

**Fathers will be proud** to have the new baby at home. Apart from breast-feeding, dads can be involved in all aspects of care, including calming the baby, changing diapers, bathing, and dressing.

**The doctor will do a checkup** before you go home to make sure the uterus has contracted; your blood loss (lochia) to ensure it isn't too heavy; and any stitches.

## SPONGE BATHS

**Babies don't need frequent baths.** Two or three times a week is enough, or their skin can dry out. For the first week or two, before the umbilical cord stump falls off, give sponge baths. Wrap your baby in a towel and lie her on a flat surface. Get ready a baby washcloth, a bowl of warm water, and mild baby soap. Uncover only the body parts you're actively washing, then rewrap them in the towel. Start with the face, with water only, then use soap on the body and end with the diaper area.

**Using a damp washcloth,** gently clean your baby's face, using water only.

**To clean her hands,** wipe the backs and palms and between the fingers.

**Wash the diaper area** last, making sure to clean between the creases in the skin.

Life with your new baby

# First outing

**YOUR BABY TODAY**

The pediatrician will examine your baby today. She will ask if he is alert and check for any signs of jaundice (see p.477). She will also weigh him and will ask how he is getting along with feeding and whether there are any problems.

Your body is gradually recovering from the birth, and you may be starting to feel like facing the world once again.

**Your breasts should be** feeling a bit more comfortable by now as feeding becomes established, and your uterus will be steadily reducing in size, but can still be felt by pressing on your abdomen.

Your blood loss will have started to ease off by now, although you may find that it's heavier first thing in the morning and also while you're breast-feeding.

**You'll visit the pediatrician** today for the baby's first in-office checkup. She will look for any signs of dehydration, such as your baby not having plenty of wet diapers and any feeding problems. She'll also measure your baby's weight, length, and head circumference. The measurements will be plotted on a graph to track your baby's own growth curves at all of his subsequent appointments. The doctor willl also examine the soft spots (fontanelles) on your baby's head; look into his ears, eyes, and mouth; listen to his heart and lungs; and examine his abdomen, hips, legs, and genitals.

**You'll likely head home** from the hospital today If you had stitches or staples these will likely be removed today before you're discharged, although many obstetricians now use subcuticular stitches (just under the skin layer) that do not need to be removed since they gradually absorb over a few weeks.

**A properly installed** baby car seat is a legal requirement when traveling with your baby in a car.

**AS A MATTER OF FACT**

**By day four about a third** of all babies are visibly jaundiced.

Jaundice in newborn babies is usually harmless and is due to an elevated level of the waste product bilirubin in the blood, caused by the baby's immature liver. Very high levels of bilirubin can cause problems and are treated with light therapy (see p.477).

**CHECKLIST**

## Taking your baby out

If you haven't been out yet, cabin fever may be setting in. Make sure you have everything you may need before venturing out on a trip.

■ **Pack a diaper bag with** two diapers, wipes or cotton pads, a spare onesie, a cloth, and a bottle of formula if you're bottle-feeding.

■ **Take layers of clothing** on outings, including an undershirt, onesie, and cardigan. In winter, add an all-in-one babysuit and a blanket in a carriage.

■ **A third of a baby's heat is lost through his head,** so on cool days, add a hat or hooded top. Socks and booties are easy to lose, Footed onesies are more practical; mittens are only needed in cold weather.

■ **In hot weather, make sure your baby is covered** and protected from direct sunlight at all times.

■ **Figure out how to use a baby sling.** If traveling by car or public transportation, learn how to fold and unfold a stroller.

■ **Do not carry your baby far in a car seat** because it's bad for your back.

# Feeding your baby

Breast-feeding provides your baby with the best nutritional start in life and has a range of other benefits, outlined here. If you decide to bottle-feed, you can also be confident that your baby will thrive. The key to both methods is preparation.

## QUESTIONS AND ANSWERS

**How often should I feed my baby?**

If you have a healthy, full-term baby, you should feed her on demand, which means feeding her when she cries and seems hungry. This can mean that sometimes she'll be fed every couple of hours and sometimes she'll go for four to six hours without a feeding. Although you may not feel as if you're producing much milk initially, your baby only needs small quantities of colostrum, the first watery milk. Her demands will grow after the first few days, which will coincide with your milk coming in (see right).

**Will I be able to breast-feed my twins?**

Milk is produced on a supply and demand basis, so it's perfectly possible to breast-feed twins and more. If your babies are born early, breast milk is beneficial since it protects against infections, which premature babies are more susceptible to, so it's worth breast-feeding, even for a few weeks, but you'll need rest and ample nutrition. Start by feeding your twins separately. If you then want to feed them together, take time to position them well. An under-arm hold works well (see p.449) and cushions and a willing helper are useful. Expressing (see p.449) means the babies can be fed together, alternating on the breast. If you think that they aren't getting enough milk, consult your doctor. A lactation consultant, La Leche League, or the local chapter of the National Organization of Mothers of Twins Clubs can offer support too.

## The benefits of breast-feeding

Breast-feeding is the perfect first food for your baby; it contains all the nutrients your baby needs and works on a supply and demand basis, so that as your baby feeds, your body responds by producing more milk. Breast milk is thought to reduce a baby's risk of developing an allergic condition, such as asthma and eczema, to make childhood obesity and diabetes less likely, and it may reduce the long-term risk of heart disease.

Breast-feeding also provides benefits for you. It helps your uterus contract to its pre-pregnancy shape more quickly. It helps you get back into shape quicker since your body uses additional energy to produce breast milk, and it reduces your risk of getting breast and ovarian cancer.

Lastly, and importantly, breast-feeding helps you and your baby to be close both physically and emotionally.

## When your milk comes in

In the first few days your breasts produce colostrum, a watery substance that contains essential nutrients and antibodies that help your baby to fight off infections such as those of the ear, chest, and gastrointestinal tract.

At around day three, or sometimes a bit later, you will start to produce milk, which contains all the nutrients your baby needs. Your breasts may feel uncomfortably full

## THE RIGHT TECHNIQUE

## Latching on

**Taking the time to ensure that your baby is latched on** properly before a feeding is important because you could otherwise develop sore nipples. A baby that is properly latched on has her mouth wide open, with the whole areola (the area surrounding the nipple) in her mouth; her bottom lip will be curled back and she will be noticeably sucking. You'll feel a sucking effect over the entire area.

**Once you've positioned your baby** so that she is level with your breast, hold her with her nose and mouth facing your nipple.

**When your baby opens her mouth wide,** bring her to the breast, ensuring that she takes all of the nipple and the areola into her mouth.

**To remove your baby from the breast** insert your finger into the corner of her mouth to break the seal so that she doesn't pull the nipple.

**Holding your baby tummy-to-tummy** is a comfortable position for you both, enabling your baby to latch on well (top, left). **An under-arm "football" hold** can help keep a restless baby still (bottom, left). **Lying side by side** is often recommended after a cesarean (right).

and tender at this time, and you'll need to make sure they're properly emptied at each feeding to prevent them from becoming engorged (see p.456).

## Successful breast-feeding

Despite the fact that breast-feeding is a natural process, it can sometimes prove difficult. Getting comfortable before a feeding, positioning your baby well, and ensuring that she latches on properly (see box, left), are all prerequisites for successful feeding.

For your baby to latch on properly, it's important that you're both positioned well. Ensure that you're comfortable and that your back is well supported; using cushions for support may be helpful. You may find sitting and cradling your baby at chest level is comfortable with her tummy facing your tummy. Or you could try a football hold with your baby under your arm. Some women find it helpful to lie on their side to latch their baby on. You'll soon discover which positions suit you best and will gradually gain confidence in your ability to feed.

Once your baby is latched on, the "letdown" reflex is triggered. You will feel a tingling sensation as milk is released, which in turn stimulates the production of more milk. Your baby will pause during

feedings and stop when she is full. It's advisable to always have water or juice during or just after a feeding to replace the fluids lost from breast milk.

## Bottle-feeding

This involves more preparation, but your partner can help and become involved with feeding. You'll need in advance 4–6 bottles: larger 8 fl oz (250 ml) bottles, and smaller 4 fl oz (125 ml) ones; newborn bottle nipples; a bottle brush; and infant formula. If you have chlorinated tap

**Bottle-feeding helps dads** strengthen the bond with their baby and allows you to have some welcome time off from feeding.

EXPRESSING MILK

## An extra supply

**Expressing your milk boosts your milk production** and enables you to go out or have an unbroken night's sleep while your partner feeds the baby. You can express milk as soon as you like after the birth, although often women wait until feeding is established, at about four weeks. Your fresh milk can be stored in a milk-storage bag or bottle for 3–8 days in the fridge or frozen for 3–6 months and defrosted in the fridge or a bowl of warm water, never the microwave.

**Many women use a breast pump,** either electric or manual, to express milk. You can also express manually.

water, it's okay to put bottles in the dishwasher or wash by hand. Otherwise, clean all of the parts, then boil in water for 5–10 minutes. Put filtered or cooled boiled water in the bottle, then add the formula according to the manufacturer's instructions. Test the temperature of the milk by squeezing a drop on your inner wrist: it should feel warm, but not hot. Cool the milk if necessary by placing the bottle in a pitcher of cold water, or running it under cold water while shaking the bottle all the time. When ready, hold your baby half sitting with her head in the crook of your elbow and her back along your forearm. Gently put the nipple into her mouth and tip the bottle so the milk covers the nipple to stop her from swallowing any air. Discard any formula leftover in the bottle.

Feeding your baby

# Baby blues

## YOUR BABY TODAY

If you had a cesarean and your baby is healthy, he'll likely come home from the hospital with you today, after passing his final in-hospital pediatric exam. Make sure you have the correct car seat for him, and pack a blanket or two to keep him warm.

## Try to spend some time focusing on the needs of older children too and helping them to adapt to the new arrival.

**Today, you might feel** emotional and weepy, known as the "baby blues." This is caused by hormonal changes and exacerbated by fatigue and a feeling of anti-climax after the build up to the birth. The baby blues last a day or so and with rest and emotional support you will start to feel better. If the feelings fail to subside after a few days, talk to your doctor since you may be suffering from postpartum depression (see p.475).

Your breasts will still feel tender and full today. Feeding your baby on demand (see p.448) will help relieve this. Feeling tired interferes with the "letdown" reflex (see p.449), so it's vital to rest or sleep in the day to make up for broken nights. It's important to continue breast-feeding at night to prevent milk stagnation, which leads to problems such as abscesses and mastitis (breast inflammation) (see p.475).

**Your baby's arrival** is a major adjustment for an older child, but there are ways to help him welcome the baby. Give your older child a gift from the baby and encourage him to help with the baby's care as is appropriate for his age. A two year old may want to touch the baby, hold his hand, and bring diaper and other things that are needed, while a five year old can hold the baby with support and sing to him.

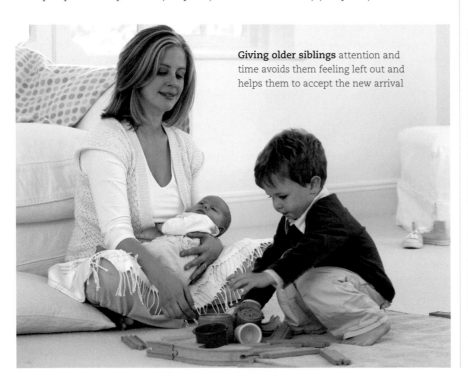

**Giving older siblings** attention and time avoids them feeling left out and helps them to accept the new arrival

### TIPS FOR COPING

## Coping strategies

Setting yourself some guidelines can help you cope with the added demands of twins or more.

■ Make time to be with your babies.

■ Prioritize activities ruthlessly, enlist practical help, and shop online.

■ Don't bathe your babies daily unless you and they enjoy it.

■ Let visitors make their own coffee.

■ Consider using pacifiers if your twins cry a lot. This helps you attend to the twin most in need.

■ Make time for yourself every day.

# Finding your way

**YOUR BABY TODAY**

It's likely that both you and your baby are becoming more confident with feeding. It's common for new babies to bring up some milk after each feeding, known as spitting up, and this is unlikely to cause any harm. Talk to the doctor if you're at all concerned.

## By now, you and your partner will be starting to feel more confident about holding, handling, and feeding your baby.

**Many parents feel uneasy** about giving their baby a bath since they worry about dropping a slippery baby. Many also find that their baby objects strongly to being undressed and immersed in water. Bathing should be fun, so if your baby hates baths at first, sponge bathe him most of the time (see p.446). Make bathtime as stress-free as possible by gathering everything you need before you start and make sure the room you undress your baby in is warm and draft-free. After the bath, dry and dress your baby immediately.

Diapers will be a part of your life for the next couple of years. There is no need to routinely change a diaper before or after feedings—just when there is a stool or it is heavy with urine. After opening a diaper, wipe away all visible feces with the diaper. Clean your baby's bottom thoroughly with wet cotton pads, wiping from front to back to avoid spreading germs. If using a cloth diaper, use a cream to avoid diaper rash. If your baby wears disposable diapers you may not need a diaper cream, but if he starts to get a diaper rash, you may find that diaper cream will clear it up.

### BATHING YOUR BABY

**Before you bath your baby,** have a towel ready to dry him and a clean diaper and change of clothes at hand so that he doesn't get cold after the bath. Half fill a baby bath with water that feels lukewarm to your elbow. After bathing, dry him quickly. Don't use talcum powder, which he could inhale.

**Wrap your baby in a towel,** and support his head and shoulders while you wet his head with the other hand.

**Wrap your baby in a towel,** and support his head and shoulders while you wet his head with the other hand.

**Still supporting his head,** wash him with a washcloth or sponge; start with the face and end with the bottom.

CHECKLIST

## Exercise basics

You will be encouraged to do some gentle exercise as soon as you feel able, although it's best to wait until the six-week checkup (see pp.462–3) before starting a strenuous program.

■ Try to maintain good posture since this will help relieve backaches.
■ Continue Kegel exercises (see p.69) after giving birth.
■ If you had a cesarean, wait until at least six weeks before starting an exercise program.
■ Start with low-impact exercises, such as walking and Pilates. Gradually increase the duration and intensity. You can also begin to strengthen your abdominal muscles (see p.456).
■ If you have any bleeding or feel faint, stop and consult your doctor.
■ Set realistic goals.

The 1st week

# Neonatal intensive care babies

Around 10 to 15 percent of all babies born in the US need to spend time in a neonatal intensive care unit (NICU). Babies most often need extra care to assist them with breathing until their lungs have matured.

There are many reasons why your baby may need special care, the most common one being prematurity (being born before 37 weeks). Babies may need to spend days, weeks, or sometimes months in a NICU until they are big enough and well enough to go home.

### Neonatal intensive care unit

If your baby is in a NICU, this is a particularly stressful time. It helps to understand a bit about who will be caring for your baby, what they will be doing, and how to make sure you're fully informed at all times.

In the US, most hospitals have a unit to provide special nursing and medical care for babies; these are divided into three levels depending on the degree of care offered. Level one is the most basic level. These units don't provide long-term ventilatory support, but they are expert at caring for babies who are slightly premature, need frequent nursing, or have previously been ventilated and are ready to be transferred to less intensive care. Level two units ventilate and give intensive care to babies from 26 weeks' gestation. Level three units offer intensive care for babies born as early as 23 weeks, and can often do neonatal surgery.

All these units are staffed by special nurses and doctors who will be happy to show you around before the baby is born if there is time.

**Ward rounds** Most units have rounds each morning, and the more intensive units will have another round later in the day. Some allow parents to be present and to ask questions during rounds, while others prefer parents to wait outside and then make time to talk to them afterward.

**Communication and visiting** You may be able to spend some time with your baby before he is sent to a NICU. However, if your baby needs to be on a ventilator, or has another serious problem, he will be sent immediately to neonatal intensive care, and you may not have any time together after the birth. You'll be encouraged to see your baby as soon as he has been transferred, and if you're unable to go immediately, you may be given a photo of your baby.

You should be able to see your baby any time of the day or night and the nurses will be happy to update you regularly. The doctors will also give you an update on an ad hoc basis or arrange to meet you for a more formal chat. Other family members may be able to visit the unit with your permission.

---

**THE ROLE OF PARENTS**

## How you can help your baby

**For most, the experience of having their baby in a NICU is extremely stressful.** Parents may feel that they have no role in the care of their baby; however, this is not the case. The most important thing you can do for your baby is to start expressing breast milk. Breast milk will nearly always be the best milk for a premature baby and can be stored in a freezer until needed.

You may be able to touch and stroke your baby and can be helped to cuddle him while he is on a ventilator. Babies thrive on skin-to-skin contact, called kangaroo care. You'll be encouraged to tuck your baby on your chest inside your shirt so that he can enjoy a close bond. Talking, reading, and singing to your baby helps him become familiar with you. You may be able to change his diaper and help with feedings, even if these are through a nasogastric tube.

Spend plenty of time with your baby, especially when breast-feeding since this may help the letdown reflex (see p.449), but save some time for yourself too so that you conserve energy for when you return home with your baby.

**Carrying your baby** close to your body and enjoying skin-to-skin contact together will help your tiny baby thrive.

**You will both be encouraged** to touch, stroke, and caress your small baby, and to spend as much time as possible talking and singing to him.

## Your baby's care

While your baby is in the NICU, he may be treated with medication and have various tests and checkups. In some cases, he will need to be on a ventilator.

**Tests and X-rays** Your baby may have blood tests to check for infection and anemia, to check kidney function, oxygen, and carbon dioxide levels, sugar levels, and to identify his blood group. The frequency of these depends on how ill or premature your baby is. In neonatal intensive care babies need blood tests periodically. Some babies need an X-ray while they're there, and very premature babies often need many chest X-rays and sometimes abdominal ones.

**Assisting your baby** Some babies need a little extra oxygen, while others need constant oxygen through a nasal tube. For very premature babies, a tube may be placed into the trachea (windpipe) and connected to a ventilator that blows oxygen into the lungs. Babies are monitored to see when they can be weaned off the ventilator.

Most babies in intensive care need one or more IVs to give fluids, blood, and antibiotics. Very small babies may be fed through a long, fine feeding tube running through the mouth or nose to the stomach. They may also need at least one blood transfusion, for some cases of conditions like anemia and jaundice.

Antibiotics are often given to prevent infection. Some babies need medicine to keep their blood pressure up, and many who are ventilated need medicine to sedate them and to prevent or treat pain.

### YOUR BABY'S CAREGIVERS

# Who's who on the neonatal unit

### Neonatal nurses
Most of the care in a neonatal intensive care unit is carried out by highly trained nurses. These include registered nurses and neonatal clinical nurse specialists who have advanced training. Some intensive care units also have neonatal nurse practitioners, who have advanced education and training and can perform many procedures.

### Doctors
Neonatologists are the doctors who run the neonatal intensive care units. These are the doctors who will coordinate your baby's daily care plan. They are pediatricians who have received advanced training to care for sick and premature newborns. The neonatologist in charge of the department is known as the attending doctor. In addition to neonatologists, there are often neonatology fellows and pediatric residents, as well. Neonatology fellows are pediatricians who are getting advanced training to care for sick newborns. Pediatric residents are doctors who are being trained in the specialty area of pediatrics.

### Other members of staff
A neonatal intensive care unit depends on a number of other staff members. These include a registered dietitian, physical and occupational therapists, technicians (who can draw blood or take X-rays), pharmacists, and, in some neonatal intensive care units, a psychotherapist to offer much needed emotional support to parents.

Neonatal intensive care babies

# Tuning in

**YOUR BABY TODAY**

Some "tummy time" is good for infants as long as they are awake and being observed. But don't lie your baby down on her stomach for bed—it's dangerous and can lead to Sudden Infant Death Syndrome (SIDS).

## As the bond between you and your baby continues to grow, you will start to feel more intuitive about his needs.

---

**CHECKLIST**

### Your baby's cries

Follow the checklist below to help you identify the cause of your baby's cries. If your baby cries for three hours or more a day, consult your doctor.

■ **Hunger is the main reason** for crying; he will stop once he is offered the breast, a bottle, a finger, or a pacifier.

■ **A cry of pain** is easy to interpret since your baby may be inconsolable, draw up his legs in pain, or arch his back. If you're unsure how to remedy the pain, consult your doctor.

■ **A wet or dirty diaper** can be uncomfortable and cause crying.

■ **Your baby may want to be held** if you can see no other reason for his crying. Babies can't be spoiled by too much cuddling. Carrying him in a sling while you do chores may comfort him.

■ **Your baby may be overstimulated.** If nothing else works, put him down in a quiet room; in our anxiety as new parents, it can be easy to forget that babies need quiet time.

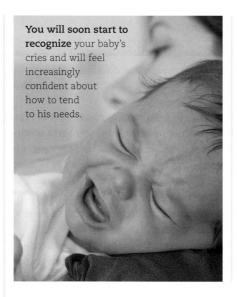

**You will soon start to recognize** your baby's cries and will feel increasingly confident about how to tend to his needs.

**Crying is the only way** your baby can get your attention. Parents-to-be often worry about how they'll know what their baby wants. Although his cries may seem indistinguishable at first, you'll soon start to interpret them (see box, left).

**Ideally, you'll have continued** Kegel exercises (see p.69) in this first week. It's important to continue doing these since they strengthen the muscles that support your bladder, helping to prevent stress incontinence (see p.475). They also help promote healing and ease discomfort if you've had stitches since they increase the blood flow to your perineum.

---

**SWADDLING**

**Swaddling: If your newborn cries a lot, is fussy, or has trouble sleeping, try swaddling her.** Being wrapped tightly in blankets, with the arms bound, makes babies feel the way they did in when they were in the uterus, and it calms them. In fact, some babies sleep an extra hour or two when swaddled and may even need to be unswaddled to wake up for their feedings. Be sure that any blankets you use for swaddling are tightly wrapped around the baby, because loose blankets can cover a baby's face and so become a factor for Sudden Infant Death Syndrome (SIDS). You may have learned how to swaddle your baby in the hospital. If not, your pediatrician should know how to do it. There are also simple swaddling products on the market that use Velcro tabs for a snug fit, thus eliminating the need to learn how to properly swaddle. These products can be found online or in stores.

# Healthy living

## YOUR BABY TODAY

Whether you're breast-feeding or bottle-feeding can have an effect on your baby's stools. The stools of breast-fed babies tend to be slightly runnier and can have a fairly sweet aroma, while bottle-fed babies may have firmer, stronger smelling stools.

## A healthy lifestyle benefits your physical and mental well-being and helps you deal with the demands of parenthood.

**It's important to eat** a well-balanced diet (see pp.14–17) to help you deal with the demands of motherhood. If you're breast-feeding, you'll need an extra 500 calories a day. Drink plenty of clear fluids, being careful to limit your caffeine intake. If you were anemic during pregnancy, or had a heavy blood loss after the birth, eat lots of iron-rich foods, such as broccoli or spinach. Foods and drinks rich in vitamin C will help you absorb iron.

If you smoke and didn't manage to stop during pregnancy, this is an ideal time to try to stop. Ask your doctor to refer you to a local smoking cessation group. Limiting your alcohol intake is also wise, and drinking while breast-feeding isn't recommended.

**It can be easy to** take over your baby's care, but it's important that your partner is involved too and doesn't feel left out. Your partner is adjusting to fatherhood and may have his own anxieties and concerns. Sharing the practical care will help him forge his own bond with the baby. As his confidence grows, you'll be able to take some time out while he cares for the baby. Keeping the lines of communication open is vital since this is a time of huge change for you both. It takes time to adjust to being a family, but if you work together you'll manage the transition more smoothly.

**Eating a variety of fresh produce** will ensure a good intake of vitamins and minerals.

### AS A MATTER OF FACT

**You'll fill out your baby's birth certificate** in the hospital

Your doctor or hospital will file this with the appropriate government agency. You'll probably also receive paperwork to apply for a Social Security number for your baby, but you can also get the forms at ssa.gov.

### YOUR BABY'S DIAPER: WHAT'S NORMAL AND WHEN TO WORRY

**The color and consistency of a baby's stools** are highly variable, but most are normal and not a cause for concern. However, some types of stool can indicate a problem and it's important that you know what to look for. A change in the color of urine or the presence of blood might also alert you to a problem.

#### What's normal
- Once your baby has passed the first dark meconium (see p.444), stools may become dark green, green-yellow, bright yellow, orange, or brown; all are normal and may vary in the same day.
- If your baby is breast-fed, stools may be loose and seedy.
- If your baby is bottle-fed, stools tend to be smooth and firmer.

- Frequency of stools varies from after every feeding to every 2–3 days.
- Urine may be yellow or clear.
- A pink or red-orange stain on the diaper due to urate crystals (which form from concentrated urine); these are common in the first few weeks, especially in breast-fed babies and are nothing to worry about.

#### What's not normal
- White or putty-colored, which could indicate a liver problem.
- Blood mixed in the stools, which could suggest a milk allergy.
- Dark urine could be a sign of dehydration or jaundice.
If you notice any of these signs, ask your doctor for advice.

The 2nd week

# Focus on you

### YOUR BABY TODAY

If your baby vomits large amounts and isn't thriving, this may suggest a problem such as gastroesophageal reflux (see p.477). This is caused by the immaturity of the stomach muscles and does resolve over time and with treatment.

Now that you've begun to adapt to the topsy-turvy world of motherhood, try to carve out some time for yourself each day.

**To help you deal** with broken nights and constant demands, you need to develop coping skills, such as taking an afternoon nap. You may also be dealing with feelings of isolation and may even find it hard to keep track of what day it is as days and nights merge into one. To revive your spirits, arrange for a friend or relative to take care of your baby while you have a break. You and your partner also need to make more of an effort to make time for each other.

### TIPS FOR MOM

## Tummy-flattening

Strengthening your abdomen enables your body to work more efficiently during any activity and helps you regain your pre-pregnancy tone.

■ Sit up straight; pull in your tummy for 60 seconds at least once each hour.

■ Stand tall and straight to keep you abdominal muscles firm.

■ Massage your abdomen with oil or body lotion in circular movements.

■ When you feel able, you can start doing gentle sit-ups to strengthen your abdomen, but wait for at least six weeks after a cesarean.

### BREAST-FEEDING PROBLEMS

**For some women, breast-feeding is a straightforward process** that both mother and baby take to without a hiccup. However, for many women breast-feeding can be surprisingly hard and extra support is needed to overcome problems. Engorged (swollen) breasts and sore nipples are a common complaint; knowing how to avoid or treat these problems can be the difference between continuing with breast-feeding or giving up.

The secret to avoiding sore nipples is to make sure that your baby latches on to your breast properly (see p.448).

Engorged breasts can make it hard for your baby to latch on, so try expressing a little milk before a feeding to relieve some pressure. Whenever possible, let the air get to your nipples, and use breast pads at other times to keep the nipples dry.

You can relieve engorged breasts by continuing with breast-feeding and expressing milk frequently inbetween feedings to relieve the pressure. Placing a warm, clean washcloth on your breast or putting a chilled cabbage leaf inside your bra can also be soothing.

**Positioning your baby** well at the breast and ensuring that he latches on properly will help to avoid sore, painful nipples.

**Putting a chilled cabbage leaf** inside your bra can be surprisingly soothing, especially if your breasts are feeling inflamed.

# Getting checked

**YOUR BABY TODAY**

Sometimes babies develop skin rashes or irritations and sore bottoms around this time and, if this is the case, you can call your pediatrician for advice on how to relieve these minor problems, which may require a prescription.

## If you find that you need some additional help with the baby, there are several options to consider.

**Adjusting to life** with a newborn is difficult for some mothers, especially those recovering from cesareans. Sleep deprivation may make it hard to handle all of the new responsibilities. If your husband took time off during the first week, you may want another pair of hands to take his place. If you're able to hire a babysitter or visiting nurse for a few hours a day, you'll get some relief. If not, consider asking a good friend or relative for assistance. But before calling in any favors, make sure that the person you ask will actually provide the type of help you need. Do you want someone to care for the baby so you can nap, make dinner, or run errands? Do you want someone to cook or clean while you tend to the baby? Do you need someone to get groceries and pick up your preschooler? Be clear about your needs so your helper isn't upset that she won't get to hold the baby the whole time she's helping.

**Your baby loves to be stimulated.** He can focus about a foot away and will watch a simple object such as a mobile. Babies soon recognize familiar faces and he will love to watch you talk. Being part of your daily life provides plenty of stimulation. Tell him what you are doing and your plans for the day, read him stories, and listen to music together. When he is awake, give him time on his tummy to develop strength in the arms and prevent a "flat" head, a common problem in babies who spend a lot of time on their back. Always supervise your baby while he is on his tummy.

### SLEEPING BABES

**Newborn babies have a least two naps each day** and many simply rotate sleeping and eating throughout the day. In the early days, you'll find that there is little routine to your baby's sleep pattern since he can't go for a long period without being fed.

You will probably find that your baby isn't fusssy about where he naps and that this can be wherever it's convenient for you, whether this is in the car, the stroller, or baby sling. If you're at home, you may prefer to put your baby somewhere quiet for a nap, such as in his crib, or you might want to keep him close by in a playpen or on a towel on the floor, if this is safe.

**Many babies find being carried close** in a baby sling deeply comforting and may sleep happily while being transported.

### TIPS FOR BABY CARE

## Nails and scratching

Babies' nails grow quickly and are also very tricky to cut! However, to stop your baby from scratching her face, you'll need to keep them trimmed. Be careful not to rip the edge of the nails since this can cause infection.

■ You can buy special baby scissors, although these may not cut the nails short enough to prevent scratching.

■ Using a soft emery keeps them short.

■ You may want to put mittens on your baby until she is past the scratching stage.

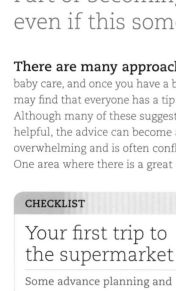

# Taking stock

### YOUR BABY TODAY

Many babies have spots known as milia, or "milk spots." These tiny whitish yellow spots appear on the face in the first two days and disappear by four weeks. Occasionally babies have spots resulting from the mother's hormones that take longer to disappear.

## Part of becoming a parent is learning to trust your own instincts, even if this sometimes means ignoring the advice of others.

**There are many approaches** to baby care, and once you have a baby you may find that everyone has a tip to offer. Although many of these suggestions are helpful, the advice can become a bit overwhelming and is often conflicting. One area where there is a great deal of advice is breast-feeding (see p.448). If you are struggling with breast-feeding and wondering why it all seems so much harder than it looks, you may find that advice from professionals, friends, family, and books is increasingly unhelpful. It can help to take a step back, decide which of your friends or relatives has a similar approach to yours in other areas of life and pay most heed to their advice. Above all, have confidence in your own ability and trust your instincts, reminding yourself that there are many right ways to do things.

### CHECKLIST

## Your first trip to the supermarket

Some advance planning and management can help to take the stress out of a supermarket shop.

■ Giving your baby a good feeding **before setting out** may mean that he sleeps peacefully at the supermarket.

■ **Supermarkets can be very cold,** so dress your baby appropriately.

■ **Check to see if your car seat clips onto a cart** since this can make life easier. Otherwise, use the supermarket's own cart with a baby seat or put your baby into a sling while you walk around the supermarket.

■ **Make a shopping list before you go** so that you don't forget essentials if you're distracted by your baby crying.

### BABY MASSAGE

**Babies love to be touched and massaging your baby** can be a great way to bond with your baby. All you need is some olive oil (avoid nut or aromatherapy oils) and a towel on the floor or bed. Ensure the room is warm and that your baby isn't hungry or too full. Undress your baby, rub some oil into your palms, and gently rub his tummy, limbs, fingers, and toes, watching his face to check that he is enjoying the massage. A baby massage class is a good way to make friends with other moms in your area.

**Lay your baby on a soft towel** and then use the tips of your fingers to gently stroke your baby's head, avoiding the soft area, or fontanelles, at the top of the head.

**With gentle downward strokes** massage your baby's chest and then use your fingertips to rub his tummy with outward circular strokes.

# Looking back

**YOUR BABY TODAY**

By now, you may feel that your baby is begining to interact a bit more as you notice that he loves to gaze at faces and enjoys watching you talk and smile. However, he won't be able to smile back for a few weeks yet.

For some, reliving a traumatic birth is painful and you and your partner may need support to work through difficult memories.

---

**ASK A ... DOCTOR**

**My baby's eye is constantly sticky. What can I do about this?** Many newborn babies wake up with sticky eyes. This is due to a temporary blockage of the tear ducts, which are tiny in newborn babies. Clear his eye by wiping it with a cotton pad soaked in cooled, boiled water, using a fresh piece for each wipe. The problem usually resolves with time, but if the secretions become yellow and look infected, tell your doctor because your baby may need antibiotic eye drops.

---

**FOCUS ON... YOUR BABY'S SENSES**

## Your baby's world

**Your baby will focus on your face when being fed.** He has been able to hear since he was in the uterus, and loves the sound of voices and music. He is startled by sudden noises, but can't locate them yet. He can taste; he loves the sweetness of breast milk and can tell if you've eaten something different! He can recognize your smell, and loves being cuddled, stroked, and carried close to you in a sling.

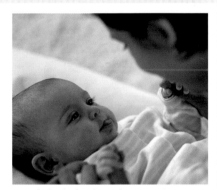

**Your baby is fascinated** by your face and loves making eye contact with you.

---

**Once the acceptance** and realization that you have had a baby sinks in and you are beginning to adapt to your new role as a mother, you may start to reflect on your birth experience and may want to share this with your relatives and friends. You will remember your birth story for the rest of your life and later share it with your baby.

Sometimes the labor and birth may not have gone as you wanted or anticipated. For example, you may have gone over your due date and had to be induced, and this may have led to interventions and possibly an instrumental delivery or an emergency cesarean section. You may feel some disappointment and be unsure about why certain things happened and whether you could have been able to do anything to prevent them from happening.

Occasionally some women, and their partners, who had a particularly difficult birth experience can suffer from post-birth trauma. If the birth was traumatic and you feel upset and unsettled, make an appointment with your doctor to discuss your birth experience. She will be able to explain events that you are unsure about and, if necessary, may be able to arrange for you to see the obstetrician who cared for you during labor, although this isn't standard, or recommend a mental health professional for you to speak with. If your partner feels traumatized by your birth experience and felt helpless during the process, he can also talk to the doctor, or if he prefers, to a mental health professional.

**Talking to your partner** about the labor and birth can help you relive good memories and to come to terms with the more unsettling ones. Your partner is one of the best placed people to reassure you about how you managed during labor, and talking together can help you open up and express your feelings about the birth.

# Feeling close

### YOUR BABY TODAY

It's inevitable that your baby will be exposed to viruses and some believe this reduces the risk of allergies later on. However, small babies can be quite sick with a cold so try to avoid people with colds at first. Breast-feeding provides protection against viruses.

## Now that you and your partner are adapting to your new roles, you can start to think about how to make time for each other.

**Finding time alone together** can be hard and resuming your love life can take time. Some women resume their love life without any problems, but for many it takes a little longer, especially if they had stitches and are sore. Also, a difficult birth can affect you emotionally, as can fatigue from lack of sleep. It's recommended that you wait two to three weeks after giving birth before sexual intercourse to let your uterus reduce in size and for the bleeding to stop. Many women prefer to wait until after their six-week checkup (see pp.462–3). Initially, cuddling and nonpenetrative sex can help you and your partner experience closeness. When you both feel right you can resume sex, but the first time needs to be gentle and you may need a lubricant since your hormones can cause vaginal dryness, especially when breast-feeding. If intercourse is painful, talk to your doctor who can make sure you're healing.

You will need to consider contraception now. If you're undecided as to what to use and want to resume intercourse, it's a good idea to use condoms until your six week checkup when you can discuss the issue further.

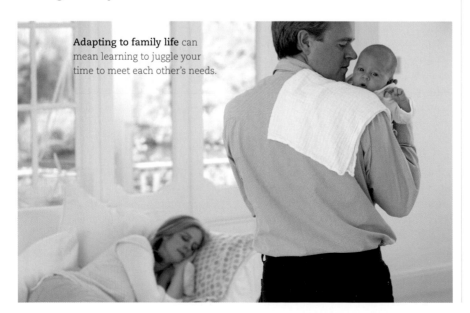

**Adapting to family life** can mean learning to juggle your time to meet each other's needs.

### GETTING YOUR FIGURE BACK

**Most women lose around 10–15 lb (4–7 kg) in the first two weeks after the birth** since, in addition to the loss of the weight of the baby, placenta, and amniotic fluid, you will lose the water that you retained in pregnancy. This water will be mobilized from your tissues and reabsorbed back into your bloodstream, and you'll eliminate it through your urine. Often women can feel more swollen after the delivery than they were before, but this extra fluid will be eliminated naturally in the next two weeks since you will probably pass large amounts of urine.

After two weeks, your weight loss will slow down. It's important to not try to lose weight too quickly after the birth, especially if you're breast-feeding, when you need around 500 extra calories each day. If you don't meet these extra nutritional needs, you will probably find that your energy will be low from a lack of calories. Eat a balanced diet that consists of whole grains, fruits, vegetables, and protein and drink plenty of fluids to avoid constipation.

# New beginnings

**YOUR BABY TODAY**

Now that you are getting the hang of being a new mom, seek out other new parents for some exercise or socializing. There should be many options available to you in your local area.

## Life will never be the same again and by now you will understand the unconditional love of a parent for their child.

**Babies like to suck,** even when they're not hungry anymore. Some suck their fingers or thumbs, but others do nicely with pacifiers. Some parents have strong feelings about whether or not to give a baby a pacifier, but they won't hurt your baby at all and have been linked to a reduction in Sudden Infant Death Syndrome (SIDS) when used during sleep. If you decide to use pacifiers, look for models with soft nipples and a one-piece design that are dishwasher-safe. Have several on hand, since pacifiers tend to fall on the floor. Keep in mind that if a baby depends on a pacifier to sleep, he may wake up and cry if it falls out of his mouth. If you are breast-feeding, many experts recommend waiting one month before introducing a pacifier, to avoid nipple confusion.

**You may now be getting out more** by yourself since your partner may be back at work. Ask your pediatrician about times and venues for support groups in you local area and any carriage-walking groups or baby massage classes since these are excellent ways to meet other moms.

At two weeks, you'll be getting the hang of being parents. Life will never be the same again, and although this means that you will always have to put your baby first and will not have as much time for yourself, in return you have the most beautiful, fascinating child with her own personality who you will always love unconditionally. There is nothing that compares with the love of parent and child, and by now, you will understand exactly what that means.

---

**ASK A... DOCTOR**

**Should I try to get my baby into a routine?** In the first few weeks, it's too early to establish routines. To establish breast-feeding, newborn babies need to be fed on demand and most, in time, will figure out their own routine. If you want to try to establish set feeding times, you will have to consider how you will cope with a screaming baby. However, it's worth starting a nighttime routine early on. Bathing your baby, singing to him, feeding him, and putting him down in his crib to sleep will help him develop good sleep patterns later on.

**RECORDING YOUR BABY**

**It's tempting to take photos and videos almost constantly when your first baby is born.** Subsequent children often remark on how relatively few photos there are of them! Digital photography means that you can email family and friends immediately with new baby photos, however, try not to go overboard since, although you will never tire of looking at your own baby, other people's baby photos are of more limited interest.

**The first pictures** together provide precious memories.

**You'll be fascinated** by your new baby's every moment.

**Don't forget to include** pictures of the proud dad.

# Your six-week checkup

At about four to eight weeks following the birth, you will have a postpartum checkup with a doctor at your ob/gyn's practice. This checkup is to see if you are physically and emotionally well. Your baby will also have a physical and developmental checkup around this time.

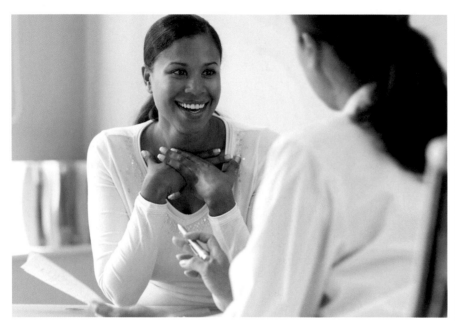

**Your six-week postpartum checkup** is the ideal time to talk to your doctor about any problems or concerns you have, and to receive reassurance that you have recovered well after the birth.

### Your assessment

In the first couple of months following the birth of their baby, the majority of women don't experience any major health concerns and will revert back to their prepregnant health status. However, it's good practice to have a general assessment to reassure you that you are well and coping with the early transition to motherhood.

Your postpartum checkup is an ideal opportunity for you to consult your doctor about any concerns you have following the birth of your baby. Any worries about yourself can be discussed at this appointment, from your mood to any apprehensions about having sex again. Your doctor will offer you advice and possibly treatment, and will also be able to refer you to a specialist for further treatment if necessary.

### Your physical checkup

Your doctor will do routine checkups, such as taking your blood pressure. He or she will also ask if you have any concerns, how you're feeding your baby, and, if you are breast-feeding, whether you've had any problems with your breasts and lactation.

Your uterus will have returned to nearly its prepregnancy size (about the size of the palm of your hand) and will not be able to be felt. However, your doctor may check your abdomen to see if the muscles are returning to normal since occasionally the abdominal muscles separate after birth, known as "diastasi

recti." If the muscles are more than four fingers apart, you may be referred to a physical therapist. Pilates and core conditioning exercises (see p.250) can help and your doctor may talk to you about these exercises.

Backaches can be a problem after the birth, exacerbated by the pregnancy hormone relaxin (see p.197), which softens muscles and ligaments and remains in the body for a few months after pregnancy. If you're suffering from backaches, your doctor may talk to you about your posture, particularly when you're carrying or feeding your baby, and about the benefits of exercise.

If you had a cesarean, the incision will be looked at to check that it has healed well. You may still feel numbness around the site of the incision, but sensation should gradually return as the nerve endings renew themselves.

If you haven't had a Pap smear in the last three years, you will likely be given one on the spot, unless you're bleeding heavily.

**Checking your bladder** You will be asked if you have problems urinating, and may be asked for a urine sample if you have symptoms such as frequent urination or stinging when passing urine. Stress incontinence, or leaking urine (see p.475), is common after childbirth, so don't feel embarrassed to mention this to your doctor. He or she may encourage you to do Kegel exercises (see p.69), and if the problem persists you may be referred to a physical therapist for bladder-training exercises.

**Your stitches** If you're still sore from stitches, your doctor will check that these are healing properly. Although most stitches are absorbable, they can take up to three months to completely absorb. Bathing can sometimes help the stitches absorb, but if you continue to have problems your doctor may recommend Sitz baths two or three times a day or a topical anesthetic cream (see also Perineal problems, p.475).

## Your emotional well-being

In addition to checking you physically, the doctor will also assess your emotional and mental health. Many women feel extremely tired in these early weeks, as night feedings and constant demands begin to take their toll. However, if you are feeling low, overly tired, or depressed a lot of the time, you may be suffering from postpartum depression (see p.475), so it's important not to ignore these symptoms. Talk to your doctor about how you are feeling; he will be able to offer support and refer you to experts in treating depression.

## Looking at your lifestyle

Your doctor will advise you on healthy eating and lifestyle measures. If you smoke, you'll be given information about support groups in your local area to help you stop smoking.

Is it true that I don't need to worry about getting pregnant again while I'm breast-feeding?

If you are breast-feeding, you may not have a period for a while after giving birth. Although this means you are less likely to conceive, you can still ovulate, so you shouldn't assume that you don't need to use contraception. The doctor or nurse will discuss contraception and sexual health with you and may recommend the progesterone-only pill, which can be prescribed from 21 days if you're breast-feeding.

I'm bottle-feeding my baby and am worried about getting pregnant again. How soon could this happen?

If you decided to bottle-feed, you will probably have had your first period prior to this checkup and so certainly could become pregnant again. Although your doctor will have already discussed contraception with you, this will be addressed again at your six-week checkup. The doctor or nurse will want to check that you have contraceptive measures in place; if not, he or she will offer you guidance and advice.

I had stitches and have felt too anxious to have sex since the birth. Is this normal?

Yes, plenty of women feel this way and many wait to resume sex until after their postpartum checkup. During this checkup, the doctor or nurse will be able to confirm that your incision has healed, and offer reassurance about resuming sex. On the other hand, there is nothing wrong with having sex before this checkup as long as you have stopped bleeding. When you do have sex, you may need to use a lubricant (KY jelly), particularly if you're breast-feeding since your hormones can cause some vaginal dryness.

# Your baby's checkup

**A pediatrician will want to see your baby at around 4 days, 1 month, and 2 months** to do a physical checkup and look at how your baby is growing and developing.

The doctor will perform a similar examination to the newborn checkup (see p.443). He or she will examine your baby's hips, spine, eyes, heart, and the pulses at the top of the legs. In boys, it's important to check that the testes are located in the scrotum. This is also a chance to look for subtle problems such as a heart murmur, which can develop after birth. Your baby will be weighed and his head circumference measured. The doctor will ask how your baby is feeding and check for signs of jaundice. Your baby's development will be checked too: whether he has head control, is starting to smile, and can focus on an object or face a foot away, and follow a moving object. Your baby should receive some immunizations during these early visits. All of these findings will be recorded in a record of your baby's growth and development.

**The head circumference** is taken and the fontanelles, the soft areas on your baby's head, are checked.

**Your baby's heart rate** will be listened to and the doctor will monitor and check his breathing.

**To check head control,** your doctor will gently lift your baby up by his arms to see how he holds his head.

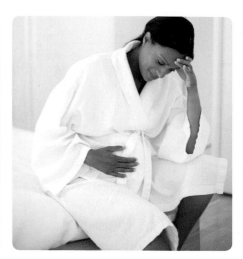

Rarely does pregnancy pass without some complaint. The majority of problems are minor and due to normal pregnancy changes. Some, however, are more serious and require medical attention. Today, high-quality prenatal care means that potentially serious conditions are usually successfully managed, both during pregnancy and in labor. Problems after the birth, either in the baby or the mother, may need medical attention with careful follow-up and sometimes referral to a specialist.

# Concerns and complications

# Common concerns in pregnancy

Pregnancy hormones affect every system in your body. In this section, you will find a list of common concerns with an explanation of the adaptation process that may cause these symptoms, information on whether medical help is likely to be required, and advice on measures you can take yourself to alleviate symptoms.

## General symptoms

### Fatigue

An overwhelming feeling of fatigue is often one of the earliest signs of pregnancy. Such feelings usually subside during the second trimester, but are likely to return in the third trimester.

**CAUSES** The main causes of extreme fatigue in early pregnancy are massive hormonal changes and the extra demands on the body made by an increase in blood volume of up to 50 percent. It's this increase in blood volume that helps the lining of the uterus to thicken and the placenta to develop. In the second trimester, energy levels usually return to normal as hormone changes settle down. Late in pregnancy, fatigue may recur because your extra size and weight and the demands of the growing baby means that your body systems need to work harder. In both early and late pregnancy, difficulty sleeping (see p.95) can contribute to feelings of fatigue. Fatigue in pregnancy can also be caused by anemia (see p.472).

**WHAT TO DO** If you are working, take regular breaks and get some fresh air at least once a day. Ensure that your fluid intake is adequate; caffeine is not helpful because it dehydrates your body and will leave you feeling worse. Take more time for sleep if you need to; housework can wait and you may need to cut back on social commitments.

### Difficulty sleeping

It's very common to have sleeping difficulty in pregnancy, especially in the first and third trimesters.

**CAUSES** A common cause of disturbed sleep is the need to urinate frequently. Early in pregnancy, this is due to the amount of blood in your body, leading to the kidneys filtering out more fluid, which ends up in your bladder. As pregnancy progresses, another factor is expansion of the uterus within the pelvic cavity, so that it competes for space with the bladder. This leads the bladder to require more frequent emptying, which will interrupt your sleep. Many women also feel hungry during the night and need to snack, while others find that nausea and vomiting interrupt their night or lead to early waking. From about 20 weeks of pregnancy, the uterus moves up out of the pelvis, taking pressure off the bladder, and nausea often subsides, which means that sleep improves. Toward the end of pregnancy, sleep patterns can once again be disturbed. Unborn babies are often active just when you want to rest; your body is bulky and finding comfortable sleeping positions becomes difficult; and as the baby becomes bigger and heavier pressure on the bladder may return.

**WHAT TO DO** If frequent urination is keeping you awake, don't drink large quantities of fluid close to bedtime, and to avoid waking up hungry include foods high in unrefined carbohydrates, such as whole-wheat bread, in your evening meal. If you do wake up, don't lie there for long periods, since this is frustrating and may lead to habitual sleeplessness. Get out of bed and engage in a simple activity that won't overstimulate your brain, have a warm, caffeine-free drink, and return to bed when you're sleepy. Later in pregnancy when you find it difficult to get comfortable, experiment with different sleeping positions: use plenty of pillows, under your head and belly and between your knees. A rest during the day is essential during late pregnancy, but limit this to a 20-minute power nap or an hour reading or watching television with your feet up. If you sleep for long periods during the day, you will further lessen your ability to sleep at night.

## Headaches

Headaches are common in pregnancy, especially in the first trimester.

**CAUSES** Most headaches are unlikely to be a cause for concern and are probably due to hormonal changes and the need for additional fluids. Headaches occurring in the third trimester that are accompanied by other symptoms, such as abdominal pain or nausea, may be a sign of preeclampsia and should be assessed by a doctor (see p.474).

**WHAT TO DO** Making sure you drink enough clear fluids (around five cups a day) and avoiding caffeine should help reduce the number and severity of headaches. If you're working or concentrating on a task, have a break every two to three hours, and get some gentle exercise in fresh air. For a sinus headache, apply a warm compress to the front and sides of your face. For tension headaches, place a cool compress on the back of your neck. If you suspect your headache is due to lack of sleep, get more sleep. And make sure you're eating enough, since hunger and low blood sugar can cause headaches. Relieve stress—another headache trigger—with deep breathing, meditation, yoga, or massage Always discuss your symptoms with your doctor before taking medication.

If you have a headache in late pregnancy that is accompanied by swelling of the legs and ankles, generalized body swelling, abdominal pain, or nausea and vomiting, contact your doctor immediately.

## Swollen feet and ankles

Some women experience a small amount of swelling in their feet, ankles, hands, and wrists, which can be particularly pronounced in hot weather.

**CAUSES** Swelling is the result of fluid retention, which in turn results from the extra blood produced during pregnancy to provide for the growing baby.

**WHAT TO DO** This is best managed by alternating light activity with periods of rest during which your feet are elevated. However, staying in bed or sitting in a chair for very long periods may increase the risk of deep vein thrombosis (DVT) (see p.186). DVT is a potentially serious condition in which a blood clot forms in a vein; if the clot breaks off, it may travel to the lungs and block a major blood vessel. Swollen feet and ankles can also be a sign of other problems such as preeclampsia (see p.474), so should always be reported to your doctor who can check for other symptoms.

## Skin changes

### Itching and dry skin

Many pregnant women suffer from itchy, dry patches of skin that worsen in late pregnancy. Such skin irritation is a reaction to hormonal changes and can be eased by a perfume-free moisturiser. Rarely, itching in late pregnancy may be due to a serious condition called obstetric cholestasis (see p.473). Itching caused by this condition is much more severe, usually constant, and often concentrated on the hands and feet.

### Spider veins

Clusters of broken capillaries (tiny red blood vessels) called spider veins may appear during pregnancy, mainly on the cheeks. These occur as a result of increased blood circulation and the softening effect of pregnancy hormones on blood vessels. Spider veins are painless, but if you are worried about their appearance you can cover them with makeup. They usually disappear soon after the birth.

### Increased pigmentation

An increase in skin pigmentation is common in pregnancy, probably due to the increased production of hormones. Most women notice a darkening of the area around the nipple (the areola), and a dark line, called the linea nigra, forming vertically through the middle of the belly from the umbilicus to the pelvis. Also common are dark patches on the cheeks, nose, and chin, known as melasma (also known as chloasma, or the "mask of pregnancy.") On women with dark skin, the patches may apppear lighter than surrounding skin. Exposure to sunlight can make the patches more obvious, so use a high-protection sunscreen on your face.

### Stretch marks

Rapid stretching of the skin during pregnancy often leads to the development of pink or purple lines, known as stretch marks. These marks, which can look quite alarming, with a scarlike appearance, usually appear in late pregnancy, commonly on the abdomen, hips, thighs, and upper breast. There is no clear evidence that any cream will prevent or remove stretch marks, although a light unscented moisturizer can help keep the skin supple, as will staying well hydrated and avoiding excessive weight gain. As time passes after the birth, stretch marks become silvery and almost invisible.

## Breast problems

### Breast tenderness

For many women, breast tenderness and an increase in the size of their breasts are the first signs of pregnancy. Sometimes breasts are so painful that you can't bear them to be touched, and they may also throb and feel hot. Breast tenderness usually subsides by the end of the first trimester.

**CAUSES** Tenderness is a sign that the breasts are preparing for their role of feeding your baby after the birth: the milk ducts are starting to enlarge and blood flow increases.

**WHAT TO DO** Wearing a properly fitting bra will help support your breasts and reduce discomfort. An ill-fitting or tight bra will be uncomfortable and may put pressure on the milk ducts. You may also find it helpful to wear a soft sleep bra at night. If your breasts feel hot, applying a cool washcloth to them may bring relief.

If you have a painful or red patch on a breast, you should report this to your doctor because it could be a sign of mastitis (see p.475).

### Nipple problems

Each woman has breasts and nipples individual to her. Women who have flat nipples that do not protrude or whose nipples are inverted (concave) may worry that they may not be able to breast-feed. However, all healthy women can breast-feed because babies feed by taking in a mouthful of breast, not just the nipple.

**CAUSES** Inverted or flat nipples are thought to be due to shorter ligaments in the underlying breast tissue that pull the nipples inward.

**WHAT TO DO** If you have any concerns about the suitability of your nipples for breast-feeding, talk to your doctor who can refer you to a lactation consultant. There are also products available that will draw out nipples in preparation for breast-feeding. However, these are by no means essential because when babies latch on to the breast they are able to draw out even a flat or inverted nipple (although you may eventually need help by a lactation consultant to show you the best way to help your baby do this).

## Digestive problems

### Nausea and vomiting

Approximately 80 percent of women are troubled by the unpleasant symptoms of nausea and vomiting in early pregnancy. During this period it can be difficult to eat large meals, and strong smells and tastes can become unbearable. Many women also find some vegetable and acidic foods more difficult to digest and worry that their usually healthy eating pattern has deteriorated. Early pregnancy nausea and vomiting usually subside between 12 and 20 weeks; however it's not uncommon to experience some return of these problems late in the pregnancy.

**CAUSES** Early in pregnancy, the pregnancy hormones interact with hormones that control other body systems, particularly those involved with blood sugar regulation, and this results in feelings of nausea and vomiting. Late in pregnancy, problems with digestion may occur because the uterus takes up most of the space in your abdomen, displacing your intestines and stomach and leaving little room for the digestion of large amounts of food.

**WHAT TO DO** The best way to manage the nausea and vomiting of pregnancy is to drink plenty of water throughout the day and also eat small amounts of food on a regular basis, which will help to avoid long gaps between meals, and snacking on complex carbohydrates such as whole-wheat and whole-grain products, whole-grain cereals, and brown rice dishes. Avoid snacks with a high sugar content because, although these will give you a quick boost, they will soon leave you feeling worse than before because your blood sugar plummets. Reducing your overall intake of the refined sugar found in candy, cake, cookies, and sugary drinks will help reduce the symptoms of nausea and vomiting and will also lessen your risk of developing gestational diabetes.

The "little and often" principle, coupled with healthy snacks is equally good advice for the late phase of pregnancy.

## Gastroenteritis

This is inflammation of the lining of the stomach and intestines, most commonly due to infection. It causes vomiting and diarrhea that usually come on suddenly. In most cases, the condition clears up on its own and is not a cause for concern. However, if it's severe, you could become dehydrated, and this can affect blood flow to your baby through the placenta. Infection with listeria bacteria can, rarely, cause late miscarriage.

**CAUSES** Gastroenteritis is caused by infection contracted either through contact with an infected person, or by consuming contaminated food or drink (food poisoning). Food poisoning is often the result of poor food hygiene.

**WHAT TO DO** Drink plenty of water, and try to avoid cross infection with other members of the household (see below). If you're unable to retain even small sips of water, or your vomiting and diarrhea have lasted for 24 hours, you should seek medical advice from your doctor. If you can't reach your doctor, go the nearest hospital emergency room for treatment. If you have a preexisting medical condition such as diabetes, you should seek help immediately. You may be treated with intravenous fluids if you are dehydrated, and fetal monitoring may be done to check the health of your baby. Infection with listeria is treated with antibiotics.

**AVOIDING GASTROENTERITIS** It is important that you try to avoid gastroenteritis by practicing good food hygiene (see p.17).

If someone else in your household has gastroenteritis, avoid infection by using separate soap, towels, cutlery, and dishes. If you have more than one toilet, get the infected person to use one separate from the rest of the household. Wipe toilets, sinks, and faucets with a mild bleach solution after each use. Infected individuals should also avoid preparing food for others.

## Indigestion and heartburn

Many women start to experience episodes of indigestion and heartburn during the second trimester.

**CAUSES** Indigestion results from slower movements of the digestive tract under the influence of pregnancy hormones combined with reduced space in the stomach from the growing baby. The muscular valve at the top of the stomach is also softened by hormones and this can allow stomach acid to flow up into the esphagus, causing heartburn.

**WHAT TO DO** Avoiding large meals, especially late at night, helps prevent indigestion and heartburn. If you suffer from heartburn at night, try sleeping in a propped up position with your head higher than your feet. For relief from heartburn, a liquid antacid preparation can be helpful; ask your doctor for advice on which medications are safe. Some women find that slowly drinking a glass of milk eases the discomfort.

## Constipation

During the second trimester, constipation often becomes a problem.

**CAUSES** Under the influence of the softening effect of pregnancy hormones, the digestive tract becomes less active. As a result, fecal matter spends more time in the large intestine, allowing reabsorption of fluids and leaving solids hard and difficult to pass. Not drinking enough fluids increases the likelihood of constipation.

**WHAT TO DO** Dietary fiber in the form of vegetables and whole foods, with an increase in fluid intake usually corrects the problem. Laxatives are not recommended during pregnancy. They can stimulate contractions and lead to dehydration. Talk to your doctor if these steps don't resolve your constipation.

## Hemorrhoids

Hemorrhoids are dilated blood vessels around the inside of, or protruding from, the anus. Their constriction by the anal muscles and sensitivity to the acidic environment leads to a feeling of discomfort in mild episodes and pain in more severe cases. They are more likely to occur during the third trimester.

**CAUSES** The hormonal softening of the tissues around the anus increases the risk of developing hemorrhoids. Pressure of the baby's head on the blood vessels is also a factor, as is constipation.

**WHAT TO DO** Treatment of constipation and avoiding pushing or straining to pass a stool are important in the prevention of hemorrhoids. Ask your doctor which over-the-counter creams for relieving discomfort are safe. If hemorrhoids are protruding and causing great discomfort, it's often possible for a health professional to "reduce" them by pushing them gently back into place.

# Heart & circulation problems

## Dizziness and faintness

Throughout pregnancy, occasional dizziness or feelings of faintness can be a problem.

**CAUSES** In early pregnancy, feeling faint may occur even when you are sitting down and is likely to be due to low blood sugar. This can happen as a result of not eating enough, a common problem at this stage of pregnancy when many women suffer from morning sickness. In the second trimester, dizziness or faintness that comes on when getting up from a sitting position or as a result of standing for long periods is likely to be caused by low blood pressure. Blood pressure is lowered in pregnancy because the pregnancy hormone progesterone softens blood vessels to enable blood to flow more freely to your baby. When you stand, the low blood pressure may mean that not enough blood reaches your brain, leading to dizziness and faintness.

As pregnancy advances, you may find that you feel dizzy lying on your back. This happens because in this position the heavy uterus puts pressure on the main blood vessels running through the trunk and reduces the blood flow to the brain.

**WHAT TO DO** To help prevent low blood sugar, have small snacks of foods high in complex carbohydrates (see p.92). Staying well hydrated, taking regular breaks from work, not standing in one position for too long, and getting fresh air are also helpful in preventing faintness. If you start to feel dizzy, sit down and put your head between your legs, which will relieve the unpleasant feeling. Stay seated until you feel completely recovered and then get up slowly. Any time you feel dizzy or faint, call your doctor immediately, especially if you also have stomach pain, vaginal bleeding, blurry vision, headaches, or heart palpitations, or the dizziness is persistent. If you have fainted and bumped your head or injured any part of your body then you should go to the hospital for a checkup.

If you experience dizziness when lying on your back, turning onto your side will quickly help you feel better. Lying on your left side is preferable because this helps to pump blood around the body.

## Palpitations

A feeling that your heart is racing, or beating irregularly is common in pregnancy, particularly between 28 and 32 weeks, but can occur at any time.

**CAUSES** The reasons for palpitations remain unclear and hypotheses range from the effect that progesterone has on the heart muscle, to the heart coping with the extra blood flow needed to maintain both mother and fetus.

**WHAT TO DO** Palpitations are usually fleeting and nothing to worry about. However, if you have frequent palpitations or they are accompanied by chest pain, dizziness, or breathlessness, you should consult your doctor. If you have a history of heart disease or a heart abnormality, seek advice immediately.

## Nosebleeds

Nosebleeds occur frequently in pregnancy, and although they are a nuisance they are rarely a serious problem.

**CAUSES** As with all other blood vessels in the body, those in the nose are softened and expanded during pregnancy. In addition,

your body has an increased blood volume in pregnancy, which puts pressure on these delicate structures. You are more likely to have a nosebleed if you have a cold or sinus infection or if your nasal membrane is dry, which can happen in cold weather or air conditioned rooms.

**WHAT TO DO** To manage a nosebleed, sit down, keep your head in a normal position, and apply pressure to the bottom of the nose with your thumb and forefinger. You will need to maintain this pressure constantly for about 10 minutes before checking to see if the bleeding has stopped. Do not be tempted to tip your head back or lie down, since this will cause you to swallow the blood, leading to nausea and possible vomiting. Ice or a cold compress applied to the nose and facial area in conjunction with the nasal pressure can help constrict the blood flow and halt the bleeding. Seek medical advice if the nosebleed results from a head injury or if heavy bleeding continues for more than 20 minutes. Mention frequent small nosebleeds at your prenatal appointment to enable the elimination of more serious conditions.

## Bleeding, tender gums

Bleeding from the gums and gum tenderness are both common complaints during pregnancy.

**CAUSES** These problems occur as a result of increased blood volume coupled with the softening effect of pregnancy hormones on blood vessels. Allowing plaque to accumulate may exacerbate these symptoms and also makes the start of gum disease more likely.

**WHAT TO DO** Good dental hygiene is vital; don't be tempted to avoid brushing your teeth if they feel tender, but switch to a softer brush. Brushing your teeth and gums and flossing regularly are particularly important during pregnancy. Also, visit your dentist regularly during pregnancy and the postpartum period.

## Varicose veins and vulval varicosities

Varicose veins are enlarged, distorted veins that may develop in the legs or around the vulval area. Varicose veins in or around the anus are known as hemorrhoids (see p.468). Varicose veins may become troublesome

during the later stages of pregnancy, causing discomfort and sometimes itching; they may also be unsightly. Varicosities in the vagina or vulva areas do not inhibit a normal birth and are not at risk of rupture during the birth.

**CAUSES** The increased blood flow and softened vessels mean that many women experience varicose veins and vulva varicosities during pregnancy. The growing uterus puts pressure on veins in the pelvis which, in turn, leads to increased pressure in the legs and vulva area.

**WHAT TO DO** Support hose designed for pregnancy can be helpful, Avoid tight clothes that constrict the waist, groin, or legs As with all conditions, varicose veins should be reported to your doctor for assessment and advice. Varicose veins usually improve within three months after the birth of the baby.

# Aches and pains

## Backaches

Lower generalized backaches are extremely common during pregnancy, particularly in the third trimester; around two thirds of all pregnant women suffer from backaches.

**CAUSES** As pregnancy progresses, the increased weight of your abdomen tends to pull on the lower spine so that it curves inward and your center of gravity shifts forward. As you try to correct this, you may strain the the lower back muscles. In addition, pregnancy hormones soften your ligaments, causing them to stretch and provide less support for your back.

**WHAT TO DO** Maintaining good posture and avoiding tilting your pelvis forward helps relieve pressure on your back and helps both prevent and alleviate backaches. Regular, moderate exercise to keep your muscles toned and supple is also beneficial. See pages 90 and 250 for suggested exercise routines. Yoga, pilates, and water aerobics are also recommended.

Try to avoid standing in one position for too long and vary your daily tasks, if possible breaking them down into shorter stints. If your work involves standing or sitting for long periods, take regular short breaks, and while sitting, make sure your lower back is supported. Avoid lifting heavy objects.

Massage and warm water can help relieve backaches. If back pain is particularly troublesome, talk to your doctor about wearing a supportive maternity belt.

## Pelvic girdle pain (PGP)

Also known as symphysis pubis dysfunction, pelvic girdle pain (PGP) refers to discomfort and pain felt in the pelvic area and groin. The pain may be concentrated in the buttocks or travel down one leg, and for this reason is sometimes mistaken for sciatica (see below). PGP is often worse when doing activities such as walking or going up stairs; it may also be troublesome at night, but this is usually related to activities done during the day. PGP is most common toward the end of pregnancy and may range in severity from mild to serious enough to need a walking aid.

**CAUSES** Various factors may contribute to PGP. The pelvis is made up of three bones: the sacrum and the two iliac (hip) bones. The bones are connected at the front by the symphysis pubis joint, and at the back by the sacroiliac joints. The joints are stabilized by ligaments and usually move very little. During pregnancy, however, ligaments soften and stretch more easily so that there is more movement at these joints. This results in instability of the pelvis. In addition, postural changes due to the enlarging abdomen may mean that one joint is more mobile than the other, putting extra strain on the joints. The result is inflammation of the joints and discomfort or pain.

**WHAT TO DO** If there is increased movement in one side of your pelvis, a pelvic support belt may be recommended, which often gives instant relief. You may be referred to a physical therapist who will show you how to modify everyday activities, such as walking and getting up, in order to avoid pain, and may also recommend abdominal and Kegel exercises (see p.69). Acupuncture can help relieve pain, and prenatal water aerobic classes are helpful. Preventative measures include avoiding activities that cause pain, and avoiding heavy lifting, lying on your back, and sustained periods of activity. It's also important to get plenty of rest.

## Round ligament pain

The two round ligaments run from the top of the uterus on either side and attach to the side walls of the abdomen. As the uterus enlarges, the round ligaments gradually become stretched, which can cause an ache or brief, sharp pain on one or both sides of the lower abdomen or in the groin. Round ligament pain usually starts during the second trimester.

**WHAT TO DO** See your doctor, who will rule out other causes for the abdominal pain. Once you have been reassured, you should find it easier to deal with the pain. When you have an episode, try to rest and relax. Lying on your side and bringing your knees up toward your chest may be helpful, as can taking a warm bath.

## Sciatica

This is pain in one or both buttocks that may radiate down one leg. There may also be tingling or numbness in the legs, although this occurs only in a small percentage of women. Sciatica is most likely to occur after the second trimester.

**CAUSES** Sciatica is caused by trapping or compression of the sciatic nerve as it runs through the spinal column. The pain is termed referred pain, that is, pain felt in an area away from the problem site. Sciatica is not caused by compression of the nerve by the fetus's head. The causes of sciatica in pregnancy are the same as in women who are not pregnant and include poor posture, wear and tear on vertebral joints, and poor lifting techniques.

**WHAT TO DO** Specific exercises can help to stretch muscles gently and release pressure on the sciatic nerve. Your doctor may be able to advise you on exercises or may refer you to a physical therapist for help.

## Coccygeal pain

The coccyx, or tailbone, is the small bone found at the base of the spine. This bone is usually fairly immobile; however in pregnancy it becomes more mobile, which facilitates the passage of the baby through the birth canal during labor. Pain in this area can make sitting for long periods extremely uncomfortable, particularly at work or during travel. Coccygeal pain can occur throughout pregnancy.

**CAUSES** Coccygeal pain may predate pregnancy due to a previous injury to the area; the discomfort may then be exacerbated by the hormonal and mechanical changes of pregnancy. Alternatively, coccygeal pain may arise in pregnancy, since increased movement in the coccyx during this time makes injury more likely. Sometimes the coccyx is injured during labor by the baby's head, and coccygeal pain therefore develops after the birth.

**WHAT TO DO** Moving around frequently and gently massaging the area can help relieve discomfort. Ask your doctor which analgesics are safe for you to take. The condition usually gets better within 6 weeks of delivery.

## Leg cramps

Cramps in the legs, particularly in the calf muscles, are a common problem during pregnancy. These occur most commonly at night, but may sometimes come on when walking, and their frequency can increase as your pregnancy advances.

**CAUSES** There is debate as to the cause of leg cramps in pregnancy. They are likely to be caused by a combination of factors including maternal posture, increasing body weight, restriction in the blood flow to the legs, and the pressure of the uterus on the pelvic nerves. Some suggest that leg cramps in pregnancy may be due to a lack of salt in the diet. However, research demonstrates that low levels of salt are healthy in pregnancy, and that it is very unlikely that anyone who is eating a balanced diet will suffer from salt depletion.

**WHAT TO DO** Leg cramps may be relieved by changing position, flexing the toes of the affected leg upward, and massaging the cramped muscle. To avoid leg cramps, massage your legs before bed and avoid sitting or standing in one position for long periods. A warm bath before bed may also help. Stay well hydrated and alternate regular periods of moderate exercise with periods of rest.

If you have persistent pain, redness, or swelling in your calf, this may be a sign of deep vein thrombosis (DVT) (see p.186), which requires prompt medical attention.

## Restless leg syndrome

Restless leg syndrome is an uncomfortable feeling or unpleasant tingling that creates an overwhelming desire to move your legs, or causes legs to jerk uncontrollably, especially during sleep. Sufferers describe the sensation as being like an electric current passing through the legs or like having itchy bones. During pregnancy, the problem is most likely to occur during the third trimester.

**CAUSES** Restless legs syndrome is frequently triggered or aggravated by pregnancy. The cause is unknown, but some studies indicate that it might be related to low iron levels. Many sufferers have a family history of the condition.

**WHAT TO DO** If you're suffering from restless leg syndrome, talk to your doctor about having a blood test to check your iron levels. If levels are low, a simple iron supplement may be prescribed. Some women find it helpful to exercise or stretch their legs, to use hot or cold compresses, or to have a leg massage. If the condition occurs for the first time in pregnancy, there is a very good chance that it will disappear after the baby is born.

## Carpal tunnel syndrome

The carpal tunnel is a small tunnel in the wrist through which nerves run from your forearm into your hands and fingers. Carpal tunnel sydrome occurs when the nerves are compressed, resulting in tingling and pain in the fingers, which is often worse at night. In severe cases, there may be considerable discomfort and a reduced grip. In pregnancy, this is most likely to occur in the second and third trimesters.

**CAUSES** Carpal tunnel syndrome is caused by pressure on nerves running through the tunnel due to swelling of surrounding tissues. During pregnancy, swelling in the hands and feet is common as a result of the extra fluid and blood volume.

**WHAT TO DO** If you think you may have carpal tunnel syndrome, talk to your doctor. You may be referred to a physical therapist for treatment, who will recommend specific exercises to help relieve the discomfort. You may also be advised to wear a lightweight splint to support your wrists, which can be especially beneficial if the pain is disturbing your sleep. Carpal tunnel syndrome usually disappears after the birth. However, if it persists, a simple surgery can be performed to relieve the pressure on the nerves.

# Urinary and vaginal problems

## Yeast infections (candidiasis)

During pregnancy, an increased vaginal discharge is normal. However, if the discharge is creamy and thick, and you have some soreness and itching in your vaginal area, you may have yeast, a fungal infection. If you have a vaginal discharge with an odor, you could have trichomoniasis or bacterial vaginosis, which are sexually transmitted infections that can lead to premature delivery if not treated with antibiotics. You are more prone to yeast during pregnancy, particularly during the third trimester.

**CAUSES** A yeast infection is caused by a fungus called *Candida albicans*. The organism exists normally in small numbers in the intestines and vagina, and doesn't cause problems. However, during pregnancy, the environment in the vagina changes, causing overgrowth of the fungus. If you are under stress, feeling generally unwell, taking antibiotics, or have diabetes, you may be more likely to develop a yeast infection.

**WHAT TO DO** If you think you have a yeast infection, contact doctor, who can take a vaginal swab to confirm the diagnosis. He or she may recommend an over-the-counter vaginal cream. Yeast infections can be harder to control during pregnancy, and may take up to two weeks to go away. To prevent additional infections, wear cotton underwear and always wipe from front to back after a bowel movement.

## Stress incontinence

If you have stress incontinence, you pass small amounts of urine unintentionally, particularly when coughing, sneezing, or laughing, and when exercising or lifting heavy objects. Stress incontinence can happen at any time during pregnancy, but is most common in the last trimester.

**CAUSES** The pelvic floor muscles are under additional strain during pregnancy and are also affected by hormonal changes. Therefore any increase in abdominal pressure caused by coughing, sneezing, laughing, or other activities that puts these muscles under pressure may result in leakage of a small amount of urine.

**WHAT TO DO** Stress incontinence can be embarrassing and distressing; however, you should mention the problem to your doctor who will be able to advise you on Kegel exercises (see p.69), which should help reduce the problem if you practice them regularly. It's important too to empty your bladder whenever you need to. You may want to wear a sanitary pad for additional reassurance.

## Urinary tract infections

During pregnancy, you're more susceptible to urinary tract infections. Most commonly, such infections are confined to the badder, when they are known as cystitis. Symptoms of cystitis include a frequent, urgent need to urinate and a painful burning sensation when passing urine; there may be some blood in your urine. Occasionally, an infection can travel up from the bladder to the kidneys. In this case you may also have pain in your lower back on one side (over the kidney area), have a high temperature, and may feel nauseous or vomit. Sometimes a urinary tract infection is present but causes no symptoms. Prompt treatment of urinary tract infections is especially important in pregnancy because if an infection reaches the kidneys, it can trigger early labor.

**CAUSES** Urinary tract infections are caused by bacteria entering the body through the urethra (the outlet from the bladder) and multiplying. Such infections are probably more common during pregnancy because the effect of hormones on the urinary tract slows the passage of urine.

**WHAT TO DO** If you have any symptoms of a urinary tract infection, see your doctor right away. The doctor will take a mid-stream urine sample and the sample will be sent to a laboratory to identify the type of bacteria that is causing the infection. Your doctor may prescribe a seven to ten day course of antibiotics that are safe for both you and your baby. Symptoms usually improve in a few days after the start of treatment. Because some urinary tract infections are asymptomatic, all pregnant women have urine tests at prenatal doctor's visits, and if bacteria are found, appropriate antibiotics are prescribed.

# Complications of pregnancy & labor

Certain conditions that are specific to pregnancy and some that occur more commonly in pregnancy mean that a pregnancy is classified as high risk. A high-risk pregnancy is closely monitored with more prenatal appointments and possibly additional scans. In labor, certain complications require immediate intervention.

## Pregnancy complications

### Miscarriage

The loss of a fetus before the baby can survive outside of the uterus is the most common complication during early pregnancy, affecting up to a third of pregnancies (see p.94).

### Ectopic pregnancy

This occurs when a fertilized egg implants outside of the uterine cavity. The vast majority of ectopic pregnancies are in the fallopian tube, but they can occur on an ovary, in the cervix, or in the abdominal cavity at the site of a previous cesarean.

**CAUSES** Any woman can have an ectopic pregnancy. However, the risk of an etopic pregnancy is increased if you have had a pelvic infection; became pregnant with a progesterone-releasing IUD in place, while taking the mini-pill, or as a result of fertility treatment; have endometriosis; have had abdominal surgery such as a cesarean section; or a previous ectopic pregnancy.

**SYMPTOMS** Most women who have an ectopic pregnancy will notice pain and light bleeding at 6–8 weeks (2–4 weeks after a missed period). The pain is usually felt on one side of the lower abdomen and it may be severe and persistent. If an ectopic pregnancy is not recognized early and an embryo growing in the fallopian tube ruptures the tube, you may feel sudden severe pain that spreads across the abdomen. Internal bleeding from a ruptured tube can also irritate the diaphragm, causing shoulder pain. If you have severe lower abdominal pain, call your doctor and go immediately to the emergency room.

**WHAT MIGHT BE DONE** If the tube has ruptured, then you will be taken straight to surgery. Usually, an ectopic pregnancy is suspected before this stage. In this case you will have an ultrasound scan, usually performed through the vagina, which often diagnoses the problem; there will be no baby in the uterus; blood may be seen in the abdomen; and sometimes the ectopic pregnancy itself can be seen. You may also have blood tests taken over a period of 48 hours to monitor the levels of hCG (the pregnancy hormone); if levels of hCG plateau or rise slightly, this indicates an ectopic pregnancy. If an ectopic pregnancy has not been confirmed by these investigations, you will probably be taken to surgery for a laparoscopy, a procedure where a telescope is inserted through a small incision in the abdomen, allowing the surgeon to see exactly what is happening. If there is an ectopic, and if the tube is still intact, the surgeon may make a tiny hole in it and remove the embryo or, if the tube has burst, he may remove part or all of it. Occasionally, ectopics may be treated medically with a drug called methotrexate, which stops the pregnancy from developing. This is only appropriate if the hCG levels are low and the tube hasn't ruptured. The advantage is that surgery is avoided; however, the treatment doesn't always work, can be associated with significant pain, and close follow-up is vital.

### Hyperemesis gravidarum

Most women experience some nausea during pregnancy. Occasionally, vomiting may be very severe, known as hyperemesis gravidarum. If you are unable to hold down any food or drink for more than 24 hours, you should see your doctor.

**WHAT MIGHT BE DONE** Your urine may be checked to ensure there is no infection, and you may have a scan to check that all is well with the pregnancy. You should be weighed, since if you lose more than 10 percent of your body weight, you're at risk of complications. If you're very dehydrated, your doctor may advise a short hospitalization so that you can receive intravenous fluids, and you may be given anti-nausea drugs and a vitamin supplement. Hyperemesis usually disappears by 13 weeks.

### Anemia

Anemia is a low level of hemoglobin, the oxygen-carrying component of red blood cells. Mild anemia is common in pregnancy because the extra fluid content of blood dilutes the number of red blood cells. Also, the baby uses some of your iron reserves. If you have anemia you may feel tired and breathless and look pale.

**CAUSES** Usually, anemia is due to iron deficiency. Occasionally, it's due to a lack of folic acid, vitamin B12, or rarer other problems. An analysis of your blood test result will help identify the cause.

**WHAT MIGHT BE DONE** Anemia is usually remedied with an iron supplement. These can have side effects, including constipation and black stools, so some women prefer to boost iron intake through diet (see p.154).

### Weakened cervix

Rarely, a woman may have a weakened cervix, sometimes known as cervical incompetence, which can lead to a miscarriage after 13 weeks. Usually, these miscarriages are relatively painless: you may feel well and perhaps notice some extra vaginal discharge, and then quite quickly miscarry the baby.

**CAUSES** Risk factors include a previous late miscarriage; cervical surgery (such as a cone biopsy for an abnormal smear); or a previous late termination of pregnancy.

**WHAT MIGHT BE DONE** If you are thought to be at risk, your doctor may suggest you have a scan to check the length of your cervix since a shortened cervix makes miscarriage more likely. However, the interval between shortening and miscarriage can be very short, so relying on scanning alone for deciding on treatment is not always helpful. The doctor may recommend that you have a cervical cerclage (stitch) put in at around 14-16 weeks to sew the cervix closed, preventing early labor. It's usually done under anesthesia and is usually successful in preventing miscarriage. It is left in until you're about 37 weeks; removal is straightforward and does not require anesthesia.

## Obstetric cholestasis

This is a rare condition affecting liver function that causes a buildup of bile acids in the bloodstream. The main symptom is severe itching without a rash that is usually most intense on the palms and soles of the feet. It usually occurs after 28 weeks.

**CAUSES** The exact cause of obstetric cholestasis is not clear, but genetic factors are probably involved since the condition tends to run in families and a woman who has the condition in one pregnancy will usually develop it in future pregnancies. Increased senstivity to pregnancy hormones, which effect the way bile is processed, is also thought to play a role.

**WHAT MIGHT BE DONE** If a woman has itching without a rash, the doctor will usually do a blood test to check her liver function and bile acids. If they're abnormal, then obstetric cholestasis will be suspected. The doctor may recommend a drug called ursodeoxycholic acid to reduce the itching and improve liver function. You may also be treated with vitamin K because levels of this vitamin, which is essential for blood to clot, are often reduced in people with liver and bile problems. Women with severe obstetric cholestasis are usually induced at around 37 weeks because there is an increased risk of late stillbirth. There is also an increased risk of postpartum hemorrhage (see p.474).

## Gestational diabetes

Diabetes that develops for the first time in pregnancy is called gestational diabetes and affects between two and seven percent of pregnant women. In this condition, the pancreas produces insufficient insulin to move glucose (sugar) from the blood to be stored, resulting in high levels of glucose in the blood. It usually begins at 20–24 weeks of pregnancy. The risk is greater if you have a family history of late-onset diabetes, or you have previously had a large baby, a stillbirth, or gestational diabetes.

**CAUSES** Insulin levels become inadequate due to the extra demands of the fetus and because hormones produced by the placenta block the effects of insulin.

**WHAT MIGHT BE DONE** Between 24 and 28 weeks, you will be tested for gestational diabetes. If you have risk factors, you may take this test earlier. The test involves having a blood test in the morning after fasting, then drinking a special sugary drink and having a repeat blood sugar check one hour later. If you have high levels of glucose, you'll have to take a similar, but longer test to confirm a diagnosis. If you do have gestational diabetes, you will be taught how to test blood glucose at home. In most cases, the diabetes can be controlled through diet and exercise. However, if these measures prove inadequate you may need insulin injections until the end of pregnancy. Extra scans may be done to check the baby's growth, and early induction (see p.432) may be advised.

If you've had gestational diabetes previously, it's important to ensure that your weight is normal before you become pregnant again.

## Amniotic fluid problems

**POLYHYDRAMNIOS** This describes an excess of amniotic fluid. Syptoms include a stretched feeling in the abdomen; breathlessness, heartburn; swelling in the legs; and constipation. This condition is more likely with diabetes; twins; with an infection; or where there is a congenital problem in the baby. Polyhydramnios increases the risk of premature labor and cord prolapse. You will therefore be carefully monitored and advised to rest. In severe cases, the fluid may be drained.

**OLIGOHYDRAMNIOS** Too little amniotic fluid may be due to a tear in the membranes; placental problems; fetal abnormalities; or problems with the baby's growth (see p.284).

A reduction of amnioic fluid is most likely toward the end of pregnancy. If a scan confirms that levels are low and there are concerns about the baby's development, an early delivery may be advised.

## Placental insufficiency

Placental insufficiency is the term used when the placenta is not functioning well enough to meet the baby's needs. The signs of this condition are a reduction in the amount of fluid around the baby, a fall off in the growth of the baby's abdomen and hence his weight, and abnormalities in an ultrasound (see p.285).

**CAUSES** Placental insufficiency is more common in women with preeclampsia, those who have an underlying medical problem, and in women who smoke. It also occurs more often in babies with a chromosomal abnormality such as Down syndrome, or a structural congenital abnormality such as a heart defect.

**WHAT MIGHT BE DONE** Placental insufficiency is usually picked up by the doctor noticing that the baby appears small and referring you for an ultrasound. If the baby isn't growing well, the doctor will follow you closely and may recommend bed rest for some or the rest of your pregnancy. Treating underlying medical problems, such as high blood pressure or diabetes can help improve your baby's growth.

## Bleeding in late pregnancy

If you experience bleeding, it's important that you and the baby are assessed immediately. If the bleeding is caused by a problem with the placenta, this can be a serious threat to your baby.

**CAUSES** The most serious causes of late bleeding are placenta previa (see p.212) and placental abruption. Placenta previa, in which the placenta lies low in the uterus, affects 1 in 200 pregnancies. The bleeding usually starts from 28 weeks; it is painless, usually recurrent, and is sometimes severe. In placental abruption, which affects 1 in 100 pregnancies, the placenta starts to separate from the uterine lining, leading to severe abdominal pain and bleeding. The bleeding may not be obvious if the blood is trapped between the placenta and uterine wall. Placental abruption is potentially very harmful for your baby because the placenta may not be functioning well.

Bleeding can sometimes be due to cervical erosion, especially after intercourse, or to a cervical polyp. In many cases, no cause is found.

**WHAT MIGHT BE DONE** If it's mild bleeding, your doctor may recommend bed rest. If your doctors think you might have abruption, he may send you to the hospital for observation. Depending on how far along you are, you may be given corticosteroids to help the baby's lungs mature in case an early delivery is necessary. Your doctor may send you home when the bleeding stops. Sometimes, delivering the baby is the safest option. If bleeding is heavy or painful, or the baby is distressed, an emergency cesarean and a blood transfusion may be needed.

## Preeclampsia

Preeclampsia (also known as toxemia, or pregnancy-induced hypertension) is a pregnancy-induced condition characterized by high blood pressure, protein in the urine, and edema (swelling). Occasionally women have symptoms such as headaches, flashing lights, abdominal pain, or nausea. If left untreated, it can lead to eclampsia, an extremely serious condition that causes convulsions and coma. If you are diagnosed with preeclampsia, your pregnancy will be watched very closely and a decision will be made as to the best time for delivery. About eight percent of women have problems with high blood pressure in pregnancy.

**CAUSES** Preeclampsia is more common in multiple pregnancies; in very young and older mothers; in women with preexisting high blood pressure or kidney disease; in women who've had severe preeclampsia before, necessitating delivery by 32 weeks; and in women who've had an egg donation.

**WHAT MIGHT BE DONE** Although the only cure for preeclampsia is delivery of the baby, the baby may need longer to mature in the uterus. The mother and baby will be closely monitored with the goal of prolonging the pregnancy as long as possible. The mother may be hospitalized or be prescribed drugs to lower blood pressure and will probably be advised to rest as much as possible. Because preeclampsia can affect blood flow to the placenta, regular ultrasound and Doppler

scans (see p.285) will be done to check the baby's growth and to look for signs of placental insufficiency (see below). If your doctor is worried that your blood pressure is dangerously high despite medication, you're losing a lot of protein in your urine, or there are anxieties about the baby, immediate delivery will be recommended. This would mean an induction (see p.432) or a cesarean.

## Group B Streptococcus

Ten to 30 percent of women carry group B Streptococcus (GBS) in their vagina, which is completely normal, and does not cause any symptoms. However, 1 in 2000 women can pass GBS to their baby once the water is broken, and the baby may develop a severe GBS-related illness.

**WHAT MIGHT BE DONE** If a woman is known to carry GBS, and if there are risk factors such as prolonged rupture of the membranes, or the baby is premature, intravenous antibiotics may be recommended once the woman is in labor, which usually prevents further problems. Women are generally screened for GBS between weeks 35 and 37. If you carry GBS, you'll be given IV antibiotics during delivery.

# Labor complications

## Premature labor

The normal length of pregnancy is 37 to 42 weeks. A baby born before 37 weeks is called premature or preterm (see p.431).

## Fetal distress

During labor, the baby is monitored for signs of distress, which can indicate that the baby's oxygen supply is reduced. One sign of fetal distress is meconium-stained water (meconium is the baby's first dark green bowel movement). However, this alone doesn't always indicate fetal distress, but if it's combined with a slowing of the baby's heart rate, fetal distress is more likely and steps may be taken for a prompt delivery. If there is thick meconium in the water, there is a danger that the baby could inhale meconium at birth, which can lead to breathing problems and lung infection.

## Failure to progress

Sometimes the cervix fails to dilate as expected during the first stage of labor. There are several factors that can hamper the progress of labor: the baby's head may be too large for the pelvis; there may be inefficient contractions; or the baby may not be in the right position (see p.336).

## Cord prolapse

Rarely, the umbilical cord lies below the baby. This is more likely in a breech birth, or where the baby lies in a transverse position. In these cases, when the water breaks, the cord can slip through the cervix. This is an emergency because the cord may be compressed and restrict or cut off the baby's oxygen supply.

**WHAT MIGHT BE DONE** Unless an immediate assisted vaginal delivery is possible, an emergency cesarean will be done.

## Shoulder dystocia

Shoulder dystocia is when the baby's head is born, but the shoulders remain stuck so the body cannot be born. It's more common if the baby is big or if the mother has diabetes.

**WHAT MIGHT BE DONE** If the head is delivered, and there are signs that the rest of the baby is not coming easily, the mother's legs will be lifted up to help the baby's shoulders down and an episiotomy may be done (see p.427). If the baby still doesn't come easily, there are maneuvers the doctor will do to help release the shoulders and aid the delivery (see also p.426).

## Postpartum hemorrhage

This condition is said to occur if a woman loses more than 1 pint (500 ml) of blood within 24 hours of birth. It can be due to the uterus not contracting quickly enough, to incomplete delivery of the placenta, or to vaginal tears. Active management in the delivery of the placenta (see p.428) makes it less likely to happen. Factors that increase the risk include a large baby or twins; prolonged labor; or bleeding before the labor.

**WHAT MIGHT BE DONE** It's often possible to control bleeding with drugs to help the uterus contract, or by correcting problems such as retained bits of placenta, or by suturing tears. If bleeding continues, arteries that supply blood to the uterus may be closed off. You may also need a blood transfusion.

# Concerns after the birth

Following the birth, you may have a range of concerns about you and your baby (see pp.441–63). However, few of these are serious and are usually easily remedied or are part of the normal development of your baby or your recovery process. The concerns in this section may require more attention from yourself or a health professional.

## Maternal problems

### Mastitis

This painful inflammation of breast tissue most commonly affects breast-feeding women. There may be localized redness, hardness, and soreness in the breast; the breast may feel swollen and hot; and there may be flulike symptoms. Research shows that 10 percent of women experience mastitis within the first three months of giving birth, although it can occur up to two years after the birth.

**CAUSES** Mastitis is either noninfectious or due to a bacterial infection. Noninfectious mastitis is caused by a blocked milk duct that allows milk to stagnate in the breast tissue. If bacteria get into the blocked duct, infectious mastitis can occur. If not treated, an infection can develop into a painful abscess.

**WHAT TO DO** It's important to continue breast-feeding to help remove the blocked milk. Massaging the breast from under the arm (axilla) toward the nipple while feeding can also help, as can expressing milk after a feeding. Rest is advised and it's important to drink lots of fluids. A warm compress on the breast and mild analgesia such as acetaminophen can relieve pain. If an infection is present, treatment with antibiotics is required. An abscess will need to be surgically drained.

### Bladder problems

After a vaginal birth, you may have problems controlling your bladder. You may leak urine when you cough, sneeze, laugh, or move around, known as stress incontinence, or you may have a sudden, intense need to urinate referred to as urge incontinence or overactive bladder.

**CAUSES** Both conditions are caused by the stretching and weakening of pelvic floor muscles and are exacerbated by excess fluid from pregnancy. Bladder problems should improve in the days and weeks after the birth as your pelvic muscles start to tone up.

**WHAT TO DO** Kegel exercises (see p.69) to strengthen and tone muscles are recommended. If problems persist, your doctor may check that you're doing the exercises properly and that there are no other symptoms, such as cloudy urine, pain on passing urine, or an odor, that could indicate an infection and require treatment with antibiotics. You may be referred to a urologist.

### Postpartum depression

This affects about 1 in 10 new mothers. It usually develops 4–6 weeks after the birth, but can come on any time in the first year after the birth. If left untreated, it can persist and have a serious effect on a woman's life.

Emotional symptoms include anxiety; irritabilty; tearfulness; panic; a prolonged low mood; an inability to cope; a lack of interest in appearance; difficulty in concentrating or getting motivated; and not bonding with the baby. There may also be feelings of inadequacy, guilt, rejection, and isolation. Physical symptoms include not sleeping; fatigue; headaches; lack of appetite; loss of libido; stomach pains; and feeling unwell.

**CAUSES** The causes are unclear, but there are several factors than may increase the risk of postpartum depression. These are having a previous history of depression or mental health problems, experiencing a traumatic birth; or having relationship problems.

**WHAT TO DO** In mild cases, emotional and practical support may be sufficient. More serious cases are often treated with antidepressants and counseling or psychotherapy may be recommended.

### Postpartum psychosis

This is a severe psychotic illness that affects 1 in 500 women and occurs in the first two weeks after the birth. The mother may be confused, unable to cope, may neglect her appearance, and forget to take care of her baby. In severe cases, she may have suicidal thoughts and could possibly harm her baby.

**WHAT TO DO** This needs treatment from a psychiatrist. The mother may be admitted to a hospital and will need follow-up care.

### Perineal problems

In a vaginal delivery, the perineum, the area between the vagina and anus, may stretch and subsequently feel sore. If you had a tear that needed stitches or an episiotomy (see p.427), this can be especially painful. If, after stitches, the area becomes red and swollen or you have throbbing pain, you may have an infection.

**WHAT TO DO** Warm baths are soothing, as are chilled witch hazel pads. Pouring warm water over stitches when urinating eases stinging, and Kegel exercises can help with healing. Your doctor may prescribe prescription medications or suggest a stool softener or over-the-counter painkillers for mild to moderate pain. Cooling gel pads can reduce swelling and bruising, and a pillow or inflatable swimming tube can make sitting easier. If your pain won't go away or you have signs of infection (the wound becomes hot, painful, and swollen or you notice pus) contact your doctor.

### Secondary postpartum hemorrhage

Excessive bleeding more than 24 hours and up to six weeks after the delivery occurs in around one percent of women with postpartum hemorrhage. The most common cause is retained tissues or bits of placenta, which may in turn become infected. The bleeding may be accompanied by symptoms such as fever, abdominal pain, and feeling generally unwell. Infection is treated with antibiotics and retained tissues are removed under anesthesia.

# Congenital problems in babies

## Down syndrome

This is the most common chromosomal abnormality, affecting 1 in 700 newborn babies. Babies with Down have some developmental delay and learning difficulties and an increased risk of other congenital abnormalities such as heart problems. Down causes a number of typical features, such as floppy muscle tone at birth; distinctive facial features such as upward slanting eyes; a single skin crease running across the palms; and a somewhat flat back of the head.

**CAUSES** Down is due to an extra chromosome 21. Increasing maternal age makes Down more likely, although most are born to younger mothers, because overall more babies are born to younger women.

**WHAT MIGHT BE DONE** Some parents who are told they are expecting a baby with Down syndrome choose to have a termination. Parents who continue with pregnancy usually find that their child has a good quality of life with advances in education meaning that many enjoy a degree of independence when older; life expectancy with Down is around 55 years.

## Clubfoot

Clubfoot describes the condition when a baby is born with one or both feet turning down and inward.

**CAUSES** doctors don't know the exact cause of clubfoot.

**WHAT MIGHT BE DONE** Treatment generally begins soon after birth. You may be referred to a pediatric orthopedist. The most common treatment is the Ponseti method, in which the baby's foot is manipulated into the right position and a cast put on. The foot is repositioned and a new cast placed every week for several weeks. More severe cases may require surgery to lengthen the tendons. The baby will wear casts and/or a brace for some time after surgery to prevent deformities from returning. The results are usually excellent, with a normally functioning foot and ankle.

## Hip dysplasia

About 1 in 1000 babies is born with a hip socket that is too shallow, meaning that the hip is easily dislocatable. It's more common in girls than boys. After birth, the pediatrician will check the hips by moving them around and making sure they're well situated within the sockets. If the condition is suspected or there is an increased risk of the condition, an ultrasound may be done.

**CAUSES** The risk is increased if there is a family history of congenital dislocation of the hip, if a baby is breech, or if a baby has clubfoot (see above).

**WHAT MIGHT BE DONE** Treatment involves placing baby in a Pavlik harness for a month or two to keep the hip in place and allow the sockets to develop properly. If the problem goes undetected until the baby is walking, she will walk with a limp and will probably require surgery.

## Cleft lip and palate

In this condition, which occurs in 1 in 700 babies, the two halves of the face don't join properly, causing a gap in the upper lip and/or palate. A cleft lip can be symmetrical or, more commonly, asymmetrical, with the cleft on one side of the lip distorting a nostril. This may be detected prenatally, but isn't always so it can be a shock initially. There's evidence that extra folic acid in pregnancy can reduce the risk of having a baby with cleft lip and palate.

**WHAT MIGHT BE DONE** Treatment may begin soon after the birth. Special bottle nipples and appliances may be used to aid feeding. Usually, at around three months, surgery is done to close the gap in the lips, and surgery to close the gap in the palate at about 6 to 18 months.

## Congenital heart disease

Any abnormality involving the structure of the heart chambers or connections between the chambers can affect the function of the heart. Some heart problems are detected prenatally and you will be given advice about where your baby should be delivered and what will happen after the birth.

**SEPTAL DEFECTS** These holes in the heart consist of a small hole between two heart chambers; some types may cause a murmur that is picked up at birth. In many babies, a hole closes on its own.

**BLUE BABY** Some babies are blue at birth because they have a major problem involving abnormal heart connections. This is an emergency. The doctor will do a series of tests and your baby may need surgery to repair the problem.

**PATENT DUCTUS ARTERIOSUS** If the duct between the lungs and the heart fails to close after birth, oxygenated and deoxygenated blood mix. Treatment may be needed in the form of medication and sometimes surgery.

## Undescended testicles

This occurs in around 3–4 percent of full-term boys. In most cases, just one testicle is undescended. Testicles often descend naturally within a year. Otherwise, surgery is advised since undescended testicles can affect sperm production and fertility and increase the risk of testicular cancer later in life.

## Syndactyly

Sometimes babies are born with two digits, either the toes or fingers, joined together. This condition, called syndactyly, is usually caused by the soft tissues fusing together and is often linked to other congenital abnormalities, such as Down syndrome. Treatment is surgical and skin grafts are used.

## Birthmarks

Marks present at birth may be long lasting, although they often fade over time.

**STORK BITES** These pink skin patches on Caucasian babies often fade by 2–5 years.

**MONGOLIAN BLUE SPOTS** Some babies, particularly of Asian or American Indian origin, have extensive gray markings on the lower back, buttocks, and other areas that resemble bruises. Known as Mongolian blue spots, they fade over a few years. They do get mistaken for bruises, so it's worth asking your pediatrician to make note of them.

**PORT WINE STAINS** These permanent marks are caused by abnormal blood vessels in the skin and may occur anywhere on the baby. If one occurs on the face, your baby may be referred to a specialist for laser treatment.

**STRAWBERRY NEVUS** This is an overgrowth of blood vessels, but is not permanent and usually needs no treatment. The nevus, or hemangioma, looks like a strawberry, and although it can be upsetting, it vanishes in a few years. It appears days after the birth and grows over a few months. If it's in a critical area, such as obstructing an eye or nose, your baby may be referred to a specialist.

# Problems in babies after birth

## Spots and rashes

Spots and rashes are common in newborns, and usually disapppear fairly quickly. Birth marks (see p.476) are longer lasting and may be of more concern.

**CAUSES** Small white spots called milia are caused by blocked sebaceous glands, while baby acne is caused by the mother's hormones remaining in the baby after the birth. Both disappear in time without treatment. Erythema toxicum is a rash of unknown cause that appears in the first day or two and disappears within a few days. It consists of red sploches with raised yellowish centers. The spots shift positions and eventually vanish with no treatment. Wash your baby's face every day with water and baby soap and avoid lotions. If your baby's acne doesn't clear up on its own within three months, call your pediatrician.

## Slow weight gain

All babies lose weight in the first days after the birth, but most are back to their birth weight by the 10th day. After that, most babies gain about 1 oz (30 g) each day. Breast-fed babies may take a little longer to regain their birth weight and generally gain weight more slowly. If a baby loses more than 10 percent of his initial birth weight or is not putting on weight as expected, you will usually need to see a doctor to check why this has happened and what you should do.

**CAUSES** Slow weight gain is occasionally due to problems with breast-feeding; for example there may be problems with positioning and latching on, which mean that both mother and baby find it hard to establish breast-feeding. Another possible cause of poor weight gain is excessive vomiting (see below).

**WHAT TO DO** If you're breast-feeding, make sure you have an adequate intake of fluids and calories (you need an additional 500 calories a day), since too little of either can affect milk supply. Getting enough rest is also important for a healthy milk supply. You may be asked to give your baby "top-up" feedings until breast-feeding is well established, and will need advice on how to do this and maintain a good supply of breast milk.

## Jaundice

This is a common condition in newborns that gives the skin a yellowish hue. Neonatal jaundice is usually caused by an excess of bilirubin, which is a substance normally produced during the breakdown of red blood cells. There are several types of neonatal jaundice: physiological jaundice, pathological jaundice, and breast-milk jaundice (see below).

**PHYSIOLOGICAL JAUNDICE** This is the most common type of jaundice in newborns and is rarely of concern. Newborn babies have an excess of red blood cells. Since the baby's liver is immature, it is unable to metabolize red blood cells quickly enough, which leads to a buildup of bilirubin. This type of jaundice often resolves on its own without treatment. However, if bilirubin levels are very high, this can damage part of the brain, so to avoid this, treatment is given with phototherapy lamps. The baby is placed, naked, under a special light or wrapped in a fiber-optic blanket. The lights help break down the bilirubin. Treatment is done for a few days, in the hospital or at home. Physiological jaundice usually appears two or three days after birth and goes away within two weeks.

**PATHOLOGICAL JAUNDICE** This is a more serious type of jaundice that can cause a rapid breakdown of the red blood cells and is usually due to an incompatibility between the mother's and the baby's blood. This may need immediate treatment in a neonatal unit.

**BREAST-MILK JAUNDICE** The most usual cause of prolonged jaundice is breast milk. This is thought to be caused by a substance in the milk that can make bilirubin levels rise. The recommended treatment depends on the bilirubin level. Your baby may not need any treatment. Doctors often recommend nursing the baby at least 8 to 12 times a day, initially, to help her body get rid of the bilirubin.

If jaundice continues beyond two weeks of age and is not thought to be due to breast milk, this should be investigated.

## Vomiting

All babies vomit to some extent in the first weeks after the birth, but you should contact your doctor if your baby has prolonged or excessive vomiting, isn't gaining enough weight, or you're concerned. Serious vomiting can have several causes, including conditions such as gastroesophageal reflux and pyloric stenosis (see below).

Other symptoms that may accompany vomiting can suggest particular conditions and will need investigating. If a baby seems lethargic or floppy, this could indicate an infection; if his abdomen is swollen, this could suggest an intestinal obstruction; if vomit is bright yellow or green, there could be a twisted bowel; and if there is also diarrhea, there may be gastroenteritis.

## Gastroesophageal reflux

If your baby is miserable, in pain, arching his back, refusing feedings, or vomiting large amounts after each feeding, he could be suffering from gastroesophageal reflux. This occurs when the valve between the bottom of the esophagus (gullet) and top of the stomach is immature, allowing the stomach contents to come back into the esophagus. Acid from the stomach can burn the lower end of the esophagus, and if the reflux is severe, a baby can refuse feedings.

**WHAT MIGHT BE DONE** Mild gastroesophageal reflux that involves vomiting but no problems with weight gain or pain, usually needs no treatment. More severe reflux will need treatment, usually with medicines to stop or prevent the acid production, and prevent the vomiting. For bottle-fed babies with mild reflux, it's worth asking your pharmacist for an anti-reflux formula.

## Pyloric stenosis

In this condition, which occurs most commonly in first-born male babies, the exit at the bottom of the stomach is thickened, meaning that milk cannot leave. It causes so-called projectile vomiting in which a feeding is vomited with so much force that it can land a foot or so away from the baby. The baby is constantly hungry and will demand another feeding immediately after vomiting. Vomiting becomes progressively more severe.

**WHAT MIGHT BE DONE** Pyloric stenosis is diagnosed with a blood test and ultrasound, and treatment is surgical. The surgery is straightforward and the improvement remarkable. Babies usually leave the hospital within two or so days.

# Glossary

**Active birth** An approach to childbirth that involves upright positions and movements during labor.

**Alphafetoprotein (AFP)** A substance produced by the embryonic yolk sac, and later by the fetal liver, which enters the mother's bloodstream during pregnancy.

**Amniocentesis** The surgical extraction of a small amount of amniotic fluid through the pregnant woman's abdomen. This procedure is usually done as a test for fetal abnormalities.

**Amnion** The thin membrane surrounding the fetus and the amniotic fluid. It's also known as the amniotic sac.

**Amniotic fluid** The fluid that surrounds the fetus in the uterus. Ultrasound scans may be done in late pregnancy to ensure that enough is present.

**Amniotomy** The surgical rupture of the amniotic sac, often done to speed up labor. This is referred to as ARM (artificial rupture of the membranes).

**Anterior position** See *Occipital anterior*.

**Apgar score** A general test of the baby's well-being given shortly after the birth to assess the heart rate and tone, respiration, blood circulation, and nerve responses.

**Areola** The pigmented circle of skin surrounding the nipple.

**ARM** See *Amniotomy*.

**Bilirubin** Broken-down hemoglobin, normally converted to nontoxic substances by the liver. Some newborn babies have levels of bilirubin too high for their livers to deal with (neonatal jaundice).

**Blastocyst** An early stage of the developing embryo when it has divided into a group of cells.

**Bloody show** A vaginal discharge of bloodstained mucus occurring before labor, resulting from the onset of cervical dilatation. A sign that labor is starting.

**Braxton Hicks contractions** Practice contractions of the uterus that occur throughout pregnancy, but which may not be noticed until toward the end.

**Breech presentation** When the position of the baby in the uterus is bottom down rather than head down.

**Catheter** A thin plastic tube that is inserted into the body through a natural channel to withdraw fluid from, or introduce fluid into, a particular part of the body. This can be used to draw off urine from the bladder after a surgery, or to maintain a constant input of fluids into a vein, or to introduce anesthetic into the epidural space.

**Cephalic presentation** (Vertex presentation) The position of a baby who is head down in the uterus. The most common presentation.

**Cephalopelvic disproportion** A state in which the head of the fetus is larger than the cavity of the mother's pelvis. Delivery must therefore be by cesarean section.

**Cervical dilation** See *Dilation*.

**Chorion** The outer membranous tissue that envelops the fetus and placenta.

**Chloasma** Pigmentation of the skin that causes darker patches, often on the face.

**Chorionic gonadotrophin** See *Human chorionic gonadotrophin (hCG)*.

**Chorionic villus sampling** A method of screening for genetic abnormality by analysis of tissue from the small protrusions on the outer membrane enveloping the embryo that later form the placenta.

**Chromosomes** Rodlike structures containing genes occurring in pairs within the nucleus of every cell. Human cells each contain 23 pairs.

**Colostrum** A kind of milk, rich in proteins, formed and secreted by the breasts in late pregnancy and gradually changing to mature milk some days after delivery.

**Corpus luteum** A glandular mass that forms in the ovary after fertilization. It produces progesterone, which helps form the placenta, and is active for the first 14 weeks of pregnancy.

**Crowning** The moment when the baby's head appears in the vagina and does not slip back again.

**CVS** See *Chorionic villus sampling*.

**Dilation** The progressive opening of the cervix caused by uterine contractions during labor.

**Dizygotic** See *Twins*.

**Doppler** A method of using ultrasound vibrations to listen to the fetal heart.

**Doula** A supportive helper who provides physical and emotional support during childbirth.

**EDD** The estimated date of delivery.

**Edema** Fluid retention, which causes the body tissues to be puffed out.

**EEG** See *Electroencephelogram*.

**Electroencephalogram (EEG)** A test where electrodes are placed on the scalp to record the electrical activity of the brain.

**Electronic fetal monitor** An electronic monitor that is used to measure the progress of the mother's contractions and the baby's heartbeat during labor.

**Embryo** The developing organism in pregnancy, from about the 10th day after fertilization until about the 12th week of pregnancy, when it is termed a fetus.

**Engorgement** The congestion of the breasts with milk. If long periods are left between feedings, or the baby is not well latched on, painful engorgement can occur. This can be relieved by putting the baby to the breast or expressing the excess milk.

**Episiotomy** A surgical cut in the perineum to enlarge the entrance to the vagina.

**Estrogen** A hormone produced by the ovary.

**External version** (External cephalic version, or ECV). The manipulation by gentle pressure on the fetus into the cephalic position. This may be done by an obstetrician at the end of pregnancy if the baby is breech or transverse.

**False labor** Braxton Hicks (rehearsal) contractions, which are so strong and regular that they are mistaken for the contractions of the first stage of labor.

**Fetal distress** A shortage in the flow of oxygen to the fetus, which can arise from numerous causes.

**Fetus** The developing child in the uterus, from the end of the embryonic stage at around 12 weeks, until the birth.

**Hormone** A chemical messenger in the blood that stimulates various organs to carry out specific actions.

**Human chorionic gonadotrophin** (hCG) A hormone released into the woman's bloodstream by the developing placenta from about six days after the last period was due. Its presence in the urine, and or blood, means that she is pregnant.

**HypnoBirthing** A type of self-hypnosis using visualization and breathing techniques to achieve a deep state of relaxation during labor.

**Hypotension** Low blood pressure.

**Identical twins** See *Twins*.

**Implantation** The embedding of the fertilized ovum or egg within the wall of the uterus.

**Induction** The process of artificially starting off labor and keeping it going.

**Intravenous drip** The infusion of fluids directly into the bloodstream by means of a fine catheter introduced into a vein.

**Intravenous injection** An injection into a vein.

**In vitro fertilization (IVF)** A type of assisted conception where fertilization occurs outside of the uterus and embryos are tranferred back into the uterus.

**Kangaroo care** A technique, adopted especially with premature babies, where baby and parent have prolonged skin-to-skin contact. This is thought to provide warmth, stimulation, and to encourage breast-feeding.

**Lanugo** The fine soft body hair of the fetus.

**Lateral position** Transverse lie or horizontal position of a fetus in the uterus (sometimes occurring if the mother has a large pelvis), where the presenting part is either a shoulder or the side of the head.

**Lie** The position of the fetus within the uterus.

**Linea nigra** A line of dark skin that appears down the center of the abdomen over the rectus muscle in some women during pregnancy.

**Lochia** Postpartum vaginal discharge.

**Longitudinal lie** The position of the fetus in the uterus in which the spines of the fetus and the mother are parallel.

**Low-birthweight baby** A baby who weighs below 5 lb 8 oz at birth.

**Meconium** The first contents of the bowel, present in the fetus before birth and passed during the first few days after birth. The

presence of meconium in the amniotic fluid before delivery is usually taken as a sign of fetal distress.

**Monozygotic** See *Twins*.

**Morula** A stage in the growth of the fertilized egg when it has developed into 32 cells.

**Nucleus** The central part or core of a cell, containing genetic information.

**Occipital anterior** The position of the baby in the uterus when the back of its head (the crown or occiput) is toward the mother's front (anterior).

**Occipital posterior** The position of the baby in the uterus when the back of its head (the crown or occiput) is toward the mother's back (posterior).

**Opioids** (Narcotics) Painkilling medications that induce drowsiness and stupor.

**Palpation** Feeling the parts of the baby through the mother's abdominal wall.

**Pelvic floor** The springy muscular structure set within the pelvis that supports the bladder and the uterus, and through which the baby descends during labor.

**Perinatal** The period from the 24th week of gestation to one week following delivery.

**Perineum** The area of soft tissues surrounding the vagina and between the vagina and the rectum.

**Posterior** See *Occipito posterior*.

**Postpartum** After delivery.

**Premature** A baby born before the 37th week of pregnancy. The baby will have a low birth weight.

**Presentation** The position of the fetus in the uterus before and during labor.

**Preterm** See *Premature*.

**Primigravida** A woman having her first pregnancy.

**Progesterone** A hormone produced by the corpus luteum and then by the placenta.

**Prostaglandins** Natural substances that stimulate the onset of labor contractions. Prostaglandin gel may be used to soften the cervix and induce labor.

**Rh immunoglobulin (RhIg)** An injection of antibodies given to women who have a Rhesus negative blood group if they may have been exposed to Rhesus positive fetal blood cells.

**Rhesus factor** A distinguishing characteristic of the red blood cells. All human beings have either Rhesus positive

or Rhesus negative blood. If the mother is Rhesus negative and the fetus Rhesus positive, severe complications and Rhesus disease (the destruction of the red corpuscles by antibodies) may occur, unless prevented by an injection of Rh immunoglobulin (RhIg).

**Rooting** The baby's instinctive searching for the breast.

**Stillbirth** The delivery of a dead baby after the 20th week of pregnancy.

**Surfactant** A creamy fluid that reduces the surface tension of the lungs so that they do not stick together when deflated. Premature babies may have breathing difficulties if surfactant has not developed sufficiently.

**TENS** See *Transcutaneous electronic nerve stimulation*.

**Transcutaneous electronic nerve stimulation** A method of pain relief that uses electrical impulses to block pain messages to the brain.

**Transducer** An instrument that translates echoes of high-frequency sound waves, bounced off the developing fetus in the uterus, to build up an ultrasound image on a monitor. See also *Ultrasound scan*.

**Transition** A phase between the first and second stages of labor when the cervix is dilating to between 7 and 10 cm.

**Trial of labor** A situation in which, although a cesarean section may be necessary, the mother labors in order to see if a vaginal delivery is possible.

**Twins** The simultaneous development of two babies in the uterus, either after two eggs are fertilized independently by two sperm—dizygotic or fraternal twins—or, more rarely, after one fertilized egg divides to produce monozygotic or identical twins.

**Ultrasound scan** A way of building up a picture of an object by bouncing high-frequency soundwaves off it. Ultrasound scans are used during pregnancy to show the development of the fetus in the uterus. See also *Transducer*.

**Vernix** A creamy substance that often covers the fetus in the uterus.

**VBAC (Vaginal Birth After Cesarean)** A situation in which a woman delivers vaginally after having a previous cesarean (in the past, if a woman had had a cesarean, any subsequent birth would be a cesarean).

# Resources

## Fertility

**www.asrm.org**
American Society for Reproductive Medicine

**www.cdc.gov/ART/**
CDC Reproductive Health: information on assisted reproductive technology

**www.plannedparenthood.org**
(800) 230-PLAN
Planned Parenthood Federation of America

**www.resolve.org**
(703) 556 7172
Resolve: The National Infertility Association

## Pregnancy, Labor, and Birth

**www.4woman.gov**

**www.americanpregnancy.org**

**www.acog.org**
American Academy of Gynecologists

**www.babycenter.com**
Information on pregnancy and childbirth

**www.babyzone.com**

**www.birthcenters.org**
(215) 234-8068
American Association of Birth Centers

**www.bradleybirth.com**
Teaching families how to have natural births

**www.childbirthconnection.org**
(212) 777-5000

**www.dona.org**
(888) 788-DONA
Doulas of North America International

**Fitpregnancy.com**

**HypnoBirthing.com**

**www.ican-online.org**
International Cesarean Awareness Network

**www.icea.org**
(919) 863-9487
International Childbirth Education Association

**www.lamaze.org**
(800) 368-4404
Lamaze International

**www.maternitywise.com**
(952) 457-6506
Information about doulas

**www.motherfriendly.org**
Coalition For Improving Maternity Services

**www.midwife.org**
(240) 485-1800
American College of Nurse-Midwives

**http://pregnancy.about.com**

**www.waterbirth.org**
(800) 641-2229
Waterbirth International

## Breast-feeding

**www.breastfeeding.com**

**www.ilca.org**
(919) 861-5577
International Lactation Consultant Association

**www.laleche.org**
(847) 519 7730
La Leche League International—breast-feeding advice and support

**www.ncsl.org/programs/health/breast50.htm**
National Conference of State Legislatures —a summary of state breast-feeding laws

## Support Groups

**www.aafa.org**
(800) 727-8462
Asthma and Allergy Foundation of America

**www.acds.org**
(516) 933 4700
Association for Children with Down Syndrome

**www.birthdefects.org**
(407) 566-8304
Birth Defect Research for Children

**www.cff.org**
(800) 344-4823
Cystic Fibrosis Foundation

**www.diabetes.org**
(800) 342-2383
American Diabetes Association

**www.fcsn.org**
(800) 331-0688
Federation for Children with Special Needs

**www.hmhb.org**
(703) 837-4792
National Healthy Mothers, Healthy Babies Coalition

**www.hopexchange.com**
(757) 826-2162
Support after miscarriage, stillbirth, or infant death

**www.marchofdimes.com**
Working against the threats of birth defects, premature birth, and infant mortality.

**www.mostonline.org**
(631) 859-1110
Support for multiple birth families

**www.ndss.org**
(800) 221-4602
National Down Syndrome Society

Index

# Acknowledgments

## Maggie Blott's acknowledgments

I would like to thank the Pregnancy and Childcare team at Dorling Kindersley for their help, guidance, and expert knowledge. In particular I would like to thank Andrea Bagg for her patience and support. I would also like to thank my children Polly, Jess, and Eddie for their love and for putting up with me and my preoccupation during this project.

## Publisher's acknowledgments

**Indexer** Hilary Bird
**Proofreader** Angela Baynham
**Additional Editorial Assistance** Suhel Ahmed, Ann Baggaley, Terry Moore, Helen Murray, Diana Vowles
**Additional Design Assistance** Isabel de Cordova, Charlotte Seymour
**Illustration Assistance** Amanda Williams
**Additional illustrations** Philip Wilson
**Picture Librarian** Romaine Werblow
**Additional Picture Research** Jenny Baskaya
**Hair & Makeup Stylist for Photography** Alli Williams
**Photographer's Assistants** Sarah Bailey and Carly Churchill
**Assistant to Art Director for Photography** Susie Sanford
**Location Agency** www.1st-Option.com

Dorling Kindersley would like to thank all the authors and illustrators for their expertise and dedication. We are grateful to the following individuals and organizations for their help:
**Dr. Mary Steen** RGN, RM, BHSc PGCRM, PGDipHE, MCGI, PhD for consultancy work and editorial assistance.
**Catharine Parker-Littler** SRN, RSCN, SCM, DPSM (Advanced midwifery), BscMid (Hons) for permission to reuse text from *Ask a Midwife*.
**Dr. Paul Moran** MD, MRCOG for consultation and expert advice on all embryonic and fetal images. His invaluable contribution provided not only the fetal text and all fetal captions, but he also sourced, scanned, and supplied images when all other image sources had been exhausted. Paul would like to thank the women who helped him to provide the images for this book and Maggie Blott for the opportunity to work on such a fascinating title.
**Dr. Pranav Pandya** BSc, MRCOG, MD for advice on embryonic and fetal images.
**The women at the Royal Victoria Infirmary** who gave permission for their scans to be used in this book.
**Nicola, Joe and Leo Hayward,** and **Reuben Marcus** for allowing us to use photographs of themselves.

A special thank you to:
**University College Hospital London** for permission to photograph in the new Elizabeth Garrett Anderson (EGA) Wing. Many thanks also to the midwives, who helped and advised during photography and who also in some cases modeled for us.

The new University College Hospital Elizabeth Garrett Anderson (EGA) Wing opened its doors to women and their babies in the first week of November 2008. The £70 million wing includes three floors dedicated to the care of mothers and babies and has been specially designed to ensure all women have ready access to the integrated care they and their babies may require. Maternity care is provided by midwifery, obstetric, neonatal, and anesthetic consultants with their teams and core midwifery staff working together to deliver up to 6,000 babies a year.

Mothers will receive care from the same team of midwives throughout their pregnancy. All women who are anticipated to have low risk pregnancies and deliveries will be offered the facilities of the Bloomsbury Birthing Centre—providing a home-from-home philosophy.

The Elizabeth Garrett Anderson (EGA) Wing houses prenatal and postpartum beds, high-dependency maternity unit beds, birthing rooms, birthing pools, special care cribs, and neonatal intensive care cribs. In addition to providing care for women with normal pregnancies, the staff also cares for women with very complicated, high risk pregnancies and treats some of the sickest and most vulnerable babies in the UK with the most modern equipment and up-to-date and highly trained medical, midwifery, and nursing teams.

## Picture credits

Most of the scans and photographs of the developing baby in this book are of the embryo and fetus live in utero, pictured using endoscopic and ultrasound technology. When this has not been possible, images have been taken by reputable medical professionals as part of research or to promote educational awareness.

Dorling Kindersley would like to thank the following for their kind permission to reproduce their photographs:
(Key: a-above; b-below/bottom; c-center; f-far; l-left; r-right; t-top)

**Alamy Images:** 322tl; Angela Hampton Picture Library 266bc; Avatra Images 33cra, 84br; Marie-Louise Avery 135cl; Peter Banos 58cr; Bubbles Photolibrary 10tr, 20br, 148br, 185cr, 233bc, 242br, 317br, 328br; Adam Burton 125br; Camera Press Ltd 255bc, 268bc; Form Advertising 338br; David J. Green 76bc; Jennie Hart 47bl; Juergen Hasenkopf 95br; Janine Wiedel Photolibrary 405bl, 438br; Martin Hughes-Jones 154cr; Medical-on-Line 381cl; Picture Partners 235c, 369br, 380c; Pregnancy Maternity And Motherhood/Mark Sykes 365bl; Profimedia International s.r.o. 3fcla; Chris Rout 119bc, 148bc, 193c, 232cr; **babyarchive.com:** MJ Kim 42cl; **Babybond® www.babybond.com:** 2clb, 146tl, 149bc, 149bl, 149fbl, 173tl, 183tl, 199tl, 206bc, 206bl, 206br, 218tl, 256bc, 257tl, 258tl, 262fcl, 262ftl, 262tl, 263bc, 281tl, 282tl, 283tl, 286tl, 287tl, 288tl, 289tl, 292tl, 294tl, 306tl, 310tl, 311tl, 320tl, 323br, 327tl, 328tl, 329tl, 330tl, 332tl, 333tl, 336tl, 337tl, 338tl, 339tl, 340tl, 353tl; **BSIP:** 166tl, 235tl, 253tl; Ramare 174tl, 240bc, 343tl, 350tl, 351tl; SGO 131tl, 270tl, 271tl, 296tl; **Bubbles:** Moose Azim 333bl; **Corbis:** Heide Benser / zefa 180br; Brooke Fasani 341bc, 382bl; Rolf Bruderer 198c; Cameron 426c; Kevin Dodge 77bl; Annie Engel / zefa 200bl, 335bc, 375bc; Wolfgang Flamisch / zefa 387c; Owen Franken (sidebar); Rick Gomez 3fcrb, 10tc, 32cra, 158bc, 177c; Ole Graf/zefa 32bc; Rune Hellestad 389bc, 438bl; A. Inden / zefa 171cl; JLP/Sylvia Torres 2fcla; Michael A. Keller 60cr, 64bc; Jutta Klee

Acknowledgments

140c; Mika / zefa 80bl, 101bc; Markus Moellenberg/zefa 2crb, 31tc; Moodboard 273cl; Kevin R Morris 314br; Peter Pfander / zefa 351bc; Shift Foto / zefa 261bc; Ariel Skelley 6fbl, 464cl; Tom Stewart 245cr; Larry Williams 6fcr, 205br, 289br, 297cr, 395cr; **Custom Medical Stock Photo:** 127tl; **Dreamstime.com:** Monkey Business Images 37br, 57bc, 65cr, 292bc; Pliene 159tl; Shahar 204br; Shipov 180tl; Starush 256bl; Studio1one 162tl; **fotolia:** Liv friis-larsen 134cl; Nyul 75cr; **Getty Images:** 83bc, 311cr, 374c; Altrendo 412bc; Altrendo Images 356bl; B2M Productions 54l; Blend Images 73cr; Blend Images/Jose Luis Pelaez Inc 6cra, 30tr; Blend Images/PBNJ Productions 33bl; Leland Bobbe 313cr; Daniel Bosler 287br; Noah Clayton 164bc; Taxi / Colorstock 157br; Donna Day 270bc; DK Stock 63br; DK Stock / Michael Rowe 172br; Dorling Kindersley / Sian Irvine 173br; Gazimal 117bl; George Doyle 339bc; Vladimir Godnik 309bc; Sammy Hart 354c; Frank Herholdt 263br; Dorling Kindersley / Ian Hooton 209br; Ian Hooton 295br; Iconica 45c; Iconica / Andersen Ross 241br; Image Bank/Tracy Frankel 263bl; Image Source 149cra; Blend Images / Jose Luis Pelaez Inc 251br; Ruth Jenkinson 306cr; Christina Kennedy 223br; Jutta Klee 169cr; The Image Bank / Bernhard Lang 115cr; Lecorre Productions 145cr; StockFood Creative / Louise Lister 114br; LWA 462c; LWA/The Image Bank 367c; Laurence Monneret 385br; Nacivet 371br, 373br; Peter Nicholson 131br; Sarma Ozols 357cr; Barbara Peacock 262bc; Iconica / Jose Luis Pelaez 110c; Photonica 97bc; Louie Psihoyos 453bl; Riser 44cr, 116br; Riser/ Frank Herholdt 3crb; Riser/Laurence Monneret 263cr; Stockbyte 86c, 263ftl, 327bc; Stockbyte/George Doyle 2cla; StockFood Creative 33ca; Stone 39c, 105br; Stone / James Baigrie 207br; Stone/Jerome Tisne 148; Jonathan Storey 246bc; Studio MPM 283c; Taxi 66br; Taxi / Bernd Opitz 252tl; Taxi / DreamPictures 106br; Jerome Tisne 151br; Titus 275bc; Tobias Titz 127cl; Paul Venning 379cr; Simon Wilkinson 139br; ZenShui / Laurence Mouton 316cr; **iStockphoto.com:** Alex Bramwell 104br; Dirk Richter 259c; **Prof. J.E. Jirasek MD, DSc.:** 3cra, 11tl, 32br, 33tc, 33tl, 68tl, 69tl, 71tl, 72tl, 73tl, 75tl, 76bl, 83tl, 87tl, 96cr, 96tl, 101tl, 104tl, 107tl, 110tl, 114tl, 115tl, 149tl, 149tr, 232tl, 242tl, 249tl; **jupiterimages:** Pixland 91c; **Lennart Nilsson Image Bank:** 33ftl, 65tl, 87cr, 91tl, 93cr, 93tl, 99tl, 100tl, 107cr, 126cr, 156cr, 219tl, 231c; **Life Issues Institute:** 125tl, 181tl, 200tr, 260tl; **LOGIQlibrary:** 113br, 138c; **Masterfile:** 191cl, 237bc; Jerzyworks 224c, 304cr; Michael A. Keller 180bc; **Mediscan:** 120tl, 211tl, 237tl; **Mother & Baby Picture Library:** 262br, 282bc, 426cl, 435cr; Dave J. Anthony 238bc; Moose Azim 307br, 427bc, 427br; Ian Hooton 6bl, 6cla, 6fcl, 6tr, 12tr, 26br, 28br, 30tc, 33br, 103bc, 122bc, 122cb, 138b, 142l, 146cl, 199c, 229bc, 230c, 243cr, 262tr, 263tl, 267cr, 278br, 279br, 286bc, 299c, 300br, 302br, 321bc, 348, 383bc, 393c, 394cl, 397c, 402cr, 411tr, 465cl; Ruth Jenkinson 3fcra, 6cl, 6crb, 11tc, 13tr, 239cr, 288br, 319cr, 331cr, 394c, 399tl, 407cr, 409bl, 416br, 432bc, 441tc; Eddie Lawrence 6cr, 395cl, 399b; Paul Mitchell 8-9, 31tl, 149cl, 203cr, 320br; James Thomson 13tc, 19; **Dept of Fetal Medicine, Royal Victoria Infirmary, Newcastle upon Tyne:** 97tl, 111, 140tl, 161tl, 165tl, 167tl, 170tl, 187tl, 188tl, 274tl, 275tl, 276tl, 277tl, 278tl, 279tl, 297tl, 299tl, 300tl, 304tl, 305tl, 314tl, 316tl, 317tl, 325tl, 370tl, 374tl, 375tl, 377tl, 378tl, 379tl, 380tl, 381tl, 382tl, 383tl, 385tl, 386tl, 388tl, 389tl, 392tl; **Dr. Pranav P Pandya:** 143c, 143cr, 285c, 285cr; **Photolibrary:** Banana Stock 2fclb, 103cl, 429b, 464c; Pierre Bourrier 133cr; Brand X Pictures 167bc; Neil Bromhall 226bl; OSF / Derek Bromhall 190tl; OSF / Neil Bromhall 221tl, 223tl, 229tl, 233tl, 255tl; OSF / Densey Clyne 193tl, 194br, 194tl, 203tl; Fresh Food Images/Robert Lawson 32tl; Henry Horenstein 366tl; Robert Lawson 322c; Graham Monro 430; Andersen Ross 323bc; Joy Skipper 332cr; **Phototake:** Dr Benoit/Mona Lisa 365tl; Sovereign 355tl; **PunchStock:** 442; **Reflexstock:** Agencja Free / Rafal Strzechowski 221br; **Rex Features:** 309tl; Prof Stuart Campbell 105tl, 106tl, 151tl, 154tl, 172tl, 189tl, 198tl, 209tl, 216tl, 217tl, 225tl, 226tl, 245tl, 252, 261tl, 269tl, 293tl, 295tl, 307tl, 321tl, 345tl, 361tl, 363tl, 387tl; **Science Photo Library:** 21tl, 77tl, 120bc, 169tl, 207tl, 240tl, 262c, 284tl; AJ Photo 335tl; Anatomical Travelogue 49tl, 63tl, 64tl, 67cl, 79tl, 81tl, 84tl, 86tl, 89tl, 92tl, 117tl, 129tl, 133tl, 145tl, 158tl, 174c, 197tl, 291tl, 344tl, 362tl, 364tl, 371tl; Samuel Ashfield 343br, 364c; Bernard Benoit / Kretz Technik 341tl; Thierry Berrod, Mona Lisa Production 354tl; Biophoto Associates 36tl; Neil Borden 215tc, 215tl; Neil Bromhall 230tl, 241tl, 243tl; Neil Bromhall / Genesis Films 227tl; BSIP Estiot 57tl; BSIP VEM 40tl; BSIP, ASTIER 395c, 434bl; BSIP, ATL 324tl; BSIP, Cavallini James 124bl; BSIP, Laurent 418br; John Burbridge 47tl; CIMN, ISM 266tl, 273cr; Clouds Hill Imaging Ltd 10tl; Clouds Hill Imaging Ltd. 53cr; CNRI 428c; Kevin Curtis 378bl; Dopamine 135tl, 163tl, 175tl, 178tl, 179tl; Dr Keith Wheeler 43tl; Du Cane Medical Imaging Ltd 367tl, 386c; Edelmann 41c, 72cr, 100c, 109tl, 119tl, 124tl, 132tl, 134tl, 144tl, 148ftr, 148tr, 155tl, 157tl, 166bl, 171tl, 182br, 185tl, 213tl, 222tl, 234tl, 238tl, 239tl, 256tl, 347tl, 369tl; Simon Fraser 141tl, 370br; GE Medical Systems 372tl, 373tl; Steve Gschmeissner 37tl, 41tl, 46tl, 48tl; Ian Hooton 1c, 2cra, 2fcrb, 3cla, 4-5c, 6fbr, 14, 24bc, 46br, 103bl, 129c, 149cb, 149ftl, 188cl, 214bc, 263c, 398cl, 455c, 464cr, 465cr; Dr Isabelle Cartier, ISM 45tl; Jean-Claude Revy-A. Goujeon, ISM 66tl; K.H. Kjeldsen 60tl; Mehau Kulyk 186tl, 246tl, 251tl; Dr Najeeb Layyous 95tl, 116tl, 121tl, 126tl, 130tl, 137tl, 156tl, 182tl, 186bc, 204tl, 208tl, 212tl, 222bl, 231tl, 267bc, 268tl, 274br, 313tl, 357tl, 358tl, 359tl; Living Art Enterprises, Llc 215c, 215cl; Cecilia Magill 6fcra, 31tr; Manfred Kage 39tl; Matt Meadows 346tl, 391tl; Hank Morgan 206tl; Dr Yorgos Nikas 50bl, 50br, 50fbr; Dr Yorgos Nikos 59bc, 59tl; Susumu Nishinaga 44tl; Lea Paterson 20bc; D. Phillips 50fbl, 53tl; Photo Researchers, Inc / Nestle / Petit Format 205tl; Alain Pol, ISM 248tl; Prof. P. Motta / Dept. of Anatomy / University 56tl; Prof. P. Motta / Dept. of Anatomy / University "LA SAPIENZA", Rome 49bc; Professors P.m. Motta & J. Van Blerkom 32tl; Professors P.M. Motta & S. Makabe 35tr; R. Bick, B. Poindexter, UT Medical School 67tl; P. Saada / Eurelios 138tc; Sovereign, ISM 139tl, 177tl, 178cr; James Stevenson 259tl; BSIP, Kretz Technik 319tl; Tek Image 310br; Alexander Tsiaras 132cr, 162cr; Zephyr 38tl, 331tl; **University College London Hospitals:** 271cr; **Wellcome Library, London:** 80tl, 164tl, 190br, 191tl, 195tl, 224tl, 265tl; Yorgos Nikas 61tl; Anthea Sieveking 429tr; **Wikipedia, The Free Encyclopedia:** Acaparadora 43bl

All other images © Dorling Kindersley
For further information see: www.dkimages.com